The Columbia Guide to Basic Elements of Eye Care

Daniel S. Casper • George A. Cioffi
Editors

The Columbia Guide to Basic Elements of Eye Care

A Manual for Healthcare Professionals

Illustrated by Daniel S. Casper, MD, PhD

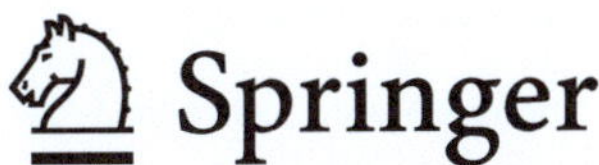 Springer

Editors
Daniel S. Casper
Columbia University Irving Medical
Center
New York, NY
USA

Department of Ophthalmology
Edward S. Harkness Eye Institute
Columbia University Vagelos College of
Physicians and Surgeons
New York, NY
USA

Naomi Berrie Diabetes Center
Columbia University Irving Medical
Center
New York, NY
USA

George A. Cioffi
Columbia University Irving Medical
Center
New York, NY
USA

Department of Ophthalmology
Edward S. Harkness Eye Institute
Columbia University Vagelos College of
Physicians and Surgeons
New York, NY
USA

ISBN 978-3-031-16871-0   ISBN 978-3-030-10886-1   (eBook)
https://doi.org/10.1007/978-3-030-10886-1

This Springer imprint is published by the registered company Springer Nature Switzerland AG
The registered company address is: Gewerbestrasse 11, 6330 Cham, Switzerland

Foreword

Perhaps no other medical or surgical specialty is as highly differentiated and poorly understood by other physicians as ophthalmology. Ophthalmology is not a required clinical rotation in many medical schools, and even electives in it are often no longer than 1 or 2 weeks. Ophthalmology patients are rarely admitted to hospitals, and the ophthalmologic equipment used for routine examinations requires expertise that other physicians do not have.

Nonetheless, ophthalmological abnormalities, ranging from the bothersome to the serious, to the sight- and even life-threatening, are among the most common problems faced throughout the world. With the aging of the population, disorders of vision—including glaucoma, cataracts, and macular degeneration—are increasing causes of disability. In the developed world, the epidemic of obesity and type 2 diabetes is already leading to an analogous epidemic of diabetic retinal disease. In the developing world, where hypertension has emerged as a leading cause of death and disability, hypertensive eye disease is a growing concern.

The increasing gap between the rising incidence and prevalence of ophthalmological disease and practicing physician's limited understanding of even the basics of ophthalmology highlights the need for a book such as *The Columbia Guide*. The Columbia Guide emphasizes the common problems that are encountered by non-ophthalmologists, as well as how to diagnose their cause, initiate treatment, and make appropriate referrals to an ophthalmologist. In doing so, *The Columbia Guide* demystifies the lingo, measurements, abbreviations, drawings, and images that often make the reading of an ophthalmic consultation note impenetrable to the non-ophthalmologist.

The Columbia Guide to Basic Elements of Eye Care: A Manual for Healthcare Professionals is a straightforward, practical, and easy-to-use aid that will help every non-ophthalmologist healthcare provider who encounters patients with eye complaints or potential eye problems.

Lee Goldman, MD
Harold and Margaret Hatch Professor
Executive Vice President
and Dean of the Faculties of Health Sciences
and Medicine, Chief Executive
Columbia University Irving Medical Center
New York, NY, USA

Preface

Recent decades have seen significant modifications in medical education, reminiscent of the changes brought about in the early twentieth century by the *Flexner Report*. That document introduced groundbreaking changes to physician training, including a national homogenization of curricula and an emphasis on requiring the study of human anatomy, physiology, and biochemistry.

We learned medicine in a structured format that almost universally consisted of 2 years of didactic training in the sciences and pharmacology, followed by 2 years of clinical study, primarily in inpatient hospitals. Ophthalmology residencies were done in eye hospital settings, where surgical patients were typically admitted the night before surgery and often remained as inpatients for a period of days, or even longer, postoperatively.

The changes that have occurred in the practice of, and training in, ophthalmology and all of medicine in the short time since we trained are staggering. Medical school curricula have undergone significant reorganizations, favoring more time devoted to learning clinical arts rather than basic science. In some schools, the result has been the almost complete abandonment of any anatomical training outside of computer-assisted dissection simulations; areas of medicine considered peripheral to primary care or general surgery—ophthalmology, otolaryngology, dermatology, and neurology—have been relegated to elective status. It is possible for a student to finish their medical training with minimal or no exposure to some or all of these disciplines.

Ophthalmology, as well, has undergone dramatic changes. The number of patients currently admitted to hospitals for ophthalmic general care or surgery is vanishingly small, as the field has transitioned almost entirely to an outpatient specialty. In many centers, ophthalmology residents no longer take overnight call in-house, so emergency room staff are required to provide initial care and appropriately triage off-hour cases. Patients admitted to hospital for other medical problems who are followed by interns or hospitalists, and during the course of their hospitalization experience ophthalmic problems, are similarly cared for, initially, by covering non-ophthalmologists. Emergency physicians, pediatricians, family practitioners, internists, hospitalists, neurologists, physician assistants, and nurse practitioners, among others, are routinely asked to evaluate eye pain, visual changes, "pink eye," and a host of other ocular complaints. This puts the burden of initial diagnosis, and possibly treatment, on healthcare providers who may have had little or no experience dealing with ophthalmic maladies.

This text is designed to provide a foundation of basic eye anatomy and physiology, functional analysis, pathology, and concepts in eye care. It is not designed to be a comprehensive course in ophthalmology. Rather, it presents basic principles of eye health and disease that will guide the non-ophthalmologist in the evaluation of eye complaints. It provides a framework to appreciate normal versus abnormal, which will help determine when and which patients need referral to an eye care specialist, and to identify which conditions are emergent, urgent, or can be routinely followed. It is hoped that students and practitioners who have limited exposure to ophthalmology find this book useful and that it might prompt them to delve further into this fascinating and all-encompassing area of medical care.

New York, NY, USA   Daniel S. Casper, MD, PhD
                                                          George A. Cioffi, MD

Acknowledgments

As digital publishing becomes the de facto mode of disseminating information, how refreshing and heartening to find people and institutions dedicated to learning material that is, actually, material.

I thank Springer for encouraging and aiding the creation of real books, the ones that can be grabbed from a shelf, flipped through, bookmarked, annotated, and even savored.

At Springer, editors Rebekah Amos, Caitlin Prim, and Asja Parrish delivered invaluable support and counsel, and throughout a long gestation, Margaret Burns was patient and helpful at every stage.

Ophthalmology is largely a visual specialty, and that is not meant flippantly; patterns of eye disease vary from subtle to severe, and recognizing them is often key to understanding and recognizing abnormalities, which enhance accurate and timely diagnosis. High-quality, representative images are one of the best ways to view, and review, typical phenotypic alterations seen in disease. The photographic staff at the Edward S. Harkness Eye Institute have been tireless in obtaining the best images possible in every case that we have illustrated here, and sincere thanks go to David McMahon, Noelle Pensec, Noelle Vallet, Eileen Frommer, Katherine Broderick, Philip Tang, April Ellis, Lanyi Zhao, Dina Yang, Alex Hannan, and Daniel Jones.

While my opening statement might suggest a blanket aversion to technology, in truth, I am something of a fan. The acquisition and storage of large numbers of high-resolution photographic images and the creation of illustrations required a great deal of sophisticated computer power, all of which was kept alive and behaving by David Wentsler and Thad Mangar, both of whom seemed to be able to materialize in seconds, for any crisis, large or small. Their assistance has been invaluable.

In the early stages of this book, our colleague, Dr. Harry Lodge, author of the *Younger Next Year* books, was extremely generous with his time and offers of assistance. Very sadly, Harry passed away last year, and we gratefully acknowledge his help and deeply miss his incomparable warmth and clinical acumen.

Numerous chapter authors have graciously provided their time and expertise throughout the development of this project, while the Harkness Eye residents have also contributed, particularly Dr. Thalmon Campagnoli.

Sincere appreciation is owed to Gaby Novak and Denisse Bejaran for their assistance throughout and to Valerie Williams-Sanchez and Suzanne Daly, who were often the involuntary sounding boards for book-related ramblings and rants, which they graciously absorbed and defused.

Finally, we owe an immeasurable debt to patients of the Harkness Eye Institute at Columbia, who have entrusted us with the care and maintenance of their vision and have taught us all so much along the way.

Contents

Contributors

David H. Abramson, MD Ophthalmic Oncology Service, Department of Surgery, Memorial Sloan Kettering Cancer Center, New York, NY, USA

Lama A. Al-Aswad, MD, MPH Associate Professor of Ophthalmology at the Columbia University Irving Medical Center, Department of Ophthalmology, Edward S. Harkness Eye Institute, Columbia University Irving Medical Center, New York, NY, USA

James Auran, MD Professor of Ophthalmology at the Columbia University Irving Medical Center, Department of Ophthalmology, Edward S. Harkness Eye Institute, Columbia University Irving Medical Center, New York, NY, USA

Srilaxmi Bearelly, MD, MHS Assistant Professor of Ophthalmology at the Columbia University Irving Medical Center, Department of Ophthalmology, Edward S. Harkness Eye Institute, Columbia University Irving Medical Center, New York, NY, USA

Dana Blumberg, MD Assistant Professor of Ophthalmology at the Columbia University Irving Medical Center, Department of Ophthalmology, Edward S. Harkness Eye Institute, Columbia University Irving Medical Center, New York, NY, USA

Steven E. Brooks, MD Professor of Ophthalmology (in Pediatrics) at the Columbia University Irving Medical Center, Department of Pediatric Ophthalmology, Jonas Children's Vision Care, Columbia University Vagelos College of Physicians and Surgeons, New York-Presbyterian/Morgan Stanley Children's Hospital, New York, NY, USA

Thiago Cabral, PhD Department of Ophthalmology, University Federal of Sao Paulo, Sao Paulo, Brazil

Ashley A. Campbell, MD Assistant Professor of Ophthalmology, Wilmer Eye Institute, Johns Hopkins School of Medicine, Baltimore, MD, USA

Daniel S. Casper, MD, PhD Professor of Ophthalmology at the Columbia University Irving Medical Center, Department of Ophthalmology, Edward S. Harkness Eye Institute, Columbia University, Director of Ophthalmology, Naomi Berrie Diabetes Center, Columbia University Irving Medical Center, New York, NY, USA

Jonathan S. Chang, MD Assistant Professor, Department of Ophthalmology and Visual Sciences, University of Wisconsin School of Medicine and Public Health, Madison, WI, USA

Royce W.S. Chen, MD Assistant Professor of Ophthalmology at the Columbia University Irving Medical Center, Department of Ophthalmology, Edward S. Harkness Eye Institute, Columbia University Irving Medical Center, New York, NY, USA

Wendy Chung, MD, PhD Kennedy Family Professor of Pediatrics and Medicine at the Columbia University Irving Medical Center, Department of Pediatrics, Columbia University Irving Medical Center, New York, NY, USA

George A. Cioffi, MD Jean and Richard Deems Professor of Ophthalmology at the Columbia University Irving Medical Center, Department of Ophthalmology, Edward S. Harkness Eye Institute, Columbia University, Edward S. Harkness Chair & Professor, Columbia University Irving Medical Center, New York, NY, USA

D. Jackson Coleman, MD, FACS, FARVO Professor of Ophthalmology at the Columbia University Irving Medical Center, Department of Ophthalmology, Edward S. Harkness Eye Institute, Columbia University Irving Medical Center, New York, NY, USA

Karina Conlin, OD, FAAO Clinical Optometrist, Department of Ophthalmology and Visual Sciences, University of Wisconsin School of Medicine and Public Health, Madison, WI, USA

Carlos Gustavo De Moraes, MD, MPH Associate Professor of Ophthalmology at the Columbia University Irving Medical Center, Department of Ophthalmology, Edward S. Harkness Eye Institute, Columbia University Irving Medical Center, New York, NY, USA

Joaquin O. De Rojas, MD Department of Ophthalmology, Johns Hopkins Medicine, Baltimore, MD, USA

Kristen E. Dunbar, MD Department of Ophthalmology, NYU Langone Health, New York, NY, USA

Jonathan Fay, MD Klamath Eye Center, Klamath Falls, OR, USA

George J. Florakis, MD Clinical Professor of Ophthalmology, Department of Ophthalmology, Edward S. Harkness Eye Institute, Columbia University Irving Medical Center, New York, NY, USA

Jasmine H. Francis, MD, FACS Ophthalmic Oncology Service, Department of Surgery, Memorial Sloan Kettering Cancer Center, New York, NY, USA

Pamela F. Gallin, MD, FACS Clinical Professor of Ophthalmology (in Pediatrics), Department of Ophthalmology, Edward S. Harkness Eye Institute, Columbia University Irving Medical Center, New York, NY, USA

Larissa K. Ghadiali, MD Department of Ophthalmology, Loyola University Medical Center, Maywood, IL, USA

Lora Dagi Glass, MD Assistant Professor of Ophthalmology at the Columbia University Irving Medical Center, Department of Ophthalmology, Edward S. Harkness Eye Institute, Columbia University Irving Medical Center, New York, NY, USA

Emre Göktas, MD Research Fellow, Department of Ophthalmology, Edward S. Harkness Eye Institute, Columbia University Irving Medical Center, New York, NY, USA

Quan V. Hoang, MD, PhD Singapore National Eye Centre/Duke-NUS Medical School, Singapore Eye Research Institute, Singapore, Singapore

Adjunct Assistant Professor of Ophthalmology at Columbia University Medical, Department of Ophthalmology, Edward S. Harkness Eye Institute, Columbia University Irving Medical Center, New York, NY, USA

Albert J. Hofeldt, MD AMA Optics, Miami Beach, FL, USA

Ahmet M. Hondur, MD Associate Professor of Ophthalmology, Department of Ophthalmology, Gazi University Medical School, Ankara, Turkey

Jason Horowitz, MD Assistant Professor of Ophthalmology at the Columbia University Irving Medical Center, Department of Ophthalmology, Edward S. Harkness Eye Institute, Columbia University Irving Medical Center, New York, NY, USA

Steven A. Kane, MD, PhD Associate Clinical Professor of Ophthalmology, Department of Ophthalmology, Edward S. Harkness Eye Institute, Columbia University Irving Medical Center, New York, NY, USA

Michael Kazim, MD Clinical Professor of Ophthalmology and Surgery, Edward S. Harkness Eye Institute, Columbia University Irving Medical Center, New York, NY, USA

Gene Kim, MD Assistant Professor, Department of Ophthalmology and Visual Sciences, Albert Einstein College of Medicine, Montefiore Medical Center, Bronx, NY, USA

Ariana M. Levin, BS Ophthalmic Oncology Service, Department of Surgery, Memorial Sloan Kettering Cancer Center, New York, NY, USA

Jeffrey Liebmann, MD Shirlee and Bernard Brown Professor of Ophthalmology at the Columbia University Irving Medical Center, Department of Ophthalmology, Edward S. Harkness Eye Institute, Columbia University Irving Medical Center, New York, NY, USA

Michelle M. Maeng, MD Postdoctoral Residency Fellow, Department of Ophthalmology, Edward S. Harkness Eye Institute, Columbia University Irving Medical Center, New York, NY, USA

Brian Marr, MD Professor of Ophthalmology at the Columbia University Irving Medical Center, Department of Ophthalmology, Edward S. Harkness Eye Institute, Columbia University Irving Medical Center, New York, NY, USA

Irene Maumenee, MD Professor of Ophthalmology at the Columbia University Irving Medical Center, Department of Ophthalmology, Edward S. Harkness Eye Institute, Columbia University Irving Medical Center, New York, NY, USA

Peter Michalos, MD Associate Clinical Professor of Ophthalmology, Department of Ophthalmology, Edward S. Harkness Eye Institute, Columbia University Irving Medical Center, New York, NY, USA

Victoria North, MD Department of Ophthalmology, Harvard Medical School, Boston, MA, USA

Jeffrey G. Odel, MD Professor of Ophthalmology at the Columbia University Irving Medical Center, Department of Ophthalmology, Edward S. Harkness Eye Institute, Columbia University Irving Medical Center, New York, NY, USA

Nailyn Rasool, MD Assistant Professor of Neurology and Ophthalmology, Department of Ophthalmology, University of California, San Francisco, San Francisco, CA, USA

Hermann Schubert, MD Professor of Clinical Ophthalmology, Department of Ophthalmology, Edward S. Harkness Eye Institute, Columbia University Irving Medical Center, New York, NY, USA

Tarun Sharma, MD Associate Research Scientist, Department of Ophthalmology, Edward S. Harkness Eye Institute, Columbia University Irving Medical Center, New York, NY, USA

Ronald Silverman, PhD Professor of Ophthalmic Science (in Ophthalmology), Department of Ophthalmology, Edward S. Harkness Eye Institute, Columbia University Irving Medical Center, New York, NY, USA

Janet R. Sparrow, PhD Anthony Donn Professor of Ophthalmic Science (in Ophthalmology) and Professor of Pathology and Cell Biology, Departments of Ophthalmology and Pathology and Cell Biology, Edward S. Harkness Eye Institute, Columbia University Irving Medical Center, New York, NY, USA

Gregory Stein, MD Uptown Retina and Vitreous of New York, New York, NY, USA

Leejee H. Suh, MD Miranda Wong Tang Associate Professor of Ophthalmology at the Columbia University Irving Medical Center, Department of Ophthalmology, Edward S. Harkness Eye Institute, Columbia University Irving Medical Center, New York, NY, USA

Linus D. Sun, MD, PhD Instructor in Neurology (in Ophthalmology), Department of Ophthalmology, Edward S. Harkness Eye Institute, Columbia University Irving Medical Center, New York, NY, USA

Tongalp H. Tezel, MD Chang Family Professor of Ophthalmology, Department of Ophthalmology, Edward S. Harkness Eye Institute, Columbia University Irving Medical Center, New York, NY, USA

Danielle Trief, MD, MSc Assistant Professor of Ophthalmology at the Columbia University Irving Medical Center, Department of Ophthalmology, Edward S. Harkness Eye Institute, Columbia University Irving Medical Center, New York, NY, USA

Stephen L. Trokel, MD Professor of Ophthalmology at the Columbia University Irving Medical Center, Department of Ophthalmology, Edward S. Harkness Eye Institute, Columbia University Irving Medical Center, New York, NY, USA

Stephen Tsang, MD, PhD Laslo Z. Bito Associate Professor of Ophthalmology, Associate Professor of Pathology and Cell Biology, Departments of Ophthalmology and Pathology and Cell Biology, Harkness Eye Institute, Columbia University Irving Medical Center, New York, NY, USA

Stephen P. Walters, MD Instructor in Ophthalmology at the Columbia University Irving Medical Center, Department of Ophthalmology, Columbia University Irving Medical Center, New York, NY, USA

Michael Jay Weiss, MD, PhD Clinical Professor of Ophthalmology, Department of Ophthalmology, Edward S. Harkness Eye Institute, Columbia University Irving Medical Center, New York, NY, USA

Bryan J. Winn, MD Associate Professor of Ophthalmology at the Columbia University Irving Medical Center, Department of Ophthalmology, Edward S. Harkness Eye Institute, Columbia University Irving Medical Center, New York, NY, USA

Lauren Yeager, MD Assistant Professor of Clinical Ophthalmology, Department of Ophthalmology, Edward S. Harkness Eye Institute, Columbia University Irving Medical Center, New York, NY, USA

Christine Zemsky, BS Research Assistant, Department of Ophthalmology, Edward S. Harkness Eye Institute, Columbia University Irving Medical Center, New York, NY, USA

Part I

Introduction

Orbital and Ocular Anatomy

Daniel S. Casper and Janet R. Sparrow

Overview

The eyes ("globes") are housed in bilateral orbital cavities, two symmetric, pear-shaped depressions in the anterior mid-skull, with large openings anteriorly to permit vision and small ones posteriorly for communication with the cranial cavity. Each orbit is formed by seven interconnected bones (Fig. 1.1). Three of these are single bones that extend across the midline (frontal, ethmoid, and sphenoid), shared equally by the two orbits; the other four (maxillae, zygomas, lacrimals, and palatines) are separate and duplicated, present individually on each side.

The small, box-shaped ethmoid sits behind the root of the nose and separates the orbits. It houses the ethmoid sinus, and its thin, fragile, lateral walls make up a large part of the medial orbital walls. The sphenoid, a large bone that traverses the entire skull from side to side and can be seen externally in the infratemporal fossae, is a complex bone, and in addition to constituting much of the lateral walls, it contains a deep, central sinus, as well as the sella turcica, which houses the pituitary gland. The sphenoid wings serve a crucial role as the boundary between the orbit and middle cranial fossa.

The orbits are arbitrarily divided into four orbital walls (Fig. 1.2a, b): the roof, medial wall, floor, and lateral wall. The floor and medial wall are thinnest and accordingly tend to fracture more commonly with trauma, while the roof and lateral wall are more substantial and less likely to break. The lateral wall is recessed about a centimeter at the orbital opening, affording greater peripheral vision but also leaving the lateral portion of the eye more susceptible to injury.

The main orbital portal to and from the medial fossa, the posteriorly located apex. The smaller and more medial opening is the optic canal, which carries the optic nerve, ophthalmic artery, and sympathetic autonomic nerve fibers. Just temporal to the optic canal is the larger, superior orbital fissure which carries almost all other neurovascular structures of importance in orbital and globe functioning (Fig. 1.3a, b). Passing through the superior orbital fissure are cranial nerves III (oculomotor), IV (trochlear), V (the first division, ophthalmic), and VI (abducens), as well the superior ophthalmic vein and parasympathetic nerve fibers.

D. S. Casper, MD, PhD (✉)
Columbia University Irving Medical Center,
New York, NY, USA

Department of Ophthalmology, Edward S. Harkness
Eye Institute, New York, NY, USA

Naomi Berrie Diabetes Center, Columbia University
Vagelos College of Physicians and Surgeons,
New York, NY, USA
e-mail: dsc5@cumc.columbia.edu

J. R. Sparrow, PhD
Departments of Ophthalmology and Pathology
and Cell Biology, Edward S. Harkness Eye Institute,
Columbia University Vagelos College of Physicians
and Surgeons, New York, NY, USA

© Springer Nature Switzerland AG 2019
D. S. Casper, G. A. Cioffi (eds.), *The Columbia Guide to Basic Elements of Eye Care*,
https://doi.org/10.1007/978-3-030-10886-1_1

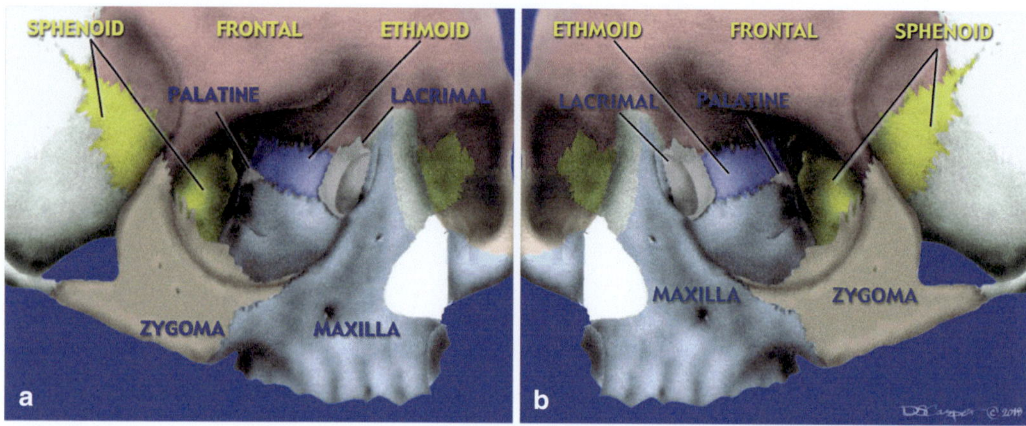

Fig. 1.1 Seven bones form each orbit, three of which are single bones that cross the midline; the remaining four contribute separately to each orbit

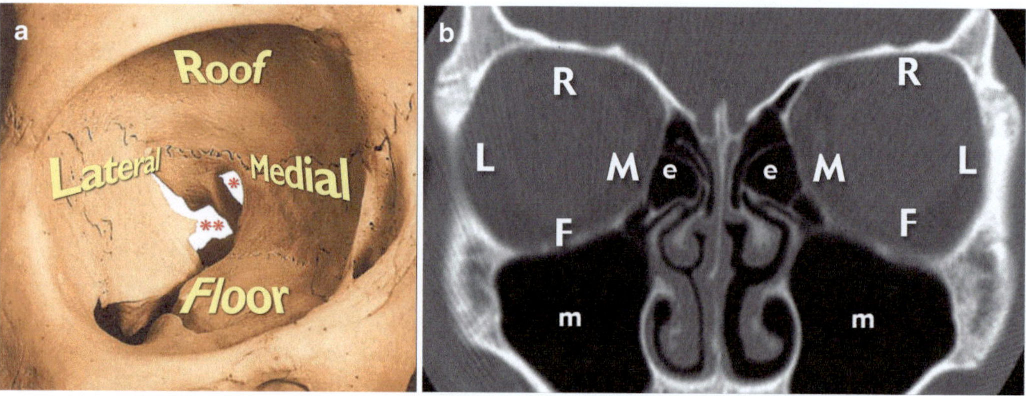

Fig. 1.2 The orbit is described as having four walls (**a**), the superior and lateral being thicker and the medial and inferior being thinner and more delicate (**b**). The openings found at the orbital apex, the more medial optic canal (*) and the larger, more lateral superior orbital fissure (**), both connect orbit with the middle cranial fossa. *L* lateral; *R* roof; *M* medial; *F* floor; *e* ethmoid sinus; *m* maxillary sinus

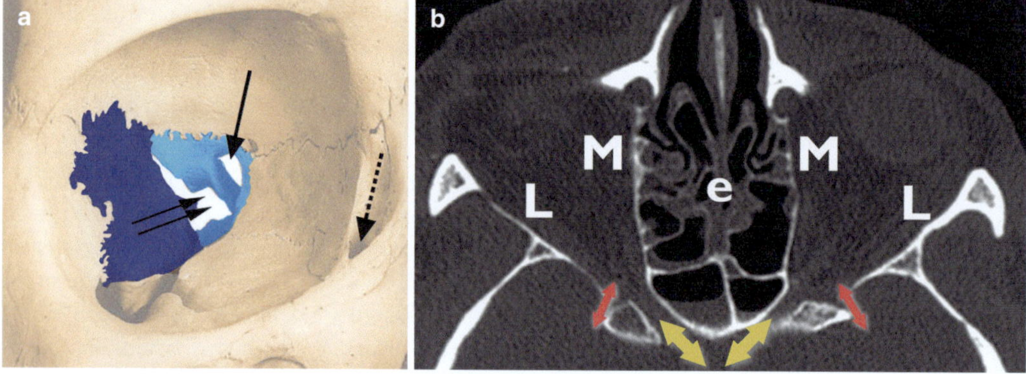

Fig. 1.3 The optic canal (single arrow) transmits the optic nerve, ophthalmic artery, and sympathetic fibers. All other structures (cranial nerves III, IV, V {first division}, and VI and the superior ophthalmic vein) travel through the superior orbital fissure (double arrows). The medially-located nasolacrimal canal (dashed arrow) contains the tear drainage system, and the gap in the orbital floor, the inferior orbital fissure, carries the second division of the trigeminal nerve (**a**). Dark blue, greater sphenoid wing. Light blue, lesser wing. In an axial CT scan, the optic canals (yellow arrows) are seen located medially to the superior orbital fissures (red arrows) (**b**). *M* medial orbital wall; *L* lateral orbital wall; *e* ethmoid

Located along the orbital floor and contiguous with the superior orbital fissure is the inferior orbital canal, which carries the second division of the trigeminal nerve (maxillary), infraorbital vessels, and the inferior ophthalmic vein. Its main components exit the orbit via the inferior orbital fissure and contribute relatively little to the orbit itself.

Two single periorbital sinuses have already been mentioned (ethmoid, located between the two orbits, and sphenoid, located posterior to the orbits, beneath the pituitary gland), and there are two additional aerated sinuses adjacent to the orbits: the large, bilateral maxillary sinuses, located just beneath the orbital floors, in the maxillae, and the frontal sinuses, located medially above the brows in the frontal bone (Fig. 1.4; see also Fig. 32.1). Periorbital sinuses are clinically significant, as commensal bacteria commonly found within them can traverse orbital walls and cause orbital infections (preseptal and postseptal cellulitis). In adults, such infections are frequently associated with antecedent traumatic wall fractures into adjacent contiguous sinus cavities; in children, however, with incomplete bone maturation, pathogens may spontaneously traverse an otherwise intact wall and enter the orbital space. Although aggressive antibiotics are usually sufficient to eradicate cellulitis, inadequately treated orbital infections can progress into orbital abscesses, which frequently require surgical intervention.

Orbital space is for the most part enclosed and limited, with the small, posterior apical opening densely packed with structures entering or exiting the middle cranial fossa and the large anterior aperture shielded only by the movable eyelids. If a retro-ocular space-occupying lesion, such as an abscess, hemorrhage, or tumor, were present, normal structures (e.g., nerves, blood vessels, orbital fat, the eye) would be displaced away from the lesion (Fig. 1.5a, b). The only real outlet to accommodate this increase in

volume is the anterior aperture, and typically the globe will be pushed outward, resulting in a prominent, bulging eye, a condition known as proptosis or exophthalmos. If the mass is situated directly behind the eye, then proptosis would be along the visual axis, whereas a superiorly located lesion would force the globe downward, and an inferior one would do the reverse. Similarly, medial masses would deviate the eye laterally and vice versa. If this process progresses rapidly or the lesion is large, there may be serious visual consequences, as well as cosmetic issues.

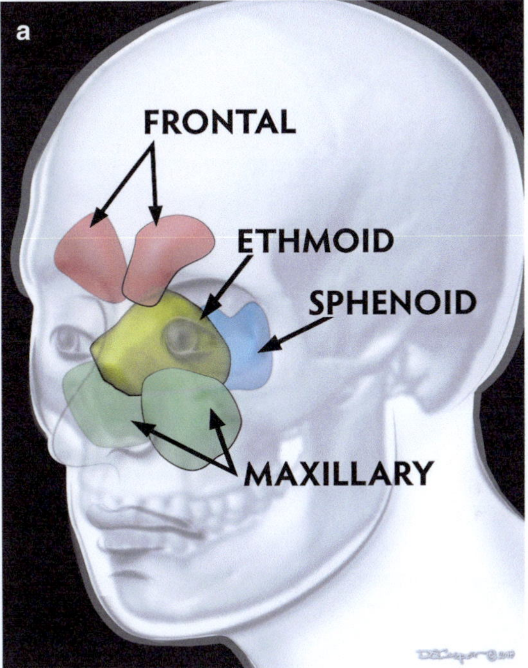

Fig. 1.4 Sinuses almost entirely surround the orbits, with frontal above, maxillary below, ethmoid in between, and sphenoid posterior and inferior. The sinuses harbor bacteria that can cause orbital cellulitis infections. (**a**) A schematic three-dimensional image of sinus locations; (**b**) a series of cadaver axial sectioned human specimens, from superior to inferior, shows the sinuses surrounding the orbits. Axial images 1 to 6, superior to inferior (Images from the Visible Human Project® courtesy of the National Library of Medicine)

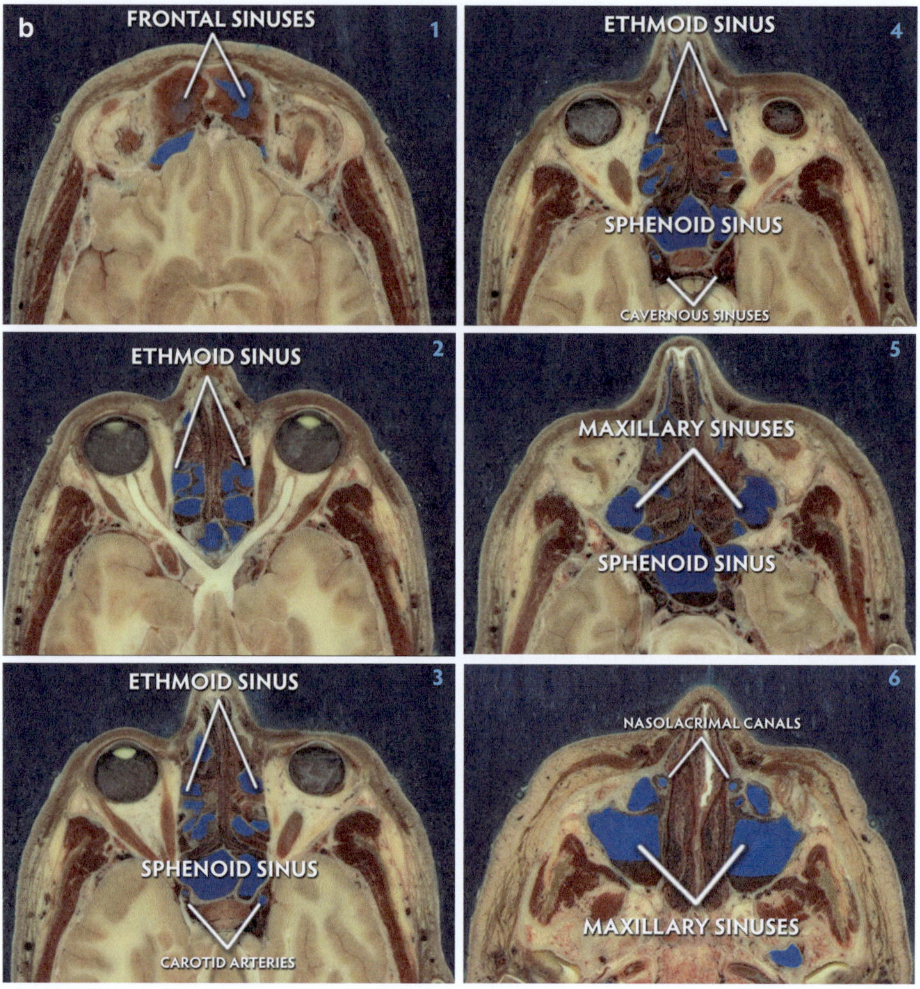

Fig. 1.4 (continued)

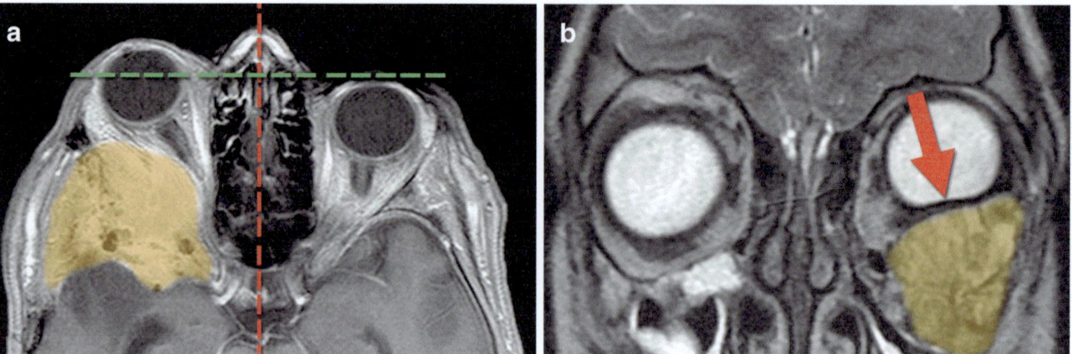

Fig. 1.5 Because the orbits are essentially closed posteriorly, space-occupying lesions will usually force the eye outward, a condition called proptosis or exophthalmos, as seen in this sphenoid wing meningioma (**a** the tumor has been highlighted in color). A line drawn perpendicular to the anatomical axis across the cornea on the normal side shows the degree of ocular displacement. In some cases, a mass may even distort the shape of the eye, thereby reducing vision, as in this case of a cavernous hemangioma pushing the globe upward and distorting its normal spherical shape (arrow) (**b**). (Courtesy of Michael Kazim, MD)

Extraocular Muscles

Six extraocular muscles control movement and the position of each eye (Fig. 1.6):

Lateral and medial recti control horizontal movements.
Superior and inferior recti control primarily vertical actions.
Superior and inferior oblique muscles bring about mostly oblique (i.e., non-vertical or horizontal) movements.

Five of these six muscles originate directly from, or adjacent to, a tough fascial ring at the orbital apex, the annulus of Zinn; the inferior oblique muscle, however, originates from the floor of the anterior orbit, adjacent to the nasolacrimal duct opening.

The actions of the horizontal recti are "pure," meaning that they will deviate the eye solely in the horizontal plane, left or right. The vertical recti, however, attach to the globe at an angle of about 22.5° lateral to the anteroposterior axis, because the orbits deviate outward from the

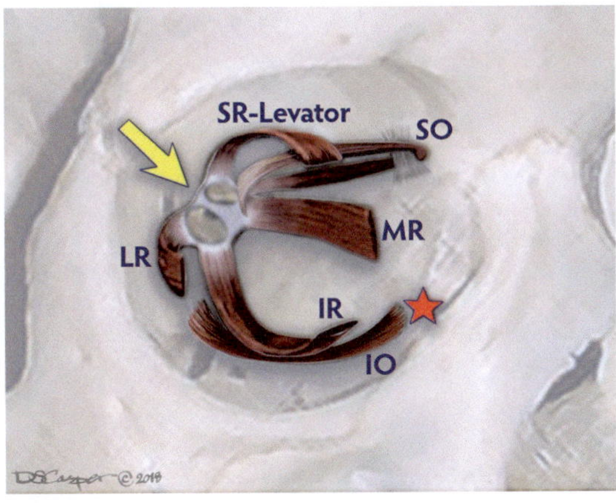

Fig. 1.6 Six extraocular muscles control movements of the eyes, five of which originate from an apical connective tissue ring, the annulus of Zinn (yellow arrow), and the remaining inferior oblique originates from the orbital floor anteriorly (red star). *SR-Levator* superior rectus levator complex; *SO* superior oblique traversing trochlea; *MR* medial rectus; *LR* lateral rectus; *IR* inferior rectus; *IO* inferior oblique

medially located apices. Because of this off-axis alignment, vertical muscle contraction does not simply elevate or depress the eye; instead, there is a lateral component in addition to the main vertical direction. The superior rectus directs the eye up and out, and the inferior directs the eye down and out. The oblique muscles attach to the globes at approximately 51° off primary axis. The superior oblique, unlike other extraocular muscles, does not attach directly to the globe but instead travels through a fascial sling, the trochlea, located in the superior medial orbit; the tendonous muscle portion then reverses direction, travels over the globe, and attaches to the posterior, superior part of the eye, close to where the optic nerve exits. The inferior oblique, originating from the orbital floor, follows the same course as the superior oblique tendon, only below the globe, and attaches directly to the posterior, inferior portion of the eye (Fig. 1.7b). Because of their posterior insertions and fascial connections which suspend the globe within the orbit, oblique muscle action is counterintuitive: the superior deviates the eye *downward* and medially, and the inferior deviates the eye *upward* and medially. The consequence of this anatomic configuration is that straight vertical, upward (90°) eye movement requires the combined vector action of the superior rectus and inferior oblique; conversely, combined inferior rectus and superior oblique actions are required to produce straight downward movement (Fig. 1.7a, b).

Innervation

Visual data processed by the neural retina is transmitted to the brain via cranial nerve II, the optic nerve (Fig. 1.8). This nerve, which is actually a bundle of approximately one million axonal fibers from individual retinal ganglion cells, can be directly visualized at its origin with ophthalmoscopy as the optic disc, located at the posterior pole of the eye. After exiting the eye, it follows a sinuous course (which allows for free movement of the eye within the orbit) medially through the

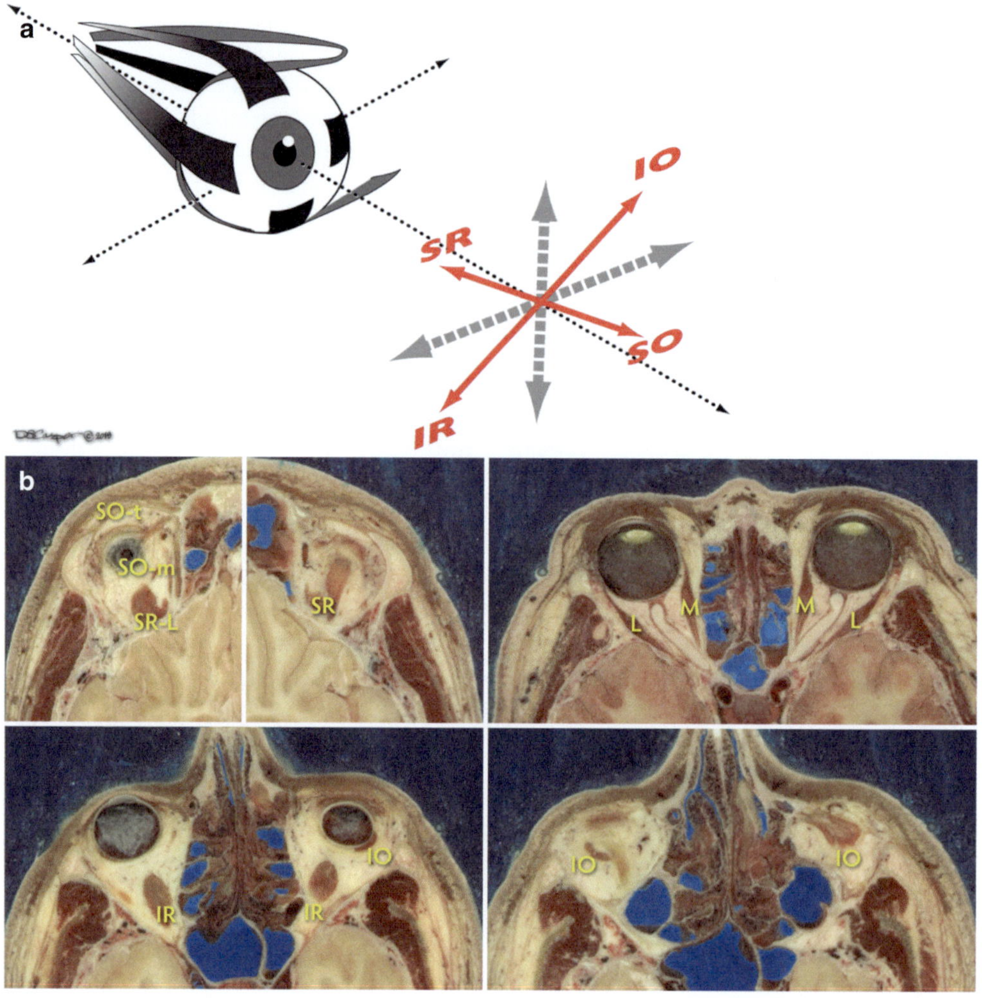

Fig. 1.7 Because the superior and inferior muscles are not aligned perfectly in the anteroposterior plan, they do not rotate the eye either straight upward or downward. Therefore, in order to elevate or depress the eye in the vertical plane, a combined action is required with the oblique muscles (**a**). In a composite image of cadaver axial sectioned human specimens, the extraocular muscles are seen within the orbit (**b**) (Images from the Visible Human Project® courtesy of the National Library of Medicine) (*SO-t* superior oblique tendon, *SO-m* superior oblique muscle body, *SR-L* superior rectus-levator complex, *SR* superior rectus, *IR* inferior rectus, *IO* inferior oblique, *L* lateral rectus, *M* medial rectus). Note that the extraocular muscles and globes are all encased in orbital fat. (Images from the Visible Human Project® courtesy of the National Library of Medicine)

orbit toward the apex, where it enters the optic canal, and is conveyed into the middle cranial fossa, just anterior to the pituitary gland. Right and left optic nerves join there to form the optic chiasm, adjacent to the pituitary, above the sphenoid sinus. Post-chiasmal optic tracts, comprised of combined fibers from both eyes, carry information derived from the contralateral visual hemifield. These nerve fiber bundles proceed posteriorly to the lateral geniculate nuclei in the thalamus. From there, the optic radiations proceed posteriorly to terminate in the optic cortex region of the occipital lobes, where visual perception occurs (see Chap. 38).

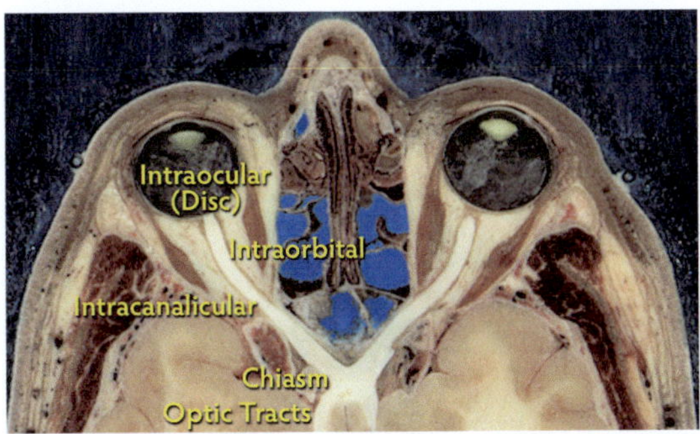

Fig. 1.8 The segments of and intraorbital course of the optic nerve and the intracranial optic chiasm. (Image from the Visible Human Project® courtesy of the National Library of Medicine)

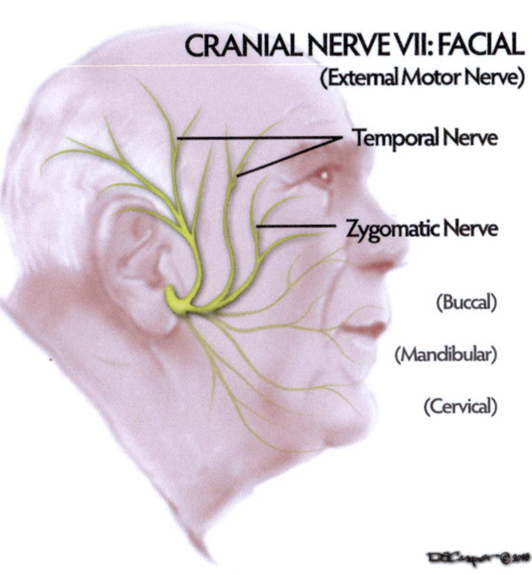

Fig. 1.9 The divisions of the facial nerve serving the orbital region

All other orbital and ocular sensory innervation is supplied by cranial nerve V, the trigeminal nerve. The majority of sensory input is via the first division of the trigeminal (V1), the ophthalmic nerve, which provides sensory fibers to the forehead, nose, upper lid, lacrimal gland, and the globe. The second division of the nerve (V2) provides sensation primarily to the lower lid and cheek.

Motor innervation to the muscles of the eyelids and upper face is provided by cranial nerve VII, the facial nerve, through the two superior divisions, the temporal and zygomatic branches (Fig. 1.9). The three inferior divisions supply the lower face.

Orbital autonomic nerve fibers control pupillary muscular action and also provide innervation to muscle fibers in the upper and lower lids. Preganglionic parasympathetic fibers enter the orbit through the superior orbital fissure, traveling on cranial nerve III (oculomotor nerve), and its branches synapse in the ciliary ganglion, located in the orbit between the optic nerve and lateral rectus muscle. Postganglionic fibers enter the eye via short ciliary nerves.

Postganglionic sympathetic fibers (which synapse in the superior cervical ganglion in the neck) travel to the orbit on the arterial system as a plexus, eventually entering the optic canal with the ophthalmic artery. Most sympathetic fibers pass through the ciliary ganglion to enter the posterior globe via long and short ciliary nerves, although some fibers proceed instead to the eyelids via the oculomotor nerve.

Autonomic innervation also plays a role in regulation of the lacrimal tear glands.

Vascular System

The common carotid arteries supply blood to the orbits; in the neck, at approximately the level of the fourth cervical vertebra, they split into external and internal carotids (Fig. 1.10). The external remains superficial, continuing upward anterior to the ear, giving off the facial artery, which curves around the jaw, prior to terminating near the medial canthus of the eye, and the maxillary artery that runs deep within the cheek and exits via the inferior orbital fissure. The external carotid terminates as the superficial temporal arteries (the usual site for biopsies to diagnose giant cell arteritis {temporal arteritis}). Anastomotic branches given off from external branches connect with the deeper orbital arterial system.

The internal carotid artery enters the skull, where it follows a sinuous course known as the

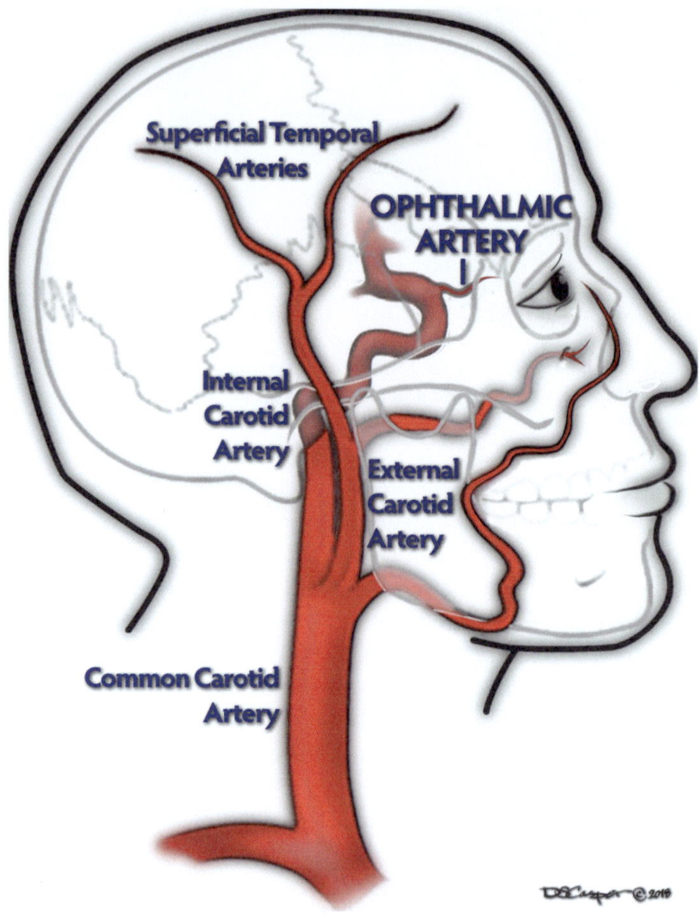

Fig. 1.10 Orbital arterial supply. The ophthalmic artery is the main supplier of arterial blood to the eye and orbit; additional contribution is from anastomotic connections with extra-orbital vascular channels

carotid siphon, before dividing into terminal branches in the middle cranial fossa, adjacent to the sella turcica: anterior, middle, and posterior cerebral arteries (which contribute to the circle of Willis) and the ophthalmic artery, which is the main supplier of blood to the orbit and eye (other sources being anastomotic connections mentioned above and below). The ophthalmic artery is a relatively small branch that enters the orbit via the optic canal, beneath the optic nerve. Numerous intraorbital branches supply the extraocular muscles, lacrimal region, lids (palpebral branches), ciliary branches to the globe, and the central retinal artery, which enters the optic nerve and can be seen with ophthalmoscopy as it divides at the optic disc (Fig. 1.11a–c). Terminal arterial branches anastomose with external carotid branches as noted above and supply superficial tissues.

Apex and Cavernous Sinus

The orbital apices, deeply set within the sphenoid bone, serve as conduits for all major neurovascular structures that connect the orbits with the middle cranial fossa. As noted above, seven of the eight extraocular muscles originate from the annulus of Zinn, located at the apex.

Just posterior to the apices, located in the middle cranial fossae, are the bilateral cavernous sinuses. These venous-filled cavities, formed by a dural cleft, are located on either side of the body of the sphenoid bone. All of the neurovascular structures entering and exiting the orbits (except the optic nerves) pass through these venous sinuses, which also contain the terminal portion of the carotid artery (Fig. 1.12a, b).

Because of the densely packed anatomical configuration of this region, even small lesions located

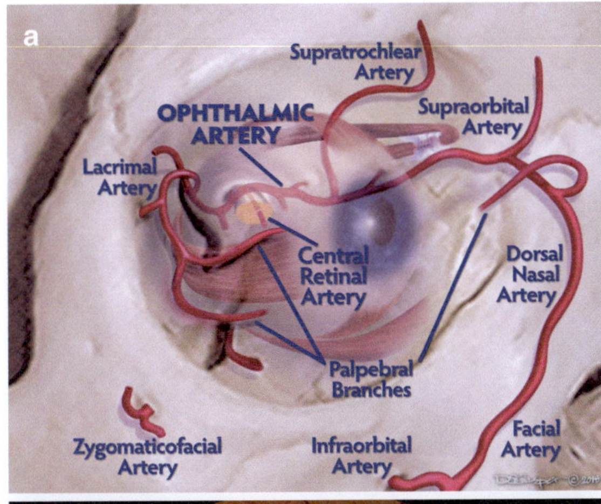

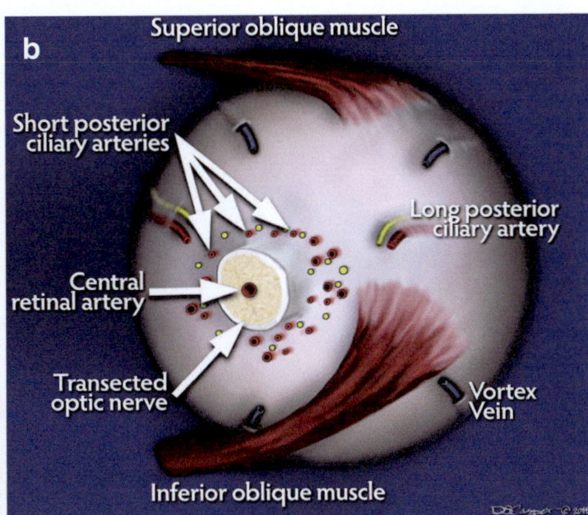

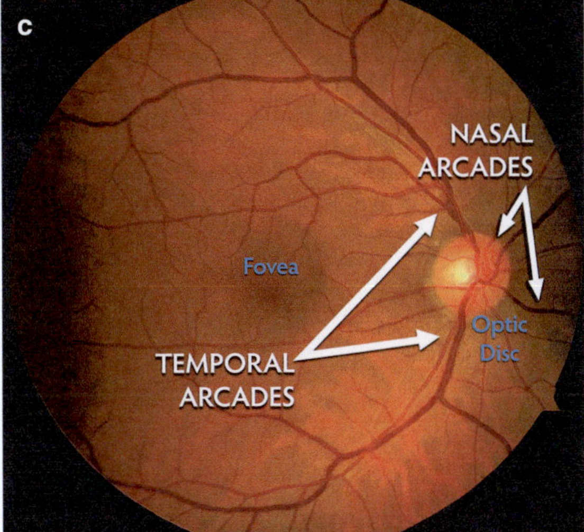

Fig. 1.11 The course of the ophthalmic artery after entering the orbit beneath the optic nerve, before wrapping around and over it, to eventually follow the medial orbital wall (**a**). The arterial supply of the globe (**b**): 2 long posterior ciliary arteries and approximately 20 short posterior ciliary arteries enter the posterior globe, and the central retinal artery travels within the optic nerve. This artery can be visualized with ophthalmoscopy (**c**) after it enters the eye and divides into temporal and nasal arterioles (arcades). The central retinal artery, a branch of the ophthalmic artery, enters the eye through the optic nerve and usually divides into four main arterioles, two temporal and two nasal, to supply the inner retina. The temporal arterioles are the largest and encircle the macula. The central fovea is approximately the same size as the disc (1.5 mm)

within, or adjacent to, the apices and the cavernous sinuses can have devastating effects on ocular neurovascular support and ultimately on vision as well.

Lacrimal System

The cornea and conjunctiva must be constantly lubricated, and this function is served by the lacrimal secretory system (Fig. 1.13a), which is comprised of two separate arms that independently provide an ocular "tear film." One, the *basal* component, is produced by microscopic glands located within the conjunctiva and lids, as well as the large lacrimal gland. This system operates continuously, producing a trilaminar fluid consisting of lipid, aqueous, and mucin layers, supplemented with electrolytes, enzymes, antibodies, and immunoglobulins. A separate system produces *reflex* tears, which, as the name implies, are made as a result of insult (foreign body, wind, heat, etc.) or emotional episodes (resulting in crying). Reflex

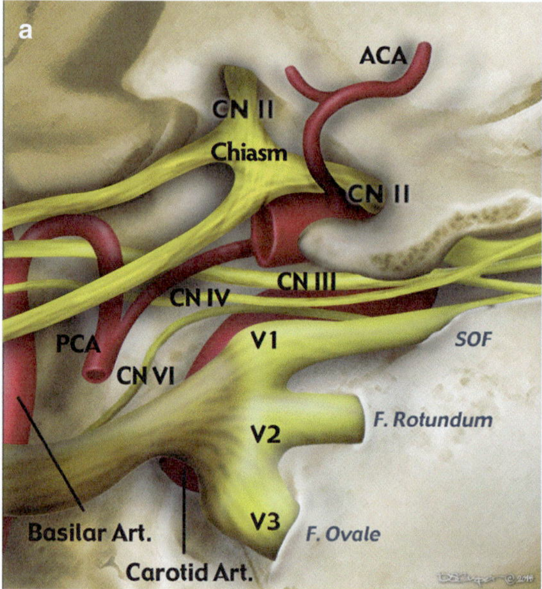

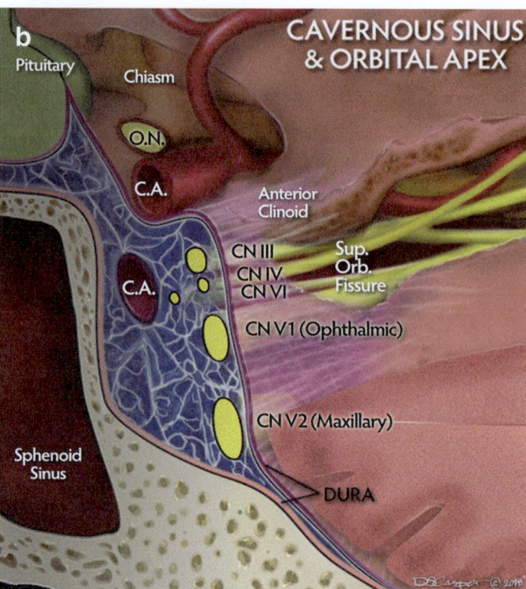

Fig. 1.12 The orbital apex (**a**) lies just anterior to the cavernous sinus (**b**), located in the middle cranial fossa on either side of the sphenoid sinus. All the important neurovascular structures supplying the eye, except the optic nerve, travel through this venous sinus before entering the orbit. Therefore, pathology in this region (such as cavernous sinusitis or carotid aneurysms) can have devastating effects on the visual system. *ACA* anterior cerebral artery; *PCA* posterior cerebral artery; *CN* cranial nerve; *C.A.* carotid artery; *SOF* superior orbital fissure; *O.N.* optic nerve

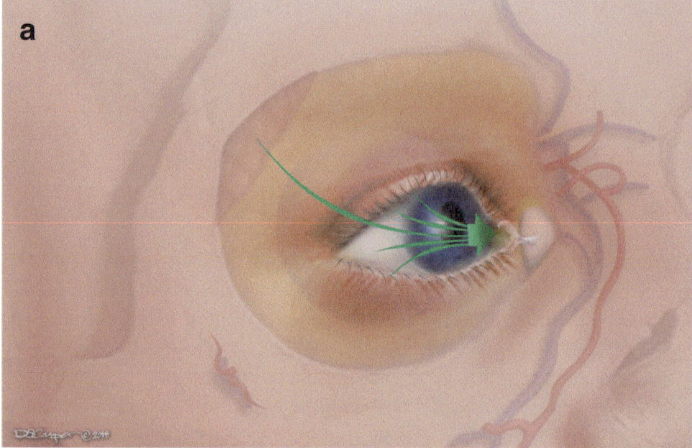

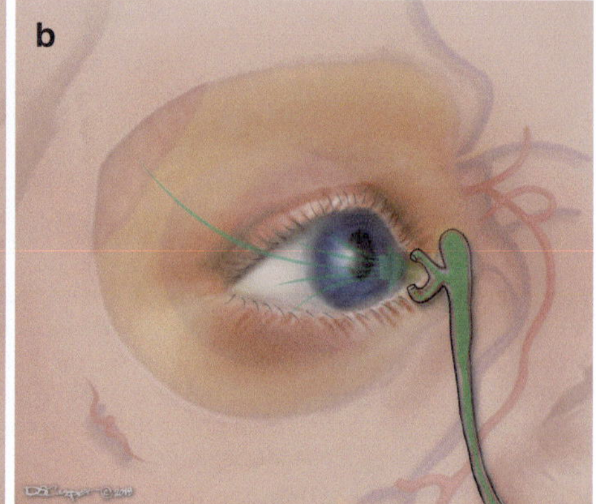

Fig. 1.13 Both basal tears and reflex tears travel inferonasally to drain into the small punctal openings in the lids (**a**) and then enter the nasolacrimal duct system, to eventually reach the pharynx after emptying under the inferior turbinate (**b**)

tears are comprised almost entirely of aqueous fluid made by the lacrimal gland.

The lacrimal system also includes a drainage component, so that excess tears do not overflow and cause irritation and maceration of lid and cheek skin. Small openings, the punctae, are located in the medial portion of the upper and lower lids and lead into canaliculi which carry tears toward the nasolacrimal sac and duct. Tears then flow down the nasolacrimal canal, to empty into the nasal cavity and pharynx beneath the inferior turbinate (Fig. 1.13b).

External Anatomy: Lids

Lids protect the underlying eye, the upper being much more mobile than the lower. The aperture is known as the interpalpebral fissure, which, in the adult, is usually about 30 mm wide by 10 mm high in relaxed, primary gaze (Fig. 1.14). Near the nose, the eyelids join adjacent to the lacrimal drainage ducts, at the medial canthus; the temporal attachment is the lateral canthus.

Deep to the skin layer is the orbicularis muscle, which brings about lid closure (Fig. 1.15a, b). Deep to the orbicularis is a fascial sheet, the orbital septum, which originates off the periosteum of the skull at the orbital opening and acts like a diaphragmatic sheet which partitions the anterior orbit into "preseptal" and "postseptal" compartments. Pathology located in the preseptal space (inflammatory, traumatic, infectious, neoplastic, etc.) is usually more easily treated and less vision-threatening than disease processes located in the postseptal segment, which are deeper in the orbit and usually of greater clinical concern (Fig. 1.16a–d).

Deep to the septum are the tarsal plates, cartilaginous "skeletons" of the lids, which contain Meibomian glands, sebum producers which empty along the lid margin, and are responsible for lipid secretions in basal tears. Also at the tarsal margins are the lashes (or "cilia"), which filter out debris.

Retractor muscles open the lids, acting as antagonists of the orbicularis. As would be expected since lower lid movement is limited, upper lid musculature is anatomically more complex. Typically, retractors can raise the upper lid approximately 15 mm; for additional opening (or if the normal retractor system is impaired), brow musculature (the frontalis) can further elevate the lid by about 2 mm.

Sympathetically innervated fibers are also found in the lids; their ascending path from the superior cervical ganglion has been described above. In Horner's syndrome, which is frequently caused by a mass lesion in the upper chest impinging on the superior cervical ganglion, findings reflect a sympathetic disturbance: the pupil on the affected side is small (miosis), the upper lid droops (ptosis), and sweating is reduced (anhydrosis) on the affected side.

The innermost lid layer is the conjunctiva, a thin, vascularized membrane which lines the

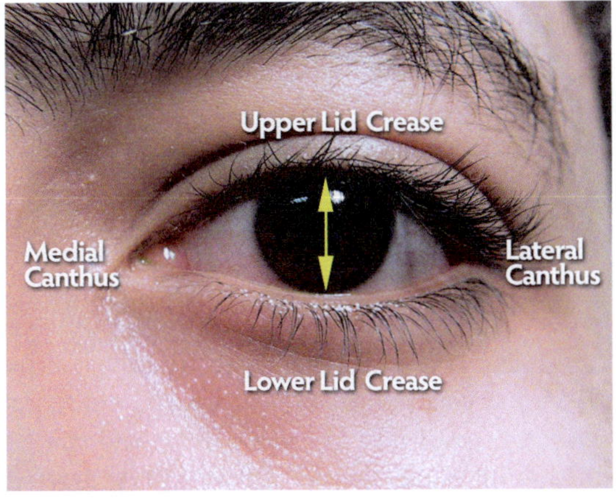

Fig. 1.14 External eyelid anatomy

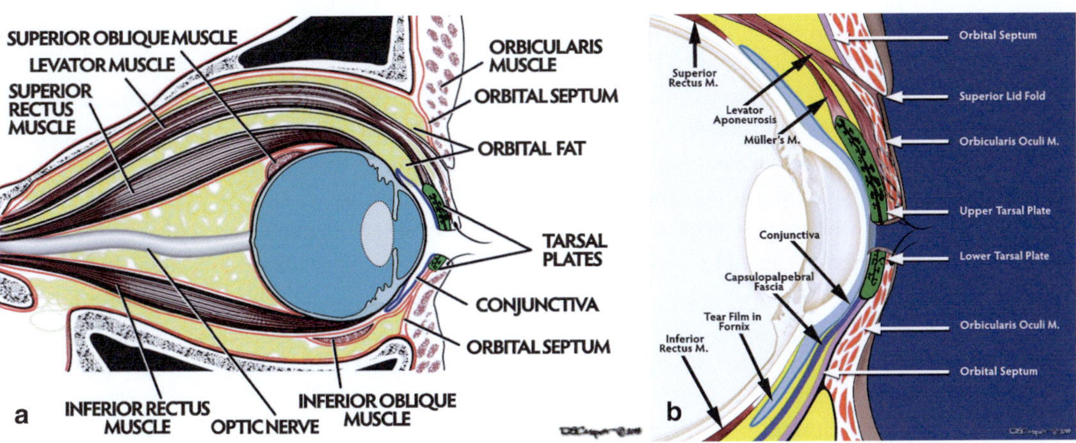

Fig. 1.15 A sagittal section through mid-orbit, showing the periorbital structures (**a**). The diaphragm-like orbital septum, which originates off the periosteum of bones of the orbital rim, defines pre- and postseptal compartments in the orbit (**b**)

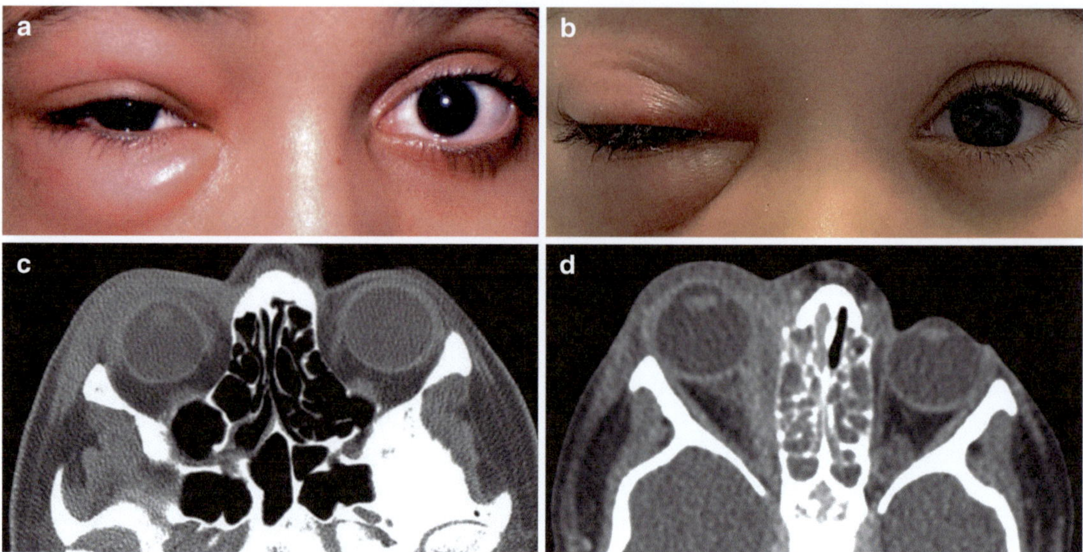

Fig. 1.16 Pathologic processes occurring superficial to the septum (such as a preseptal cellulitis, here showing lid edema [**a**, external photograph and **c**, axial CT]) are generally less severe, and more easily treated, than postseptal ones (such as orbital cellulitis, here showing intraorbital involvement with proptosis [**b**, external photograph and **d**, axial CT])

inner lids, and then reflects back, at the fornix, to cover the globe, merging with the clear cornea at the limbus.

The lids are anchored at the canthi, and an externally or internally directed force can cause the lid to rotate either outward (ectropion) or inward (entropion), respectively. The normal equilibrium of the skin, muscle, septum, and conjunctival forces keeps the lids positioned properly in the vertical plane. Should there be some disturbance in this balance (e.g., a muscle palsy, a lid tumor, conjunctival scarring, normal aging changes with tissue laxity, etc.), then a lid malposition may result. Inward rotation of the lid margin, particularly the lashes (trichiasis), results in persistent corneal irritation and epithelial breakdown, with secondary infection (keratitis), scarring, and loss of vision due to loss of corneal transparency (see Chaps. 9 and 31).

The Globe

The average, normal human eye (Fig. 1.17) is approximately 24 mm in diameter, a size that is usually achieved by the late teenage years. The anteriorly placed cornea has a smaller radius than the overall globe, so its curvature bulges out slightly from the front of the eye.

The eye can be viewed as a composite of three concentric layers or tunics (Fig. 1.18a–c). The outermost layer is the thick, corneoscleral tunic, formed primarily of collagen fibers, and can be thought of as the skeleton of the eye, providing structural support to the spheroid shape.

The innermost layer of the globe is the photosensitive retina, which receives light information focused at the posterior pole of the eye, particularly at the macula, and its central foveal area. Retinal neurons process and refine image signals before they are collected at the optic nerve for transmission to the visual cortex of the occipital lobe of the brain.

Sandwiched between the outer sclera and inner retina is the uvea, the vascular tunic of the eye. The uvea has three contiguous components: the anteriorly placed iris; posterior to the iris is the ciliary body; and behind the ciliary body, beneath the retina, is the choroid. Although these structures also have secondary functions (the iris's central variable opening is the pupillary aperture; the ciliary body produces aqueous fluid

Fig. 1.17 The main parts of the eye. The globe averages 24 mm in diameter, with the anteriorly bulging clear cornea having a smaller radius of curvature. *CB* ciliary body

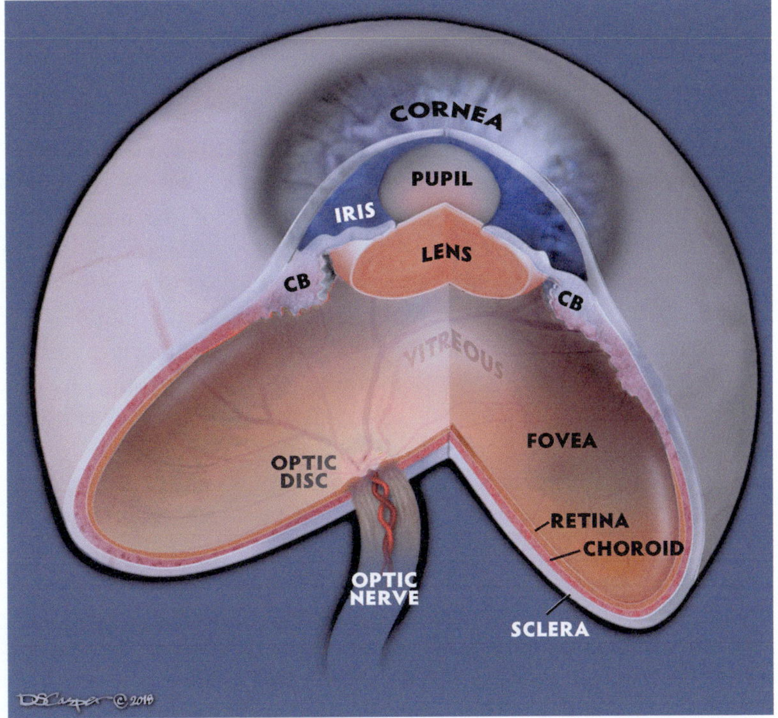

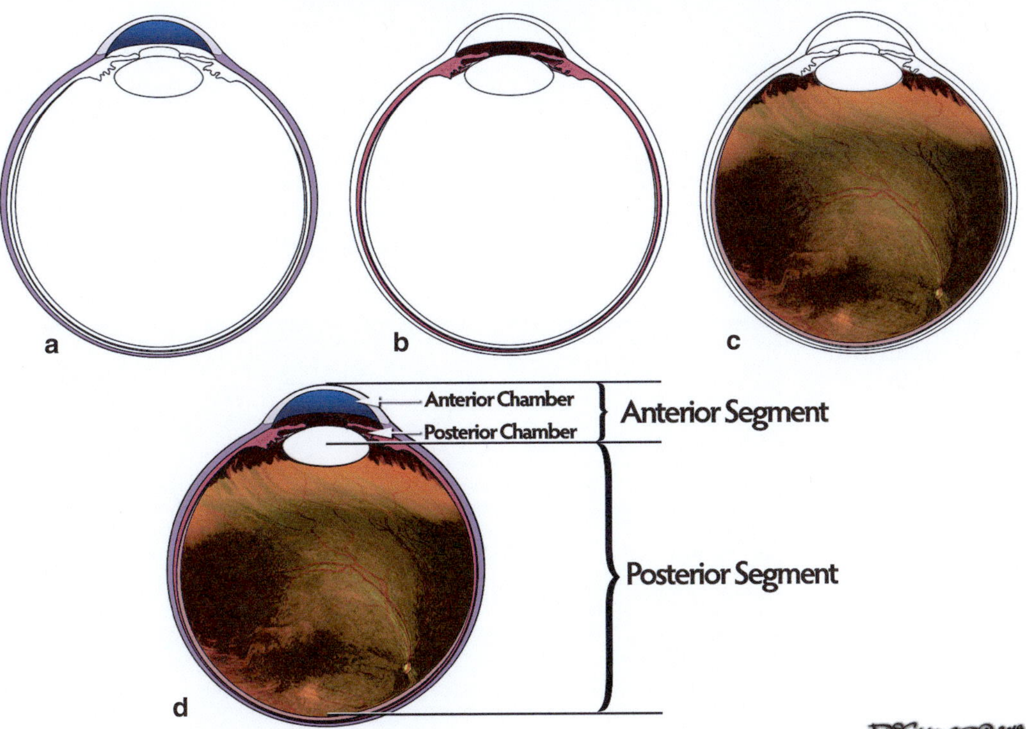

Fig. 1.18 (**a–d**) The globe has three main layers or tunics: the outer, supporting sclera-corneal tunic (**a**); the middle, vascular uvea (**b**); and the innermost retina (**c**), the photosensitive layer of the eye

and controls the shape of the lens within the eye; the choroid controls thermoregulation and may participate in image focusing), the uvea's primary function is nourishment of the eye.

The front part of the eye, anterior to the vitreous, is known as the anterior segment (Figs. 1.18d and 1.19) and consists of the cornea, iris, ciliary body, lens, and zonular fibers.

The clear cornea, located anteriorly, fuses with the portion of the transparent conjunctiva that overlies the sclera. The delicate, highly vascularized conjunctiva extends up to the corneoscleral junction, an area known as the limbus, but does not cover the cornea. When the conjunctiva becomes engorged with blood (e.g., with infection or inflammation), one is said to have "bloodshot" or "pink" eyes.

The cornea, the eye's main focusing element, bends or refracts light so that images focus on the retina (see Chap. 7). Two-thirds of the light bending that is required to produce a focused retinal image is performed by the cornea. This refractive power is possible because of the convex surface of the cornea and the difference in refractive index of air and the corneal tear film. Corneal transparency, which facilitates light reaching the ocular interior, is enabled by the highly ordered architectural arrangement of its collagen fibers; the contiguous sclera, with the same histologic makeup, has no such regularity and is therefore opaque.

The cornea is multilayered (Fig. 1.20). Beneath the air-tear film interface is the corneal epithelium, which consists of approximately five

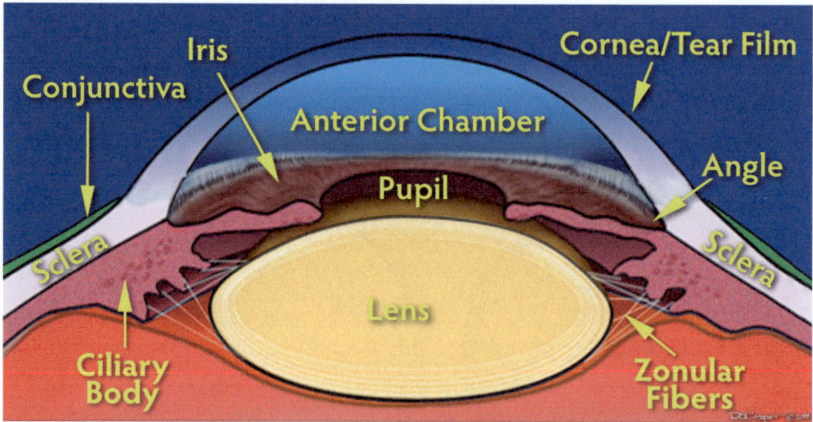

Fig. 1.19 The anterior segment, consisting of the cornea, clear aqueous fluid within the anterior chamber, the iris, and the lens of the eye

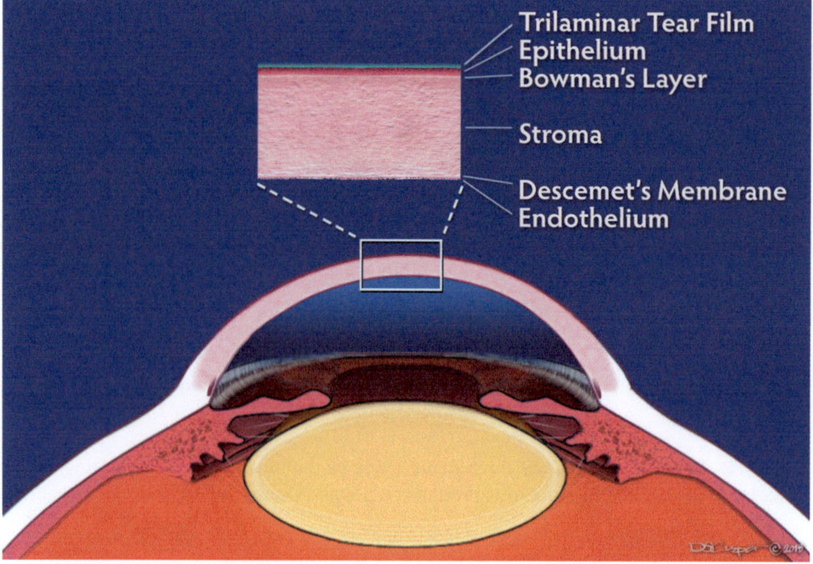

Fig. 1.20 The cornea, showing its multilayered construction, with superficial epithelium overlying Bowman's layer; the stroma, making up the bulk of the cornea; and inner Descemet's membrane, underneath which is the innermost layer, the endothelium

layers of cells. A single-layered corneal endothelium is innermost and is bathed and nourished by aqueous humor in the anterior chamber. Between the epithelium and endothelium is the corneal stroma, consisting of flattened fibroblast cells (keratocytes) and fine collagen fibers. The corneal epithelium undergoes mitosis and can replace damaged cells, as occurs after a corneal abrasion, a common superficial injury (see also Figs. 8.10 and 12.2). The capacity of the corneal endothelium to repair itself, however, is limited. In the normal eye, the epithelium is constantly and evenly bathed in the tear film.

The "white of the eye" is the outer connective tissue coat called the sclera, which extends all the way around the eye and in front becomes continuous with the transparent cornea at the corneoscleral junction.

The anterior chamber is the space just posterior to the corneal endothelium and anterior to the iris. The chamber contains the aqueous humor, a fluid which is constantly being produced and drained at a steady state in the normal eye.

Iris color depends on the total amount of melanin pigment in the iris cells, overlying muscles and blood vessels; it is the interplay of these different components that produces apparent eye color, as all melanin pigment is brown. The iris is a contractile diaphragm, its central opening the variable-sized pupil that controls the amount of light entering the eye. Pupillary miosis (constriction) reduces the amount of light entering the eye, and dilation (enlargement) lets in more light. Miotic smooth muscle fibers encircle the pupillary opening, while fibers of the pupillary dilator muscle are oriented radially, to enlarge the pupillary opening. Pupillary size varies (an involuntary response) because of actions of these iridial muscles, which respond to ambient light as well as autonomic nerve input.

The lens (Fig. 1.21) is a normally clear, elastic biconvex structure situated behind the pupil. It is suspended from the ciliary body (Fig. 1.19) by zonular fibers (Figs. 1.19, 2.5, and 11.1a). The lens is responsible for accommodation, the ability to focus on a near object, controlled by the ciliary muscle, which adjusts lens shape so as to manipulate its refractive power. The outermost layer of the lens is the lens capsule, under which,

anteriorly and at the lens equator, lies a layer of cuboidal cells: the lens epithelium (see Fig. 11.1a). The interior of the lens (cortex and nucleus) consists of so-called fiber cells. These unusual, densely packed cells are flattened and ribbon-like, and the innermost ones lose their nuclei and most organelles, and are instead filled with proteins (crystallins). Cytoplasmic homogeneity and the regular arrangement of lens fiber cells are responsible for lens transparency. Loss of lens transparency, which occurs normally with aging, or secondary to a variety of pathologic conditions, constitutes a cataract (see Chap. 11). Although a primary function of the cornea and lens is to enable focused light to enter the eye, they also act to block potentially harmful ultraviolet light from reaching the retina. With age, the lens also acquires yellow pigment that reduces the transmission of short wavelength (blue) light. When particularly obvious, this yellowing is referred to as "brunescence" (see Fig. 11.1b).

The ciliary body is contiguous with the iris anteriorly and the choroid posteriorly and contains the ciliary muscle that controls the shape of the lens via zonular fibers. Ciliary processes, which extend from the ciliary body into the posterior chamber, secrete aqueous humor and give attachment to the zonular ligaments (Fig. 1.22). Ciliary epithelium secretes aqueous humor by transferring ions, and secondarily water, from the stroma of the ciliary body into the posterior chamber.

Aqueous humor is a fluid that fills the anterior and posterior chambers, being continually secreted and drained, normally in equilibrium, and provides nourishment to the avascular lens and cornea. The aqueous humor also generates intraocular pressure to maintain the spherical shape of the eye. Aqueous, produced continuously by the ciliary body, flows forward over the anterior lens surface, through the pupil, and toward the junction of the iris with the anterior sclera (Fig. 1.23). This junction, known as the chamber angle, houses a sieve-like microscopic labyrinth, the trabecular meshwork, through which aqueous fluid flows and is filtered (Fig. 1.24). Filtered aqueous eventually reaches a drainage system, Schlemm's canal, which encir-

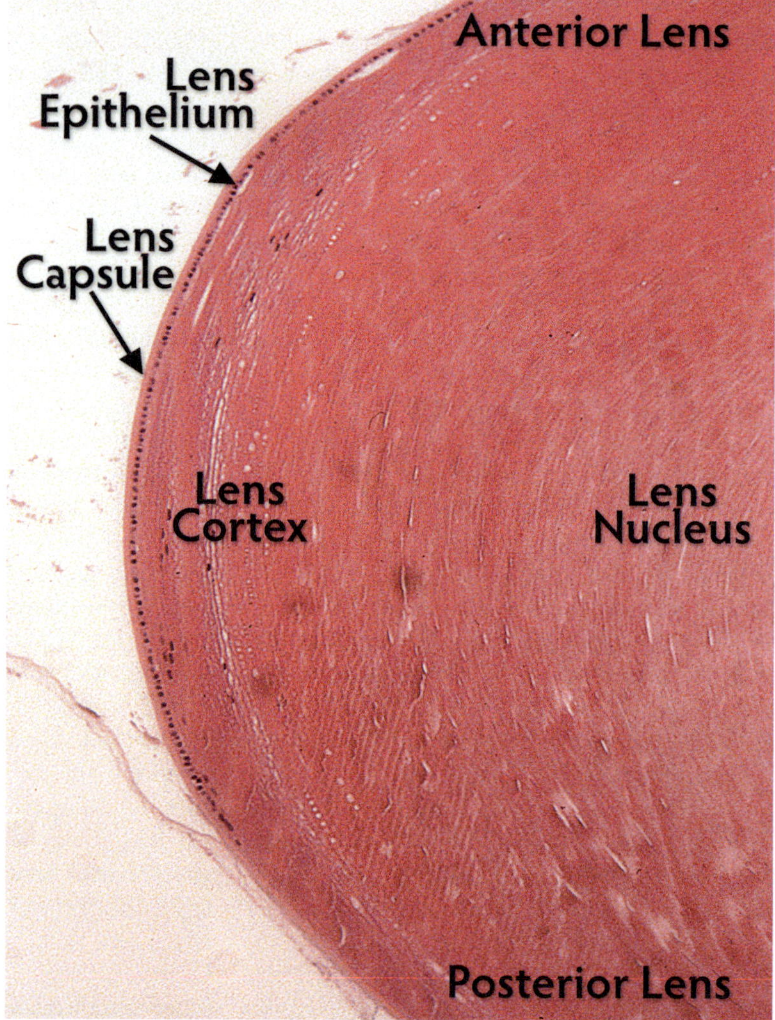

Fig. 1.21 The lens, shown here in histologic cross section, is biconvex, with an outer lens capsule overlying the epithelium and an interior structure of fiber cells which make up the cortex and nucleus. The lens can adjust its anteroposterior depth, which alters the lenticular curvature, thereby modifying its refractive power

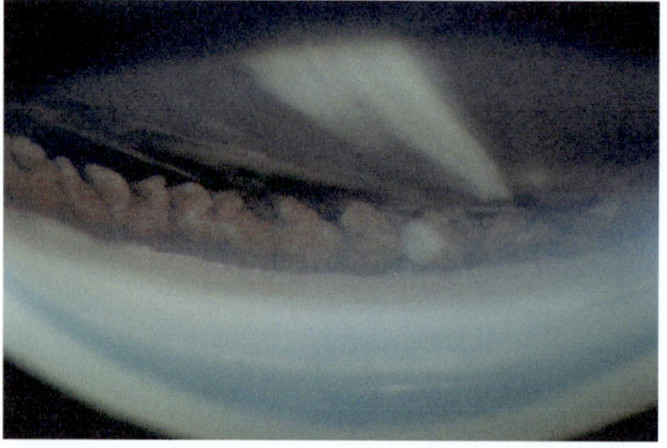

Fig. 1.22 Ciliary processes. The lens is connected to the circular ciliary body by 360° of fine zonular fibers which originate from the ciliary processes, behind the pupil, and therefore are not normally visible. In this case of congenital aniridia (absence of the iris), the ciliary processes are clearly seen, as there is no overlying iris to obscure them

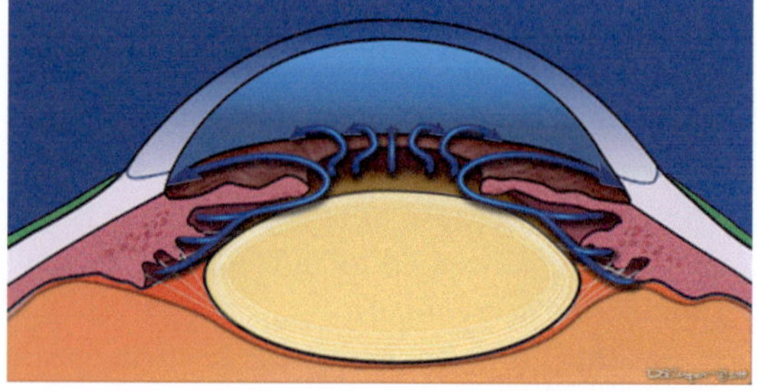

Fig. 1.23 Aqueous fluid is constantly produced by the ciliary body epithelium and flows over the lens and through the pupil to exit the anterior chamber at the region where the cornea and the iris meet, known as the angle; the angle encircles the anterior portion of the eye for 360°. If aqueous drainage decreases while production remains stable, intraocular pressure will increase

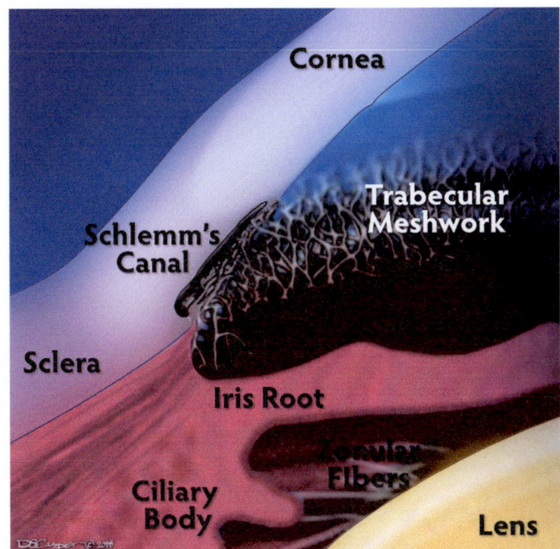

Fig. 1.24 Within the angle, a microscopic filter, known as the trabecular meshwork, is the area through which aqueous fluid exits, prior to entering Schlemm's canal for drainage. Fluid in Schlemm's canal eventually empties into the venous system for recirculation

cles the eye and ultimately empties into aqueous veins, which merge with the venous system (see Figs. 19.1 and 19.2). Abnormalities in aqueous drainage are believed to play a major role in the eye disease known as glaucoma. In open-angle glaucoma, the irido-scleral angle is grossly normal, but aqueous fluid drainage is believed to decrease slowly over many years; in narrow-angle glaucoma, the anatomical angle itself is not sufficiently wide to enable normal drainage, and aqueous outflow can decrease precipitously, leading to a rapid and potentially sight-threatening increase in intraocular pressure (Fig. 1.25).

The remaining portion of the eye is known as the posterior segment, comprised of sclera, underlying choroid and retina, and the optic nerve. Within the globe, the majority of the posterior segment is filled with the gelatinous vitreous body, a clear substance consisting predominantly of water, collagen fibers, a few

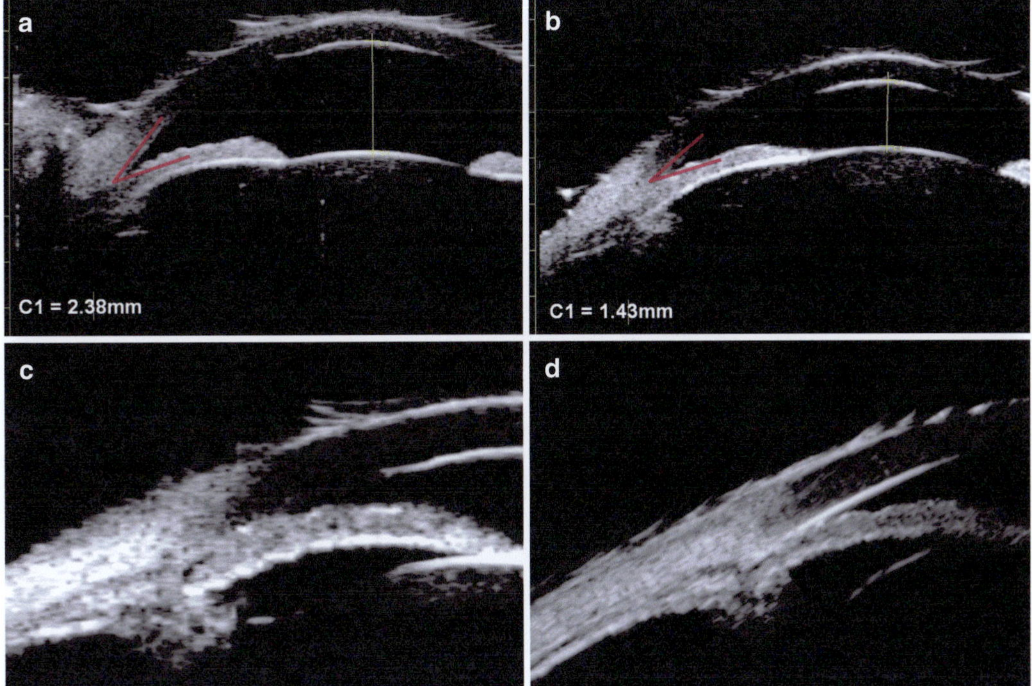

Fig. 1.25 (**a–d**) If the angle is narrower than normal (a condition usually seen with some farsighted people or occasionally as an anatomical variant and often exacerbated by cataract), aqueous drainage may be reduced, leading to fluid buildup which can force the iris forward, causing the angle to be completely occluded. This uncommon event is known as a narrow-angle attack and is an ophthalmic emergency. (**a**) Ultrasound biomicroscopy (UBM) images show an open angle, with an anterior chamber depth measurement of 2.38 mm, and (**b**) a narrow angle, with an anterior depth measurement of 1.43 mm; the red lines indicate the angles. (**c**, **d**) UBM images of narrow angles. (Courtesy of Dr. Ronald Silverman)

different types of cells, and proteins, encased within a clear membrane (Fig. 1.26).

The view into the fundus using a handheld, monocular, direct ophthalmoscope is only about 5°, which is typically a little larger than the optic disc. The binocular indirect ophthalmoscope and standard fundus photographs usually provide an image of about 45°. With the use of indirect ophthalmoscopy, special lenses at the slit lamp, or newer wide-field photography, this view can be greatly expanded to approximately 200°, enabling examination of a large amount of peripheral retina which is otherwise not easily visualized (Fig. 1.27).

There are two regions in the central retina where structural organization of the neural retina is normally altered. One is the optic disc, lying approximately 3 mm to the nasal side of the posterior pole. Here, retinal layers are interrupted by ganglion cell axons that exit the eye to travel via the optic nerve to the brain. Because of this interruption, the optic disc produces a blind spot in the normal visual field (Fig. 1.28). The central retinal artery enters the retina within the optic nerve and generally divides into four main branches (see above, Fig. 1.11c): two large arterioles course toward the ear (the temporal arcades) and two smaller ones are directed toward the midline (nasal arcades). The temporal arcades surround and define the area known as the macula, where, due to the high density of cone photoreceptor cells, the eye has its most acute vision, as well as color appreciation (photopic vision). The retina

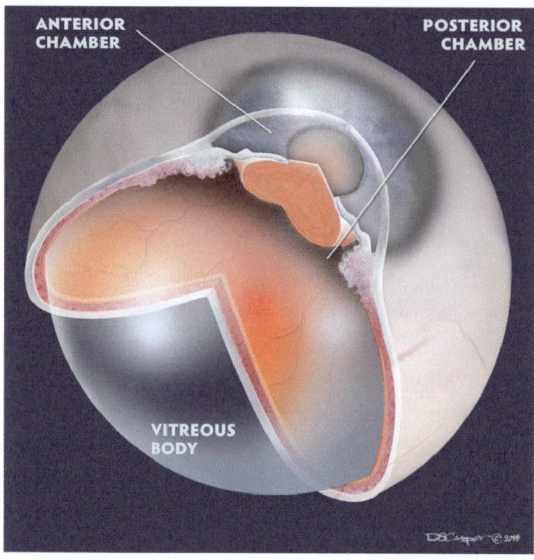

Fig. 1.26 A representation of the anterior and posterior chambers and the large, transparent vitreous body, making up the majority of the posterior segment of the globe

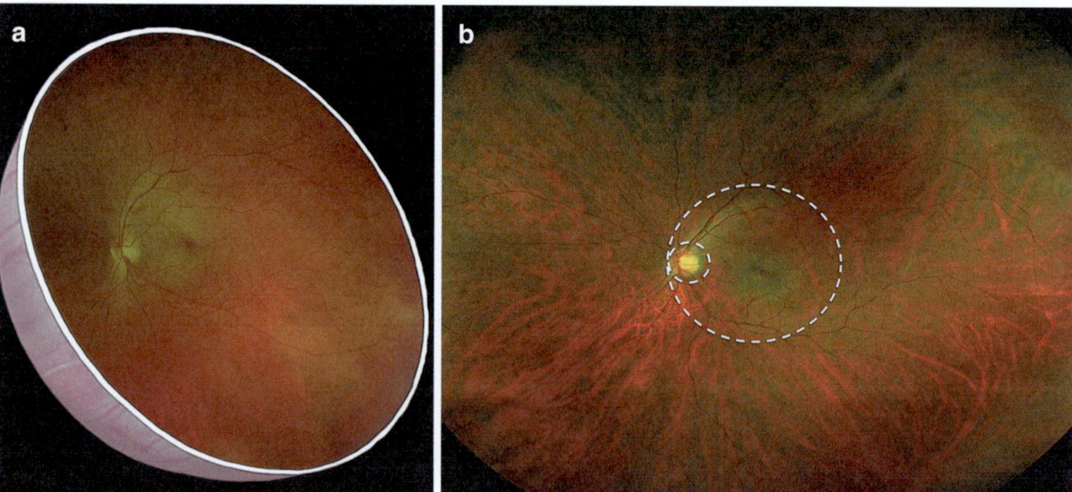

Fig. 1.27 (**a**) An illustration of the posterior half of a sectioned eye, showing how the retina follows the curvature of the globe. (**b**) A wide-field fundus image (approximately 200°) taken with an Optos camera system, showing how the retina appears "flattened" in a two-dimensional image. Note the approximate size of the examiner's fields of view, seen with a monocular handheld ophthalmoscope (the smaller dashed circle, approximately 5°) and the head-mounted indirect binocular ophthalmoscope or using slit-lamp ophthalmoscopy (the larger dashed circle, approximately 45°). Prominent choroidal vessels are seen through the transparent retina and underlying pigment epithelium

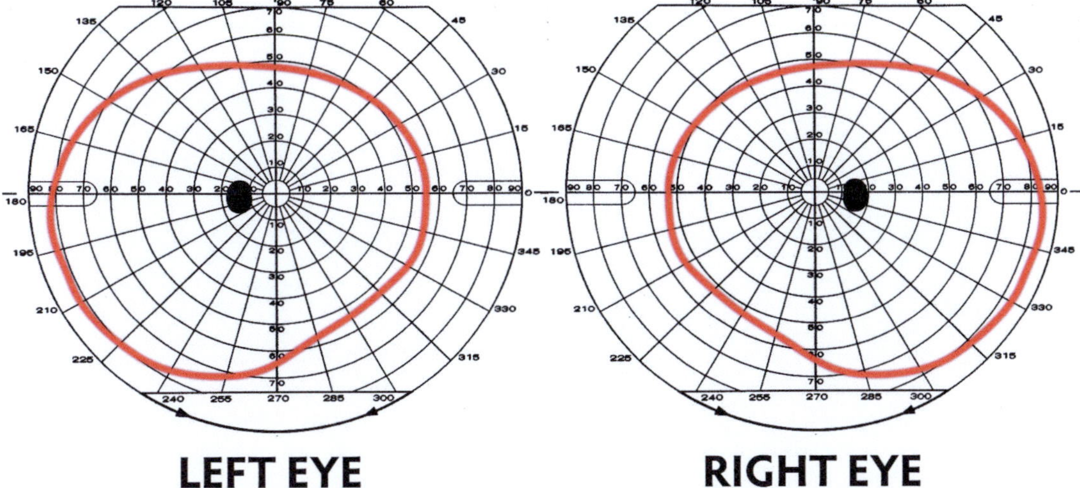

Fig. 1.28 A normal Goldmann visual field test, which analyzes optic nerve functioning. The red outlines represent the limit of the peripheral vision when looking straight ahead. Lighter areas of the field are more clearly appreciated, while dark areas are relatively unseen areas. Note the blind spots seen temporally in each eye, which correspond to the optic nerve head, which has no photoreceptors and, therefore, no visual potential. Visual field tests are used to analyze both enlargement of the normal blind spots, seen here, and the appearance of peripheral defects, indicative of optic nerve dysfunction (see Chap. 18)

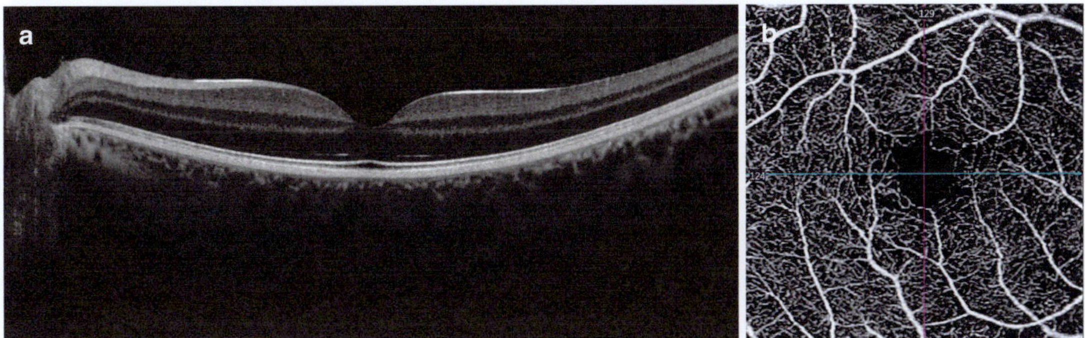

Fig. 1.29 An optical coherence tomogram (OCT), which produces a non-invasively obtained cross-sectional image, here shows how the fovea is a depression in the retina and is the thinnest area of the macula. The optic nerve is seen exiting on the left (**a**). The remarkable resolution of the OCT image clearly shows the retinal layers and demonstrates the absence of the innermost retinal layers in the central fovea, which results in the typical concavity seen here. An OCT angiogram of the foveal area (**b**) demonstrates that in addition to the absence of inner retinal layers, there is a gap in the retinal capillary net over the fovea, further permitting central light rays to fall directly on posteriorly located retinal photoreceptor cells with minimal distortion induced by overlying capillaries

peripheral to this macular region has predominantly rod photoreceptor cells, which have much less distinct acuity, and monochromatic vision (scotopic vision) predominates.

The second regional specialization is the fovea, situated directly at the central posterior pole. The fovea, the thinnest area in the macula, measures approximately 0.5 mm across, has no overlying capillaries to interfere with image focusing, and is the area which provides the highest level of visual acuity, needed to read, recognize faces, and see detail (Figs. 1.1c and 1.29a, b). Even a small lesion in this area can cause a debilitating blind spot known as a central scotoma.

The retina terminates peripherally, in the anterior portion of the eye, in an area called the ora serrata. At the ora serrata, the neural retina becomes continuous with ciliary body epithelium.

In order for vision to occur, the pathway to retinal photoreceptors must be transparent and

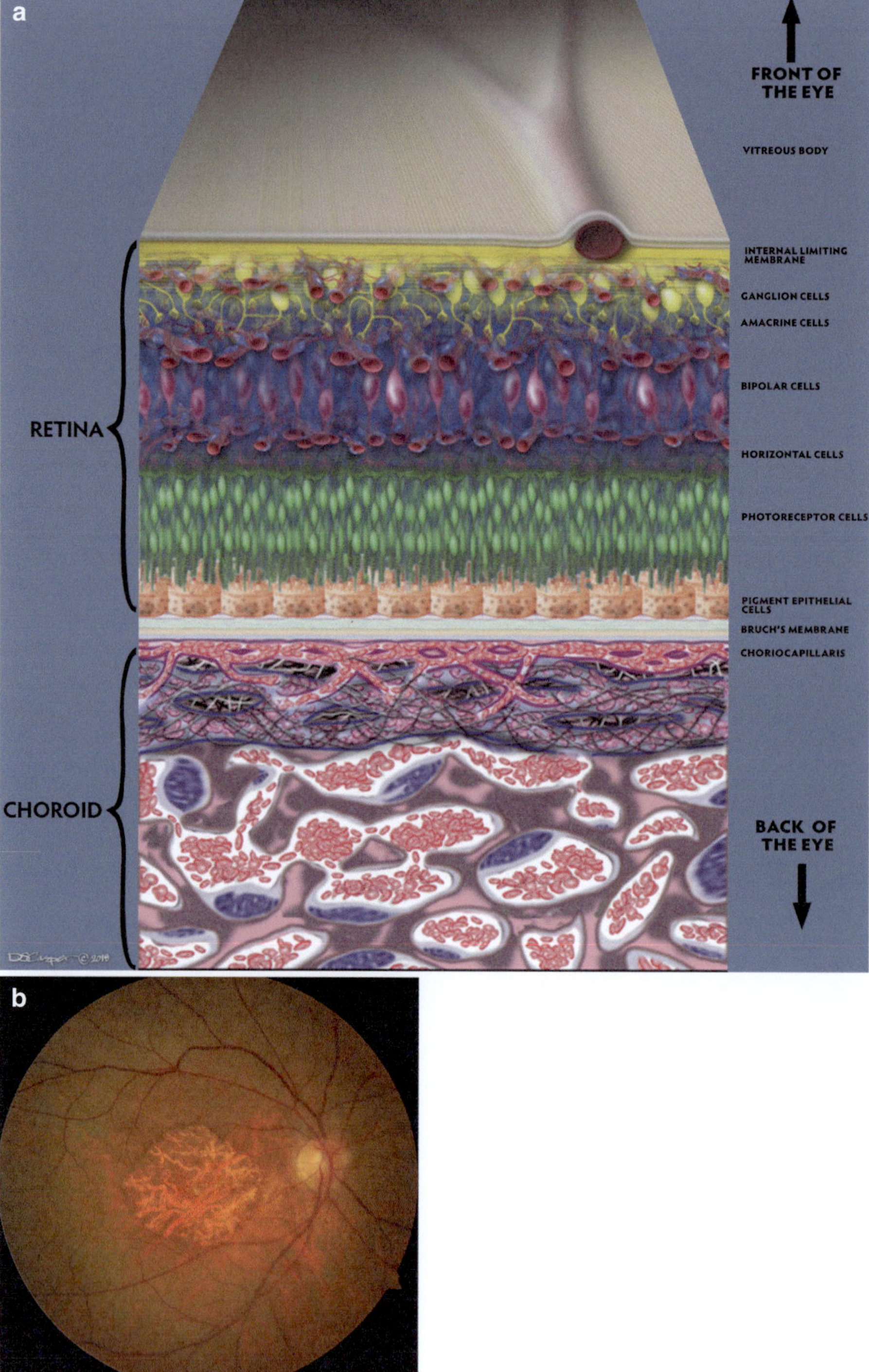

Fig. 1.30 (**a**) A schematic diagram of the retina and anterior choroid. The anterior eye is above and the posterior below. The vitreous body, not shown, is in contact with internal limiting membrane, just anterior to the retina. A retinal arteriole is shown on the inner retinal surface. Deep to the outer retina are the pigmented epithelial layer, Bruch's membrane, and the layers of the vascular choroid, with the smaller chorio-capillaris vessels anteriorly and the larger choroidal vessels more posterior. Not shown, posterior to the choroid, is the sclera. (**b**) A fundus photo of a patient with dry macular degeneration and central geographic atrophy. Degeneration of the retina, pigmented epithelium, and choriocapillaris reveals underlying large choroidal vessels made visible due to the overlying tissue atrophy

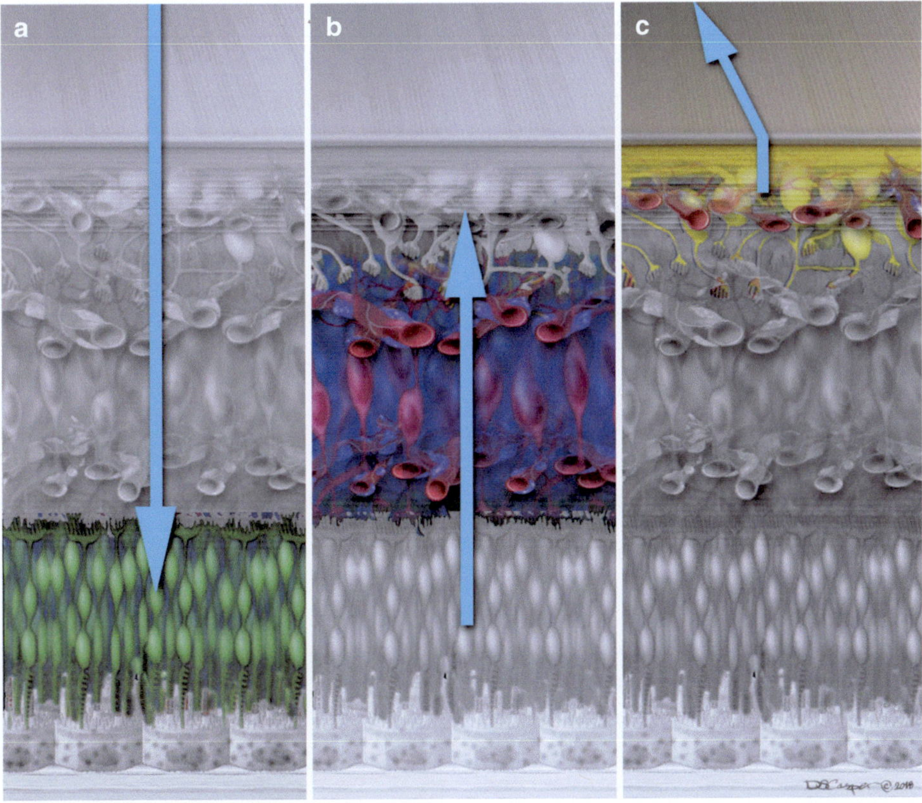

Fig. 1.31 The retina must be transparent because photo-receptor cells are located posteriorly (**a**). Light travels through the retinal stroma to reach the photosensitive rods and cones, where photic energy is converted to electro-chemical signals. This electrochemical information then reverses direction and travels anteriorly through a series of retinal neurons, to finally reach ganglion cells located in the innermost, anterior retina (**b**). Each ganglion cell axon then carries these signals centripetally, to join together and form the optic nerve (**c**)

unobstructed: an image must traverse the tear film, cornea, aqueous fluid, pupil, lens, vitreous body, anterior (or "inner") retinal surface, and middle retinal layers before finally reaching the light-sensitive photoreceptor cells at the pos-terior (or "outer") retina (Figs. 1.30 and 1.31a–c). Attenuation of inner retinal layers in the foveal region optimizes direct image access to cen-tral photoreceptor cells. Images received by rod and cone photoreceptors are transformed into electrochemical signals which reverse direction and travel back through the middle retinal layers via complex neuronal chains, where further pro-cessing occurs, to finally reach the innermost retina, where the ganglion cell bodies are located (Fig. 1.31). Each ganglion cell (which total approximately 1.25 million per eye) sends an axonal fiber centripetally across the retinal sur-face, to assemble as the optic nerve, which is a bundle of these aggregated ganglion cell axons. In their course toward the optic nerve, individual axonal fibers deviate around the central foveal area, theoretically providing light images a more direct route to foveal photoreceptor cells by diverting overlying inner retinal layers and capil-laries in the "foveal avascular zone". Normal central foveal thinning and capillary absence is clearly seen in OCT cross-sectional images and OCT angiograms (Fig. 1.29).

When viewing the interior of the eye with an ophthalmoscope or camera, one sees arterioles and venules overlying the clear retina and, due to retinal transparency, layers posterior to the retina: the pigmented choroid, and the single-layered pigmented epithelium, sandwiched between the choroid and outer retina. Normal retinal tissue is

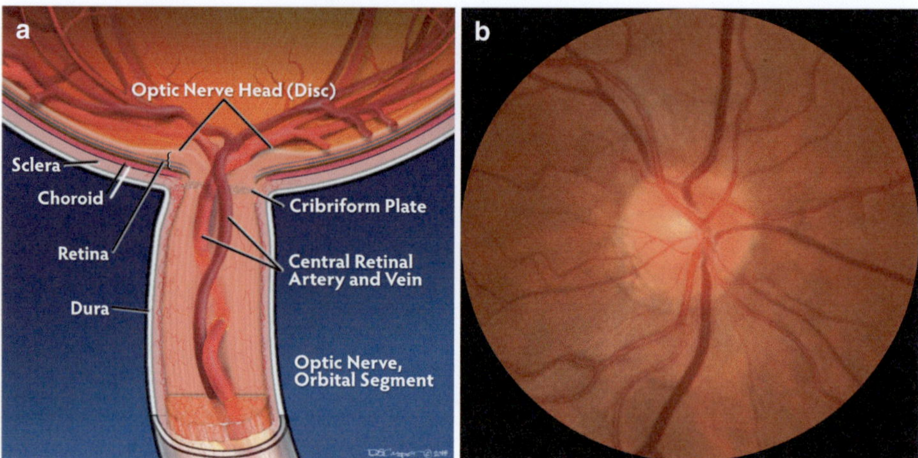

Fig. 1.32 (**a, b**) Examination of the optic nerve head (also referred to as the "disc") is a major part of any complete ophthalmic exam. Enlargement or obliteration of the central depression (referred to as the "cup"), blurring of the sharpness of the disc borders, obscuration of the arterioles or venules, or elevation of the nerve head may indicate significant pathology

not visible with standard viewing. When there is a vascular disturbance, as with an arterial occlusion, or long-standing diabetes, the retina may become ischemic and will then lose its transparency. These ischemic portions of retina become temporary yellow-white opacities that obscure the posterior layers and are known as "cotton wool spots" because of their whitish appearance with soft, feathery borders. In such cases, the opaque retinal tissue obscures the normally visible deeper layers (Fig. 1.32).

The temporal and nasal arcades, which originate at the termination of the central retinal artery at the optic disc, ramify into capillary networks which nourish inner retinal layers. The posterior, deeper retinal layers and pigmented epithelial layer are supplied by choriocapillaris, the anteriormost layer of the vascular choroid (Fig. 1.30a, b).

The orbital portion of the optic nerve has been discussed. Where the nerve exits the globe, it can be seen with an ophthalmoscope as the optic disc. The disc is circular or oval in shape and has a central depression known as the optic cup (Fig. 1.33). In diseases such as glaucoma, the size of this central cup can enlarge, which occurs due to loss of surrounding axonal tissue, known as the optic rim. This loss of rim tissue is most easily visualized as enlargement of the cup, which can

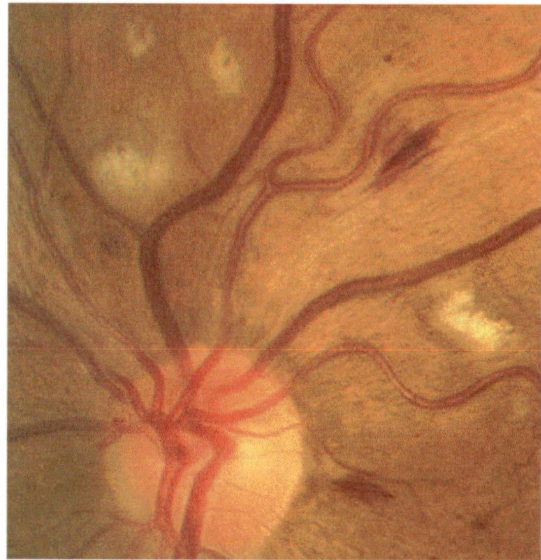

Fig. 1.33 The optic disc and adjacent area in a patient with diabetic retinopathy, showing white areas of retinal opacifiation, so-called cotton wool spots, indicative of retinal ischemia. The retina is normally transparent, permitting visualization of more posterior layers, the pigmented epithelium and choroid. Diabetes-related flame-shaped hemorrhages are also present in this image

be monitored, and helps with disease diagnosis and staging (see Chap. 16). With increased intracranial pressure, which is transmitted down the dural sheath of the optic nerve, one may see blurring and elevation of the disc with oblitera-tion of the optic cup, known as disc edema, or papilledema.

The optic nerves exit the eyes posteriorly, travel medially through the orbit to the optic canals, and join in the middle cranial fossa as the optic chiasm, adjacent to the pituitary, above the sphenoid sinus. Post-chiasmal optic tracts, comprised of combined fibers from both eyes, carry information derived from the contralateral visual hemifield. These nerve fiber bundles pro-ceed posteriorly to the lateral geniculate nuclei in the thalamus, and from there, the optic radia-tions proceed posteriorly to terminate in the visual cortex region of the occipital lobes, where perception occurs.

Suggested Reading

Hogan M, Alvarado J, Weddell J. Histology of the human eye. Philadelphia: Saunders; 1971.
Casper D, Chi L, Trokel S. Orbital disease: imaging and analysis. New York: Thieme; 1993.
Doxanas M, Anderson R. Clinical orbital anatomy. Baltimore: Williams & Wilkins; 1984.
Warwick R. Wolff's anatomy of the eye and orbit. Philadelphia: Saunders; 1976.
Oyster C. The human eye: structure and function. Sunderland: Sinauer Associates; 1999.

Adult Eye Examination Techniques

2

Quan V. Hoang

The adult eye examination is unique in medicine in that most of the pathology is directly, objectively visible to the examiner. The adult eye examination includes an analysis of the physiologic function and anatomic status of the eye, visual system, and related structures. Through the use of specialized instruments, the adult eye examination is performed in a systematic manner (See Appendix 3).

Components of the Adult Eye Exam

Components of the adult eye exam generally consist of:

- Patient and family history, including visual, ocular, and general health, medication usage, and vocational and avocational visual requirements and systemic health assessment as indicated
- Visual acuity with and without present correction (if any) at distance and near
- Best corrected visual acuity (determined by retinoscopy and refraction)
- Pupillary exam
- Ocular alignment and extraocular motility (and exophthalmometry, binocular vision and accommodation as warranted by age and visual complaints)
- Intraocular pressure
- Visual field examination
- External exam (lids/lashes, ocular adnexa)
- Anterior segment (conjunctiva/sclera, cornea, anterior chamber, iris)
- Posterior segment (dilated fundus examination of nerve, macula, vessels, retinal periphery)
- Systemic health assessment when warranted (e.g., blood pressure measurement, carotid artery assessment, laboratory testing, imaging, cranial nerve assessment)

Visual Acuity

Visual acuity, measured one eye at a time (Fig. 2.1), with and without the patient's most recent spectacle or contact lens correction, may include:

- Distance visual acuity (DVA), most commonly with a standard Snellen chart at 20 ft.
- Near visual acuity (NVA).
- Pinhole acuity, using an occluder with pinholes, in an attempt to improve the vision and estimate the eye's best potential vision. Improvement in

Q. V. Hoang, MD, PhD (✉)
Singapore National Eye Centre/Duke-NUS Medical School, Singapore Eye Research Institute, Singapore, Singapore

Columbia University Medical, New York, NY, USA

Department of Ophthalmology, Edward S. Harkness Eye Institute, Columbia University Vagelos College of Physicians and Surgeons, New York, NY, USA
e-mail: qvh2001@cumc.columbia.edu

© Springer Nature Switzerland AG 2019
D. S. Casper, G. A. Cioffi (eds.), *The Columbia Guide to Basic Elements of Eye Care*,
https://doi.org/10.1007/978-3-030-10886-1_2

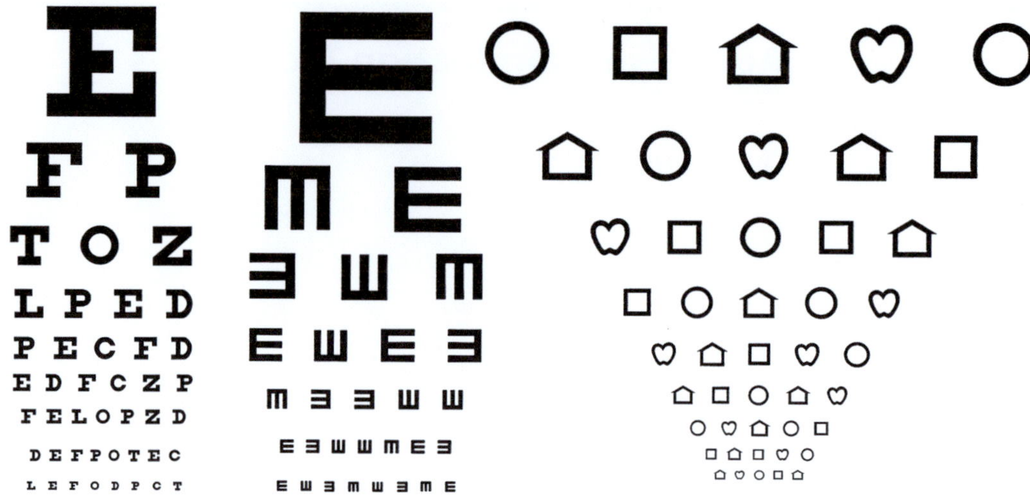

Fig. 2.1 Typical acuity measurement charts, showing, left to right, Snellen, Tumbling E's, and pictographs

acuity with a pinhole occluder is accomplished by a reduction in diffraction of the image presented to the macula. If vision improves with pinhole, uncorrected refractive error or cataract is typically present. Conversely, if vision does not improve, it suggests that a more serious cause for decreased vision may be present.

- Visual acuity at identified vocational or avocational working distances.

Vision worse than 20/400 is recorded as:

- Counting fingers (CF at the test distance) if the patient can identify the number of fingers held up by the examiner
- Hand motion (HM) if the patient can only identify movement of the examiner's hand
- Light perception (LP) with or without projection, depending if the patient can determine the direction of the incoming light
- No light perception (NLP)

Eye charts for nonverbal or patients who cannot read English letters include a Tumbling E chart and an eye chart with pictures.

Refraction

Assessment of refractive error incorporates objective and subjective assessment of the patient's refractive error to determine the lens correction necessary to provide optimal visual acuity. The refractive analysis may include:

- Measurement of the patient's current spectacle correction.
- Objective measurement of refractive error.
- Subjective measurement of refractive error performed with a phoropter or trial frame to allow the patient to decide on preferred lens. Sometimes, the patient wears the prescription in a trial frame while walking, reading, or doing other tasks to ensure that the spectacle correction will provide an improvement in vision and also be well–tolerated.

Generally, a manifest refraction is performed (without dilation). Cycloplegic refraction can be performed on eyes after dilation with cycloplegic drops to prevent accommodation (which is particularly important in children and hyperopic patients).

Initial Examination

Preliminary examination evaluates aspects of the patient's visual function, ocular health, and related systemic health status. Although elements may vary, the following areas are typically assessed:

- General observation of the patient
- External examination of eye and adnexa
- Pupil size and pupillary responses
- Eye movements and ocular alignment
- Stereopsis
- Color vision
- Amsler grid

The size, shape, symmetry, and reactivity of the pupils are assessed, while the patient fixates on a distant target with both direct and consensual responses that are observed. The swinging flashlight test (also known as the Marcus Gunn or afferent pupillary defect test) is done to identify a relative afferent pupillary defect. A positive test (usually indicated in the chart as either "APD" or "RAPD") suggests an intracranial or intraorbital lesion which requires additional study. Normal pupils should be equal, round, and briskly reactive to light (usually abbreviated in the chart as "PERRL" or "PERRLA," if accommodation is also tested). The swinging flashlight test should be negative.

Ocular Motility, Binocular Vision, and Accommodation

Appropriate tests of ocular motility, binocular visual function at distance and near, and accommodation are incorporated into the examination depending on patient age and visual complaints. Assessment may include evaluation of:

- Ocular motility
- Vergence amplitude and facility
- Suppression
- Accommodative amplitude and facility

The alignment of the eyes in primary gaze is observed, and the movement of the eyes is assessed as the patient looks in all directions of gaze, following an object moved by the examiner. Several methods are used to characterize ocular misalignment, vergence, suppression, and accommodation, which are covered in the pediatric section of this text.

Visual Field Testing

Confrontation visual field (CVF) testing consists of subjective description of the examiner's face and quadrant finger counting. It is a simple method of identifying substantial loss in visual field. However, CVF is not very sensitive in detecting significant disease such as glaucoma, compressive optic neuropathies, and tumors, suspicion for which should warrant more sophisticated and/or, computerized tests for visual field, such as Goldmann and Humphrey visual field testing.

Anterior Segment Examination

In order to ensure a thorough examination, the anterior segment examination proceeds from anterior to posterior and from a low magnification, gross anatomic view, to a higher magnification, detailed view. To allow for such a detailed examination, a specialized biomicroscope called a slit lamp is used (Fig. 2.2). The slit lamp consists of a moveable illuminating arm (containing the light source and many of its controls) and a moveable viewing arm (containing the binocular eyepiece and magnifying elements) that are parfocal, meaning the image of the source of illumination and the image viewed are both in focus at the same location.

Many of the ocular structures (including, from anterior to posterior, the tear film, cornea, aqueous fluid, lens, vitreous, and retina) are transparent, making their direct examination difficult. The broad range of slit lamp illumination characteristics allows viewing of both translucent and non-translucent tissues of the eye with varying angles of incident light, when the subject is placed in the patient-positioning frame. In the slit lamp examination (SLE), the illuminating arm, height, width, angle, and intensity of the light beam can all be controlled, and various filters can be changed to enhance visualization. Six main illuminating options are offered, each with its own special properties and particular uses: diffuse illumination, direct focal illumination, specular reflection, transillumination (retroillumination), indirect lateral illumination, and specular scatter.

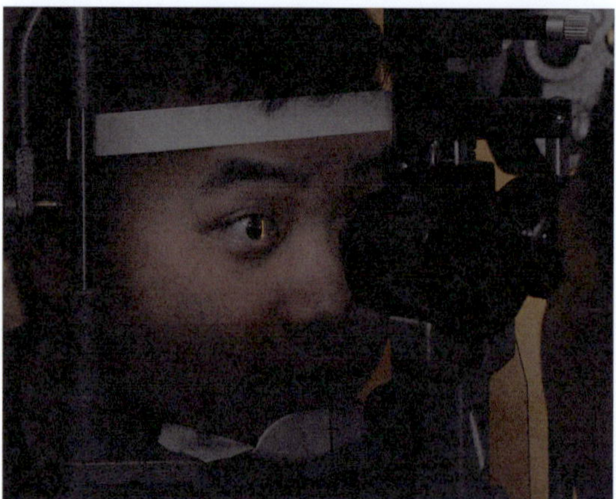

Fig. 2.2 Slit lamp examination

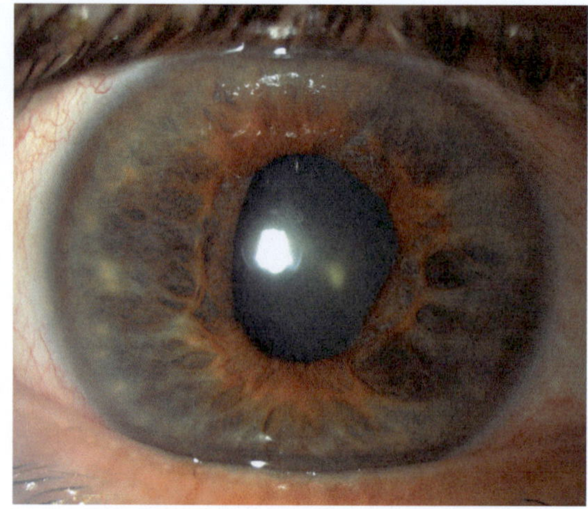

Fig. 2.3 Direct illumination: a vertically distorted pupil which appears otherwise normal

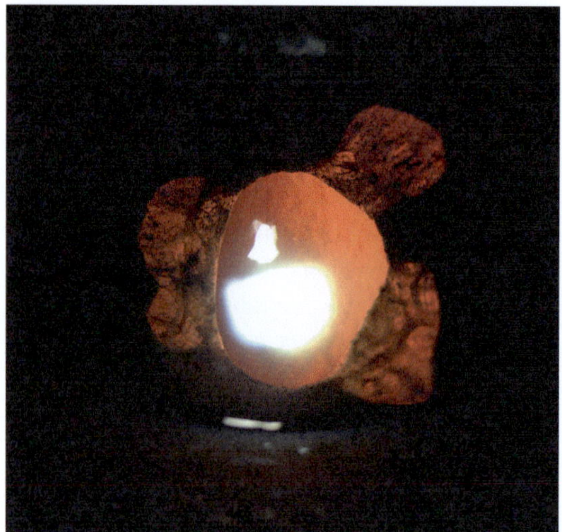

Fig. 2.4 Retroillumination of the same patient as seen in Fig. 2.3 shows areas of segmental iris atrophy where areas of iris pigment loss allow reflected light to transmit through atrophic areas. The slit lamp filament is seen centrally as bright reflections

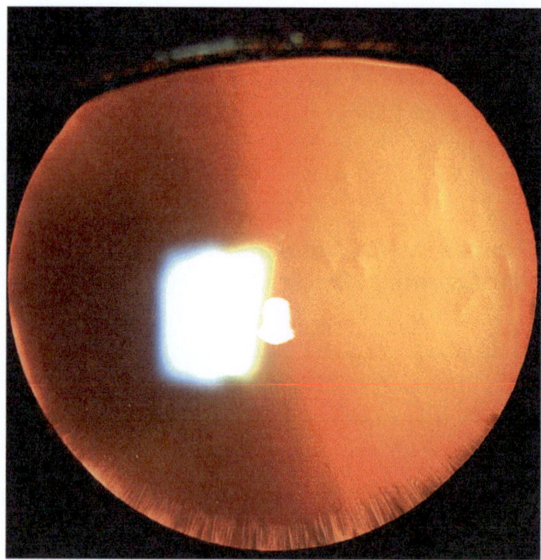

Fig. 2.5 Retroillumination through a widely dilated pupil shows peripheral, fine, fibrillar zonular fibers extending from the ciliary body to attach to the inferior lens, which would normally not be visible with standard axial illumination. The lamp filament is seen centrally as bright reflections

Specifically, retroillumination (coaxial alignment of the light bean with the oculars) uses the red reflex from the retina to backlight the cornea, iris, and lens, making some abnormalities more easily visible (Figs. 2.3, 2.4, and 2.5). Furthermore, anterior segment lesions can be accurately measured by recording the height of the slit beam from the millimeter scale on the control knob. In the viewing arm of the slit lamp, a wide range of magnification (10–500×) can be used. A thin beam directed through the clear ocular media (cornea, anterior chamber, lens, and vitreous) acts as a scalpel of light illuminating a cross-sectional slice of optical tissue (Fig. 2.6). This property of the slit lamp allows precise localization of pathology. Additionally, using specialized attachments and lenses, the slit lamp permits applanation tonometry and viewing of the posterior segment of the eye.

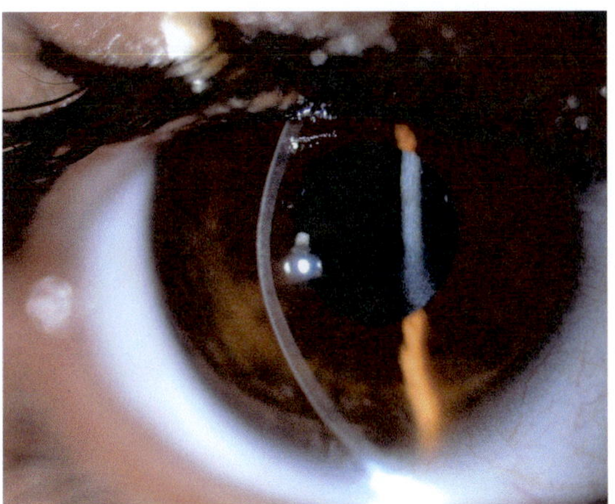

Fig. 2.6 The slit lamp beam is set on thin and angled to show corneal thickness and contour in this patient with the condition keratoconus, an abnormality of corneal structure and curvature

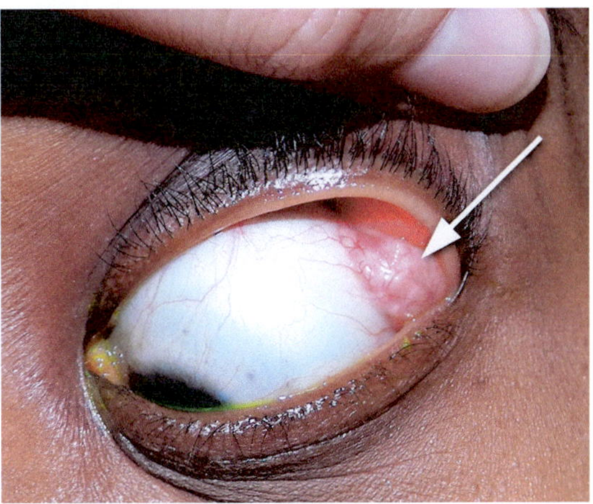

Fig. 2.7 Palpebral lobe of left lacrimal gland visible on downward and nasal gaze. (Courtesy Dr. Lora Dagi Glass)

Components of the slit lamp exam (SLE) include:

Lids, Lashes, Lacrimal Glands, and Skin

The lid, lashes, puncta, and Meibomian gland orifices are inspected. The medical canthus or lid margin can be palpated to express discharge or secretions from the inferior punctum or Meibomian glands, respectively. Mass lesions (styes, chalazia, or neoplastic) and blepharitis (inflammation of the lid) are the most common findings of the lid and are visible with low magnification and broad lighting on the slit lamp examination. A chalazion is a subacute or chronic granuloma surrounding lipid due to a blocked sebaceous gland resulting in a dome-like elevation of the skin with or without erythema. Oftentimes the blocked gland can be located on SLE. The superotemporal palpebral lobe of the lacrimal gland can be examined by lifting the temporal edge of the upper lid upward and having the patient look down and nasal (Fig. 2.7).

Conjunctiva, Episclera, and Sclera

The patient is asked to look in the horizontal and vertical directions to observe the entire bulbar conjunctiva, and the lids can be everted to observe the tarsal conjunctival surface. The tarsal conjunctival can be assessed for the presence of papilla or follicles (signs of inflammation). The caruncle and plica semilunaris are also inspected. The upper eyelid can be double everted to evaluate the superior fornix, and a moistened cotton-tipped applicator can be used to sweep the fornix to remove suspected foreign bodies. The sclera can be assessed for the presence of hyperemia ("injection"), pigmentation, or signs of thinning (blue discoloration).

Cornea and Tear Film

With the SLE, all five layers of the cornea can be inspected readily. The cornea is composed of (from anterior to posterior) (1) corneal epithelium and epithelial basement membrane, (2) Bowman's layer, (3) stroma (which composes 90% of the corneal thickness), (4) Descemet's membrane (the collagenous basement membrane of the endothelium), and (5) corneal endothelium (Fig. 2.8). The abnormalities of these five layers are discussed elsewhere in this text.

The tear film is evaluated for breakup time and height of the tear meniscus. Additionally, corneal "iron lines," deposits which may be normal aging phenomena or may be associated with a variety of pathologic processes, are made more visible on SLE with the use of the cobalt blue filter. Fluorescein dye is useful with the SLE since it does not stain corneal or conjunctival epithelium, but does stain the stroma in areas where the epi-

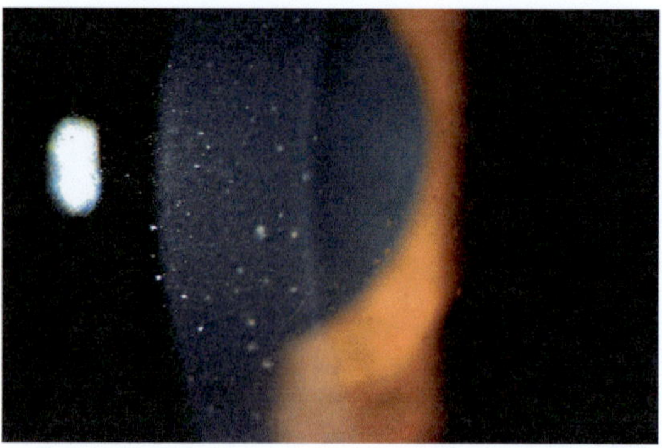

Fig. 2.8 Small white deposits consisting of old inflammatory cells (keratic precipitates, "KPs") are seen lining the corneal endothelium in this slit lamp photograph. Just to the right of the beam, some pigmented KPs are also visible, an indication of long-standing presence

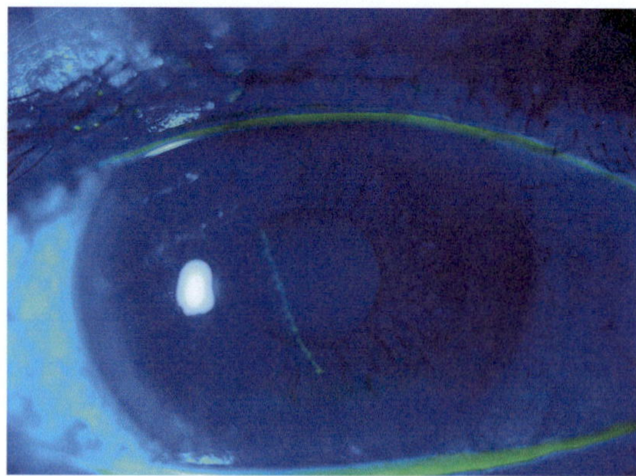

Fig. 2.9 A thin, linear corneal abrasion (from the corner of a sheet of paper) is seen with cobalt-light illumination of fluorescein stain

thelium is absent (e.g., due to corneal abrasion, recurrent erosion, or corneal ulcer).

Diffuse slit lamp lighting with the cobalt blue filter causes the dye to fluoresce bright green and enhances examination of the tear film integrity (Fig. 2.9).

Anterior Chamber

The anterior chamber (AC) is evaluated for depth (on a scale from 1+ (shallow) to 4+ (deep)) and the presence of cells (visible as minute dots in the AC) and flare (aqueous turbidity visible as a hazy, cloud-like opacity within the AC).

Normally the AC is deep and quiet, with clear aqueous fluid filling the chamber. Intraocular inflammation produces protein and inflammatory cells that leak from the normally intact vascular system in the AC. The slit lamp light beam (set at approximately 1×1 mm and at the highest light intensity) shone directly through the normally optically empty AC becomes visible as protein content (flare) increases, producing a "light beam through chalk dust" appearance. Additionally, inflammatory white blood cells are visible in the slit lamp light beam and rise and fall with convection currents of the AC (rising near the warm iris posteriorly and falling near the cooler corneal anteriorly), which can be differentiated from red blood cells and pigmentary cells that may be present in the AC in pathologic conditions (Fig. 2.10). The presence of "cell and flare" is assessed before

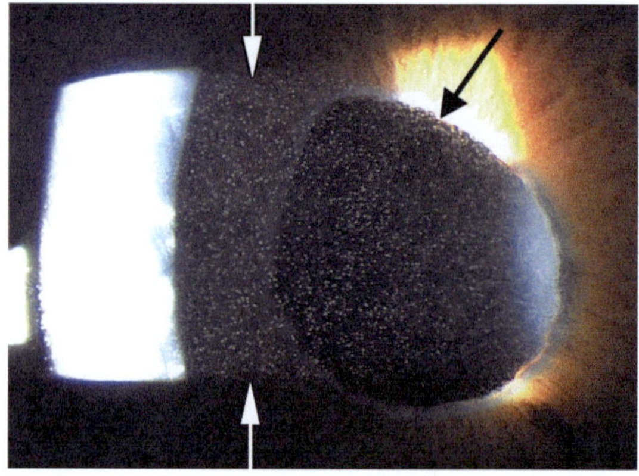

Fig. 2.10 Acute iritis: "cell and flare." The slit lamp beam is coming from the left, where it can be seen on the corneal surface, and then proceeds through the anterior chamber to illuminate the iris surface and the slightly distorted pupil (black arrow). Within the anterior chamber, numerous small white dots, which are white blood cells, can be seen suspended, and the light beam illuminates the hazy anterior chamber aqueous fluid (between the white arrows) indicating protein leakage from iris vessels which, along with the suspended white cells, now fills the anterior chamber. (Courtesy of Emmett Cunningham, Jr., MD, PhD)

instillation of any fluorescein dye, which can enter the AC and produce false flare. In extreme cases, layered white blood cells in the AC (hypopyon) (Fig. 2.11) and layered red blood cells in the AC (hyphema) (Fig. 2.12) can be visualized with a broad beam of the slit lamp or even grossly.

Progression or regression of these layered AC cells can be easily assessed by utilizing the slit

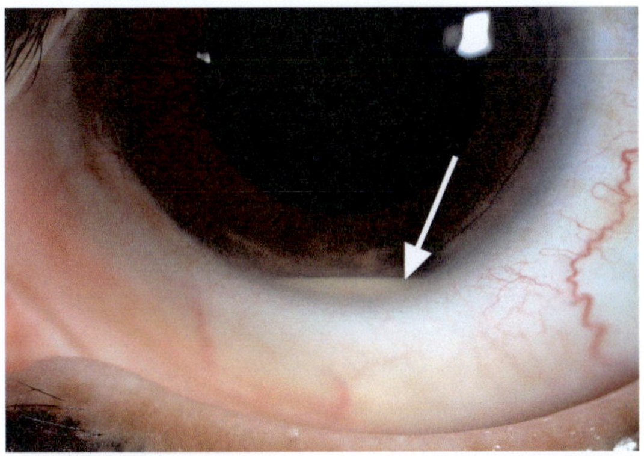

Fig. 2.11 Layered white cells (hypopyon) seen inferiorly at arrow

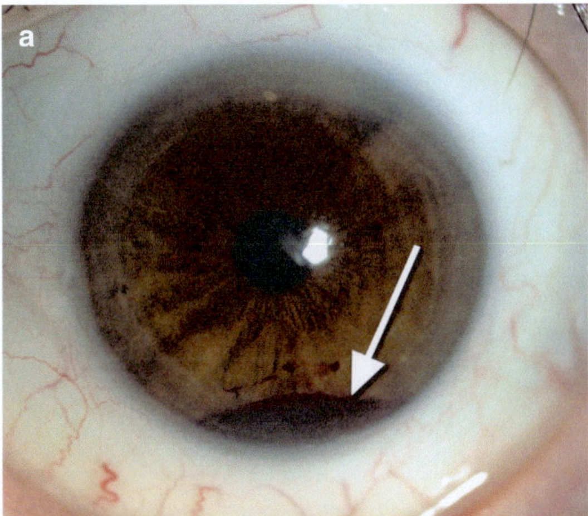

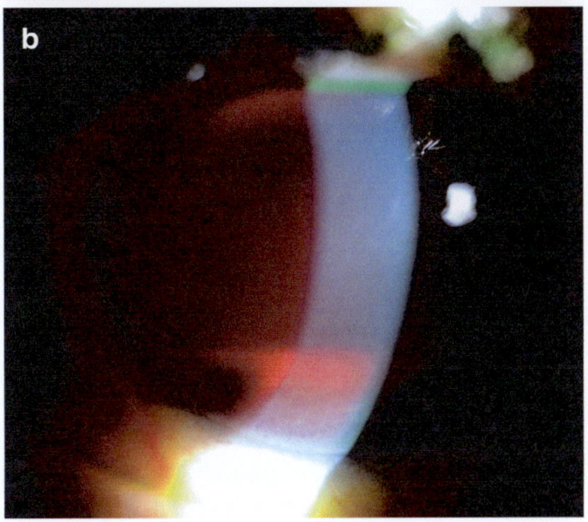

Fig. 2.12 A small layered blood clot (hyphema) is seen inferiorly at the arrow in image (**a**), which utilizes a broad light source; in (**b**), a larger, diffuse hyphema is seen utilizing the slit beam

lamp beam height with the marked dial (in mm) to make serial measurements over time.

Iris, Lens, and Anterior Vitreous

The iris can be inspected for nodules, neovascularization (rubeosis, arising from ischemic conditions, such as diabetes), cysts, tumors, as well as atrophy, displaced pupil, and iridodonesis (vibration of iris with eye movement due to aphakia or abnormality of the zonular attachments of the lens capsule). The crystalline lens is best evaluated after pupillary dilation and is composed of an enveloping capsule, outer cortex, and inner nucleus, any of which can become opacified, leading to various forms of cataract. If the eye is pseudophakic, the position and stability of the intraocular lens implant are noted, and the condition of the posterior capsule is assessed. The anterior vitreous can also be observed without the use of additional lenses and can be assessed for inflammatory cells, red blood cells, or pigmentary cells that may indicate a retinal tear is present ("tobacco dust").

Measurement of Intraocular Pressure (IOP)

The Goldmann applanation tonometer is considered the gold standard for the measurement of

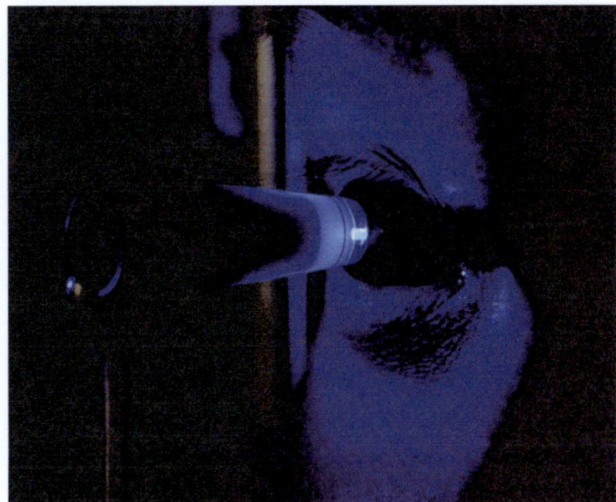

Fig. 2.13 The Goldmann applanation tonometer attachment on the slit lamp is used to obtain an intraocular pressure reading. The cornea has been briefly anesthetized with a topical anesthetic drop prior to the measurement

intraocular pressure (IOP) (Fig. 2.13). Noncontact and handheld applanation tonometers are alternatives. Consistent use of the same tonometer during clinical follow-up testing and recording of the time of day are key to detect meaningful versus spurious changes in IOP.

Posterior Segment Examination

Pharmacologic dilation of the pupil is generally required for thorough stereoscopic evaluation of the ocular media, retinal vasculature, macula, optic nerve, and peripheral retina. The posterior segment examination ("fundus examination") therefore follows the pupillary examination. Additionally, the dilated fundus examination (DFE) follows assessment of visual acuity and refraction, given the intensity of the light used and the loss of accommodation which dilation produces. The optic nerve and limited portions of the retina can be examined without dilation with a variety of instruments and lenses. Direct ophthalmoscopy provides high magnification (15×) with a narrow field of view, whereas indirect ophthalmoscopy produces a wide field of view with a lower magnification (2–3×). Images obtained by indirect ophthalmoscopy (with a 20D or 28D lens) and SLE fundus lenses are flipped and inverted, in contrast to images obtained with direct ophthalmoscopy.

The appearance of the disc, vessels, macula, and periphery are noted. Dimensions and location of lesions are compared to the size of the disc; therefore measurements are recorded as multiples of disc diameters (DD) or disc areas (DA). The optic nerve is inspected with particular attention paid to the cup-to-disc ratio, appearance of the disc rim and color, and assessment for edema (Fig. 2.14).

Retinal vessels are observed as they emerge from the optic cup and branch toward the periphery with particular attention given to signs of tortuosity, dilation, or anomalous patterns (Fig. 2.15). The macula and central macula (the fovea) are evaluated for any signs of edema, exudates or overlying hemorrhages, or abnormal tissue (Fig. 2.16). A bright light reflex, the umbo, is seen at the center of the fovea in healthy young

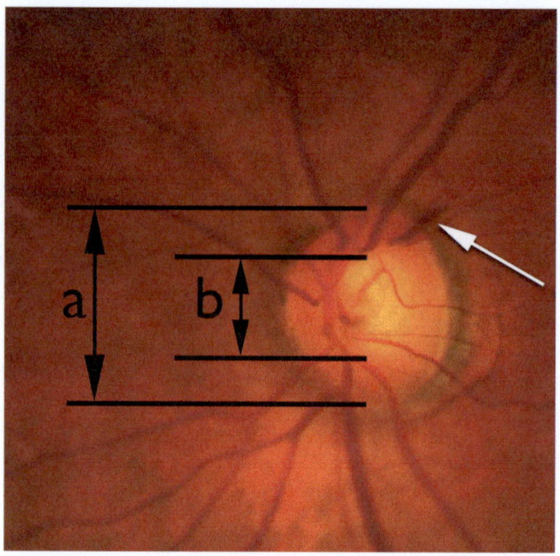

Fig. 2.14 Image of a left optic nerve. (**a**) Vertical disc size; (**b**) vertical cup size. White arrow, a flame-shaped hemorrhage at disc margin. The large cup size and disc hemorrhage make this optic nerve suspicious for glaucoma. The vasculature appears normal

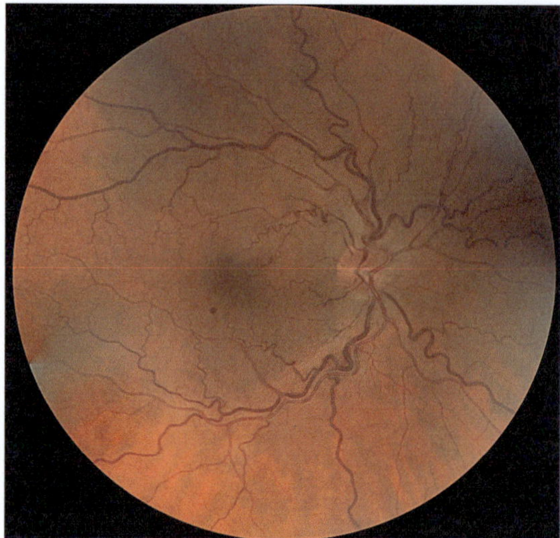

Fig. 2.15 Tortuous vessels with hypertensive changes and a parafoveal blot hemorrhage in a 69-year-old man with type II diabetes

patients. If the amount of pigment in the pigment epithelial and choroid layers is relatively sparse, then the choroidal vasculature, which is usually obscured, may be visible through the transparent retinal layers (Fig. 2.17).

The vitreous body is examined for the presence of blood, or other opacities ("floaters"),

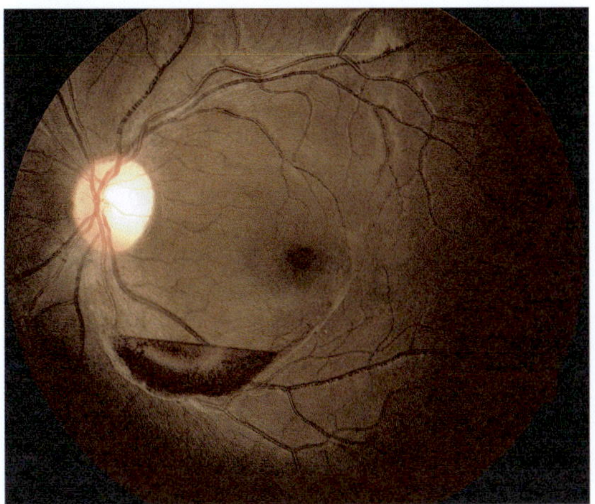

Fig. 2.16 A boat-shaped ("scaphoid") hemorrhage in the preretinal space, behind the posterior vitreous surface, overlying the inferior temporal arcade. It extends a minimal amount into the macula and does not obscure the fovea

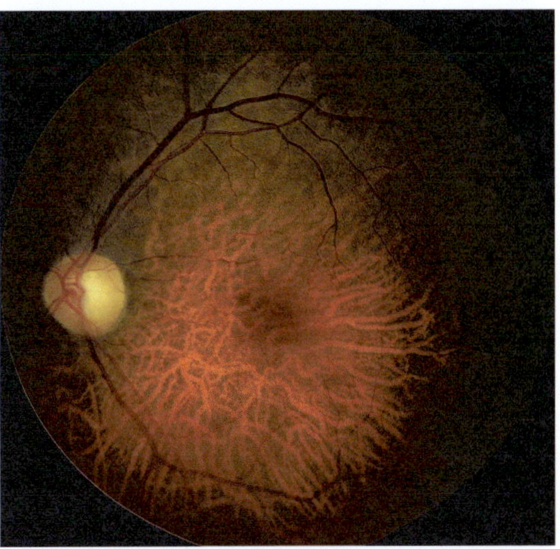

Fig. 2.17 The normally poorly seen choroidal vasculature is visualized here in the macula due to hypopigmentation of the overlying retinal pigment epithelium and choroid

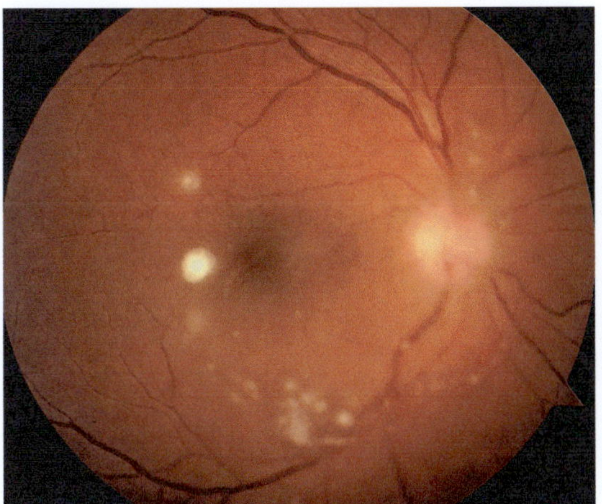

Fig. 2.18 Intraocular fungal infection (endophthalmitis), showing fungus infiltrates scattered in mid-vitreous, overlying the macula and the optic nerve. Folds in the normally smooth macula are seen radiating outward from the fovea

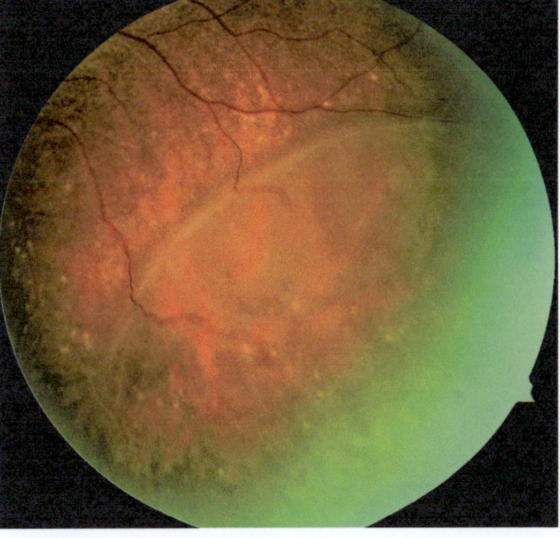

Fig. 2.19 An elevated fold of retina (notice the retinal vessels deviated over the elevation) seen on examination of the peripheral fundus, using scleral depression. This represents an area of retinoschisis, a splitting of the retinal layers

which may be indicative of a variety of pathologic processes (Fig. 2.18).

The retinal periphery is most easily seen through a widely dilated pupil with an indirect ophthalmoscope, while the subject is asked to look in all directions of gaze (Fig. 2.19). Visualization near the ora serrata in the far periphery (underlying the anterior sclera) is aided with scleral depression.

Supplemental Testing

Throughout the adult eye examination, the interpretation of subjective and objective data may indicate the need for additional testing, such as optical coherence tomography (OCT), threshold visual field testing, gonioscopy, fundus photography, keratometry, glare testing, contrast sensitivity testing, and fluorescein angiography, or referral for consultation with, or treatment by, another ophthalmologist, the patient's primary care physician, or another healthcare provider.

Suggested Reading

American Academy of Ophthalmology. Introducing ophthalmology: a primer for office staff. 3rd ed. 2013. https://www.aao.org/Assets/ee65c92c-838e-45f9-922c-e703fda56714/635653348833100000/introducing-ophthalmology-a-primer-for-office-staff-3rd-ed-pdf?inline=1.

Bagger N, Wajda B. The Wills eye manual: office and emergency room diagnosis and treatment of eye disease. 7th ed. LWW; 2016. ISBN-13: 978-1496318831.

Carlson N, Kurtz D. Clinical procedures for ocular examination. 4th ed. McGraw-Hill Medical; 2015. ISBN-13: 978-0071849203.

Cunningham E, Riordan-Eva P. Vaughan & Asbury's general ophthalmology. 18th ed. New York: McGraw-Hill Medical; 2011.. ISBN 978-0071634205

Leitman M. Manual for eye examination and diagnosis. 9th ed. Hoboken: Wiley-Blackwell; 2016.. 13: 978-1119243618

The Pediatric Eye Examination

Lauren Yeager

The physician must take a unique approach to the pediatric eye examination, as children are not simply small adults and vision issues they face vary with age. The adept examiner utilizes a distinct skillset to evaluate children and understands the importance of tailoring the examination to each age group and each individual child. With proper tools, the pediatric examination can be a rewarding and enjoyable experience that provides information that may be critical in ensuring the development of normal, binocular vision.

Preparation

If possible, the waiting room has a defined area that is designated for children, complete with toys and children's furniture. This creates a comfortable space for families and keeps the child occupied during wait times. It is also more favorable and accommodating to adult patients in the waiting room.

Equipment for the non-ophthalmologist who performs pediatric eye examinations in a primary care setting includes:

1. Penlight or other light source
2. Near fixation targets (finger puppets, stickers, other small, fine detailed objects)
3. Age-appropriate distance acuity charts, including Snellen letters, tumbling Es, and Allen pictures
4. Near reading card with age-appropriate optotypes
5. Direct ophthalmoscope
6. Dilating eye drops

Optional but helpful equipment for the primary care office includes a portable slit lamp and fluorescein eye drops. Many offices employ photoscreeners, which are cameras that take multiple images of a child's undilated eyes to detect amblyogenic risk factors including high refractive errors, anisometropia, anisocoria, and strabismus. Photoscreeners may be very useful for vision screening in the primary care setting and can aid in guiding referrals to the pediatric ophthalmologist.

History

A thorough history is critical to the examination of a child. The chief complaint and history of present illness is obtained, and if possible, an attempt is made to have the child explain the chief complaint in his own words, with subsequent confirmation and any additional history

L. Yeager, MD (✉)
Department of Ophthalmology, Edward S. Harkness Eye Institute, Columbia University Vagelos College of Physicians and Surgeons, New York, NY, USA
e-mail: ly2292@cumc.columbia.edu

© Springer Nature Switzerland AG 2019
D. S. Casper, G. A. Cioffi (eds.), *The Columbia Guide to Basic Elements of Eye Care*,
https://doi.org/10.1007/978-3-030-10886-1_3

obtained from the parents. It is important to note, however, that young children will rarely complain of vision loss, and therefore one should not interpret a lack of eye complaints as an affirmation that vision is normal. The past medical history in infants includes prenatal and perinatal problems, gestational age at birth, birth weight, complications during birth, and use of forceps or cesarean delivery. A maternal history during pregnancy including travel, illness during pregnancy, and use of alcohol or illicit substances are reviewed. Early development is also assessed by inquiring about specific developmental milestones, such as rolling over, sitting up, walking, and speaking.

Past ocular history, including history of retinopathy of prematurity, ocular surgery or procedures, use of glasses, patching, eye or head trauma, or other ophthalmic diagnoses, is necessary, and medications and allergies are reviewed. Any family history of blindness, childhood eye disease, strabismus, amblyopia, "lazy eye," and genetic disorders is also sought.

As children have a limited attention span, it is often helpful to obtain a focused history initially, and then pertinent aspects of the examination are immediately performed before the child becomes restless. A complete, thorough history can then be supplemented subsequent to the actual exam.

Examination

The pediatric examination begins the moment the examiner spots the child in the waiting room. By observing the child from afar as he interacts with the environment, the physician gains valuable knowledge about the patient's overall alertness, development status, and gross visual ability. These observations are extremely valuable, because young patients may become scared and difficult to examine when they are in the formal examination room with the physician.

Once the patient enters the examination room, every effort is made to furnish an atmosphere that is comforting and engaging to the child, and the examiner must tailor his approach to the age of the patient. By putting the patient at ease and creating an initial bond, it becomes easier moving forward with the evaluation. The examiner sits at eye level with the child, introduces himself to the child and the parents, and calls the patient by the preferred name. It helps to be playful, and the examiner may tell the patient a joke or compliment a toy or article of clothing. Small children are frequently scared of the white coat, and it is often beneficial to dispatch with this unwelcome piece of clothing.

Noninvasive portions of the examination are easily performed and usually completed before moving on to more uncomfortable parts of the evaluation. However, it is important to perform the most vital aspects of the examination upfront in case the child becomes upset and the opportunity to perform a thorough exam is lost. If a child becomes too difficult to examine, it is always an option to schedule them for another visit. At times, an evaluation under anesthesia may be required.

External Examination

The external examination includes an assessment of the child's head posture, noting any face turn or tilt. Assessment of head and facial symmetry as well as facial features helps identify any signs of dysmorphia. The examiner should appraise the orbits for depth, fissure size, and shape and look carefully for any ocular asymmetry.

Red Reflex Examination

Red reflexes are evaluated in the newborn nursery and at all subsequent routine visits. It is a critical element of the pediatric examination, and one that is very easy to perform. The red reflex test is performed by holding a direct ophthalmoscope at the examiner's eye with the ophthalmoscope lens power set at "0." In a darkened room, the ophthalmoscope is projected onto both of the baby's eyes simultaneously from approximately 18 in. away. To be considered normal, there should be a bright red reflex seen that appears symmetric in each eye. Asymmetry of the reflexes, a darkened reflex,

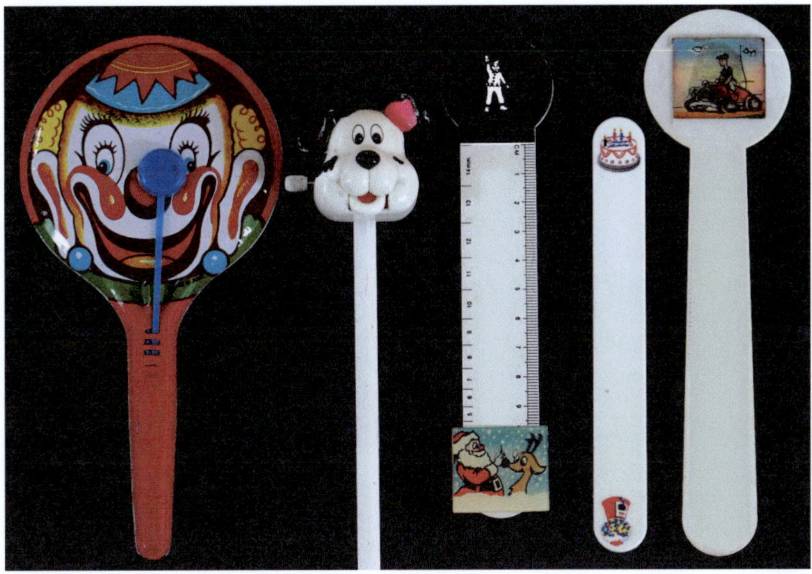

Fig. 3.1 Small, fine detailed objects are used as fixation targets to test motility in patients as well as visual acuity in infants and young toddlers

a dark spot within the reflex, or a white reflex are all considered abnormal and require further evaluation (See Fig. 40.5).

Visual Acuity Testing

When testing visual acuity in children, the examiner must account for a variety factors. Age of the child, education, developmental status, primary language spoken, and language abilities can all impact the visual acuity test.

Visual Acuity Testing in Preverbal Children

Infants aged 0–2 months are tested for a blink to light response in each eye. Interestingly, the blink response to a bright light is generally observable even in children who are asleep. By 2 months of age, most children have developed fixation. Monocular fixation testing assesses whether the patient fixates with each eye individually. In order to perform the examination, each eye is occluded in turn, using whatever works with each child, usually an open hand, or an occlusion spoon, and the smallest possible target that elicits a fixation response is used. In a newborn, the

examiner's face may be an appropriate target to hold the patient's attention. Finger puppets and other fine-detailed objects make good fixation targets for older infants and children closer to 1 year of age (Fig. 3.1). Although it may be helpful to initially attract a child's attention to an object by making a noise, accurate fixation and tracking must be assessed without noise, relying solely on visual function.

Binocular fixation testing, which compares the vision of one eye to the other, detects amblyopia in preverbal children. In large-angle strabismus, the examiner looks for spontaneous alternation in visual fixation between the two eyes, which implies that there is no strong preference for either eye, making amblyopia less likely (Fig. 3.2a, b). A lack of spontaneous alternation suggests amblyopia in the non-preferred eye. In straight eyes or with small-angle strabismus, a test which utilizes a vertical prism is used to determine fixation preference. A child who consistently objects to occlusion of one eye but not the other can be assumed to have decreased vision in the eye that he allows to be covered, which requires further investigation and likely treatment as well.

In difficult cases, ophthalmologists may have to assess visual acuity in the preverbal population by employing visual evoked potentials,

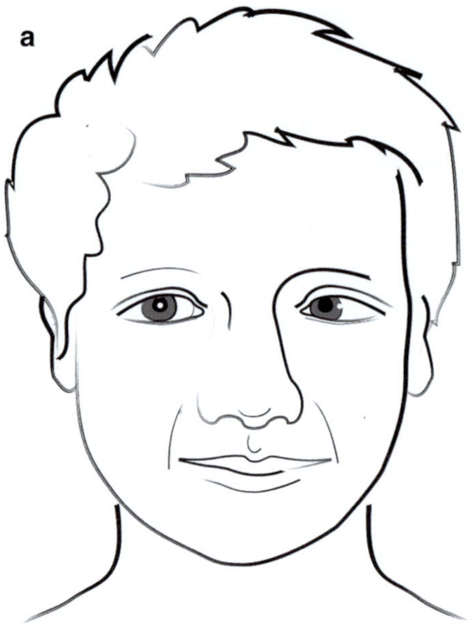

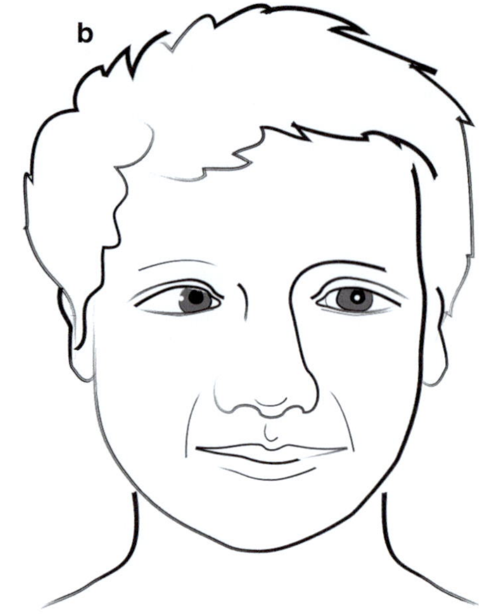

Fig. 3.2 Patient with large-angle strabismus and spontaneous alternation in visual fixation. (**a**) The patient fixates with the right eye. (**b**) The patient fixates with the left eye. This spontaneous alternation implies there is no strong preference for either eye and makes amblyopia unlikely

preferential looking with Teller acuity cards, and optokinetic testing.

Visual Acuity Testing in Verbal Children

By 4 years of age, most children can cooperate with chart acuity testing, and this is sometimes seen in children as young as 2 years of age. Chart testing optotypes should reflect the ability of the patient. Allen figures and tumbling Es are appropriate for children who do not yet know how to read letters. Special pediatric eyecharts using only the letters HOTV are a good option for children who do not know the entire alphabet. Commonly used Snellen optotypes are the gold standard and should be introduced as early as possible, usually by age 5 (see Fig. 2.1). Visual acuity testing with linear optotypes is at times more accurate than single letter testing and is therefore preferred. A child who is barely verbal or too shy to talk may use pointing games to match a sheet of pictured figures to the displayed cards.

Each eye is tested separately, and the examiner carefully occludes the eye that is not being tested. Children who do not see well from one eye can easily fool examiners as they discreetly peek around a cover in order to please the examiner and their parents. Oftentimes, children may lose attention before reaching their best visual acuity endpoint. To shorten testing time and avoid distraction and fatigue, vision testing may be initiated with moderate-sized, rather than large, optotypes.

Pupillary Examination

Pupils are examined using a penlight and are evaluated for size, shape, symmetry, reactivity to light, reactivity to accommodation, and afferent pupillary defect. The pupillary light reaction is present at 30-week gestational age. Reactivity to light in infants may be difficult to assess secondary to natural miosis and an uncontrolled near response in this age group. When testing light response in older children, fixation is directed toward a distant target in order to control the misleading near (accommodative) response.

Visual Fields (Peripheral Vision)

Once a child can steadily fixate on an object, the examiner can obtain a rough estimate of visual fields. It is useful to occlude one eye with a patch in order to test monocularly, but if the child objects to occlusion, binocular visual fields still provide useful information and can be performed. In infants and young children, visual fields are evaluated by having the patient fixate centrally on an interesting target held by the examiner. The examiner then brings another fixation object in from the periphery, watching for the child to switch fixation from the central to the peripheral object. Infants with good fixation will usually switch to a peripheral target when it comes into view. This test is performed in the four peripheral quadrants. Older children, often starting around 5 years of age, can focus on a central target while accurately counting fingers held by the examiner in the periphery. Assessment of peripheral vision can reveal potentially serious pathologies that might not be apparent on visual acuity testing, such as CNS lesions, glaucoma, or early retinal detachments.

When necessary, formal visual field testing, such as Goldmann perimetry, may be performed in children as young as preschool aged, whereas automated visual field testing is usually not reliable until at least 10 years of age.

Motility (Extraocular Movements and Eye Alignment)

Eye alignment and motility are monitored at every pediatric eye examination. To evaluate for strabismus, the examiner first inspects the patient from afar to observe for any obvious ocular deviation. The red reflex is then used to perform the Hirschberg and Bruckner tests. The Hirschberg test assesses the white light reflex that reflects off the cornea. With normal (orthotropic) alignment, the light reflexes appear slightly decentered nasally but are symmetric in each eye (Fig. 3.3a–c). The Bruckner test employs the direct ophthalmoscope to obtain a red reflex from both eyes simultaneously. The examiner compares the quality and symmetry of the red reflex between the two eyes; if a strabismus is present, the Bruckner test will show asymmetrical reflexes with a brighter reflex coming from the deviated eye.

Cover and alternate cover testing are the gold standards for assessing eye alignment. In order to

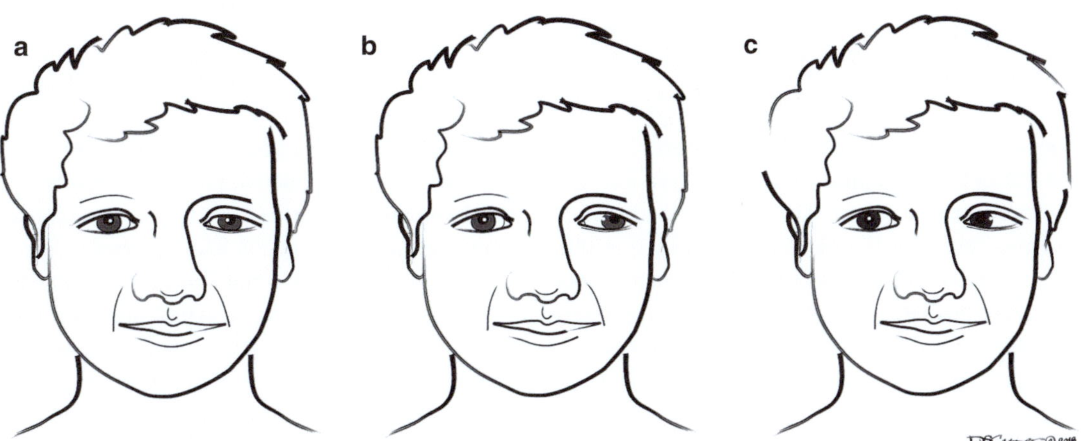

Fig. 3.3 The Hirschberg test utilizes the light reflex to assess for manifest strabismus. (**a**) The patient is orthotropic and the light reflex falls slightly nasal on each eye. (**b**) The light reflex is seen nasally on the exotropic eye. (**c**) The light reflex is seen temporally on the esotropic eye

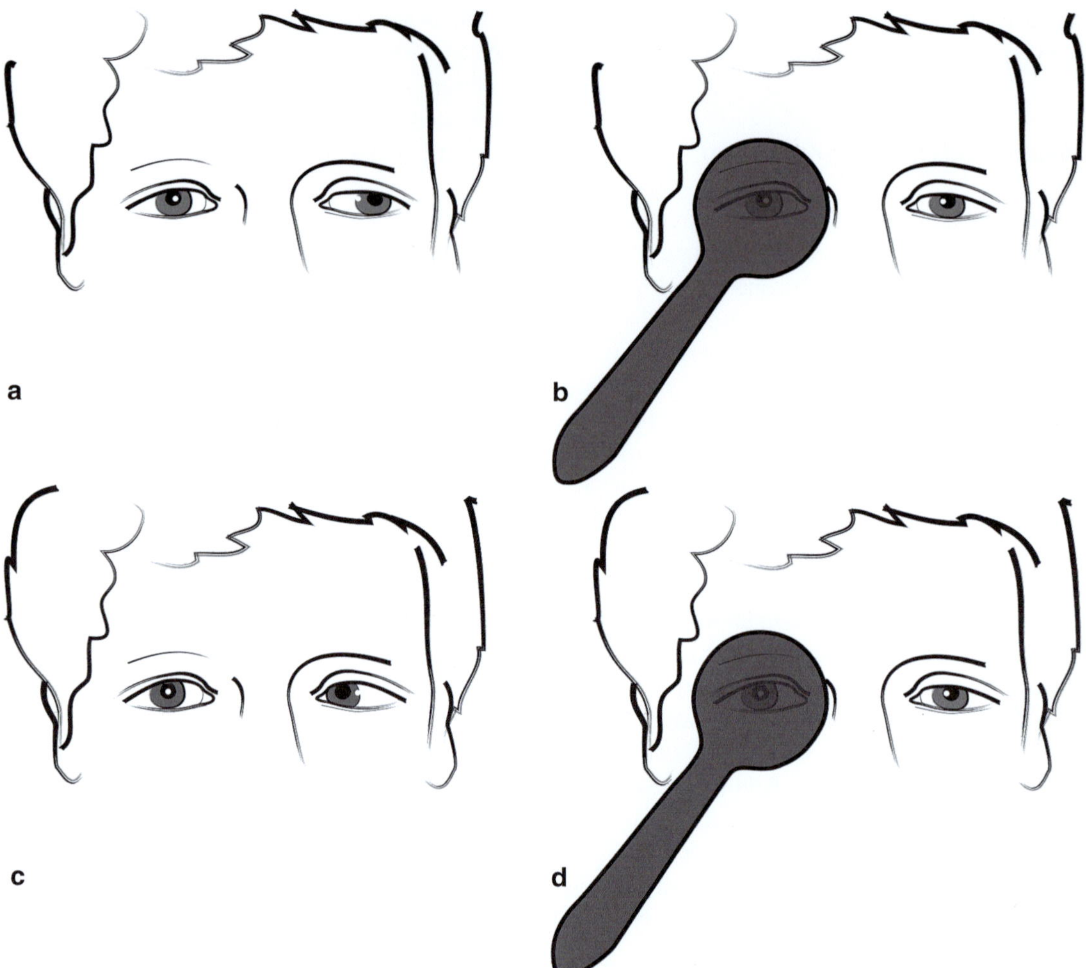

Fig. 3.4 The cover test is used to determine if a manifest strabismus is present. (**a**) There is a manifest exotropia. (**b**) The fixating eye is covered, and the examiner observes a refixation movement nasally of the uncovered eye. (**c**) There is a manifest esotropia. (**d**) The fixating eye is covered, and the examiner observes a refixation movement temporally of the uncovered eye

cooperate with cover and alternate cover testing, the patient must demonstrate good fixation and be attentive to a target. The cover test identifies manifest eye misalignment, i.e., a deviation that is constantly present, while the alternate cover test identifies latent eye deviations, such as intermittent eye misalignment or phorias, deviations that intermittently occur when binocularity is disrupted.

To perform the cover test, the patient focuses on an accommodative target. One eye is covered, and the uncovered eye is observed for resulting vertical or horizontal movement toward the midline (Fig. 3.4a–d). A refixation movement toward the midline in the uncovered eye confirms eye misalignment in that eye. If there is no movement, the uncovered eye is fixating on the object. The test should be performed on each eye, always assessing the uncovered eye. Alternate cover testing is performed in a similar manner, but the examiner alternates cover between the two eyes while assessing for any refixation movement toward the midline in the uncovered eye. Prisms may be used to quantify the size of the deviation in each eye for better quantification, monitoring, and management planning.

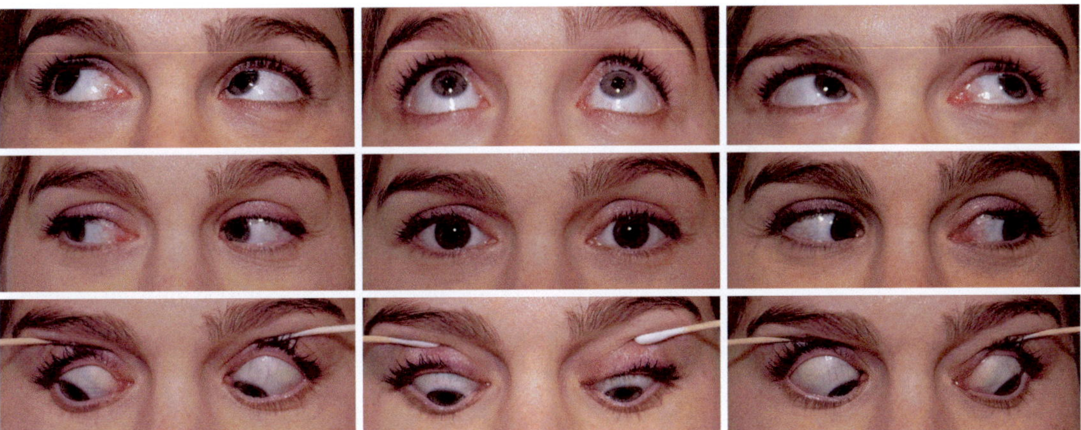

Fig. 3.5 The examiner tests version movements in the nine cardinal positions of gaze

Ductions/Versions

Ductions and versions are tested at each examination. Ductions measure the ability of the eye to move into far positions of gaze and are tested in each eye separately while one eye is occluded. A numerical scale is used to indicate any limitation of an eye's movement. Versions detect subtle eye movement imbalances and oblique muscle dysfunction; both eyes are tested together in the nine cardinal positions of gaze (Fig. 3.5). A numerical scale is also used to grade muscle dysfunction, indicating overaction or underaction.

Intraocular Pressure

Formal measurement of intraocular pressure using tonometry may be extremely difficult or even impossible to obtain in children. Some children may cooperate with handheld devices such as the Tono-Pen or I-care tonometer. If a child is crying, squeezing the eyelids, or holding his breath, the intraocular pressure will likely be falsely elevated. It may be possible to distract a child with fixation targets or conversation so that an accurate pressure can be obtained. Ocular palpation ("finger tension") does not provide quantitative data but may be useful for a gross assessment to distinguish between normal and abnormal pressures. If there is concern for increased intraocular pressure or glaucoma and accurate pressures cannot be obtained in the office, an examination under anesthesia may be required.

Anterior Segment Examination

The anterior segment examination evaluates the anterior portion of the eye, including the eyelids, eyelashes, adnexa, conjunctiva, sclera, cornea, anterior chamber, and lens. The examiner uses a bright light source, such as a penlight, to perform the examination, and if necessary, handheld lenses or even a direct ophthalmoscope can be used for magnification. If available, a slit lamp provides a stereoscopic, magnified, well-illuminated and more detailed view of the anatomy. The eyelids are examined for normal anatomical structure and positioning, noting approximation to the globe and any lash loss. Ptosis, asymmetry between the lids, and fissure height and length are all noted, as are any masses or lesions present on or near the lids. Conjunctiva and sclera should appear white without injection or discharge. The cornea is examined for clarity, and the presence of abnormal blood vessels. If there is concern for a corneal abrasion, the examiner can place a small amount of fluorescein into the cul-de-sac of the eye and shine the blue (cobalt) light from the direct ophthalmoscope. If the epithelium is compromised, the corneal surface will fluoresce green in those areas (see Fig. 9.10). Under normal conditions, the anterior chamber may be difficult to adequately assess with only a penlight exam. However, pathology in the anterior chamber, such as a hypopyon (inflammatory cells; see Fig. 2.11) or hyphema (blood, see Fig. 2.12), can usually be visualized. The iris is evaluated for texture, color, and symmetry and the lens for clarity.

Posterior Segment (Fundus) Examination

In the primary care setting, the posterior segment is usually viewed through an undilated pupil using a direct ophthalmoscope. In an ophthalmologist's office, the posterior segment examination is performed through a pharmacologically dilated pupil with the use of an indirect ophthalmoscope and a 28D or 20D lens. A complete posterior segment assessment includes evaluation of the vitreous, optic nerve, macula, retinal vessels, and retinal periphery. However, in infants and very small children, a quick view of the posterior pole is often all that is possible and is in most cases sufficient. The Retcam is a wide angle pediatric retinal imaging system and can be extremely useful in photographing posterior and peripheral retinal conditions. The images can be shared electronically for immediate evaluation or tracked longitudinally over time. Concern for abnormal findings or an incomplete evaluation in vision threatening cases may require an examination under anesthesia.

Suggested Reading

Nelson LB, Olitsky SE. Harley's pediatric ophthalmology. 6th ed. Philadelphia: Lippincott Williams & Wilkins; 2013.
Simon J, et al. Pediatric ophthalmology and strabismus, basic clinical science series. San Francisco: American Academy of Ophthalmology; 2008–2009.
Wright KK, Ning Y, Strube J. Pediatric ophthalmology and strabismus. New York: OUP; 2012.
Wright WW, Spiegel PH, Thompson LS. Handbook of pediatric strabismus and amblyopia. New York: Springer; 2006.

Sudden Vision Loss

4

Jason Horowitz

History of Present Illness for Patients with Sudden Visual Loss

Sudden visual loss, whether unilateral or bilateral, is an ophthalmic emergency that necessitates a history including the patient's age, time course, laterality, character of the symptoms, associated symptoms, prior ocular history, and concurrent medical conditions.

Age is a critical component of the history – one of the most important entities, GCA (giant cell arteritis), is extremely rare under age 50, while optic neuritis associated with demyelinating disease usually presents before age 35. Clarifying the time course is of paramount importance: the meaning of the word "sudden" can vary greatly – from fractions of a second to weeks. The more acute the presentation, the greater the urgency of potential intervention that can prevent progression of disease and/or restore vision. Persistent severe sudden visual loss most commonly results from retinal or optic nerve infarction, retinal detachment (RD), or intraocular hemorrhage. Monocular and transient visual loss is most commonly caused by carotid artery and cardiac disease, migraine auras, intermittent angle closure with resultant intraocular pressure increase, and GCA. If the loss is both bilateral and transient, it is more likely to represent transient hypoperfusion of the brain and/or optic nerves, papilledema, or ophthalmic migraine. An inquiry should be made into the quality of the visual loss: a fixed, profound darkness is more indicative of neuronal infarction or massive hemorrhage; myriad small opacities are suggestive of red blood or inflammatory cells; halos around lights suggest corneal edema and high pressure; and having some element of visual distortion is suggestive of retinal topographic alteration brought on by RD or exudative macular degeneration. Associated symptoms can be helpful in guiding one to a preliminary diagnosis; scalp tenderness and jaw claudication are hallmarks of GCA, flashes and floaters often precede visual loss from RD, and intermittent mild ocular pain may stem from angle closure attacks.

Concurrent medical conditions can be major determinants of significant ocular disease. Diabetic patients are frequently prone to retinopathy and associated vitreous hemorrhage, tractional retinal detachment, and neovascular glaucoma (NVG). Patients with known risk factors for atherosclerotic disease are more likely to suffer from retinal vascular occlusions. Patients with sickling hemoglobinopathies are prone to peripheral retinal neovascularization and vitreous hemorrhage. Immunocompromised patients are

J. Horowitz, MD (✉)
Columbia University Irving Medical Center,
New York, NY, USA

Department of Ophthalmology, Edward S. Harkness
Eye Institute, Columbia University Vagelos College
of Physicians and Surgeons, New York, NY, USA
e-mail: jh3177@cumc.columbia.edu

© Springer Nature Switzerland AG 2019
D. S. Casper, G. A. Cioffi (eds.), *The Columbia Guide to Basic Elements of Eye Care*,
https://doi.org/10.1007/978-3-030-10886-1_4

more vulnerable to severe intraocular opportunistic infections.

A history of prior ocular conditions can provide important clues as well. Diabetic eye disease frequently progresses to severe complications such as hemorrhage and NVG. RDs often become bilateral; myopes are especially prone to RDs, especially if they have undergone cataract surgery. Glaucoma patients are more prone to central retinal vein occlusion (CRVO). Patients with stable mild macular degeneration can suddenly develop hemorrhage or severe exudation.

The Basic Examination for Patients with Sudden Visual Loss

A basic ocular exam is crucial to correctly triage the patient. This includes visual acuity, visual field testing, assessment of pupil reactivity, extraocular motility testing, and direct ophthalmoscopy to assess red reflexes and fundus visibility. Measuring the visual acuity of each eye, even if only a rough estimate (from a near card downloaded on a smartphone), is immensely useful. Confrontation visual field testing is invaluable when considering possible stroke or RD. Accurate examination of the pupils can reveal a wealth of information useful for assessing sudden visual loss. Seeing the pupil clearly in an eye with visual loss helps rule out many anterior segment entities, such as severe corneal disease or blood in the anterior chamber (hyphema). Assessing direct and consensual pupil reactivity, especially when combined with testing for afferent pupillary defects, is invaluable for distinguishing retinal or neuronal disease from media opacities or an ongoing glaucoma attack. Basic extraocular motility testing helps rule out simultaneous brain stem, skull base, or posterior orbital disease. The direct ophthalmoscope can be used to check for and/or compare red reflexes and fundus visibility and thereby establish the presence or absence of a significant media opacity as being the cause of the vision loss.

An afferent pupillary defect combined with a normal red reflex in an eye with sudden severe visual loss is of utmost importance because neuronal visual pathway dysfunction is essentially a certainty, and in a person over 50 years of age –

unless the presentation strongly suggests RD – one is obligated to manage the patient without delay as if they had GCA that could at any moment cause bilateral permanent blindness.

Conversely, if the poorly seeing eye has normal pupillary responses but lacks a red reflex, one can be reasonably certain that a media opacity is the cause of the visual loss. This conclusion suggests that referral to an ophthalmologist's office would be more appropriate than an emergency room.

Ischemic Optic Neuropathy (ION) and Giant Cell Arteritis (GCA)

Giant cell arteritis (GCA) is a terrifying entity because of its propensity to produce bilateral visual loss. Its granulomatous, inflammatory effect on the posterior ciliary arteries – the main blood supply to the optic nerve head – can be sudden and devastating. There may be little or no time to attempt to intervene to save the sight in the contralateral eye; there is literally a race against time to prevent a lifetime of blindness. High-dose corticosteroids are usually successful in controlling the disease, but they require hours to days to take effect, and if the inflammatory process has already involved the contralateral eye, it can be too late to prevent further visual loss.

Patients with GCA will often experience a succession of episodes of transient visual loss (amaurosis fugax) preceding the main event. The ultimate visual loss is often near total, stemming from optic nerve head infarction caused by thrombosis in the posterior ciliary arteries, resulting in an acute, arteritic, anterior ischemic optic neuropathy (AION) (Fig. 4.1). Headache, jaw claudication, scalp tenderness, and constitutional symptoms such as weight loss or malaise are common, but not universal. An afferent pupillary defect is usually present in the affected eye. As mentioned above, this observation, combined with the presence of a red reflex on direct ophthalmoscopy, obligates one to consider the patient as having giant cell arteritis until proven otherwise. Urgent consultation with an ophthalmologist should be pursued and blood drawn for sedimentation rate (ESR) and C-reactive protein (CRP), but neither should delay immediate initiation of systemic corticosteroid therapy (intravenous solumedrol or oral prednisone, whichever can be given faster) that is the absolute priority to prevent permanent blindness.

Definitive diagnosis by temporal artery biopsy (preferably within several days, but no later than 2 weeks) is important since GCA is a relatively rare disorder – it represents only about 10% of IONs – and the long-term treatment with systemic steroids that it necessitates generates considerable morbidity in a population with an average age of 76 years. A positive temporal biopsy will show loss of the internal elastic lamina, most characteristically associated with narrowing of the vascular lumen by concentric intimal hyperplasia caused by an infiltrate featuring multinucleated giant cells. The more common, non-arteritic ischemic optic neuropathy (NAION) can occasionally also cause severe visual loss but usually produces only sectoral or altitudinal optic nerve infarction and accordingly results in an eye with at least ambulatory vision in most patients. Patients tend to be an average of 10 years younger than those with GCA and generally lack the associated constitutional symptoms and markedly elevated ESR/CRP of GCA. Noting the loss of vision upon awakening in the morning is a typical observation with NAION, which is thought to be caused by anatomical compromise of intraneural branches of the posterior ciliary artery related to having a "disc at risk" – one with a relatively tight vascular compartment (Fig. 4.2). A vicious cycle is generated, triggered by reduced optic nerve per-

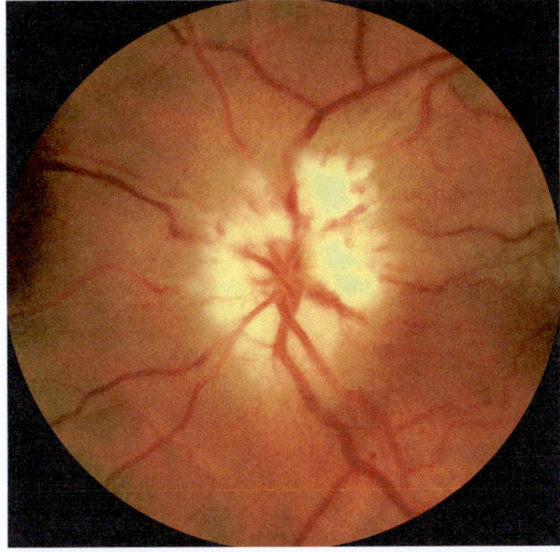

Fig. 4.1 Optic nerve head showing pallor and edema associated with giant cell arteritis (Courtesy of Dr. Jeffrey Odel)

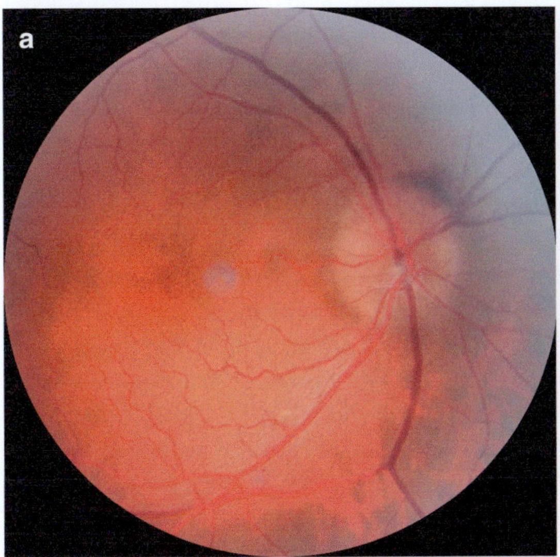

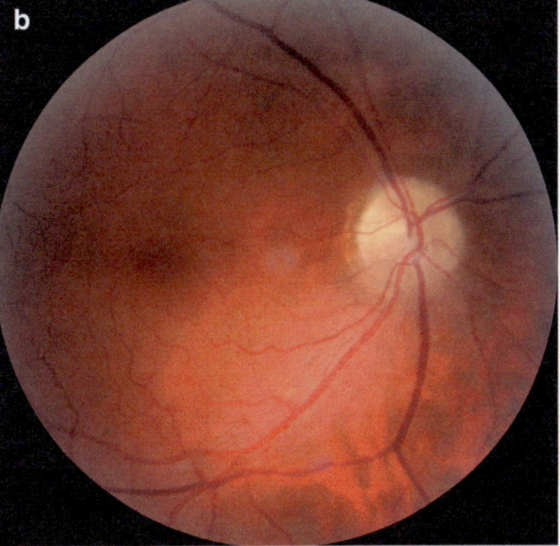

Fig. 4.2 (**a**) A "disc at risk" with small, crowded anatomy and absent cup. The disc is slightly swollen, and there is a subretinal hemorrhage just superonasal to the disc border. (**b**) Post-NAION, the disc is no longer swollen, and optic pallor (i.e., atrophy) is now present. (Courtesy of Dr. Jeffrey Odel)

fusion caused by nocturnal hypotension followed by ischemia-induced edema, which further compromises optic nerve perfusion.

Bilateral involvement only occurs in about 15% of cases of NAION, as compared to 55–95% of patients with GCA. Temporal artery biopsy will usually be definitive in case of doubt.

While there is a significant association between NAION and hypercoagulable states as well as systemic hypertension, there is no proven treatment for NAION, although weak evidence has been reported for modest benefits from systemic steroids while the optic nerve is clinically swollen.

Retinal Artery Occlusion

Central retinal artery occlusion (CRAO) is a more common cause of severe visual loss than GCA but fortunately is much less likely to become bilateral (Fig. 4.3). An embolus from an atheromatous plaque – usually in the ipsilateral internal carotid artery – is the most common

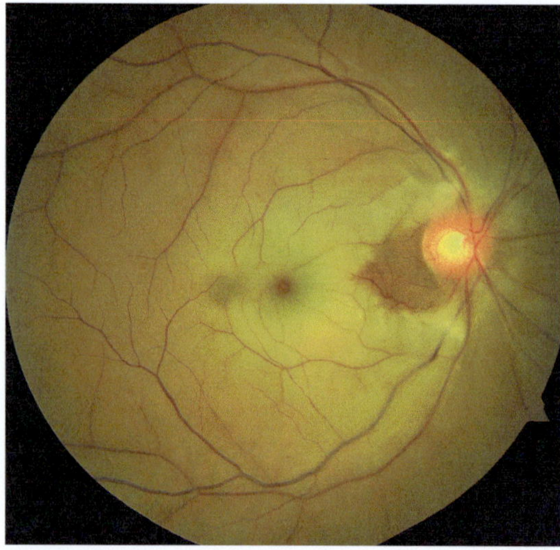

Fig. 4.3 Central retinal artery occlusion. Note the small peripapillary wedge of normal-appearing retina, still perfused because it is supplied by a cilioretinal artery which comes directly off the posterior ciliary artery and not the central retinal artery. The underlying intact choroidal circulation is seen through the thin fovea as a classic "cherry red spot"

cause, followed in frequency by a cardiac source usually related to valvular abnormality or atrial fibrillation.

A CRAO is a form of "ischemic stroke," thereby necessitating an urgent complete physical and neurological evaluation, diagnostic imaging both to identify the likely embolic source and to evaluate the CNS for other signs of ischemic damage, and medical/surgical interventions based on the workup to prevent future cardiac and cerebrovascular damage.

Interruption of blood flow to the retina results in neuronal cell death in 1.5–4 h. Not only is it rare for patients to present for treatment within that time span, there is no evidence supporting the efficacy of the traditional interventions of ocular massage, paracentesis (removal of fluid from the anterior chamber), pharmacologic lowering of intraocular pressure, and/or breathing in of increased carbon dioxide. However, it is possible that intravenous tissue plasminogen activator – started within a few hours of the event – may have a beneficial effect on final visual outcome while having a favorable safety profile. Another reason to act promptly is that GCA is the underlying etiology in 2–4% of CRAO patients. The presence of pale optic nerve swelling and/or "no light perception" vision might in particular suggest GCA, which tends to affect patients about 7 years older than non-arteritic CRAO patients. Prompt fluorescein angiography might demonstrate choroidal filling defects that would further raise the index of suspicion for GCA and necessitate the initiation of high-dose systemic steroids until GCA had been ruled out by temporal artery biopsy.

For a primary care provider, there may be considerable overlap between the clinical picture presented by CRAO and GCA. The fundus findings in CRAO of emboli, retinal vascular "boxcar" formation, and "cherry red spot" appearance of the macula amidst a retina whitened by ischemic edema can be subtle, even for experienced clinicians. It deserves emphasis that unless ophthalmological consultation can be obtained in extremely short order – and/or when in doubt – it is prudent to use GCA as the temporary working diagnosis since, if not immediately treated with

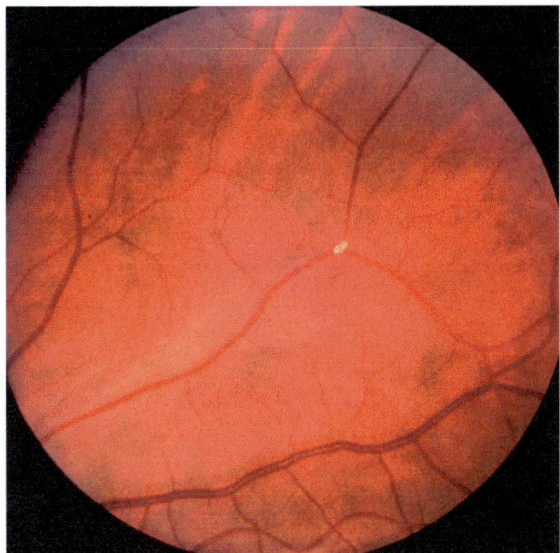

Fig. 4.4 A refractile embolus seen at an arterial branch point, known as a Hollenhorst plaque. These are typically cholesterol emboli which arise in the internal carotid artery

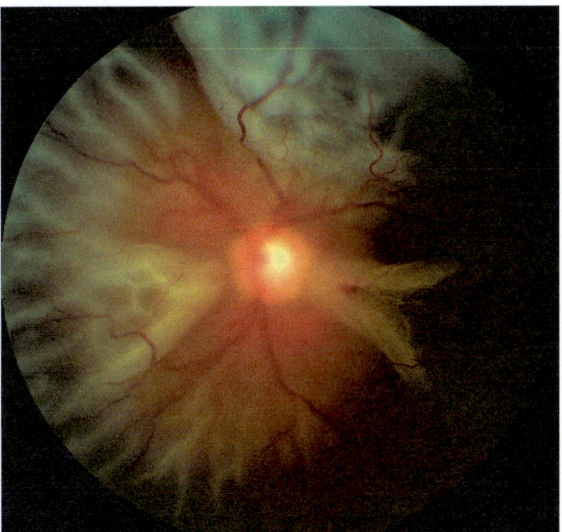

Fig. 4.5 Total bullous retinal detachment

high-dose systemic corticosteroids, it poses the greatest risk of giving rise to a bilaterally blind patient.

Branch retinal artery occlusion (BRAO), also usually embolic (Fig. 4.4), may cause severe sudden visual loss if it involves the circulation of the macula; if so, as with CRAO, rapid ophthalmic intervention to decompress the globe to improve retinal perfusion or move the embolus might have occasional efficacy. If the macula is spared, one could dispense with local measures and focus on a systemic workup similar to that for CRAO. One important difference is the exceedingly unlikely chance of GCA being the underlying diagnosis in the setting of BRAO.

Retinal Detachment (RD)

In order to function and maintain viability, the retina must be attached to – in fact remain in intimate contact with – the retinal pigment epithelium (RPE). The RPE provides metabolic support to the photoreceptors and is essentially inseparable from the high blood flow choriocapillaris layer and wall of the eye. The most common cause for a retina to detach is (middle) age-related involutional deterioration of the collagen and mucopolysaccharide structure of the vitreous. As the vitreous degenerates, it shifts anteriorly and sometimes pulls on and rips the retina. Once a retinal tear has occurred, highly liquefied portions of the vitreous can rapidly flow through the tear (or tears) and dissect the retina off of the RPE. This may cause a near total rhegmatogenous RD (from the Greek word "rhegma" meaning "crack") – and therefore severe vision loss – in a span of hours (Fig. 4.5). Some RDs remain outside the macula so that the patient sees fine straight ahead but notices that the peripheral or side vision is impaired. In others, the macula is only slightly detached so that it functions partially but results in distorted vision, termed metamorphopsia (Fig. 4.6).

The lifetime risk of RD is about 1 in 300. The mean age is about 65 but younger in myopes, who are also at higher risk for RD. The fellow eye tends to eventually get an RD about 10–15% of the time. Other risk factors for RD include cataract surgery, significant ocular trauma, and family history of RD.

If the detachment has not involved the macula, then surgery to prevent extension of the detachment – sometimes necessary within hours – can make a permanent difference in the patient's quality of vision in that eye. On the

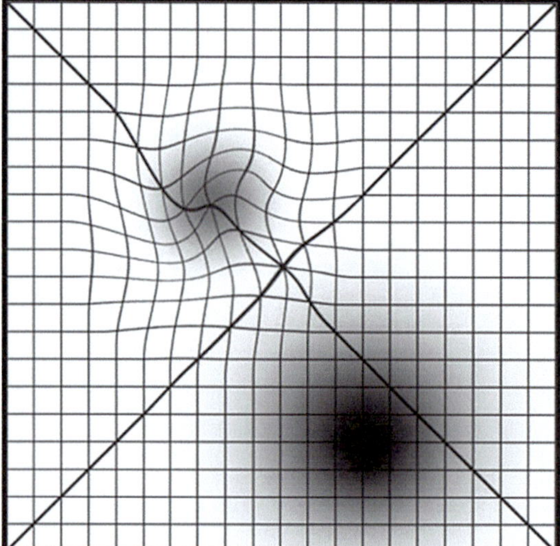

Fig. 4.6 Metamorphopsia shown superiorly on an Amsler grid card, with a small scotoma (localized area of relative or total visual loss) seen inferiorly

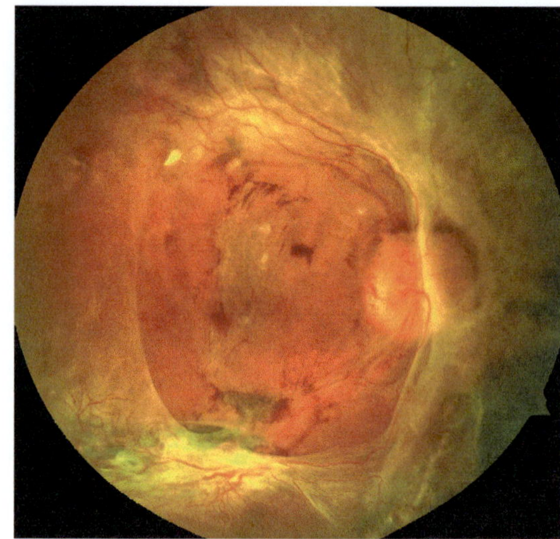

Fig. 4.7 Total tractional retinal detachment, diabetic

other hand, if the detachment has already involved the macula, there will likely always be some permanent alteration of central visual function; the timing is hence less critical, but surgical repair within 3–7 days has been shown to render a better chance of restoring high-quality vision than further delay. Repair of a more chronic RD, while still potentially very useful, is accordingly less urgent.

Diabetic tractional RD occurs when scar tissue – most commonly resulting from the involution of retinal neovascularization caused by severe diabetic retinopathy – distorts and pulls the retina off the RPE without ripping it (Fig. 4.7). The vision loss is usually not quite as sudden as the rhegmatogenous variety; very complex vitrectomy surgery is required to restore somewhat normal retinal anatomy and is best performed within a few weeks if the detachment has involved the macula.

Intraocular Hemorrhage

Clarity of the aqueous humor and vitreous cavity is essential for good vision; bleeding into the anterior chamber or vitreous cavity in an other-

wise sighted eye will immediately be apparent to a patient.

Vitreous hemorrhage (VH) is a common cause of sudden visual loss. Patients will describe numerous black dots, cobwebs, swirls, or near total loss of vision (Fig. 4.8). The most common causes of VH are middle-age-related posterior vitreous separation (with or without the occasional accompanying retinal tear or RD) and proliferative diabetic and sickle cell retinopathy (Fig. 4.9). These critical entities are discussed further in Chap. 3 entitled "Flashes and Floaters."

Hyphema – blood in the anterior chamber – when not caused by trauma is most commonly caused by neovascularization of the iris (NVI) secondary to severe diabetic retinopathy or central retinal vein occlusion (Fig. 4.10). In turn, NVI often leads to neovascular glaucoma (NVG). In the patient with NVG, the trabecular meshwork – the tissue in the anterior chamber angle that is responsible for outflow of aqueous humor – is mechanically clogged first by blood cells and the abnormal new vessels and finally by adhesions that form between the peripheral cornea and iris. Saving vision is sometimes possible if both the secondary pressure elevation and neovascular process are promptly treated by pharmacologic glaucoma and anti-vascular endothelial growth factor (VEGF) therapy; surgical

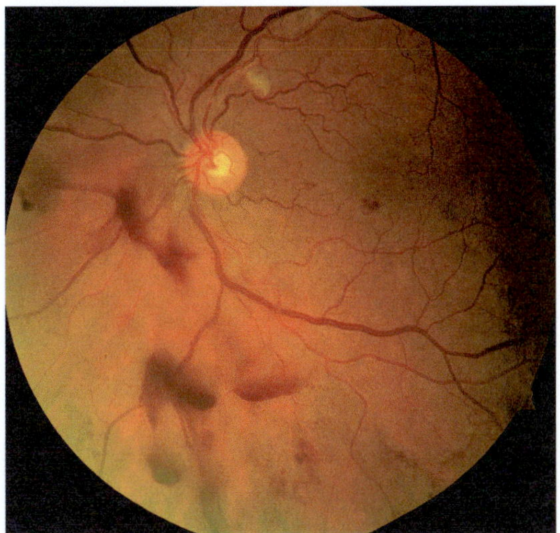

Fig. 4.8 Vitreous hemorrhage associated with diabetic retinopathy

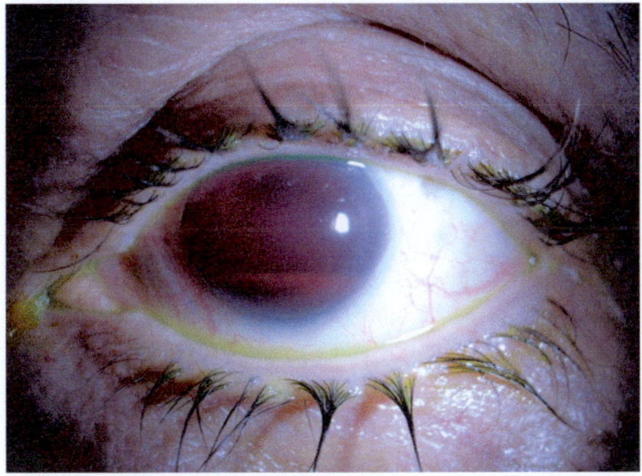

Fig. 4.10 Hyphema, post-trauma

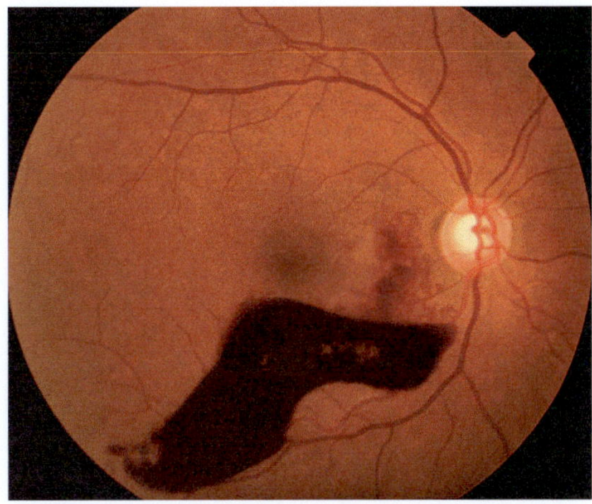

Fig. 4.9 Pre-retinal and intravitreal hemorrhages associated with posterior vitreous separation

intervention is also possible. Difficulty in seeing the pupil or the red reflex – especially if one could discern blood in the anterior chamber – as well as variable ocular pain and redness provides clues to a primary care physician that this dire process is in need of immediate management by an ophthalmologist.

Subretinal hemorrhage, especially when involving the macula, can produce painless, sudden, and sometimes severe visual loss, most commonly in the form of a central scotoma or blind spot. Peripheral vision is usually unaffected. The most common cause is choroidal neovasculariza-tion (CNV) that is most often secondary to age-related macular degeneration. Other causes include high myopia, presumed ocular histoplasmosis, angioid streaks, and traumatic choroidal ruptures. Prompt anti-VEGF intravitreal injection can prevent the growth and even induce involution of the offending CNV; rarely, urgent surgical intervention for the purpose of debulking submacular hemorrhage is undertaken.

Retinal Vein Occlusion

Occlusion of the central retinal vein (CRVO) (Fig. 4.11) or one of its branches (BRVO) (Fig. 4.12) can produce significant visual loss with a time course of hours to days. The severity of visual loss – while it can vary widely – is usually not quite as profound as in occlusions of the central retinal or posterior ciliary artery. Much more common than ION and CRAO, retinal vein occlusions damage – even destroy – capillaries; the subsequent ischemia, edema, and hemorrhage lead to loss of retinal function.

The most important local cause of the actual occlusion is a tight connective tissue compartment that contains the artery and vein at their crossing points in the optic nerve (for CRVO) or retina (for BRVO). Increasing age is an important risk factor as are hypertension, hypercoagulable states, and diabetes complicated by end organ

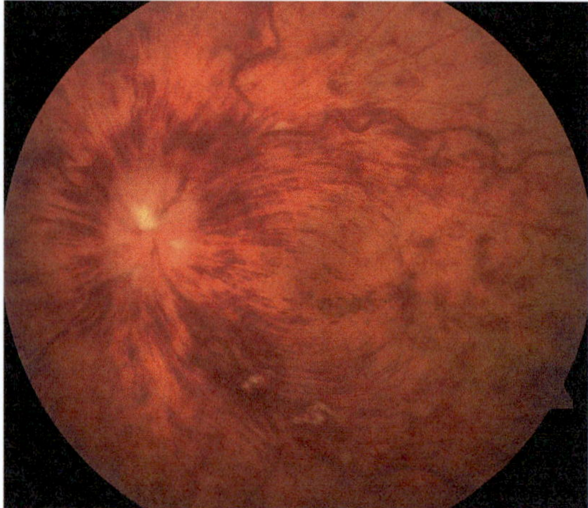

Fig. 4.11 Central retinal vein occlusion

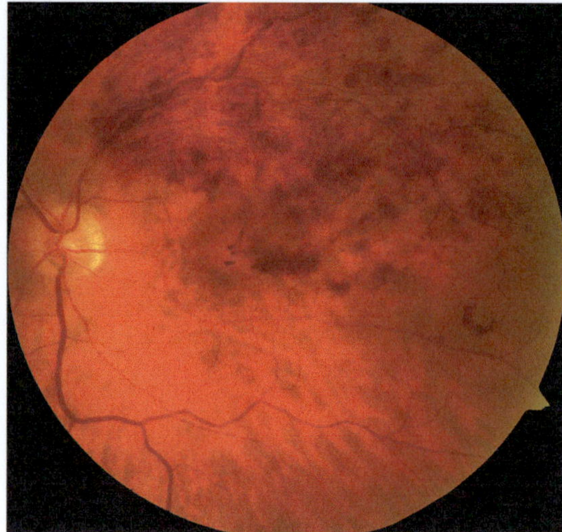

Fig. 4.12 Superior temporal branch retinal vein occlusion

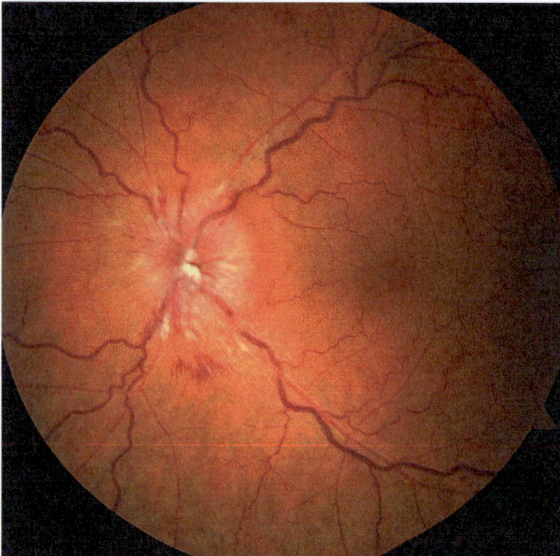

Fig. 4.13 Acute optic neuritis

damage. Glaucoma is significantly associated with CRVO. There is no established treatment to relieve the actual venous obstruction, but ophthalmic intervention for macular edema and NVI can be sight-saving; accordingly, referral within a few days to an ophthalmologist is indicated.

Optic Neuritis

Acute optic neuritis can produce profound vision loss in young people; the typical patient is a 30-year-old woman with vision that progressively declines over hours or days (Fig. 4.13). There will often be pain on eye movement despite an absence of external sings of inflammation. The most common cause is acute demyelinating disease, and roughly half of new cases will turn out to be associated with multiple sclerosis. Neuromyelitis optica, which tends to produce more severe permanent visual loss along with spinal deficits (paralysis and loss of bladder control), is a less common etiology. Rarely, other infectious or autoimmune diseases, such as syphilis, bartonella, and sarcoidosis, may cause optic neuritis. The lifelong implications of the condition are profound, and the management options differ markedly and depend upon accurate diagnosis, so the patient with optic neuritis requires detailed ophthalmologic evaluation, serologic and possibly cerebrospinal fluid studies, and extensive neuroretinal and central nervous system diagnostic imaging.

Amaurosis Fugax (AF): Transient Visual Loss Caused by Ischemia

Amaurosis fugax (from the Greek/Latin for "fleeting blindness") refers to transient monocular visual loss lasting anywhere from seconds to hours. The spontaneous restoration of vision to completely normal can easily mislead one into assuming that it "can't be too serious."

AF can occasionally be caused by GCA and accordingly may be an ominous harbinger of permanent optic nerve infarction. Most commonly it is caused by an embolus from the carotid artery or heart that breaks up or repositions itself, allowing reperfusion of the retina before actual cell death occurs. Another possible explanation is transient relative systemic hypotension aggravated by arterial stenosis leading to reduced ocular perfusion. AF is a form of transient ischemic attack (TIA), and therefore if the patient presents within 72 h of the event, it is important to consider hospitalization especially if the patient (1) has systemic risk factors such as diabetes, age greater than 60, or current elevated blood pressure; (2) had non-ocular neurological symptoms such as focal weakness or speech impairment; and (3) had symptoms lasting more than an hour or (4) if the workup would not otherwise be completed in 48 h. The workup must include appropriate history and physical, laboratory testing for GCA, diabetes and dyslipidemia, and imaging for carotid artery stenosis and/or ulceration and cardiac valvular disease. While endarterectomy is usually only performed for significant internal carotid artery

stenosis, it is more often the case that an atheromatous plaque – in an artery without critical stenosis – is the source of the emboli that produce damage to the retina downstream. Initiation or augmentation of antiplatelet, anticoagulant, antihypertensive, and/or antilipid therapy, as well as endarterectomy, is frequently indicated.

Papilledema and Transient Visual Obscurations

"Transient visual obscurations" – very brief losses of vision, usually lasting from 5 to 30 seconds and bilateral – are commonly caused by papilledema. The temporary visual loss probably results from transiently reduced perfusion to the optic nerves brought on by activities such as rising or Valsalva maneuvers in combination with compromise of small vessels in the optic nerve head caused by mechanical compression (Fig. 4.14). These symptoms – however innocuous given their fleeting nature – should not be ignored in any patient, young or old, and should prompt referral for evaluation for possible papilledema and its critical central nervous system implications, including possible brain tumor.

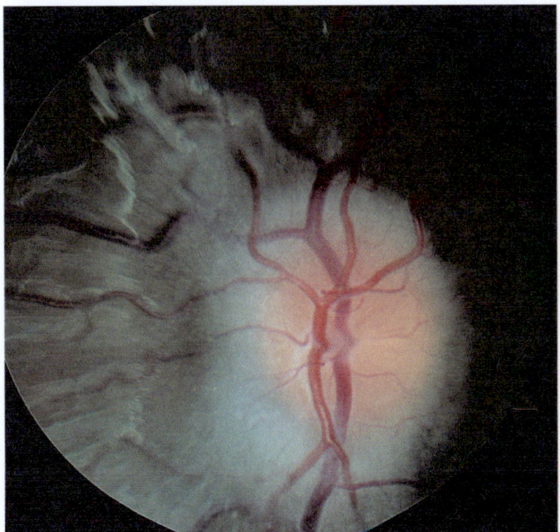
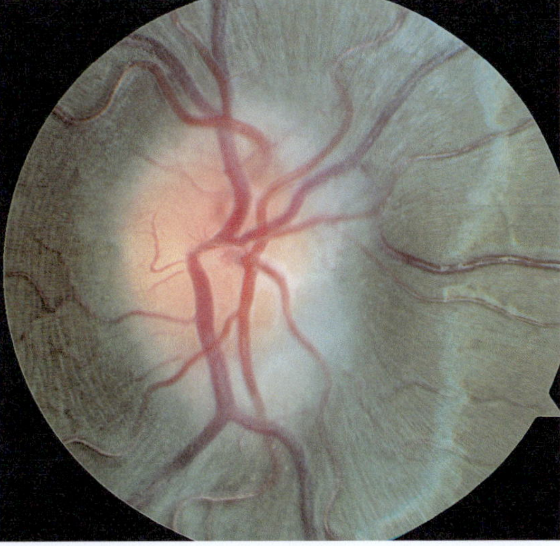

Fig. 4.14 Bilateral acute papilledema in a 7-year-old boy with a history of mild retinopathy of prematurity, found on follow-up to have idiopathic intracranial hypertension (pseudotumor cerebri). Concentric and radial folds are seen in the left peripapillary area

Intermittent Angle Closure Glaucoma Attacks

In ophthalmology, the term "angle" has two closely related meanings. "Angle" can refer to the structures at the junction of the iris and cornea – especially the trabecular meshwork, which is the tissue that is critical for proper outflow of aqueous humor from the anterior chamber. Or "angle" can refer to the actual geometric angle made by the iris and cornea as they converge (see Chap. 1). Narrow angles can intermittently lead to angle closure, in which iris tissue sticks to the peripheral cornea, thereby blocking flow to the trabecular meshwork with consequent marked elevation of intraocular pressure, which in turn produces loss of vision from reduced optic nerve/retinal perfusion and corneal edema. These episodes are sometimes spontaneously aborted by a bright light which produces a strong pupillary constriction reflex that pulls the iris off the trabecular meshwork or by a strategically placed massage of the eyeball that produces a fluid wave that moves the iris to a more fortunate configuration. Although the high pressure may become painful – which certainly assists in differential diagnosis – some patients never volunteer that they ever have ocular pain and consequently only report temporary vision loss. The proper diagnosis is therefore sometimes missed, even by seasoned ophthalmologists. When the proper diagnosis is made, laser iridotomy can prevent future attacks and thereby likely prevent permanent visual loss.

Migraine

Ophthalmic migraine can produce alterations of vision that sometimes appear purely monocular to the patient and occur without associated headache. The duration of these episodes is usually about 20 min, and there is a characteristic scintillation and evolution of the area of visual loss. Atypical migraine can sometimes be difficult to distinguish from the more ominous causes of AF, and, because of potential dire consequences, it is better in these cases to proceed on the side of caution and pursue an AF workup for potential life- and sight-threatening etiologies, unless the history and exam are entirely reassuring.

Conclusion

This chapter has focused on the many causes of predominantly painless acute visual loss. Those causes of visual loss that are associated with trauma or are external and immediately apparent to the casual observer are discussed in other chapters. From the standpoint of seriousness of visual and systemic impact and actionability, GCA-associated ION, CRAO, RD, AF, and diabetic VH should be foremost in the mind of the healthcare professional.

Suggested Reading

Cugati S, Varma D, Chen C, Lee A. Treatment options for central retinal artery occlusion. Curr Treat Options Neurol. 2013;15:63–77.

Hayreh S. Pathogenesis of optic disc edema in raised intracranial pressure. Prog Retin Eye Res. 2016;50:108–44.

Hayreh S, Zimmerman M. Amaurosis fugax in ocular vascular occlusive disorders: prevalence and pathogeneses. Retina. 2014;34:115–22.

Hayreh S. Prevalent misconceptions about acute retinal vascular occlusive disorders. Prog Retin Eye Res. 2005;24:493–519.

Sacco R, et al. An updated definition of stroke for the 21st century: a statement for healthcare professionals from the American Heart Association/American Stroke Association. Stroke. 2013;44:2064–89.

Floaters and Flashes

5

Jason Horowitz

Floaters and flashes are common visual symptoms that can signal sight- or life-threatening disease but most often represent no significant morbidity. Determining the etiology, therefore, is of critical importance. Retinal tears and retinal detachments (RD), for example, which sometimes require emergency intervention, must be differentiated from benign etiologies such as uncomplicated vitreous detachment and migraine.

A patient will generally use the term "floater" to refer to a visually discernable opacity, interruption, or imperfection that is not perfectly fixed within the patient's visual field; such a complaint is explained by some optical flaw of the vitreous body. A patient reporting "flashes" is typically perceiving rapid alterations of brightness generated internally in an eye; these visual disturbances are termed photopsia. Flashes are usually generated by shifting tension on retinal structures or by abnormally rapid acceleration/deceleration of the retina caused by excess mobility. This makes sense when one considers that there are no nociceptive or proprioceptive neurons in the retina; all of its neural output travels to visual processing areas of the brain. Any abnormal stimulation of the retina's neuronal output results in perceived alteration of light or visual pattern. Visual migraine auras often have a "scintillating" quality and can sometimes be difficult to distinguish from retinal-generated flashes.

Primary Evaluation of the Patient with Flashes and Floaters

A careful history can greatly assist in unraveling the cause and impact of a patient's symptoms of floaters and/or flashes. Are they in one eye (more likely intraocular pathology) or both eyes (more likely to be migraine or other intracranial phenomena)? Are the symptoms persistent (as in posterior vitreous detachment (PVD) or RD), or did they completely disappear at a certain point in the episode (another typical feature of migraine auras, which are usually limited to less than 30 min in duration) (Fig. 5.1)? Is there associated eye pain (indicative of intraocular inflammation or secondary glaucoma) or subsequent headache (typical of classic migraine)? Are they more apparent in the dark (more likely to be "flashes") or in bright ambient illumination (more likely to be "floaters")? The direction, location, and pattern of the flashes should be determined (a "dinosaur's back" pattern is typical of migraine aura). Are the floaters numerous small black dots

J. Horowitz, MD (✉)
Columbia University Irving Medical Center,
New York, NY, USA

Department of Ophthalmology, Edward S. Harkness
Eye Institute, Columbia University Vagelos College
of Physicians and Surgeons, New York, NY, USA
e-mail: jh3177@cumc.columbia.edu

© Springer Nature Switzerland AG 2019
D. S. Casper, G. A. Cioffi (eds.), *The Columbia Guide to Basic Elements of Eye Care*,
https://doi.org/10.1007/978-3-030-10886-1_5

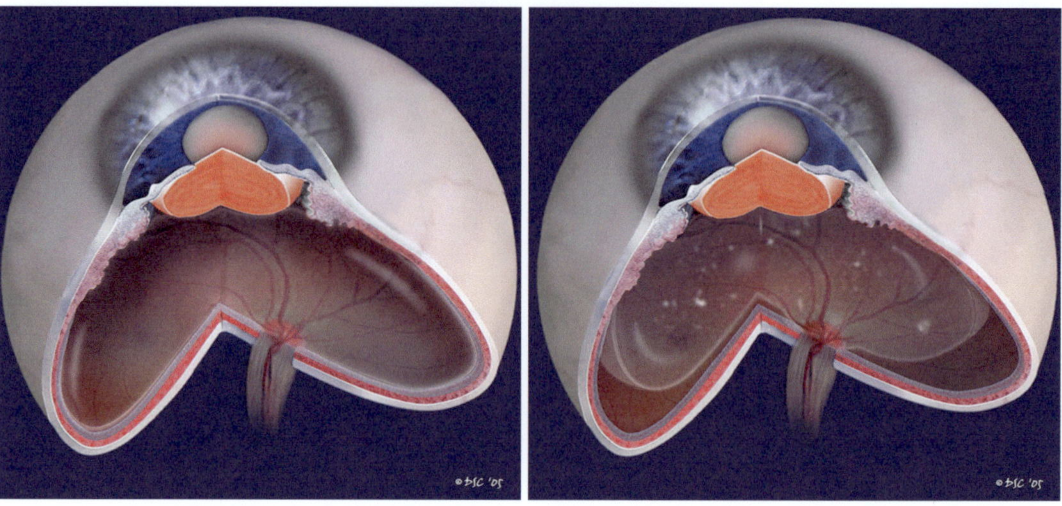

Fig. 5.1 Illustration of normal vitreous body on the left and an incomplete posterior vitreous separation (or detachment) on the right, showing shrinkage of vitreous, seen with syneresis

(suggestive of red blood cells) or a highly translucent amorphous oval (suggestive of a PVD)? Is there a history of diabetes or sickling hemoglobinopathy that can lead to retinopathy and intraocular bleeding, or is the patient pregnant, which can bring on gestational diabetes and retinopathy or preeclampsia and exudative retinal detachment? Is there a history of past migraine? Has there been recent ocular trauma or a family history of retinal detachment? Is there any significant immunological disease or cancer that can lead to uveitis or masquerade syndromes? The medication history can uncover important medical issues that may seem irrelevant to a patient, such as gastrointestinal or rheumatologic disorders, or reveal the use of drugs that can aggravate bleeding and/or impact management such as antiplatelet or anticoagulant agents.

Even a very basic ophthalmic examination can be helpful in framing a rudimentary diagnosis. Floaters and/or flashes combined with a quadrantic loss of confrontation visual field testing in one eye – despite maintenance of central vision – would be most concerning for a macula-threatening RD, while loss of central vision could be due to hemorrhage and/or RD, as well as many other serious pathologic entities. In both instances prompt referral to an ophthalmologist is critical. Conversely, an examination that reveals normal visual acuity and normal visual fields with complete absence of any residual symptoms after a well-defined twenty minute episode of "flashing zigzag lines" points to acephalgic (also referred to as retinal or ophthalmic) migraine, which does not merit urgent referral.

Benign Floaters

The term "floaters" is widely used in several different contexts. When healthy, asymptomatic young people are specifically asked about floaters, they will often recount translucent ameba-like images frequently seen as a child or teenager when exposed to a bright sky or very bright screen. These images are instinctively assumed to be normal visual phenomena because of their reproducibility under similar bright backgrounds, the minimal or absence of visual functional impairment, and the lack of associated ocular symptoms.

By early middle age, an increasing majority of people, especially myopes, will develop symptoms that are described as floaters or blobs, dots, spider webs, strands, or films. These optical phenomena arise from age-related loss of homogeneity of the three-dimensional microskeletal matrix of the vitreous humor; its new heterogeneity becomes optically observable to the patient. This vitreous degeneration is termed syneresis.

Although annoying, these early middle age floaters are only rarely associated with serious ocular pathology, and most patients increasingly become unaware of the symptoms, once they have had a thorough and reassuring confirmatory dilated fundus examination. Patients must, however, be instructed to return if the pattern of floaters changes as it may indicate a progression of vitreous degeneration to PVD.

Posterior Vitreous Detachment (PVD): Flashes and Floaters

Collagen fibers that make up the three-dimensional microskeletal matrix of the vitreous body insert into, and are utterly inseparable from, glial cells of the vitreous base which are integral to the anterior-most retina. Posterior to the vitreous base, the attachment of the vitreous to the retina is normally relatively weak but slightly stronger at the peripapillary border and the perifoveal region; in addition, in some patients, there are a few other isolated areas where – by reason of heredity, sporadic developmental anomaly, and vascular or inflammatory pathology – the vitreous is abnormally adherent. As vitreous syneresis progresses, repetitive tugs on the flimsy attachments of the vitreous body result in separation – or detachment – of the posterior vitreous from the retina (Fig. 5.2). PVD is common and normal; it will occur in a majority of people by the age of 60. The onset of PVD is often rapid and dramatic. The sudden peeling of the vitreous off of the retina produces considerable mechanical stimulation of the visual neurocircuitry and may thereby generate alarming photopsia. The drastic change in vitreous configuration in the wake of PVD often renders floaters much more apparent. After the initial fusillade, flashes usually gradually subside over a period of hours to weeks. The combination of sudden-onset flashes and floaters often causes a patient to seek medical attention. Often patients fear that their symptoms are the warning signs of any impending stroke or other intracranial pathology.

In most cases, the posterior vitreous peels off the retina cleanly so that the mechanical pulling on the retina – and its accompanying photopsia –

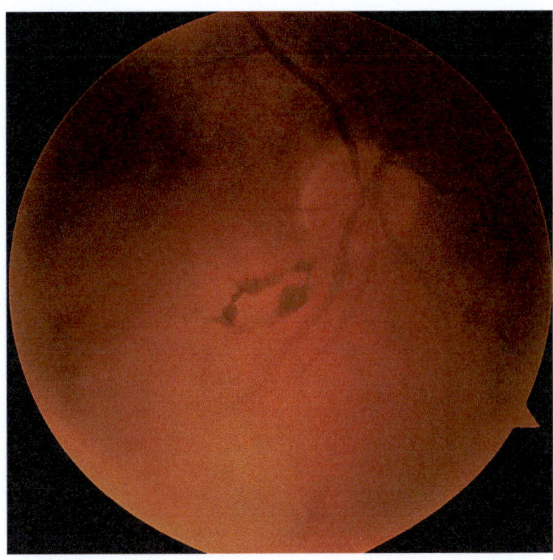

Fig. 5.2 A prominent vitreous floater (known as "Weiss's ring") associated with a PVD

ceases and the patient gradually habituates to the new floater configuration. Visual acuity remains unaffected, and PVD eventually becomes a distant memory. Sometimes, however, the separation from the retina is hindered by an area of abnormally increased adhesion of the vitreous face to an underlying retinal blood vessel. When the vitreous exerts traction, or pulling on a blood vessel, secondary bleeding into the vitreous cavity can occur and cause symptoms that – depending on the amount of blood – can range from minimal aggravation of the floaters to complete obscuration of vision. In the absence of coincident proliferative retinal vasculopathy or retinal tear, the blood will eventually resorb without treatment.

Retinal Tears and Retinal Detachment (RD) Caused by PVD

Sometimes, otherwise normal peeling of the vitreous off of the retina will, because of tenacious vitreoretinal adhesions, result in one or more retinal tears. Retinal tears are commonly associated with a variable degree of bleeding that becomes visible to a patient in the form of additional floaters.

Most importantly, retinal tears that are caused by a PVD are typically the critical intermediary

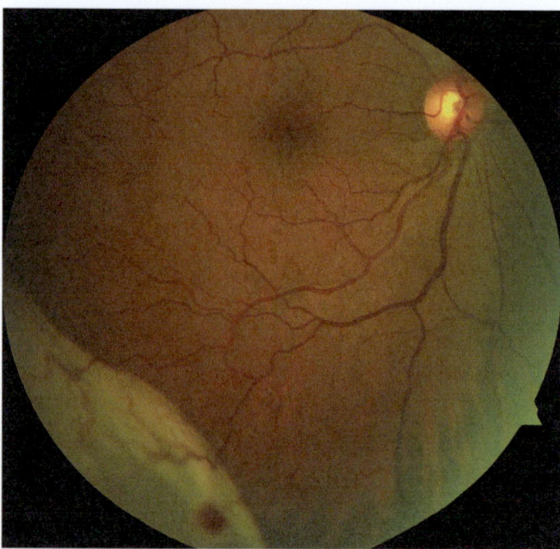

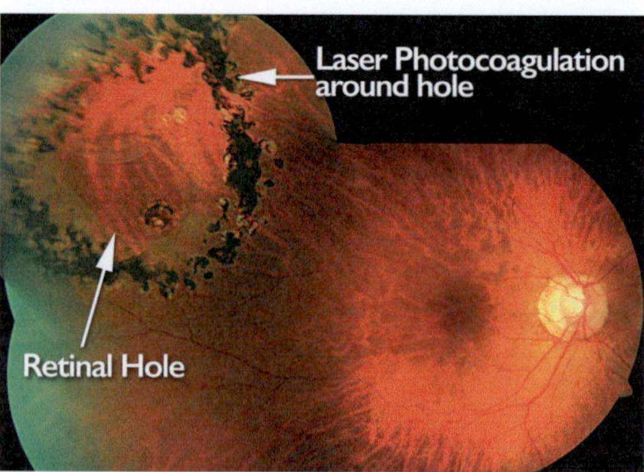

Fig. 5.4 A peripheral retinal tear, with partially trimmed flap, surrounded by laser burns to prevent retinal detachment

Fig. 5.3 Bullous peripheral inferior temporal retinal detachment sparing the macula. A small round hole is noted in the detached portion of the retina

step in the development of RD. The newly formed breaks in the retina allow vitreous cavity fluid to enter the subretinal space and float the retina off the wall of the eye (Figs. 5.3 and 5.4). Rods and cones of the neurosensory retina normally remain in intimate apposition to the retinal pigment epithelial (RPE) layer directly posterior only by means of an active metabolic pumping mechanism. This pumping mechanism can be overwhelmed by the perfect storm of vitreous cavity fluid seeping into the subretinal space through a new break and inward traction forces generated by still adherent vitreous collagen fibers. RDs that are caused by tears are often called "rhegmatogenous" (from the Greek word for "crack" or "rift").

The portion of the retina that is detached will not function properly because the rods and cones, which lack a conventional blood supply, will not receive their required metabolic support from the normally closely apposed RPE cells. The patient's visual field will have a dead zone, or scotoma, in the sector corresponding to the area of detached retina. If the retinal detachment only involves the peripheral retina, sparing the macula, the central vision may be unharmed and remain so if the RD is repaired successfully before macular detachment has occurred. Occasionally, a patient will be

unaware of a small, peripheral scotoma, particularly if the fellow eye has normal acuity that may help mask the visual defect.

Symptomatic PVD-induced retinal tears can often be stabilized by laser treatment alone, if detected before progression to RD, sparing the patient the pain, risk, and inconvenience of incisional surgical repair.

If RD has already occurred, one of the most important tasks of the medical system is to treat a "macula-on" RD before it becomes "macula-off." A matter of hours may make a difference in some cases. Bilateral eye patching can help retard progression of a detachment, by reducing saccadic eye movements, and should be instituted until surgery is performed. Once the macula is detached, there is usually considerable visual loss, and the prognosis becomes variable and uncertain. The longer the rods and cones are separated from their nutritional support, the more likely their deterioration and the permanent loss of acuity in the corresponding visual field. Thus, even if a RD has involved the macula, prompt referral to a retinal surgeon who can restore macular attachment within a matter of days will optimize the patient's chances for maximal visual recovery.

Any patient that seeks medical attention because of new photopsia and floaters needs to have a dilated retinal examination to rule out a retinal tear or detachment, even if the visual acuity and visual fields are normal. If there is a recent decline in visual acuity and/or a new visual field deficit, the potential seriousness of the condition and the urgency of ophthalmic consultation are increased.

Floaters from Vitreous Hemorrhage in Proliferative Retinal Vascular Disease

Floaters are a frequent presenting symptom of vitreous hemorrhage (VH) in patients with proliferative diabetic retinopathy (PDR). VH is caused by bleeding of retinovitreal neovascularization, a manifestation of increased vascular endothelial growth factor (VEGF) production by the ischemic retina caused by diabetic microangiopathy (Fig. 5.5) (see Chap. 22).

These patients are at high risk for profound permanent, and frequently bilateral, visual loss on the basis of tractional RD, macular edema, and neovascular glaucoma and need be given every opportunity for comprehensive ocular and general medical intervention within 1 or 2 days of presentation. Pregnancy is sometimes associated with a significant worsening of diabetic retinopathy, and the development of VH might be an indication for early delivery. Sickle cell retinopa-

thy can also present as vitreous hemorrhage, and affected patients should be referred to retinal specialists to be monitored carefully for tractional RD. Branch retinal vein occlusions can cause symptomatic VH from retinovitreal neovascularization; not usually as profoundly sight-threatening and urgent as PDR, this condition usually responds well to treatments such as laser, anti-VEGF injections, and occasionally vitreous surgery.

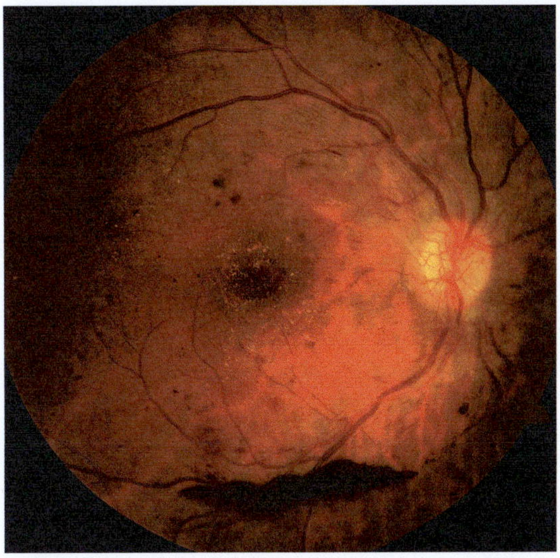

Other Causes of Floaters

Noninfectious and infectious intraocular inflammation (uveitis) can present with floaters that are due to (1) inflammatory cells in the vitreous; (2) blood-ocular barrier breakdown-induced protein exudation and clumping of collagen fibers; (3) bleeding from retinal neovascularization caused by vasculitis-induced retinal ischemia; and (4) inflammation-induced early PVD (Fig. 5.6).

The most common forms of uveitis presenting as floaters are intermediate uveitis (which is occasionally associated with multiple sclerosis) and toxoplasmosis.

Intraocular lymphoma can also produce symptomatic floaters and can masquerade as uveitis. Rare etiologies of uveitis, such as endogenous

Fig. 5.5 Proliferative diabetic retinopathy, with preretinal hemorrhage visible inferiorly

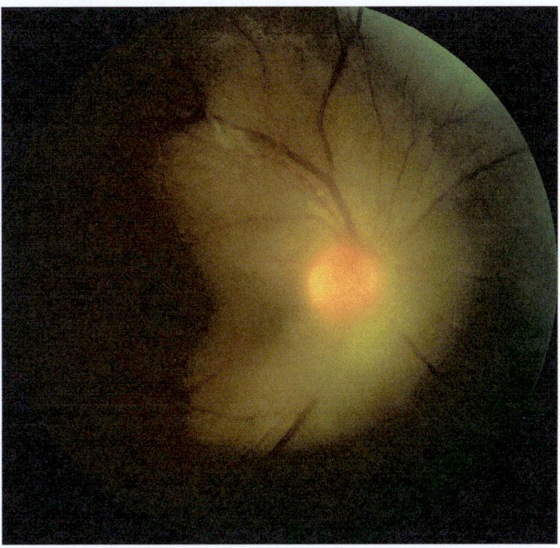

Fig. 5.6 Acute toxoplasmosis, showing vitreous haze

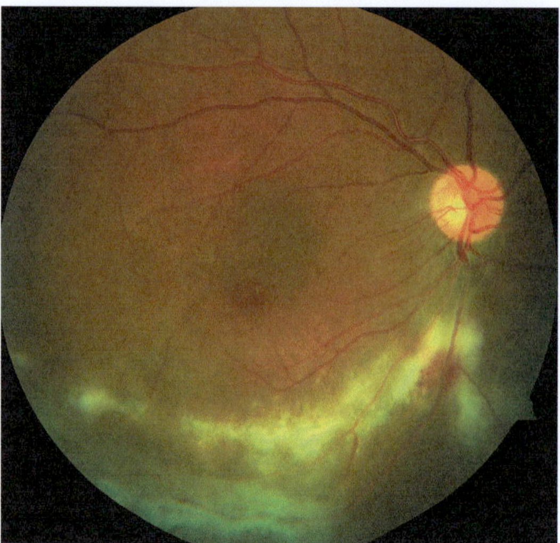

Fig. 5.7 CMV retinopathy seen along the inferior temporal arcade, associated with HIV

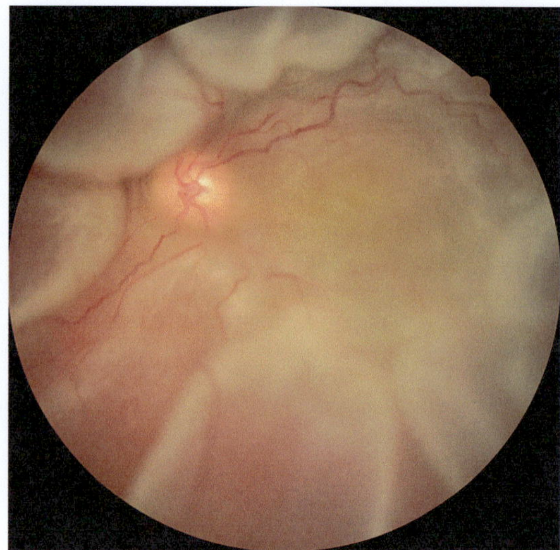

Fig. 5.8 Exudative retinal detachment in a case of uveal effusion syndrome (Courtesy Dr. Hermann Schubert)

endophthalmitis, can lead to discovery of life-threatening infections elsewhere in the patient's body. Cytomegalovirus retinitis needs to be considered in patients with human immunodeficiency virus who are not being adequately treated with highly active antiretroviral therapy (Fig. 5.7).

In general, the differential diagnoses of floaters in the setting of confirmed or suspected uveitis are often broad, requiring an exquisitely detailed comprehensive medical history, meticulous ocular examination, ocular imaging, and laboratory and radiological investigations. Even then, some cases of uveitis defy unequivocal diagnosis. Prompt referral for evaluation and treatment – emergently, in the case of severe and acute symptom onset – can improve the prognosis for these complex vision- and life-threatening disorders.

Flashes Without Floaters: Intraocular Causes

Photoreceptors in areas of the retina no longer attached to the wall of the eye will be abnormally mobile, therefore more subject to abnormally robust or rapid acceleration-decelerations and thus prone to generate photopsia. An RD that is caused by chronic holes or tears may only first become symptomatic when, after a slow increase in subretinal fluid, there is enough abnormal retinal mobility to generate photopsia.

Serous or exudative RDs differ from rhegmatogenous RDs in that no retinal breaks are present; instead, they result from a breakdown in the normal blood-ocular barriers between the subretinal space and either the underlying choriocapillaris or the retinal circulation (Fig. 5.8). Serous or exudative RDs usually result from inflammatory eye disease, preeclampsia, or tumors, such as uveal melanomas and hemangioblastomas, and can also present with symptomatic photopsia. Tension on the retina produced by the contraction of fibrovascular scar tissue in diabetic and sickle cell retinopathy often produces photopsia that is sometimes the first symptom of an incipient tractional RD.

Probably the most common cause of photopsia without floaters is typical age-related vitreous degeneration that leads to chronically increased mobility of the vitreous gel as a whole, which in turn aggravates the momentary peaks of tension exerted at adhesion sites to the retina during eye movements. (Think of the velocity at the tip of a snapping towel compared to a tight bundle). At this point, even though the vitreous has degenerated, its collagen fibers are, overall, in a sufficiently stable configuration so that the patient does not perceive floaters. Tension on the retina produced by the contraction of fibrovascular scar tissue in diabetic and sickle cell retinopathy often produces photopsia that is sometimes the first symptom of an incipient tractional RD.

Migraine-Induced Visual Auras

Migraine headache-associated visual auras often produce scintillating scotomas that many patients refer to as "flashing lights." Bilaterality, the frequent pattern of slowly enlarging "zigzag" lines and subsequent headache make the diagnosis of migraine straightforward, but these features are not universal. The most important distinguishing feature of migraine visual aura is the time course. With rare exception, the visual symptoms usually proceed with constant severity for about 20 minutes (range from 1 to 100 min) and then stop completely, without any ongoing sporadic or lingering visual phenomena. When the clinical picture fits this time course, there is little reason to proceed with any additional examination or diagnostic investigation.

Conclusion

A patient presenting with recent onset of flashes and/or floaters always needs referral to an ophthalmologist, with the exception of unequivocally classic migraine episodes. If accompanied by acute vision or visual field deficit or significant eye pain, the urgency of the referral is greatly increased.

Suggested Reading

American Academy of Ophthalmology. Basic and Clinical Science Course. Section 12. Retina and Vitreous, 2015–2016.

Milston R, Madigan MC, Sebag J. Vitreous floaters: etiology, diagnostics, and management. Surv Ophthalmol. 2016;61(2):211–27.

Ocular Emergencies

6

Royce W. S. Chen and George A. Cioffi

Two primary categories of ocular emergencies require immediate attention: those that are acute in onset and may rapidly lead to irreversible visual loss without prompt treatment and those that are acute in onset and are associated with high risk of systemic morbidity or mortality. These categories are not mutually exclusive. The following are conditions that should always be considered and never missed by any physician.

Ocular and Periocular Trauma

Ocular trauma includes eyelid and conjunctival lacerations, corneal abrasions, penetrating injuries with or without intraocular foreign body, and globe rupture (Figs. 6.1 and 6.2). In addition, ocular trauma is often associated with orbital trauma that can lead to retrobulbar hemorrhage, traumatic optic neuropathy, orbital fracture, and eye muscle entrapment. Any patient who presents with a history suspicious for globe trauma should be thoroughly evaluated with visual acuity exam, pupillary assessment, motility testing, and slit lamp evaluation with dilated exam when possible. If there is concern for globe rupture, every effort should be taken to avoid placing pressure on the globe itself, as this could lead to expulsion of intraocular contents. While corneal abrasions and eyelid lacerations generally have good visual prognoses, globe rupture and penetrating injuries may lead to severe visual loss due to corneal scarring, lens dislocation or expulsion, vitreous hemorrhage, suprachoroidal hemorrhage, retinal detachment, and direct chorioretinal injury (Fig. 6.3).

Intraocular foreign bodies may lead to infection (endophthalmitis) or toxic injury to the retina. If the globe is ruptured, the eye is initially closed surgically to preserve the integrity of the globe, achieve stability of intraocular pressure and intraocular contents, and decrease risk of infection. Secondary procedures, such as retinal detachment repair and cataract extraction, are typically performed within a few days to a few weeks. If there is concern for retained intraocular foreign body at the time of injury, computed tomography of the orbit and brain should be performed. Magnetic resonance imaging should

R. W. S. Chen, MD (✉)
Columbia University Irving Medical Center,
New York, NY, USA

Department of Ophthalmology, Edward S. Harkness
Eye Institute, Columbia University Vagelos College
of Physicians and Surgeons, New York, NY, USA
e-mail: rc2631@cumc.columbia.edu

G. A. Cioffi, MD
Columbia University Irving Medical Center,
New York, NY, USA

Edward S. Harkness Eye Institute, Columbia University
Vagelos College of Physicians and Surgeons,
New York, NY, USA

© Springer Nature Switzerland AG 2019
D. S. Casper, G. A. Cioffi (eds.), *The Columbia Guide to Basic Elements of Eye Care*,
https://doi.org/10.1007/978-3-030-10886-1_6

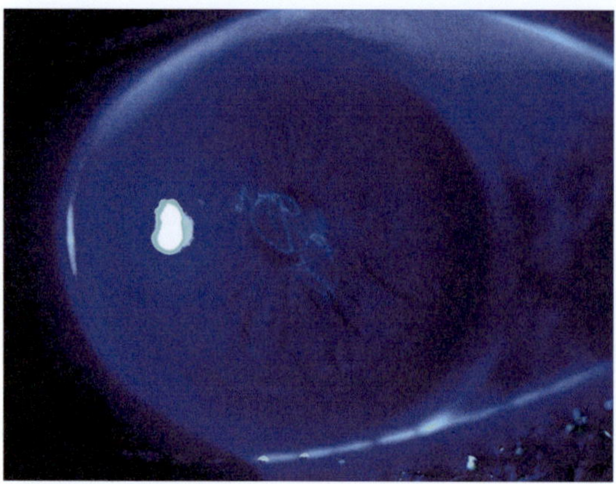

Fig. 6.1 A curvilinear series of fine corneal abrasions are seen in this patient; a small foreign body had become lodged under her rigid gas permeable contact lens. The slit lamp illumination is seen reflecting off the cornea on the left. (Image courtesy Dr Suzanne Sherman)

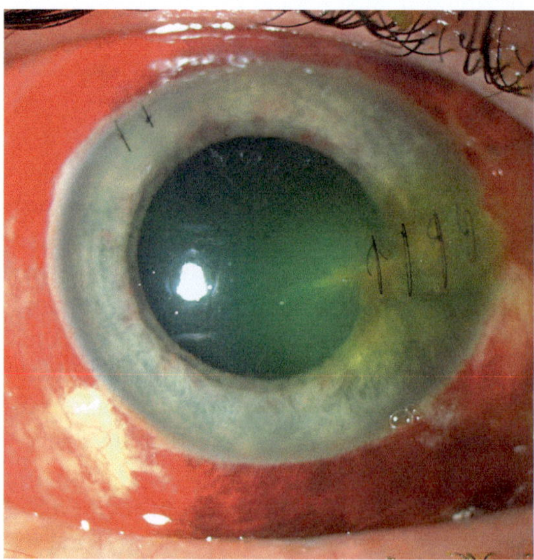

Fig. 6.3 Immediate postoperative repair of full-thickness nasal corneal laceration, showing sutures in well-aligned and apposed wound, with additional sutures noted supero-temporally where a port was inserted during surgery to maintain intraocular pressure. The anterior chamber is deep, indicating a good seal and a functioning ciliary body. A 360° subconjunctival hemorrhage is also present

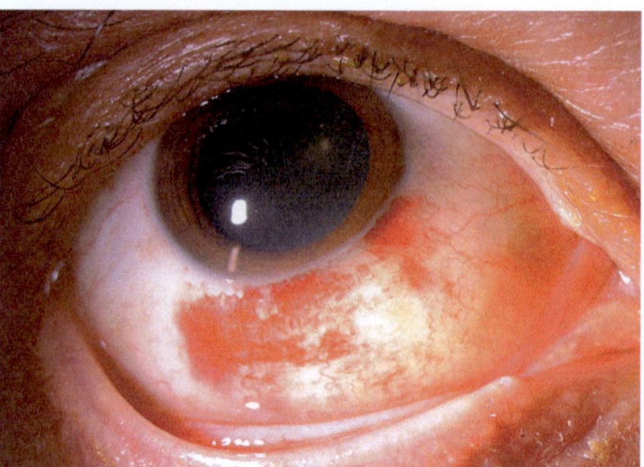

Fig. 6.2 A small inferior subconjunctival hemorrhage noted after minor eye trauma during a basketball game. No additional pathology was found

blunt trauma, with or without orbital bone fractures, may damage the optic nerve, leading to traumatic optic neuropathy (Fig. 6.4). Additionally, blunt trauma may lead to bleeding behind the eye and an ensuing compartment syndrome in the retrobulbar space that manifests as proptosis, pain, decreased vision, and decreased ocular motility. If these signs are present, the optic nerve is at risk, and intraocular pressure may be dramatically elevated, and a lateral canthotomy and cantholysis should be performed emergently to decompress the space around the globe and preserve vision.

Chemical Injury

Ocular chemical injuries affect young men most frequently and may result in serious injury. Alkali agents, which are lipophilic, may penetrate more deeply into the eye, thereby causing more severe injury than do acids. Patients generally present with a known history of a chemical exposure and typically exhibit pain, redness, photophobia, decreased vision, and discharge. The appropriate exam includes pH measurement, visual acuity, and thorough evaluation of the anterior segment, including inspection of the conjunctival fornices. The cornea may be clear or hazy, and there may be significant epithelial defects visible with fluorescein staining and cobalt light illumination. While the conjunctiva

never be used if there is concern for metallic foreign body, as MR-induced movement of metallic objects can produce additional intraocular injury; however, MRI may be more sensitive in detecting organic foreign bodies such as wood. Periocular

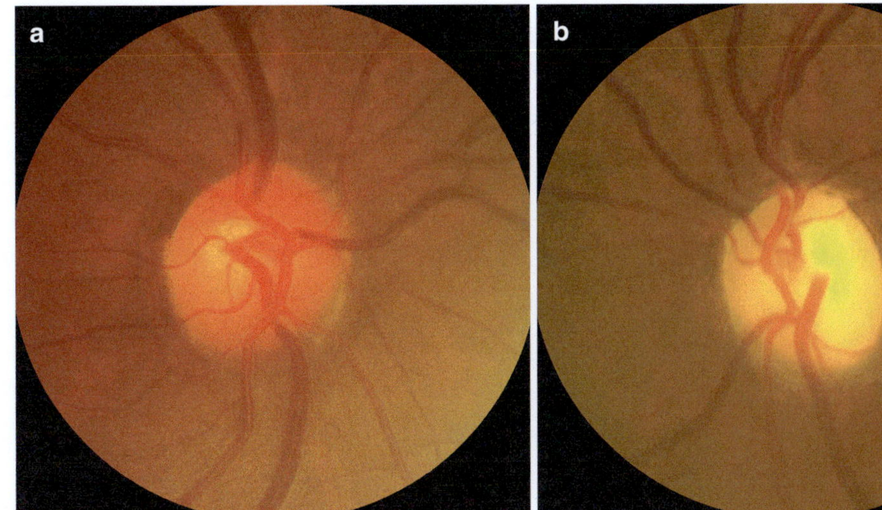

Fig. 6.4 A 57-year-old man injured in Afghanistan in 1991, shot in left orbit without direct trauma to, or severing of, optic nerve. Optic nerve contusion led to eventual left eye blindness. A, the right optic nerve is normal, while the left, B, appears pale and atrophic

is injected in mild cases, there may be a counterintuitive whitening of the eye in cases of a severe burn, which incorrectly implies minimal injury; in fact, this "quiet" appearance frequently signifies limbal ischemia and therefore a significantly worse visual prognosis. Prompt, copious irrigation of the eye is critical to remove the offending substance and restore normal pH. Topical antibiotics may be necessary to prevent superinfection, and topical steroids may be required to limit inflammatory side effects and further corneal damage. Other agents such as ascorbic acid and doxycycline may be used to promote corneal healing; surgical treatment including debridement, limbal stem cell transplant, and amniotic membrane graft may be indicated.

Infection

Extraocular Infection: Orbital Cellulitis

The majority of cellulitis cases around the eye originate from sinus disease. In adults, orbital cellulitis secondary to adjacent sinus disease often follows a fracture of the intervening orbital walls, but in children, with incompletely developed boney structures, cellulitic processes may occur in the absence of any antecedent injury in both children and adults; cellulitis can also originate from superficial skin lesions resulting from localized infections as small as a pimple or as the result of a laceration with subsequent infection (Fig. 6.5).

Broadly speaking, periocular cellulitis is divided into two categories: preseptal and orbital. Preseptal cellulitis is limited to the tissues anterior to the orbital septum (see Fig. 1.15). Edema and erythema of the lids and periorbital skin may be significant, but the globe and orbital structures are not involved. Thus, the visual acuity and ocular movements should be normal when the lids are opened and the eye is examined. Preseptal cases can typically be managed with oral antibiotics, but when cellulitis involves structures posterior to the orbital septum (orbital cellulitis), patients may experience fever, leukocytosis, proptosis, pain, ptosis, decreased vision, and restriction of ocular motility. Orbital cellulitis may be more common in children, as their orbital septum is less developed. Prompt diagnosis and treatment of orbital cellulitis are imperative to prevent permanent vision loss. As well, particularly in young children, septicemia and even meningitis may occur as the orbital infection extends. A CT scan should be performed to determine the extent of orbital involvement, and whether surgical drainage of a subperiosteal or orbital abscess is required. Intravenous antibiotics and close monitoring are indicated. If treatment is delayed, a compressive optic neuropathy may develop, with possible irreversibly impaired vision. Further progression of an untreated orbital infection may lead to cavernous sinus thrombosis, brain abscess, and death.

Ocular Infection

Infections affecting the eye itself may be exogenous or endogenous. Exogenous infections originate externally and may follow corneal ulcers (e.g., contact lens-associated infections) and trauma (e.g., injury, postsurgical, post-intraocular medication injection). Patients usually present with an acutely red eye, vision loss, pain, and photophobia. If not treated early and aggressively, corneal ulcers may cause corneal perforation and lead to infection of all the inner layers of the eye or endophthalmitis (Fig. 6.6).

Following resolution of infection with aggressive antibiotic therapy, corneal ulcers may cause visual loss because of subsequent corneal scarring. Eyes with endophthalmitis require intravitreal antibiotics and in some cases vitrectomy

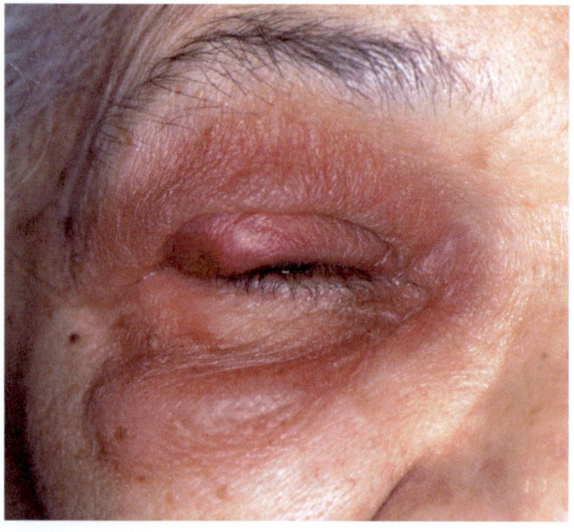

Fig. 6.5 A 77-year-old woman with a right upper lid hordeolum which progressed to a periorbital cellulitis

surgery. Prognosis is variable depending on promptness of therapy and the type of organism. For example, *Staphylococcus epidermidis* infections tend to be relatively mild, while *Streptococcus pneumoniae* infections are often severe.

The eye may also acquire infections via hematogenous spread from a distant source in the body. For example, septic emboli from an infected cardiac valve may seed in the retina or choroid, leading to one or more subretinal abscesses. If these lesions are not identified and treated early, the infection may migrate anteriorly, leading to vitritis and endophthalmitis.

Acute Diplopia

The causes of diplopia are numerous, but two bear mentioning in the context of ocular emergencies. Both *pituitary apoplexy* and *intracranial aneurysms* may present with oculomotor nerve palsy. Patients typically develop acute onset exotropia (out-turned eye) and ptosis, often with decreased pupil reactivity on the side of the lesion.

In the case of pituitary apoplexy, an acute hemorrhagic event is the cause, typically occurring within an existing pituitary adenoma. Associated symptoms may include headache, decreased vision, and possibly altered mental status. In addition to third nerve compression, such an expanding pituitary lesion may affect other cranial nerves in the cavernous sinus, including nerves IV, V, and VI. Patients with posterior communicating artery aneurysm are more likely to display an isolated oculomotor nerve palsy. In any patient presenting with an incomplete third nerve palsy, neuroimaging must be obtained to investigate for these life-threatening conditions.

Acute Angle-Closure Glaucoma

Glaucoma is defined by visual field loss secondary to optic nerve damage. In most cases, injury to the optic nerve occurs insidiously, but in acute angle closure, a sequence of events may lead to

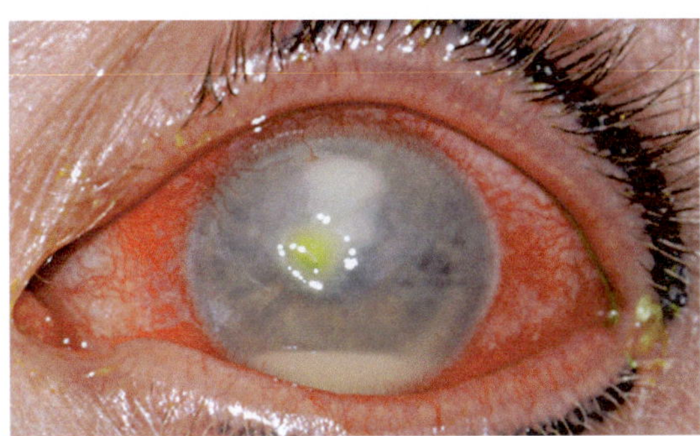

Fig. 6.6 A central corneal ulcer which eventually grew out *fusarium*. There are intense limbal injection, a large central ulcer, and layered inflammatory cells (hypopyon) visible in the anterior chamber

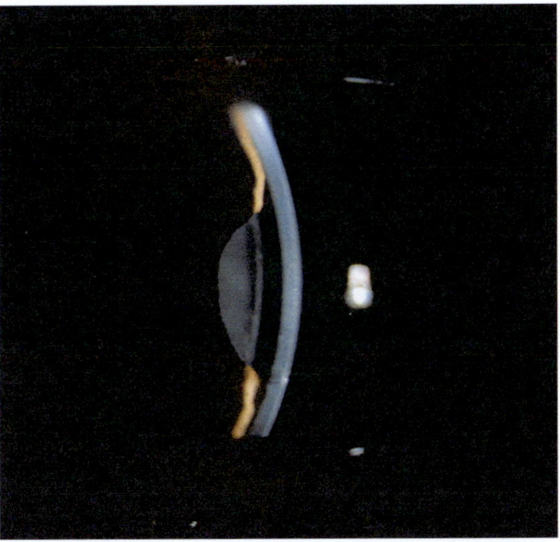

Fig. 6.7 Slit lamp image of angle-closure attack. The anterior chamber has almost fully collapsed, with the corneal endothelium almost touching the anterior iris surface. The pupil is fixed in mid-dilation

rapid visual loss. In the normal eye, aqueous fluid produced continuously by the ciliary body flows through the pupil into the anterior chamber, where it drains through the trabecular meshwork and into Schlemm's canal. Anatomically, the periphery of the anterior chamber forms an angle, composed of the internal corneal endothelium anteriorly and the iris posteriorly. Risk factors for acute angle closure include older age, shorter axial length (usually found in farsighted or hyperopic eyes), thicker crystalline lens with the development of a cataract, inflammatory scarring, and drugs that may affect the position of the ciliary body and/or dilate the pupil. In particular, any medication with anticholinergic properties should be avoided. While a variety of drug classes have been implicated, common medications that may precipitate an acute angle-closure attack include both over-the-counter and prescribed medications (such as cold and allergy medicines, sleep disorder medications, seasickness medications, antidepressants, and incontinence medications to name a few). Therefore, individuals at risk of angle closure should be cautioned to carefully read all medication labels and avoid medications with specific warnings regarding glaucoma. If the angle closes and the drainage pathway is blocked, patients present with sudden pain, decreased vision, headache, halos around lights, redness, and nausea or vomiting, all due to the sudden rise in intraocular pressure as aqueous drainage ceases. Examination reveals an injected conjunctiva; decreased acuity; a fixed, mid-dilated pupil; extremely elevated intraocular pressure; corneal edema; and a closed angle on gonioscopy (Fig. 6.7).

Treatment consists of emergent topical and systemic medications to lower the intraocular pressure and laser peripheral iridotomy as soon as possible (corneal haze from elevated intraocular pressure may initially prevent this from being accomplished during an attack). This procedure creates a hole in the peripheral iris, allowing aqueous fluid to pass into the anterior chamber via a different pathway than through the pupil. As more aqueous fills the peripheral chamber, the angle may deepen, and the acute angle-closure attack may be resolved. In more recalcitrant cases, surgical removal of the cataract with or without implantation of a glaucoma drainage device may be indicated.

Central Retinal Arterial Occlusion

A central retinal artery occlusion (CRAO) occurs when the central retinal artery is occluded by emboli, thrombi, or inflammatory disease affecting the vessel wall. Risk factors include arterial hypertension, diabetes mellitus, carotid artery

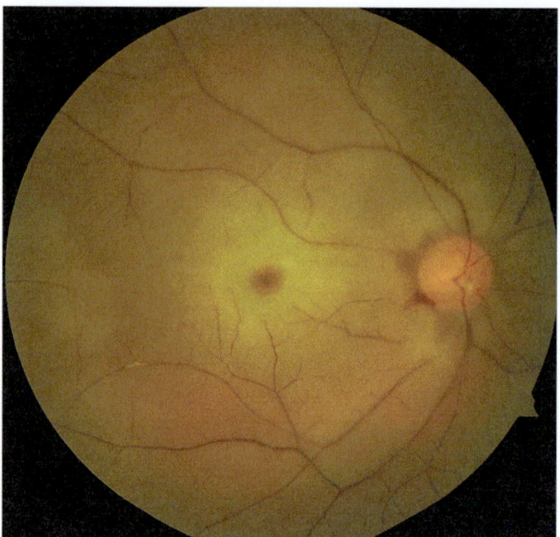

Fig. 6.8 Acute CRAO showing pale, edematous macula, with cherry red spot at the fovea. A small flame hemorrhage is also noted at the disc margin, and arterial filling is minimal and absent in some areas (e.g., inferotemporally)

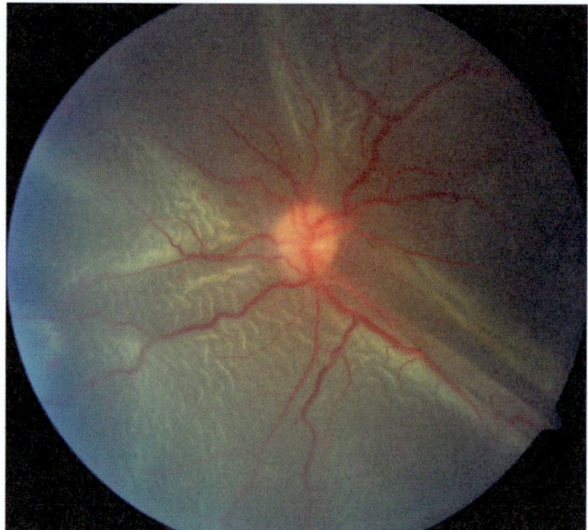

Fig. 6.9 Total rhegmatogenous retinal detachment in a patient with sickle cell disease. Undulating retinal folds are clearly visible in all quadrants; the retina remains attached only at the optic disc

disease, and coronary artery disease. Occlusion leads to ischemic injury and edema of the entire retina. Patients present with a sudden and profound painless loss of vision, often to the level of counting fingers or worse. Examination reveals poor visual acuity, an afferent pupillary defect, and normal intraocular pressure. Dilated exam reveals whitened retina with abnormal blood flow within the affected vessels. The foveal center, devoid of ganglion cells, does not experience the same swelling as adjacent retinal tissue and therefore appears strikingly red in contrast to the rest of the retina (the so-called cherry red spot), as the posterior choroidal circulation can be visualized through the relatively thin fovea, while perifoveal edema whitens the retina and diminishes the view of the underlying choroid layer (Fig. 6.8). Because giant cell arteritis (GCA) may be a cause of CRAO, it should be suspected in any patient that has characteristic symptoms, including headache, scalp tenderness, jaw claudication, fevers, malaise, weight loss, and neck or limb pain. GCA requires systemic immunosuppressive treatment in order to avoid complications of visual loss in the fellow eye, aortic aneurysm, and stroke.

Rhegmatogenous Retinal Detachment

Rhegmatogenous retinal detachments occur when the neurosensory retina is separated from the underlying retinal pigment epithelium. There is always at least one full-thickness break in the retina, typically in the periphery where the vitreous is more tightly adherent to the retina (Fig. 6.9). Patients present with the acute onset of flashes (from traction induced upon the retina) and floaters (from blood or release of pigment into the vitreous), accompanied by a dense scotoma in part of or the entire field of vision in one eye. Risk factors include age, myopia, lattice degeneration, previous intraocular surgery, trauma, and retinal detachment in the fellow eye. Without surgical treatment, rhegmatogenous retinal detachments typically progress, and the eye develops significant visual loss.

Suggested Reading

Bagheri N, Wajda B, Calvo C, Durrani A, editors. The Wills Eye Manual. Philadelphia: Wolters Kluwer; 2016.
Webb LA. Manual of Eye Emergencies. Diagnosis and management. 2nd ed. Butterworth-Heinemann; 2004.

The Refractive State of the Human Eye

7

Karina Conlin and Stephen L. Trokel

A large portion of the sensory input to the brain arises from the visual system. Many of the terms used to describe human vision at the dawn of western civilization have persisted into modern usage. It was noted in ancient Greece that some people would squint when trying to see distant objects clearly. Squinting eyes appeared narrow and were called *myopia*, a Greek term for "narrow" or "squinting" eyes. This term has persisted to this day to describe people with poor distance vision. The ancients also noted that near vision deteriorated as a person became older, and they labeled this condition, *presbyopia* or "old eyes," a term we continue to use today to describe functional visual changes that occur as people age. Hyperopia was noted in young people who had trouble reading and resembled presbyopes. This was thought to be a form of presbyopia and was know as hyperpresbyopia, a term that gave rise to the terms hyperopia and hypermetropia.

K. Conlin, OD, FAAO
Department of Ophthalmology and Visual Sciences,
University of Wisconsin School of Medicine
and Public Health, Madison, WI, USA

S. L. Trokel, MD (✉)
Columbia University Irving Medical Center,
New York, NY, USA

Department of Ophthalmology, Edward S. Harkness
Eye Institute, Columbia University Vagelos College
of Physicians and Surgeons, New York, NY, USA
e-mail: slt3@cumc.columbia.edu

Refractive States

Each person has a range of clear vision that has a characteristic near point and a far point due to the intrinsic focusing mechanism of the eye. The location, size, and range of clear vision define the optical performance of an eye and gives rise to its clinical classification. Objects closer than a person's near point or more distant than their far point will appear blurred. We all are aware that when we are young, the range of clear vision is large and the far-sighted eye will see clearly from a distant far point to a point close to the eye. This range of clear vision is known as the accommodative amplitude and gets progressively smaller with age and decreases noticeably in the fourth decade of life – hence the need for reading glasses for many patients.

Refractive Classification

The refractive state of the eye is classified according to the location of its far point (Fig. 7.1) of clear vision. If the far point is close (i.e., distant objects appear blurred), then the eye is called "nearsighted" or "myopic." Although simple myopia is common, there are forms of pathologic myopia which are usually due to a greater than average axial length of the nearsighted eye. These eyes may be associated with a variety of pathologic conditions. These include retinal tears and detachments and myopic retinal degeneration.

© Springer Nature Switzerland AG 2019

D. S. Casper, G. A. Cioffi (eds.), *The Columbia Guide to Basic Elements of Eye Care*,
https://doi.org/10.1007/978-3-030-10886-1_7

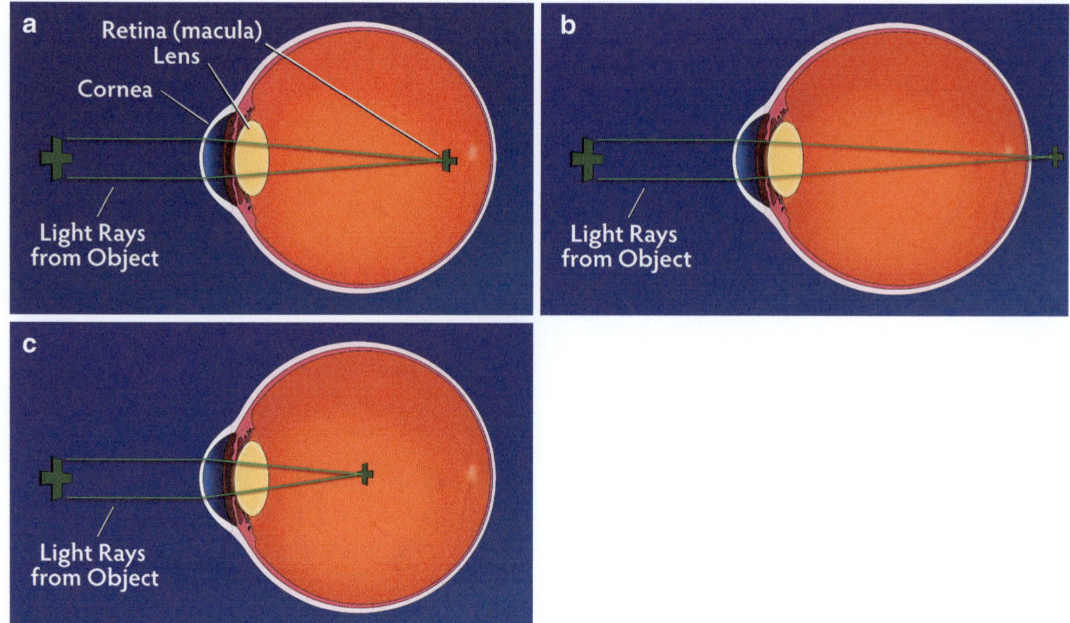

Fig. 7.1 (**a**) In an emmetropic eye with a spherical, symmetric cornea, all light rays from an object of regard are focused in a single plane, directly on the fovea. (**b**) The image focuses posterior to the fovea if hyperopic. (**c**) The image focuses anterior to the fovea if myopic. In the latter cases, the focal point misplacement is corrected with hyperopic or myopic lenses, to replace the image directly on the fovea

If, on the other hand, the far point is at or beyond infinity, then the eye is called "farsighted" or "hyperopic." A severely farsighted eye in a young person will also have a relatively remote (i.e., distant) near point, a condition that very much resembles the old or presbyopic eye. In fact, the resemblance was so close that this eye was described as "hyper-presbyopic," because, when present in a young person, it resembled the vision of an older person. If, however, the amount of farsightedness is small, hyperopic people may not need glasses until near vision fails in the fourth decade of life.

The term astigmatism means "not to a point" and occurs when the corneal surface is not spherical but rather has a toric shape. An unaided astigmatic cornea cannot sharply focus a point. The corneal surface of an astigmatic eye resembles the surface of a football with its two different curves, rather than a baseball with a single symmetric spherical curve (Fig. 7.2). The differing surface curves do not allow a point in space to be sharply focused upon the retina. As with the football surface, the corneal surface has two different curves that focus a point of light into an ellipse rather than a point, thus making images appear blurred. Astigmatism can be present in any refractive state, and its correction was first incorporated into spectacles in 1841. Astigmatism creates blurred vision at all distances and reduces the overall sharpness of visual acuity. Patients with small amounts of uncorrected astigmatism may be asymptomatic. Patients with uncorrected astigmatism notice that signs are difficult to read or letters appear stretched rather than crisp. Some will complain about ghost images, and others may be bothered by glare from car headlights and other bright light sources.

Spectacles evolved on an empirical basis at the end of the first millennium in the Venetian empire. It was recognized that nearsighted people had better vision by using lenses that were thinner in the center than at the edges. Conversely, presbyopic people saw better with lenses that were thicker in the center. It was not until 1604 that Johannes Kepler explained for the first time why lenses of different designs improve vision.

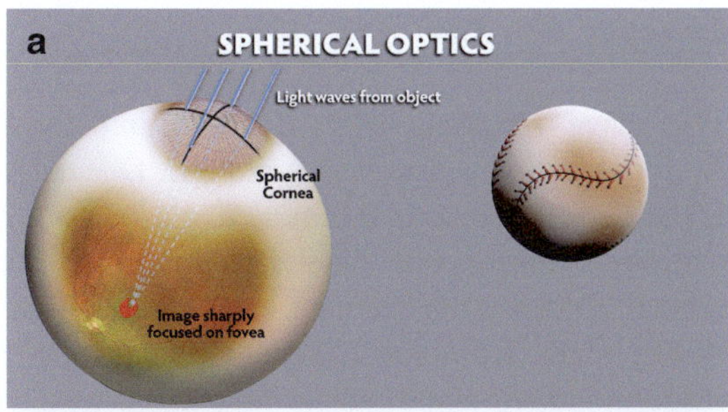

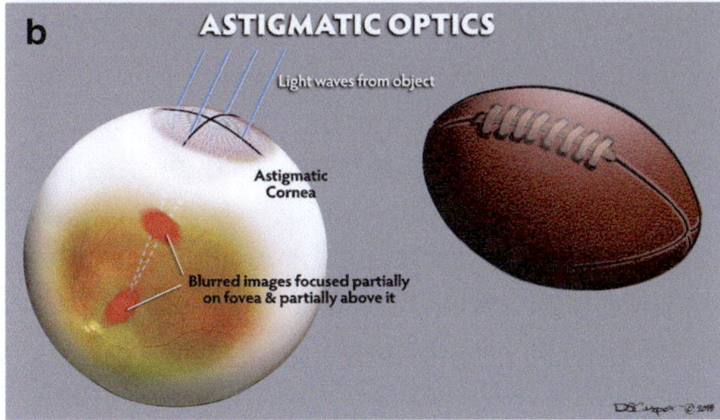

Fig. 7.2 (**a**) In the eye with a spherical, symmetric cornea, all light rays from an object of regard are focused in a single plane, directly on the fovea if the eye is emmetropic or has been properly corrected with myopic or hyperopic lenses. (**b**) The astigmatic cornea is not spherical, but rather is asymmetric, and the curvature in one meridian is different than from that in another (as with a football). Therefore, with an astigmatic cornea, when some light rays are focused on the fovea, others will either be focused in front of the retina (as shown here) or behind the retina, resulting in blurring of the image. Astigmatic lenses, with power in only one meridian, are used to correct this error

Anatomic Elements Determining the Refractive State

The Length of the Eye

The refractive state of the eye is based largely on the axial length of the globe. Nearsighted eyes are longer, and farsighted eyes are shorter than the normal average length of 24 mm.

The Shape of the Cornea

In addition to ocular length, the refractive state is also changed by the corneal shape. A steeper corneal curvature will increase myopia, while flatter corneas result in hyperopia. As noted above, a toric-shaped astigmatic cornea will focus a point of light into an ellipse rather than a point. A highly irregular corneal surface cannot focus light into a precise image, even with the use of optimally corrected spectacles. This distorted surface occurs in eyes with keratoconus, a condition where the cornea is structurally weaker than normal and bulges forward asymmetrically, creating an irregular surface that introduces severe aberrations. These aberrations significantly degrade optical function and the ability of the eye to clearly focus an image on the retina, resulting in blurred vision. Other corneal conditions that degrade visual function, include local scars that arise from injuries, infections, or genetic dystrophies. Scars and irregularities scatter light that passes into the eye and can cause disturbing glare or halos. Significant improvement in visual function can be obtained in many patients who have irregular corneas with the use of contact lenses that create a more uniform optical surface that minimize optical distortion and enhances visual clarity.

The Lens

The lens, usually called the "crystalline lens," is the third major optical component that determines the refractive state of the eye. Variation in the optical power of the crystalline lens is the physiologic basis for the variable optical power of the eye creating its automatic focus mechanism. The actual mechanism is accomplished by its ability to change both shape and position by action of the ciliary muscle. This change in lens power is a variable focus that allows the wide range of clear vision that characterizes the young eye. Age-related structural changes in the crystalline lens and its support mechanism are responsible for the receding near point (i.e., the progressive difficulty in reading) that characterizes presbyopia, becoming manifest as the accomodative amplitude shrinks with aging.

What Determines the Refractive State

Genetic factors are clearly important in determining the ultimate refractive state of the eye. However, there is compelling epidemiological evidence that environmental factors play a role as well. It is fairly well-established that multifactorial inheritance patterns are involved in the development of certain myopic errors, and most likely other refractive errors will also be shown to have environmental influences.

Correction of Refractive Errors

Spectacle Correction of Refractive Error

While the major function of spectacles is to improve visual function, its protective role should not be ignored. In addition to physical protection of the eye from foreign materials, spectacles may be designed to limit a portion of the optical spectrum that enters the eye. This is most commonly seen in sunglasses that are designed to reduce the intensity of visible light and block most UV light. Modern safety glasses may be designed to block specific portions of the optical wavelength. Laser safety glasses are an example of this protective function. While all spectacles protect the eyes from some foreign material, there are specialty spectacles with lenses and frames designed for industrial use and sports such as hockey.

Changes with Age

The range of focus is called "Accomodative Amplitude" and it decreases with age. Difficulty with reading is one of the most disturbing, normal signs that occur with the passage of time. Figure 7.3 shows the decrease in the ability of the eye to focus with increasing age. The loss of accommodative amplitude is first noted by the patient as a discomfort while reading which eventually progresses to an inability to read. Patients will often complain that their "arms are too short" to read comfortably, as their near point slowly recedes with aging. Accommodative amplitude may be affected by many external factors. Among these factors are fatigue, alcohol consumption, medications that have an effect on the autonomic system, and psychoactive drugs.

Correction of the Near Point

The oldest and simplest solution for improving near vision is the so-called reading glass (also referred to as magnifiers) that are available in prefabricated models with increasing optical power. These glasses are designed to improve visual clarity at near when the accommodative

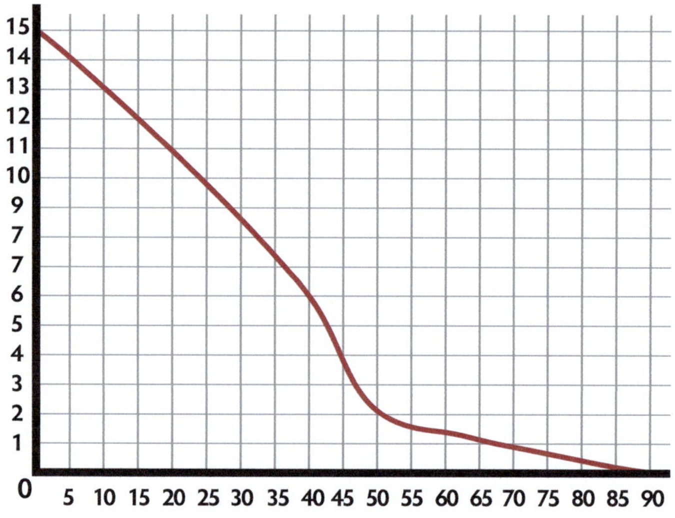

Fig. 7.3 The normal, age-related decrease in the ability of the eye to focus at near distances. This loss of accommodative amplitude usually becomes symptomatic at approximately age 40 and progresses for 10–20 years, before leveling off. Magnifier lenses of increasing power are used to overcome this predictable accommodative decrease. (Adapted from Duane [9])

amplitude is no longer able to complete this task. Because they sharpen near vision, they facilitate near visual tasks and compensate symmetrically for loss of accommodative function. They do not, however, compensate for differences between the two eyes or astigmatic refractive errors or account for pupillary distance. More complex optical states require a custom-made spectacle that considers ocular dominance, the optics of the eye, the state of the patient's general health, consideration of medications taken, and the needs of the patient for clear near vision.

Correction of the Far Point

The far point of the nearsighted eye can be moved further away with a lens that is thinner in the center than at the edge (a concave lens), enabling myopic people to see objects in the distance. If astigmatism is present, the correcting spectacle lens can incorporate a toric shape that will compensate for the asymmetric shape of the cornea.

Correction of Both Far and Near Points

In the older patient's eye, the focusing range is reduced, and different optical corrections are necessary for clear vision at distance and at near. There are several ways to achieve this. The simplest is to provide two different glasses, one designed to improve vision at distance and the other to provide clear vision at near. This is obviously inconvenient, and optical modifications that allow simultaneous clear vision at different distances have been developed. These are referred to as multifocal spectacles.

Multifocal Spectacles

There are three types of multifocal spectacles in wide use today. The bifocal, developed in the early eighteenth century, was popularized and perhaps invented by Benjamin Franklin. This spectacle variation uses two different lens powers: one for distance on the top and one for near in the lower half. Variations on this include a bifocal with an additional reading element built into the upper portion of the spectacle lens, which was first developed for pilots to use who have instrumentation placed high in the cockpit but is also employed by others, such as carpenters and painters who must do work on overhead ceilings. A variation of the bifocal is the trifocal where a lens for intermediate distances is incorporated into the lens just above the reading segment.

Normal distance vision encompasses objects located from about 20 ft and out to infinity; near vision correction for presbyopic patients is set at their most comfortable reading distance and provides very limited depth of field, usually only a few inches. Therefore, bifocals do not improve acuity in the middle or "intermediate zone" located from the reading position and out to 20 ft. Unfortunately, included in this uncorrected zone are a variety of visual tasks that are ubiquitous in modern society. Chief among these are viewing computer screens, but pictures at museums, sheet music for musicians, and schedule screens in airports are typical of activities requiring sharp vision at varying distances that are neither "near" nor "far." More modern spectacle lens designs have been developed and commercialized that use a lens with a progressively stronger correction, beginning at approximately mid-lens and increasing toward the bottom (Fig. 7.4). This enables the user to clearly see objects that are at a wide range of distances by varying the position of his line of sight by tipping the head up or down. While some people have trouble adapting to these "progressive" lenses, they have served to increase the flexibility of visual comfort for most users, enabling them to use one single spectacle for all visual tasks over a wide range of distances.

Monovision is a technique where patients use their dominant eye for distance and correct the non-dominant eye for reading. This remains a choice for a minority of patients who are able to adapt to it. Many of these patients have a preexisting optical asymmetry between their two eyes. Some degree of binocularity is sacrificed with this solution. Monovision is more commonly

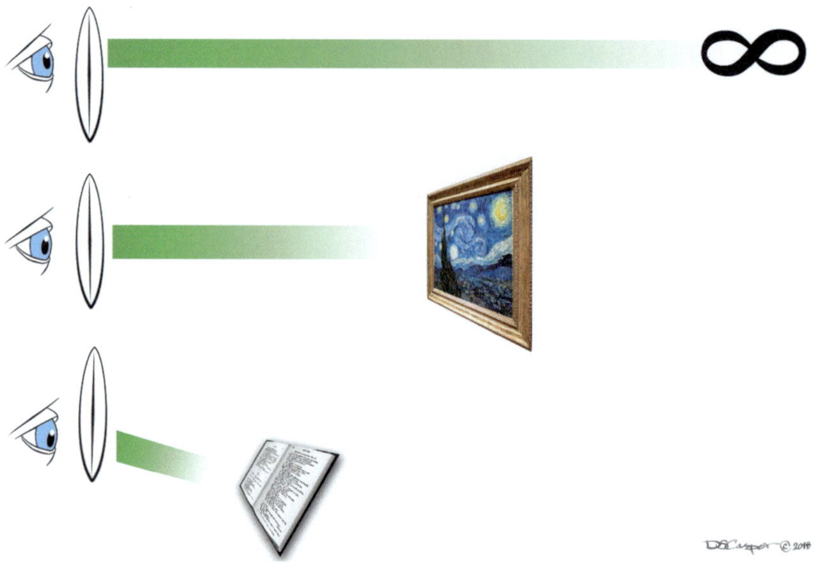

Fig. 7.4 With trifocal or progressive lenses, the lens correction becomes progressively stronger from top to bottom. Variation of the line of sight, accomplished by tipping the head up or down, allows someone wearing these lenses to view objects at a wide range of distances, enabling them to use a single spectacle for visual tasks over a wide range of distances. The upper portion of the lens allows distance clarity from approximately 20 ft out to infinity, the middle covers the "intermediate zone," and the bottom is used for reading distance

employed by contact lens wearers and after refractive surgery.

Contact Lenses

In spite of the excellent optical results and protective features afforded by spectacles, there are many situations in which they fail. They are difficult to use when it's raining, and they often fog when moving into different temperature-controlled areas. Furthermore, they are prone to slippage and loss, especially when the wearer is engaged in active sports. Spectacles are only useful if the optical quality of the cornea is high. Alternative solutions are necessary to provide the best vision possible when irregularities of the corneal surface are present. The alternative solution that has achieved wide acceptance is the use of small lenses placed directly on the eye (cornea or sclera), called contact lenses. These lenses provide a new optical surface that creates a visual experience that is, in many ways, superior to that provided by spectacles.

Contact Lens Types

A variety of contact lens types have been developed to overcome the limitations of spectacles. Among these contact lenses are scleral lenses (Fig. 7.5), small gas permeable lenses (Fig. 7.6), and a variety of lenses made of a soft plastic that is designed to better transmit fluid and nutrients to the cornea. These small lenses are made from a variety of materials designed so they cover the cornea and provide an optical surface that clarifies the retinal image in a manner similar to spectacle lenses. Initially developed in the 1930s as glass shells that covered the entire cornea and adjacent sclera, they have undergone technical transformations into a variety of solid and flexible plastics that have many advantages in terms of comfort and visual function to the user.

The wide varieties of materials that have been developed for contact lens use vary in their physical properties. Some contact lenses incorporate optical elements to combine refractive as well as cosmetic components, to enable chang-

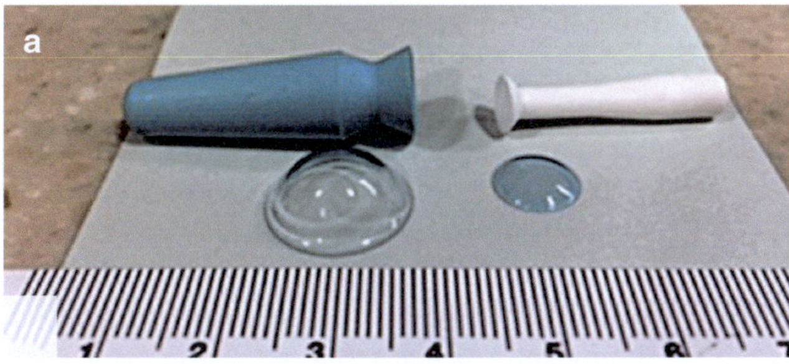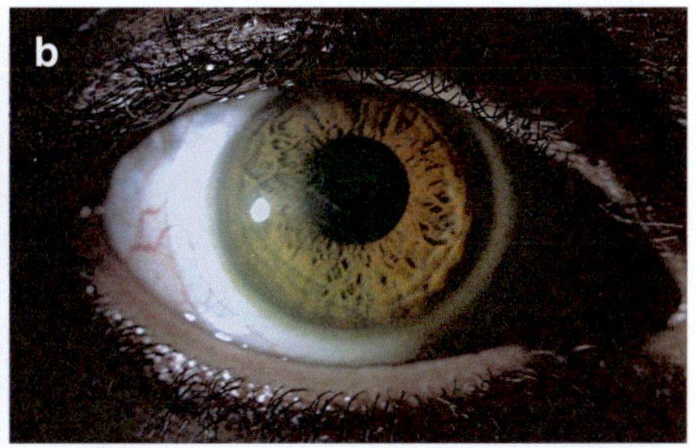

Fig. 7.5 (**a**) The size of the scleral gas permeable contact lens and applicator/remover tool, seen on the left, vs. the small corneal gas permeable lens and matching tool on the right. (**b**) An external photograph of a 16-mm-diameter spherical scleral contact lens made out of gas permeable material. Unlike with the typical corneal contact lenses in use today, these lenses extend past the limbus and come in contact with the anterior sclera

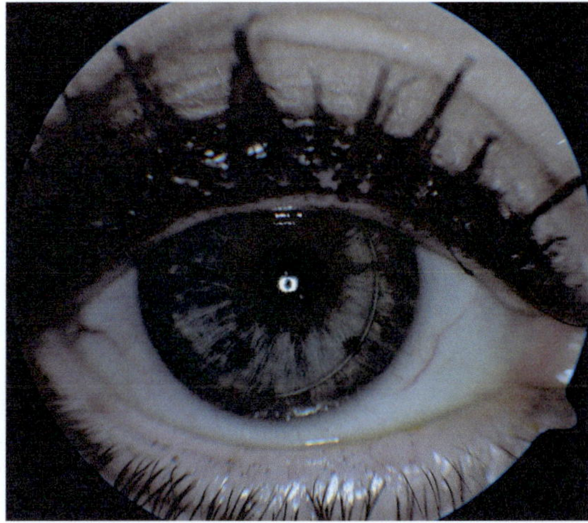

Fig. 7.6 A gas permeable (GP) contact lens centered on the cornea

ing of eye color. Lenses made of firmer material offer a better optical surface but are usually less comfortable than lenses made of softer, more flexible material. Soft plastic materials are designed to allow free passage of oxygen and fluids, so vital nutrients can reach the corneal epithelium, an avascular structure that requires exogenous nourishment and oxygen. Lenses that are less porous will rely on movement of the lens to allow nutrients and oxygen to reach the corneal surface.

Most "normal" eyes can achieve a full vision correction with soft, disposable spherical lenses for simple myopia and hyperopia. To achieve best vision, the presence of significant astig-matic error requires that the contact lens have a toric surface to compensate for the corneal toric surface.

Patients who have been using contact lenses and develop presbyopia generally have three options for seeing comfortably both at intermediate and near distances. The first option is to use contact lenses set for distance in both eyes with reading glasses added for near visual tasks. This combination generally provides the best vision, but the wearer remains dependent on carrying and using a separate pair of glasses. The second option is monovision, where the optics of the dominant eye is set for distance vision and the optics of the other eye is set for near visual tasks. This eliminates the need for glasses but sacrifices some binocularity and depth perception. The third option is the use of bifocal contact lenses, introduced in 1982, which eliminate the need for glasses and give better binocularity. However, some patients using bifocal contact lenses experience and complain about the presence of ghost images, halos around lights, and glare.

There are various types of disposable soft lenses, such as daily disposable, 2-week disposable, monthly disposable, and quarterly or annual replacement lenses. A more frequent replacement schedule is generally more acceptable and safer when patients have ocular allergies or suffer from some degree of dryness. There is no particular age that is too young for contact lenses, but for normal children, their parents should affirm that the child is fairly compliant with other responsibilities in order to properly care for their contact lenses and avoid complications from their use. Successful contact lens use decreases with age, which is attributed largely to the decrease in tear production and increasing dryness of the eye in older patients.

Advantages and Disadvantages of Contact Lenses

Among the most prominent advantages of contact lenses is the increased peripheral field of vision they provide as compared to spectacles. There is no peripheral field blockage by spectacle frames. Because they are under the lids, the contact lens surface is cleared with each blink, and they are functional in a larger number of environments than are spectacles. When properly fitted, they rarely fall out of their position even under the most strenuous of activities. These qualities make contact lenses an excellent option for many sports, although proper eye protection should always be considered when trauma to the globe is a possibility. Swimming is the one exception to contact lens use, primarily due the possibility of lens loss when the eyes are open and immersed in water. There is also an increased risk of infection when swimming in contaminated waters. Contact lenses are classified as a medical device by the FDA and should have proper fitting and assessment by an eye care provider, and the fit and health of the eye should be evaluated annually.

Contact Lens Use for Pathological Conditions

Because contact lenses create a new optical surface, they can provide significantly better vision than can be achieved with spectacles for patients with corneal diseases that create surface irregularities of the eye. This surface unevenness creates an irregular astigmatism that cannot be simply compensated for by a spectacle lens. Examples of corneal conditions that fall into

this category include keratoconus, scars following injuries or infections, Salzmann's nodular degeneration, anterior basement membrane dystrophy, granular dystrophy, post-corneal transplant, or post-refractive surgery ectasia. Sometimes soft contact lenses can achieve better vision for these patients, but more commonly lenses with a more rigid surface will produce significantly better visual results because their structure does not transmit the surface irregularity, as do soft lenses. These more rigid plastic lenses are permeable to nutrients and oxygen and are called "gas permeable lenses." The tear film created between the back surface of these gas permeable lenses and the front surface of the cornea induces a power known as the tear lens. This tear lens helps to create a more regular refractive surface, thus enabling better visual results than can be achieved with spectacle correction.

Complications of Contact Lens Wear and Their Treatment

If a contact lens wearer has pain, redness, decreased vision, discharge, burning, or photophobia, they should immediately remove the lens and have an eye examination if symptoms persist.

Corneal Abrasion

Contact lens wear may damage the corneal epithelium, causing a corneal abrasion. Patients with corneal abrasions will have sharp eye pain with associated photophobia, conjunctival injection, and tearing. No specific history may be associated, but one can suspect contact lens overwear, a possible foreign body, or a history of rubbing the eye. Clinical examination shows an epithelial defect that stains with fluorescein, and the eyelids may be swollen (Fig. 7.7). It is important to rule out associated foreign bodies, iritis, or tissue laceration.

Corneal abrasions in contact lens wearers can have a number of causes. Sometimes lens insertion, but more commonly lens removal, can pose a risk of abrasion if not handled correctly. This is why it is important that all new contact lens wearers have a proper fitting with insertion and removal training. A foreign body trapped between the cornea and contact lens can also cause a corneal abrasion. Contact lens wearers should remove their lenses immediately when there is a foreign body sensation or any ocular discomfort. This is essential to minimize risk or worsening of an abrasion. A contact lens-related abrasion usually requires fairly urgent ophthalmic consultation, both for treatment, and to rule out the presence of a coexistent corneal infection.

Infection and Contact Lens-Related Corneal Ulcers

Contact lens wear may be associated with the development of corneal ulcers, which are stromal infections commonly caused by bacteria and more rarely fungi or protozoa. Fungal and amebic ulcers are difficult to diagnose, treat, and are more sight-threatening. Corneal infections are presumed bacterial until proven otherwise. Bacterial corneal ulcers typically appear as a focal white infiltrate (Fig. 7.8) that stains with fluorescein and should be considered in any contact lens wearer with eye pain, a red eye, or upper eyelid edema. Ulcers occur more frequently when there is a history of sleeping with contact lenses in place, contact lens overwear, poor lens hygiene, or when using extended wear contact lenses. Smears and cultures are often taken if the infiltrate is greater than 1 mm in size or if fungus or acanthamoeba is suspected. Because there is serious risk of vision loss when corneal ulcers are present, they should be treated by practitioners experienced in their management.

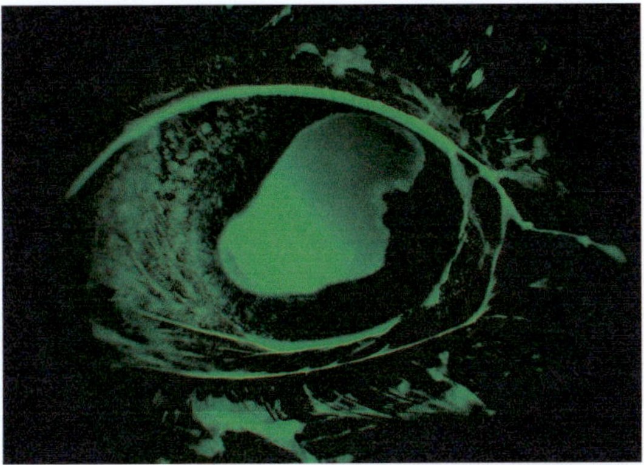

Fig. 7.7 A slit lamp photograph of a large cornea abrasion from contact lens overwear. The large, central area of fluorescein dye staining clearly shows the extent of corneal de-epithelialization. Excess dye in the tear film is also seen to be fluorescing in areas of tear pooling, which are not additional pathologic accumulations

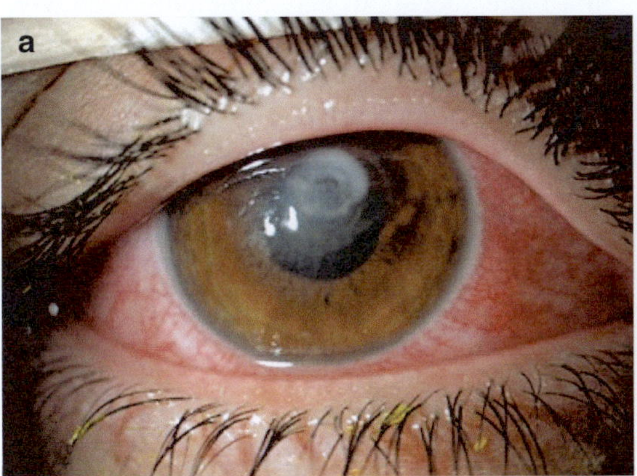

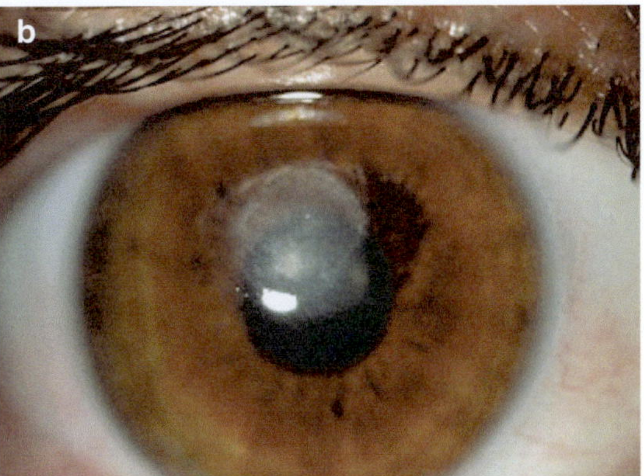

Fig. 7.8 (**a**) An acute, round corneal infectious ulcer associated with overnight contact lens wear in a poorly controlled diabetic. *Pseudomonas aeruginosa* was cultured from the lesion and successfully treated with aggressive antibiotic therapy. (**b**) The same eye as seen in Fig. 7.9a, 1 year later. Although the infection has been successfully eradicated, a paracentral corneal stromal scar persists, with accompanying visual distortion

Giant Papillary Conjunctivitis

Giant papillary conjunctivitis (GPC) is a chronic conjunctival reaction caused by a hypersensitivity reaction and characterized by giant papillae, located on the superior tarsal conjunctiva, sometimes associated with ptosis (Fig. 7.9). The upper eyelid must be everted to make the diagnosis and is part of the routine eye examination of contact lens wearers. Symptoms of GPC include itching, mucous discharge, and lens intolerance. GPC is a hypersensitivity reaction that can be related to contact lens material and/or deposits on the lenses or mechanical irritation by the contact lens edge. Giant papillae also can result from an exposed suture, the presence of an ocular prosthesis or atopic or allergic conjunctivitis. Successful treatment may be difficult, but initial steps include modifying the contact lens regimen to more frequent replacement of the lenses. This may require reduced contact lens wear time or an enzyme lens cleaner or use of a preservative-free disinfection system. GPC responds well to topical mast cell stabilizers and antihistamine combination drops, but in severe cases, short-term use of low-potency topical steroids may be required. In rare cases GPC will not respond to treatment, which will preclude further contact lens wear.

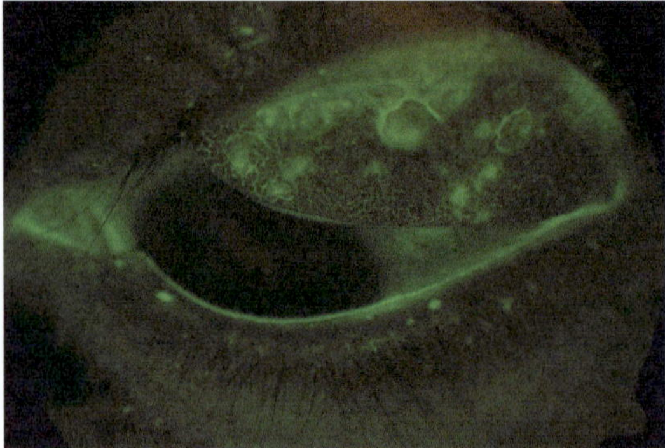

Fig. 7.9 Giant papillary conjunctivitis (GPC) from silicone hydrogel soft lens wear, seen on the surface of an everted upper eyelid. Topical fluorescein stain and cobalt lighting enhance visualization of the irregular conjunctival surface, which is normally quite smooth

Surgical Correction of Refractive Errors

History

As the refractive state of the eye is determined by axial length of the eye, optical power of the crystalline lens, and optical power of the cornea, modification of any of these properties will produce a change in the refractive state of the eye. If the globe can be shortened or stabilized, progressive myopia can be prevented from worsening or even be reduced. The crystalline lens can be removed and replaced with a prosthetic plastic optical element designed to produce a given refractive state. The cornea, eminently accessible to the surgeon, can have its shape changed to alter the refractive state.

Cornea and Refractive Surgery

Manipulation of the corneal shape has been the method utilized in most efforts to adjust the globe's refractive state. These attempts go back many years and have employed many technologies. In the no-longer commonly performed procedure known as radial keratotomy (see Fig. 12.1g), the corneal curvature is flattened with suitably placed, partial-thickness incisions. In a more successful and commonly used technique, corneal tissue is removed with a laser that can selectively reduce myopia, astigmatism, and hyperopia. Tissue removal can also eliminate contour anomalies such as scars, which create higher-order optical aberrations. Not every patient is a suitable candidate for this procedure; assessment of the integrity and thickness of the cornea is essential to assure that corneal refractive surgery can be safely done.

Two laser technologies are in wide use to alter the refractive state. One technology operating under the acronym SMILE (SMall Incision Lenticule Extraction) removes corneal stromal tissue using a high irradiance pulsed laser that allows a precisely shaped element of stromal tissue to be removed via a small incision. This has the advantage of creating minimal damage to corneal innervation and other structural elements. Another technology uses an excimer laser that produces high-energy UV pulses to remove tissue. This is done either at the surface and is called PRK (PhotoRefractive Keratectomy), or alternatively tissue can be removed beneath a thin superficial layer of tissue and is called LASIK (Laser-ASsisted In situ Keratomileusis). Both PRK and LASIK have been shown to have a high degree of accuracy and long-term stability. Both procedures, however, can cause an increase in dry eye syndrome in a minority of patients.

A variety of implanted materials have been placed into the corneal stroma to alter its optical performance and increase the depth of field. These include implants of plastic materials as intrastromal corneal rings to treat keratoconus. Another use of intrastromal rings is to reduce the diameter of the entrance pupil of the eye, which has been shown to increase the depth of field of the image at the retina, thereby improving near vision.

An innovative technology has been introduced that allows manipulation of the corneal ultrastructure using photochemical technology. This technology is based on the photochemical interaction engendered when UVA light illuminates a riboflavin-soaked corneal collagen stroma. The riboflavin undergoes molecular excitation and forms free electrons and singlet oxygen. These are chemically reactive and interact with the collagen to create additional cross-linking. The effect of this process is to increase corneal tissue strength with an associated alteration in the molecular dimensions.

This technology has proven successful in preventing the progress of corneal deformation in patients with keratoconus. In many of these patients, there is an associated marked improvement in the deformation of the cornea with a reduction in the ectasia and irregular astigmatism. This observation led to the investigative application of the cross-linking concept to refractive surgical techniques. Alternative technologies to achieve cross-linking of the corneal collagen are being investigated. A variety of pharmacologic compounds, when applied topically, have been shown to increase collagen cross-linking

and are being investigated as an alternative technology to prevent the progress of keratoconus.

More recently, direct laser interaction with collagen has been shown to create a similar, albeit localized pattern of cross-linking and anatomic change. To achieve this interaction, highpowered pulsed lasers are used which are focused within the stroma with an energy level just below the threshold for the creation of optical breakdown. The high-powered laser pulses strip electrons off the atomic orbits of corneal tissue, which creates a field of free electrons. This free electron field results in production of singlet oxygen that leads to local cross-linking. The advantage of this laser technique is that cross-linking can be achieved in a precisely defined volume of tissue. Because the tissue shape is altered by this interaction, it will produce refractive changes. This is potentially the next precise technology for corneal refractive surgery.

Axial Length Modification

While many attempts have been made to stabilize the growth of the eye with surgical procedures, theses have not found wide acceptance. There is, however, considerable research being done to develop compounds to prevent scleral growth as soon as a myopic state becomes apparent. Recently, the use of atropine topical drops has been shown to retard myopia progression. This may have significant benefit for those with pathologic or so-called malignant myopia, which is associated with significant visual morbidity over time.

Manipulation of the Crystalline Lens

The optics of the eye can be altered by removing the crystalline lens or placing a supplemental lens in front of it. A non-cataractous lens may be removed exclusively to change the refractive power of the eye. This procedure (so-called clear lens extraction) may, as with cataract surgery, involve implantation of a replacement plastic intraocular lens selected to create a desired

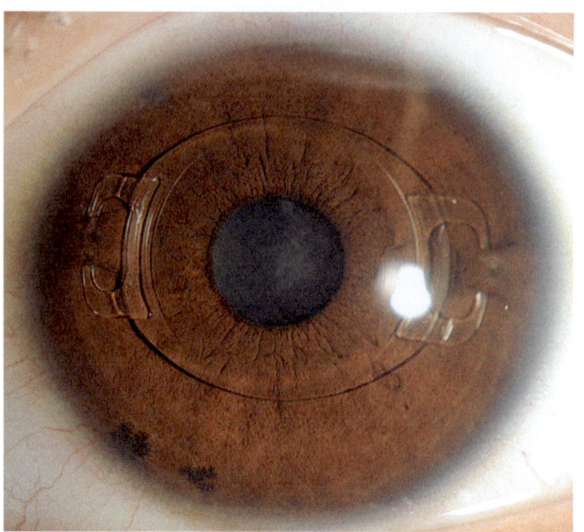

Fig. 7.10 A slit lamp photo of the right eye of a 29-year-old nurse who had approximately −11 diopters of myopia with 4 diopters of astigmatism in each eye and underwent bilateral piggyback, toric, multifocal anterior chamber, iris-fixated lens implantation procedures to correct her refractive errors. She currently sees 20/25⁻ in both eyes without correction. Of note, there are mild central congenital cataracts seen in both eyes, but apparently due to the patient's good best-corrected acuity, the crystalline lenses were not removed. Incidentally, a small peripheral iridotomy can be seen at 10:00, as well as two small nevi inferiorly

change in the refractive power of the eye, or it may only involve removal of the crystalline lens. The procedure is technically identical to standard cataract extraction. Most commonly, this option is offered to patients with high degrees of myopia, who would otherwise not be considered as candidates for other refractive surgical procedures and cannot wear contact lenses. In some cases, it may also be employed for patients with high hyperopia. Unlike the other refractive procedures discussed here or the attempts to modify axial length, clear lens extraction requires intraocular surgery, which carries a higher risk than surgical procedures that do not require entering the eye. A related procedure places a small contact lens in the eye in front of the crystalline lens. This lens may be placed in front of or behind the iris plane. It does carry the same risks associated with intraocular surgery, and it can accelerate the development of a cataract (Fig. 7.10).

Suggested Reading

Contact Lens Spectrum: monthly newsletter subscription related to clinical contact lens information on overcoming complications and new technologies. https://www.clspectrum.com/.

Duane A. Normal values of the accommodation at all ages. JAMA. 1912;59:1010–3.

Farhad H, Randleman JB, editors. Corneal cross-linking. 2nd ed. Thorofare: Slack Incorporated; 2017.

Goldschmidt E, Jacobsen N. Genetic and environmental effects on myopia development and progression. Eye (Lond). 2014;28(2):126–33.

GPLI (Gas Permeable Lens Institute) website (webinars): https://www.gpli.info/.

Tylers Quarterly: soft contact lens parameter guide. Subscription to quarterly magazine with up to date lens availability. http://www.tylersq.com/.

Young TL, Metlapally R, Shay AE. Complex trait genetics of refractive error. Arch Ophthalmol. 2007;125(1):38–48.

Walker M. Introduction to scleral lenses; GP lens institute, webinar, 2017. Gpli.info. Accessed 10 May 2017.

van der Worp EA. Guide to scleral lens fitting [monograph online]. Forest Grove, OR: Pacific University; 2010. Available from: http://commons.pacificu.edu/mono/4/.

Part II

Anterior Segment

The Red Eye

8

Danielle Trief

The "red eye" is a common finding in ophthalmological practice. In fact, one study looking at the etiology of visits to an ophthalmic emergency department found that the vast majority of visits were secondary to ocular surface issues causing "red eye," including conjunctivitis, blepharitis, and dry eye. The "red" or "pink eye" is really a wastebasket term for a myriad of eye conditions, many of which are benign and self-resolving. However, there are a few sight-threatening and even health-threatening conditions associated with "red eye." Understanding how these conditions present and are treated is critical to preventing complications.

The white sclera of the eye and inner surface of the eyelids are covered by the vascular conjunctiva, a mucous membrane composed of non-keratinized, squamous epithelium and goblet cells, which protects the eyeball and provides immune defense. The bulbar conjunctiva, which covers the globe, is rich in microvessels, and this vasculature easily dilates in inflammatory conditions (infection, allergy, toxicity, neoplasia), direct irritation (foreign bodies, chemical exposure, aberrant eyelashes), and venous obstruction and with systemic or topical vasodilators. The appearance of dilated vessels is often referred to as conjunctival "injection." From a distance, the injected conjunctiva gives the appearance of a "pink eye." Additionally, these vessels can sometimes bleed, causing a bright red appearance easily visible through the transparent conjunctiva.

The underlying sclera, a dense, fibrous, generally "white" tissue composed of type I collagen and proteoglycans, also contains blood vessels which can become dilated in the setting of ocular inflammation. Dilation of these deep scleral vessels produces a characteristic violaceous hue, typically seen in the condition known as scleritis.

Much more common is inflammation of the episcleral vessels, which lie between the conjunctiva and sclera. Episcleritis, a generally less serious condition than scleritis, can be associated with injection that is diffuse or focal.

Neoplastic growths, benign and malignant, may occur on the ocular surface. Benign growths are common and can cause the eye to appear red (e.g., pterygium). Benign growths can also cause irritation, with subsequent surface injection (e.g., conjunctival cysts). Malignant growths like lymphoma, squamous cell carcinoma, and even amelanotic melanoma can give the eye a red or pink appearance and must be identified and treated to prevent systemic complications.

D. Trief, MD, MSc (✉)
Columbia University Irving Medical Center,
New York, NY, USA

Department of Ophthalmology, Edward S. Harkness
Eye Institute, Columbia University Vagelos College
of Physicians and Surgeons,
New York, NY, USA
e-mail: dft2102@cumc.columbia.edu

© Springer Nature Switzerland AG 2019
D. S. Casper, G. A. Cioffi (eds.), *The Columbia Guide to Basic Elements of Eye Care*,
https://doi.org/10.1007/978-3-030-10886-1_8

Evaluation

A plethora of conditions can cause "red eye," and it is important to facilitate the identification of pertinent underlying pathology by obtaining a careful history and exam. For example, a red eye that is worse in the spring and is very itchy, but maintains good vision, suggests vernal/allergic conjunctivitis, while a sudden red eye associated with intense boring pain, nausea, and halos may point toward angle-closure glaucoma. The treatment for these conditions is very different; so is the urgency of treatment. Allergic conjunctivitis is a self-limited condition, while acute angle closure is vision-threatening.

History

A careful health history can help deduce etiologies. Patients with autoimmune conditions (e.g., rheumatoid arthritis, granulomatosis with polyangiitis {Wegener's}, or sarcoid) are more likely to have an autoimmune/inflammatory etiology for their red eye. These include anterior uveitis, episcleritis, and scleritis. A contact lens wearer, by contrast, may have a red eye from contact lens-associated keratitis or poor contact lens fit. Patients with recent upper respiratory infection or recent contact with sick associates are more likely to have viral conjunctivitis. Even mild ocular trauma can cause an injury such as a corneal abrasion, which may have a delayed presentation of injection and pain.

Patients should be asked about the presence and intensity of pain. Most benign causes of red eye (conjunctivitis, subconjunctival hemorrhage, episcleritis) are relatively painless, although patients may complain of mild-to-moderate discomfort. Pain should be distinguished from foreign body sensation, which is usually associated with a corneal condition (e.g., keratitis or corneal foreign body) or trauma.

It is also helpful to consider the onset of symptoms. A red eye present for "months to years" points to a chronic condition, which would include such pathologies as benign or malignant growths, structural problems of the eye leading to surface irritation (e.g., lagophthalmos), or chronic conjunctivitis. An acutely red eye typically points toward a traumatic or infectious etiology.

Other important questions to ask include: Has this ever happened before? Are you currently using any eye drops, or were you prior to onset of symptoms? Any new systemic illnesses/medications/allergens? Recent trauma? Do you have discharge from your eye other than tears? Are you sensitive to light (photophobia)? Any history of skin cancers or other malignancies? If vision is affected, is it constant or intermittent? Each of these questions can help narrow down the many etiologies of "red eye."

Examination

Visual acuity and intraocular pressure (IOP) must be assessed. These two vital signs of ophthalmology are important in triaging the severity of the condition. Most causes of red eye will have a normal IOP. However, IOP will be elevated in angle-closure glaucoma and is often decreased in anterior uveitis. The clinician should inspect the pupil and test its reactivity. Nonreactive pupils can be seen in angle-closure glaucoma or in anterior uveitis with synechiae (adhesions from the iris to the lens). Very small pupils can be seen when there is irritation of the cornea (e.g., infectious keratitis or corneal abrasion) or with the use of certain topical ocular medications, which may themselves cause ocular injection (e.g., pilocarpine).

The pattern of hyperemia should be assessed. Diffuse injection can be seen in conjunctivitis, whereas a localized injection may be associated with a growth or sectoral episcleritis. Ciliary flush (redness near the limbus, where the cornea transitions to the sclera) can be seen in angle closure or anterior uveitis. The hue of any injection should also be noted. Subconjunctival hemorrhages are bright red, whereas scleritis has a deep violaceous hue.

The cornea should be carefully inspected. An opacity on the normally clear cornea may point

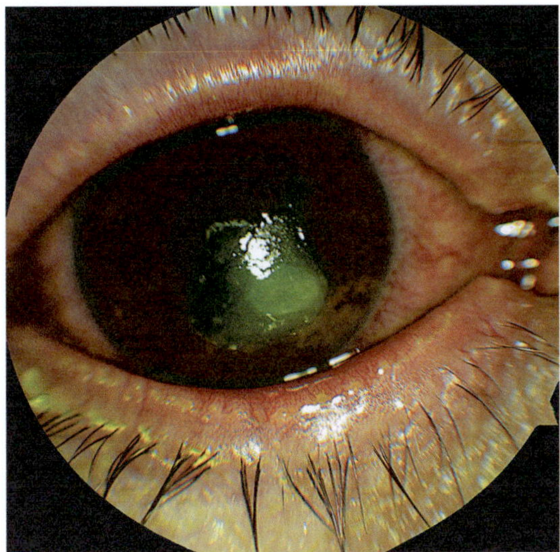

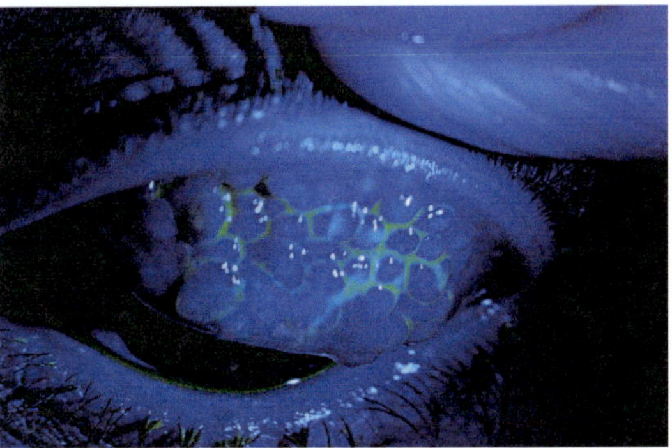

Fig. 8.2 Papillary changes of the conjunctiva. The fluorescein in this figure pools around the papillae, which can be seen here as "bumps" under the lid. Papillae are the result of vascular changes, spoke-like capillaries that are surrounded by edema, on the palpebral conjunctiva in the setting of inflammation or allergy

Fig. 8.1 Fluorescein stain disruptions in the corneal epithelium. The green area seen here is a result of an irregular epithelium stained with fluorescein. These epithelial defects are even more apparent with a cobalt blue light

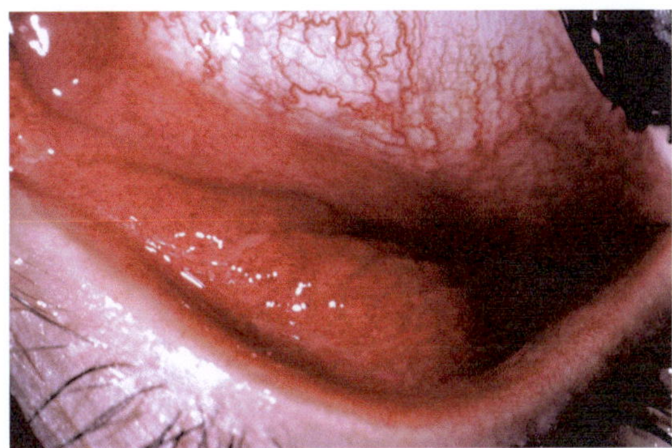

Fig. 8.3 Follicular changes of the conjunctiva. Follicles are round clusters of lymphocytes. Vessels surround the surface of the follicles but are not usually seen within the follicles themselves (distinguishing them from papillae). They are commonly seen in viral conjunctivitis

to an infectious keratitis or foreign body. Epithelial defects/abrasions can be assessed with the use of fluorescein dye and a cobalt light source. The missing epithelial area will fluoresce bright green (Figs. 2.9 and 8.1). A diffusely hazy cornea can be seen in angle-closure glaucoma, anterior uveitis, or infection. A healthy corneal surface should be smooth and reflective. A rough-appearing cornea, which will produce dull light reflections, can be seen with severe dry eye or contact lens keratitis.

The eyelids should also be examined. In healthy eyes, the lids move freely over the underlying globe, evenly spreading the underlying tear film across the cornea.

Adhesions between the globe and lid (symblepharon) can be seen in chronic conjunctivitis. Conjunctiva lining the inner lids (palpebral conjunctiva) should be inspected. Occasionally, retained foreign bodies can be seen under the lids, and eversion of both upper and lower lids is necessary to find these elusive causes of red eye. The palpebral conjunctiva itself may provide insight on the etiology of red eye.

Papillary changes of the conjunctiva (Fig. 8.2) characteristically have a central

dilated vessel surrounded by edema, giving the conjunctival surface a bumpy appearance. Each bump has a central red dot that represents the dilated capillary. They can be small and diffuse (commonly seen in allergic conjunctivitis) or very large, so-called giant papillary conjunctivitis, seen in contact lens overwear. Papillary changes can also be seen with allergy and bacterial conjunctivitis.

Follicles are another type of palpebral conjunctival change (Fig. 8.3). Follicles represent conjunctival lymphoid tissue and appear as round clusters with conjunctival vessels coursing

Table 8.1 Clinical characteristics of selected conditions that cause red eye

Etiology	Pattern of hyperemia	Pain	Vision	IOP	Discharge	Time course
Viral conjunctivitis	Diffuse	Minimal	Preserved	Normal	Yes	Acute
Subconjunctival hemorrhage	Focal, bright red	Minimal	Preserved	Normal	No	Acute
Episcleritis	Focal or diffuse, bright red	Mild tenderness	Preserved	Normal	No	Acute
Scleritis	Focal or diffuse	Yes	Usually preserved	Normal	No	Acute or chronic
Anterior uveitis	Ciliary flush or diffuse	Yes, photophobia	Reduced	Usually reduced	No	Acute or chronic
Corneal abrasion	Diffuse	Yes, foreign body sensation	Reduced	Normal	No	Acute
Corneal foreign body	Diffuse	Yes, foreign body sensation	Reduced	Normal	No	Acute
Keratitis	Diffuse	Yes	Reduced	Normal	No	Acute
Conjunctival or corneal exposure	Usually greatest inferiorly	Mild	Variable	Normal	Tearing more than discharge	Chronic
Angle-closure glaucoma	Ciliary flush or diffuse	Yes, deep pain	Reduced	Elevated	No	Acute
Pterygium	Focal	No	Preserved initially, compromised as pterygium grows	Normal	No	Chronic
Conjunctival malignancy	Usually focal but can be diffuse	No	Preserved	Normal	No	Chronic

around the clusters. Follicles can be seen in viral causes of conjunctivitis as well as chlamydia.

Lastly, the eyelid margin and lashes should be assessed. The small sebaceous glands on the eyelid margin, meibomian glands, are responsible for producing the oily component of the tear film. These glands may become clogged in blepharitis or rosacea, leading to the development or exacerbation of dry eye. Larger obstructions of the eyelid glands can produce hordeola ("styes") or chalazia. Poor closure of the eyelids (lagophthalmos), or out-turning (ectropion), or in-turning (entropion) of the eyelids can lead to chronic irritation of the ocular surface and secondary redness. Eyelashes may also be misdirected toward the globe (trichiasis), producing a chronic irritation and redness, and in severe cases, microabrasions and infection (as seen with trachoma). Table 8.1 provides a summary of common causes of red eye and some key findings on history taking or examination.

Specific Conditions Commonly Associated with Red Eye

Conjunctivitis

Conjunctivitis is a general term for any inflammation of the conjunctiva. Most often, it refers to viral conjunctivitis, typically referred to as "pink eye." Viral conjunctivitis is quite common and has been identified as the leading cause of urgent ophthalmology visits in several studies. Patients with viral conjunctivitis often have had a preceding upper respiratory infection or sick contact. The conjunctiva is usually diffusely injected, which may affect one or both eyes; if both are affected, there may be asymmetry both in severity and the timing of presentation between the eyes (Fig. 8.4). Patients usually complain of discharge, which may be copious, with crusting and "stuck" lids in the morning. Viral conjunctivitis is usually painless, although the eye may feel

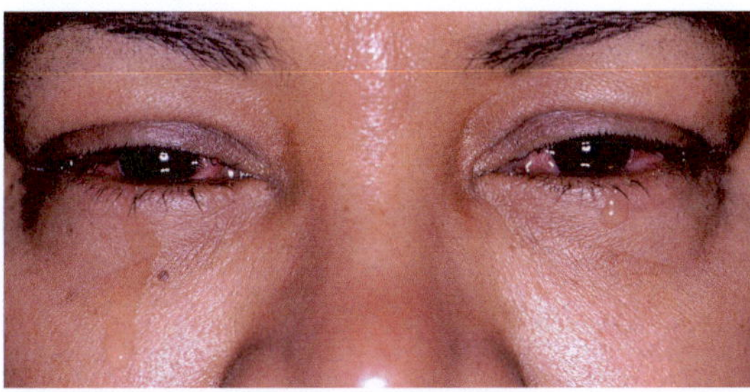

Fig. 8.4 Diffuse conjunctival injection and swelling (chemosis) in a patient with viral conjunctivitis. The eyelids appear edematous and likely have underlying follicles or papillae. Teary discharge and mucous, as seen here, are quite common in viral conjunctivitis

itchy or sore, and there may be general malaise if it is associated with a systemic viral syndrome. Vision is preserved, although discharge may cause intermittent blurring. Viral conjunctivitis usually heals without sequelae, and treatment is supportive. Patients should be informed that it is very contagious and thus practice strict hygiene. Chilled artificial tears and antihistamines can help symptomatically. In cases where there is prolonged inflammation of the eye or if the cornea becomes inflamed, a weak topical steroid can be considered, but this may prolong the disease course. Since the etiology is viral, antibiotics are not necessary.

There are many other causes of conjunctivitis. Allergic conjunctivitis is common, is usually seasonal, and is marked by pruritus, a papillary reaction, and less discharge than its viral counterpart. It may be accompanied by other typical atopic symptoms, such as nasal congestion, wheezing, or eczema. Bacterial conjunctivitis is much less common than viral but should be considered, especially in neonates. Gonorrhea and chlamydia can both cause a neonatal conjunctivitis that can be sight-threatening and must be treated with systemic antibiotics.

A chronic, noninfectious conjunctivitis, which may be quite severe, can be seen in certain autoimmune conditions, such as ocular cicatricial pemphigoid and Stevens-Johnson syndrome. Chronic inflammation can lead to bands of adhesion between the bulbar and palpebral conjunctiva known as symblepharon (Fig. 8.5). Scarring such as this is usually treated with immunomod-

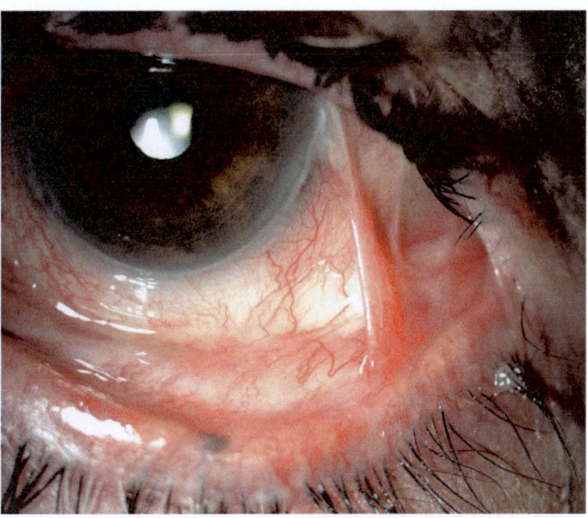

Fig. 8.5 An example of symblepharon. In healthy eyes, the lid and palpebral conjunctiva should be freely mobile from the globe and bulbar conjunctiva. Attachments between the lid and globe from chronic inflammation are called symblephara

ulators in an attempt to prevent dysfunctional lid movement and closure, which would eventually compromise vision. A chronic, unilateral conjunctivitis may be seen with adult chlamydial infection, which produces a follicular reaction. Conjunctivitis is further discussed in Chap. 10.

Subconjunctival Hemorrhage

The fine vessels of the conjunctiva can occasionally bleed, leading to the dramatic presentation of a subconjunctival hemorrhage (SCH). SCH appears suddenly, is bright red, and can be alarming to the patient, although in practice, SCH are almost always benign and resolve without consequence (Fig. 8.6). They most frequently occur spontaneously without an identifiable cause. Occasionally they occur if the patient has been straining or performing Valsalva-type maneuvers (e.g., weight lifting, straining at stool, or vomiting), particularly in patients taking anticoagulants, including aspirin. SCH can be seen in the setting of trauma, and damage to underlying (and therefore obscured by blood) ocular structures must be ruled out. Patients with recurrent SCH should be questioned about bleeding or clotting problems. In such cases, a coagulation work-up

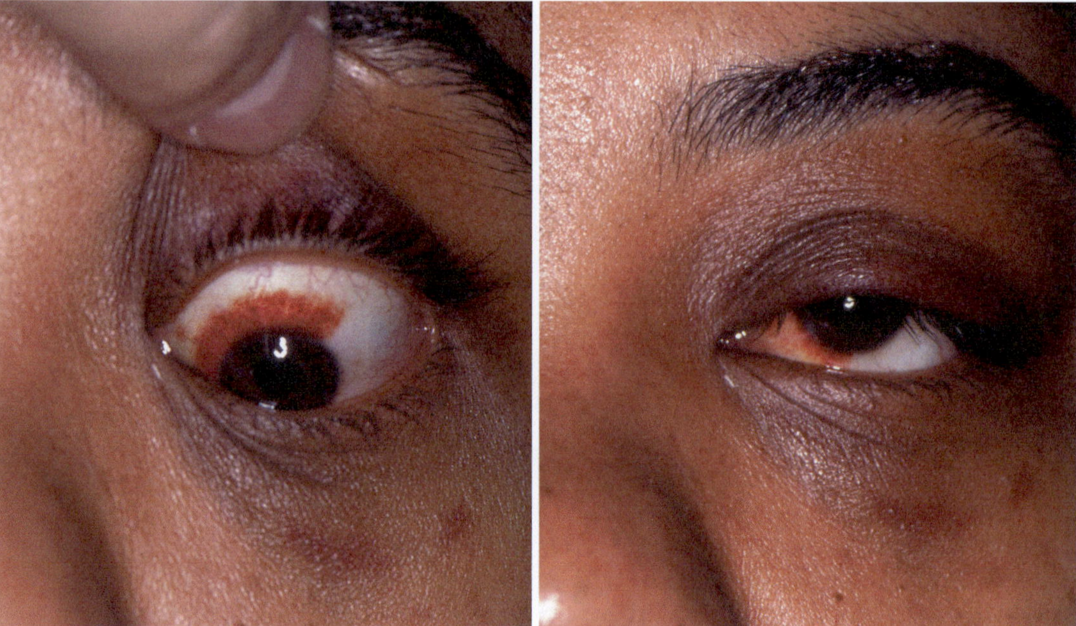

Fig. 8.6 A subconjunctival hemorrhage is a small collection of blood just under the conjunctival surface. It occurs when tiny blood vessels break and is almost always benign and self-resolving. It appears bright red as seen in this figure

should be considered. Occasionally, certain ocular conditions like hereditary hemorrhagic telangiectasia or lymphangiectasia can predispose a patient to repetitive SCH, and an ophthalmologic/cornea consultation could be considered. In first-time episodes without an inciting incident, the patient should be reassured. The hemorrhage usually resolves in 7–12 days, and patients should be forewarned that the hemorrhage may spread and change color before all blood is eventually resorbed.

Inflammatory Causes of Red Eye

Episcleritis

Inflammation and engorgement of the episcleral vessels can lead to acute sectoral (70%) or diffuse (30%) redness of the eye (Fig. 8.7). Episcleritis is a self-limited condition, usually lasting days to weeks, and is most common in young adults. It is almost always unilateral. An underlying systemic cause (such as autoimmune conditions, herpetic infections, or syphilis) is found only in a minority of patients, and work-up is unnecessary unless the

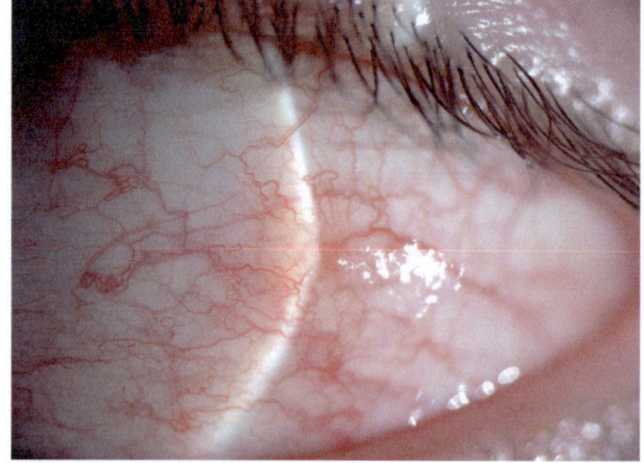

Fig. 8.7 Sectoral episcleritis. One can appreciate the superficial conjunctival and subconjunctival injection. These vessels blanch with phenylephrine. Episcleritis is usually self-limited and should be associated with minimal pain

patient has multiple recurrences. Patients usually complain of a slight tenderness, but not severe pain, and normal vision is preserved. The inflammation seen in episcleritis is superficial and should be distinguished from scleritis (see below), which is deeper. Episcleritis has a red or pink hue, and the application of 2.5% topical phenylephrine drops should blanch the engorged episcleral vessels. Treatment is generally supportive (artificial tears), but oral or topical nonsteroidals (NSAIDs) can be considered for recalcitrant cases. In unusual cases that do not respond to lubrication and NSAIDs, a short course of a mild topical steroid can be considered.

Scleritis

In contrast to episcleritis, scleritis is associated with an underlying systemic autoimmune condition in 50% of patients and is the manifestation of an immune-mediated vasculitis (Fig. 8.8). Scleritis presents with deep, boring pain, along with exquisite tenderness (if the injected area is gently touched by a cotton swab, patients flinch or withdraw). Because the inflamed vessels are deep, they do not blanch with topical phenylephrine. These vessels have a violaceous hue in natural sunlight and have a crisscross pattern. Anterior scleritis can be diffuse, nodular, or necrotizing. Recurrent episodes of scleritis can lead to thinning of the sclera (scleromalacia) and visual compromise. Given the high association with systemic conditions, a work-up is indicated unless a known underlying disease is present. Scleritis is most commonly associated with connective tissue disorders (e.g., rheumatoid arthritis, granulomatosis with polyangiitis (Wegener's), and systemic lupus erythematosus). Infectious etiologies should also be considered and ruled out. Scleritis can be seen in the setting of tuberculosis, pseudomonas, and Lyme disease. Appropriate serologies should be sent. Scleritis may be associated with other ophthalmic complications including peripheral keratitis, uveitis, and glaucoma. If no systemic etiology or infectious condition is discovered, diffuse anterior and nodular scleritis can be treated with NSAIDs or systemic steroids. If the scleritis is recalcitrant, immunosuppressive therapy should be considered. Systemic therapies are often co-managed between ophthalmology and rheumatology. In addition to immunosuppression, in necrotizing scleritis, scleral patch grafting may be necessary if there is risk of globe perforation. Posterior scleritis, which is much less common than the anterior form, is most often not associated with systemic illness and may be accompanied by other ocular complications such as retinal detachment.

Anterior Uveitis

Anterior uveitis, or iridocyclitis, occurs when the uveal track of the eye (iris and ciliary body) is inflamed. Patients typically complain of redness, deep ocular pain, light sensitivity (photophobia), and blurry vision. On slit lamp examination, white cells can be seen floating in the anterior chamber aqueous fluid; these sometimes may be numerous enough to visibly layer out inferiorly as a hypopyon (Fig. 8.9).

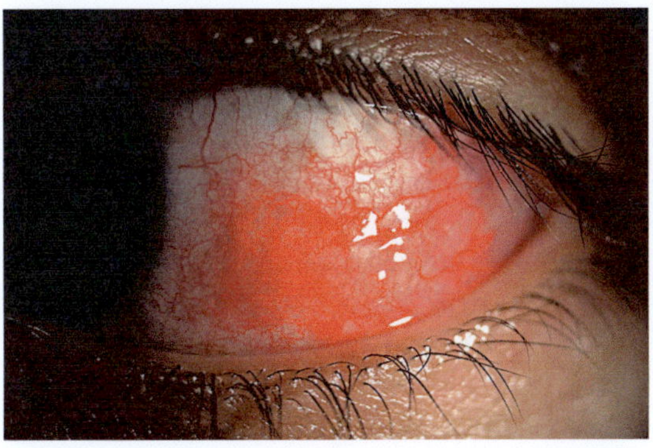

Fig. 8.8 Scleritis is characterized by deeper injection giving it the characteristic "violaceous" hue. These vessels do not blanch easily with phenylephrine. Scleritis is often associated with rheumatological conditions

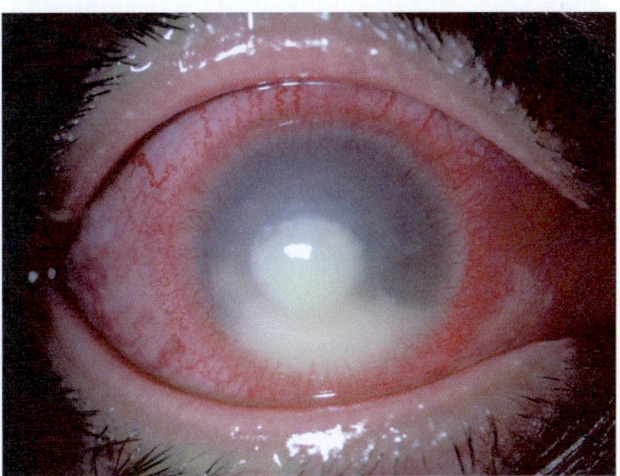

Fig. 8.9 In this example of anterior uveitis, the patient has a large hypopyon which is secondary to a central corneal ulcer. The hypopyon is caused by layered white cells inferiorly in the anterior chamber. Uveitis is an inflammatory condition, which is often autoimmune in nature. However, in this example, the inflammation is secondary to an infectious corneal ulcer. Note the marked diffusely red eye, typically found with an active uveitis

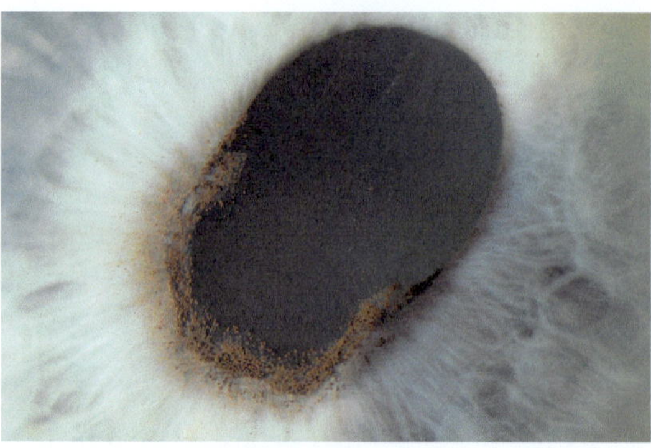

Fig. 8.10 Anterior chamber inflammation can lead to adhesions between the iris and lens, called posterior synechiae, as seen here in a 70-year-old woman with a history of rheumatoid arthritis; she was unaware of having had iritis attacks in the past. The pupil is normal above, but synechiae cause an irregular contour inferiorly, where the distorted pupillary margin is adherent to the anterior lens surface, and pigment can be seen deposited in the abnormal attachment area

Associated findings may include anterior or posterior synechiae [adhesions of the iris to the cornea or lens, respectively (Fig. 8.10, and see Fig. 27.8)], corneal edema, and corneal precipitates. First episodes of anterior uveitis are generally idiopathic. However, recurrent or bilateral episodes can be seen in autoimmune conditions, particularly HLA-B27-associated conditions, sarcoidosis, and inflammatory bowel conditions. Anterior uveitis can also be seen in infectious conditions (e.g., tuberculosis), and recurrent episodes of anterior uveitis necessitate a serologic work-up. The mainstay of treatment of idiopathic anterior uveitis is topical corticosteroids, which may be used as frequently as every hour initially. Drops that dilate the pupil (cycloplegic agents) must also be considered to prevent synechiae from developing. Patients should be followed closely until resolution of the inflammation, and they should be monitored for complications such as glaucoma. Uveitis is further discussed in Chaps. 27 and 28.

Trauma

Any injury to the globe can cause conjunctival hyperemia. Trauma necessitates a full exam, including a dilated fundus exam, to rule out damage to the globe, including any open globe injury. Superficial injuries to the cornea and conjunctiva are extremely common and almost always produce a red eye.

Corneal Abrasion

The most superficial layer of the cornea, the epithelium, is delicately adherent to the underlying basement membrane. Either sharp or blunt contact with the cornea can disrupt the epithelium and lead to an abrasion. The cornea has one of the densest populations of nerve endings in the body, and even a small irregularity in the corneal epithelium can produce pain, foreign body sensation, tearing, and hyperemia. Pain is usually more pronounced with eyelid movement (due to rubbing of the posterior surface of the lid against the loose epithelium) and is relieved by sustained lid closure. Disruptions of the corneal epithelium can easily be seen on slit lamp examination with the aid of fluorescein, which will stain denuded areas of epithelium green when viewed with a cobalt light source (see Fig. 8.1). Abrasions usually heal over the course of days without consequence, but topical antibiotic drops or ointments should be considered if the abrasion was caused by a potentially contaminated object (e.g., a fingernail).

Corneal Foreign Body

Foreign material can become embedded within the corneal epithelium and stroma. Often, the patient will report a preceding incident (e.g., a construction worker using a power tool who noted a piece of metal fly toward the eye). Patients will complain of foreign body sensation, pain, and may have decreased vision and tearing. Full-thickness lacerating and penetrating injuries should first and foremost be ruled out. Fluorescein can again be useful here. In full-thickness corneal injuries, the fluorescein may highlight a stream of aqueous from the anterior chamber (so-called Seidel test). The eyelids should be everted and the entire conjunctiva inspected for retained foreign bodies. The corneal foreign body can usually be identified at the slit lamp and should be removed if possible (Fig. 8.11a–c). Metallic foreign bodies may have associated rust rings, which should also be removed if superficial. If the foreign body is deep, additional curettage may be necessary if not all of the material can be removed on first encoun-

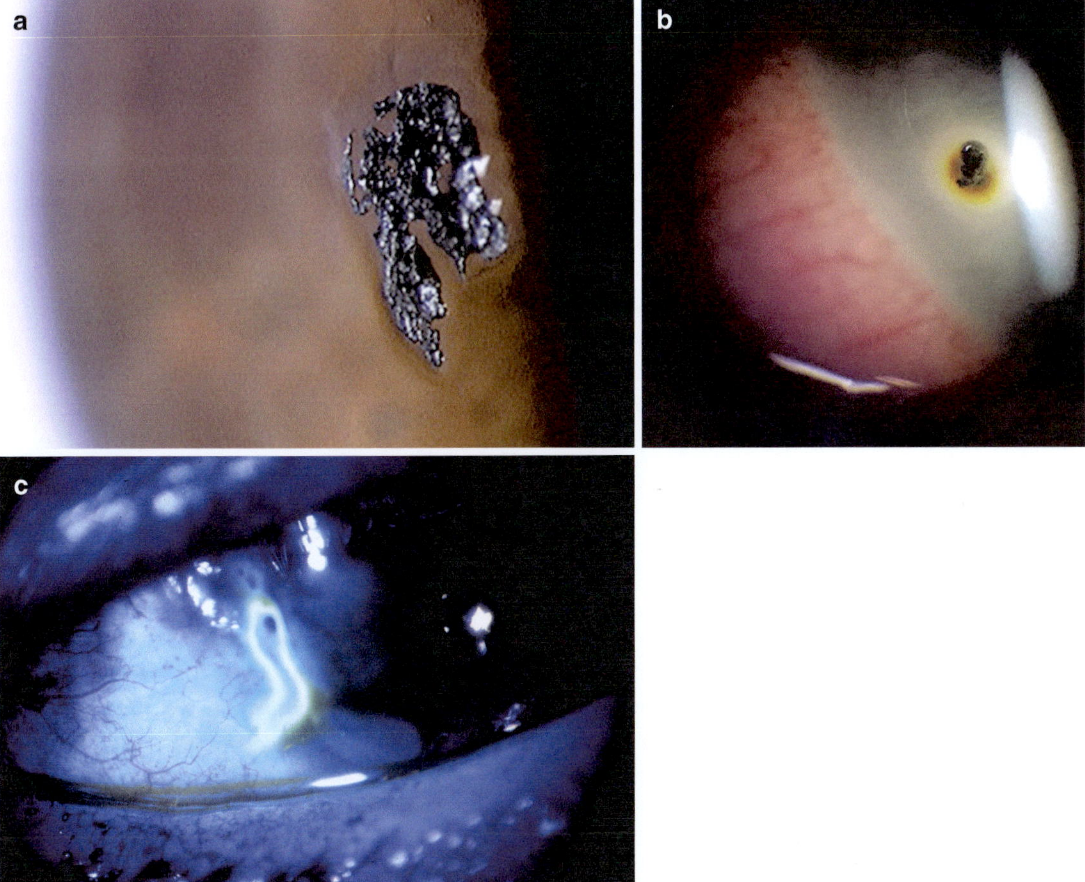

Fig. 8.11 (**a**–**c**) A metallic foreign body (**a**) (solder) is seen superficially embedded in the cornea. Such material should be debrided and removed if possible, and care should be taken to assess the depth of the foreign body. The majority of foreign bodies are superficial, but full-thickness foreign bodies often need to be surgically removed and the perforated cornea repaired. In (**b**), a metallic foreign body with a classic rust ring (produced as the FB interacts with the tear film and oxidized iron stains the cornea) is seen adjacent to the limbus. The patient was grinding metal without safety goggles in place (Courtesy of Dr. Peter Michalos). Aqueous leakage revealed by dilution of fluorescein stain (**c**) demonstrates an anterior chamber leak, indicating a full-thickness corneal perforation. Given the temporal location here, this is most likely a leaky surgical wound. Fluorescein-stained tears appear as bright green in a cobalt blue light. With an anterior chamber aqueous leak, as seen here, the green color is disrupted by a stream of fluid, referred to as a positive Seidel test

ter. Patients are treated post-procedure with topical antibiotic coverage and cycloplegia (to reduce effects of any secondary iritis).

Chemical Burn

Chemical injuries to the eye are ophthalmic emergencies, and delay in treatment can result in permanent vision loss. Alkali injuries are generally more severe than acid injuries as alkali is lipophilic and therefore penetrates the ocular surface more rapidly than acids. Acids, by contrast, precipitate proteins in the tissues they contact, and these coagulated proteins act as a barrier to deeper penetration. Patients will complain of pain, tearing, reduced acuity, and foreign body sensation. Copious irrigation of the eye (with water or balanced salt solution, whatever can be instituted most quickly) should be undertaken immediately, even before an initial exam, until the eye is restored to physiologic pH (by testing of tear pH with pH paper strips). The eye is generally very injected. However, areas of conjunctival whitening are concerning for limbal ischemia and are associated with much worse outcomes. Areas of limbal ischemia should be measured and documented in clock hours. Eyelids should be everted, and the fornices should be inspected for any retained material or chemicals. Initial treatment of chemical burn to the eyes usually includes antibiotics, cycloplegic agents, and steroids. Placement of amniotic membrane graft may also be considered if large areas of ischemia are present. Patients with severe chemical injuries should be emergently referred to an ophthalmologist.

Iatrogenic

The eye is often red following surgical or laser procedures. This can be secondary to inflammation or subconjunctival hemorrhage. Patients should be reassured that this is almost always temporary. If there is persistent hyperemia, the clinician should rule out any complications.

Topical ophthalmic drops used in the treatment of a variety of eye conditions can also cause hyperemia. Notable are some of the glaucoma medicines. Brimonidine, for example, can cause hyperemia in as many as 1/4 of patients, and latanoprost is also associated with hyperemia, which may lessen over time. Although patients will typically be quite concerned and often resistant to treatment in such a setting, conjunctival hyperemia alone is not necessarily a reason to discontinue an otherwise effective medicine.

Structural

A healthy conjunctiva requires proper positioning of the lids and eyelashes. If the eyelids do not close adequately (lagophthalmos), the ocular surface will become dry (exposure) and lead to conjunctival and corneal damage. The eyelids should closely appose the globe. Out-turned eyelids (ectropion) can lead to conjunctival exposure and hyperemia, while in-turned eyelids (entropion) can cause lashes and lids to abrade the globe (Fig. 8.12a–c). Eyelashes may be misdirected against the globe (trichiasis), producing irritation, and in severe cases, areas of de-epithelialization and subsequent infection (e.g., trachoma).

The conjunctiva, like the cornea, is normally coated by the tear film, which provides continuous lubrication, antimicrobial protection, and nutrition to the underlying ocular surface. Deficiencies in the tear film, either through inadequate tear production (aqueous deficiency) or early evaporation, can produce ocular surface irritation and a "red eye." Dry eye is a multifactorial disease. Patients complain of discomfort, foreign body sensation, and occasional visual disturbance. Treatment depends on etiology, but lubricating drops (artificial tears, gels, or ointments) or treatments that help improve the quality and stability of the tear film are often employed. Dry eye syndrome is further discussed in Chap. 11.

While contact lenses can provide great benefit to patients in correcting refractive error, if they do not sit properly over the cornea and globe, they can rub against the conjunctiva and produce surface irritation. Additionally, poorly fitting contact lenses can damage the cornea over time by inducing hypoxia or even by direct epithelial injury.

Contact lens wear can also lead to contact lens keratitis or inflammation of the cornea. Patients may be sensitive to the preservatives in contact lens solutions or may develop corneal and conjunctival irritation from deposits on the contact lenses themselves. Patients may complain of pain, photophobia, red eye, and contact lens wear intolerance.

Normally, a healthy corneal epithelium serves as a barrier to bacterial, fungal, and parasitic infection.

Contact lens-wearing patients are at risk for infectious keratitis (Fig. 8.13). Large corneal infiltrates should be cultured, and empiric therapy, usually with a broad-spectrum antibiotic, should be rapidly initiated. Patients must be monitored closely until resolution of the infiltrate. Clinicians should maintain a high suspicion for infectious keratitis in any contact lens wearer presenting with a red eye and should inquire about additional risk factors such as sleeping or swimming in contact lenses, extending contact lens wear beyond the recommended exchange time (e.g., extending daily contact lens wear to weekly), and any history of previous infections.

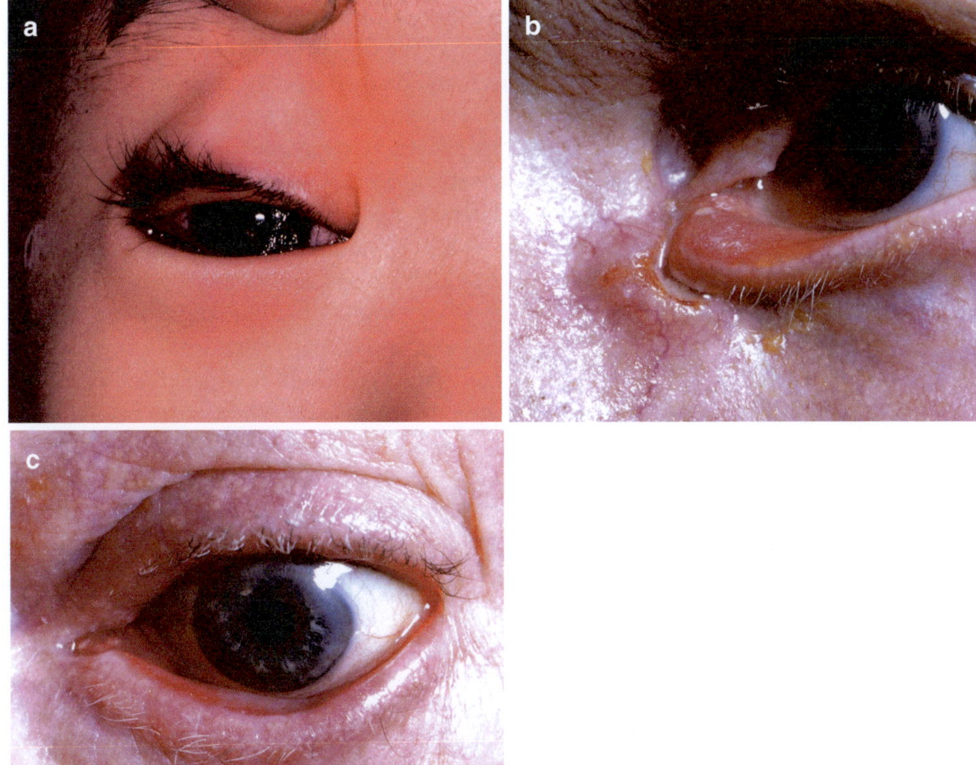

Fig. 8.12 (**a**) A child with inferior entropion and a medial epicanthal fold. (**b**) Severe medial ectropion caused by an adjacent basal cell carcinoma, with secondary palpebral conjunctival keratinization and epiphora due to the outwardly turned inferior punctum. (**c**) Senile ectropion, with mild secondary red eye

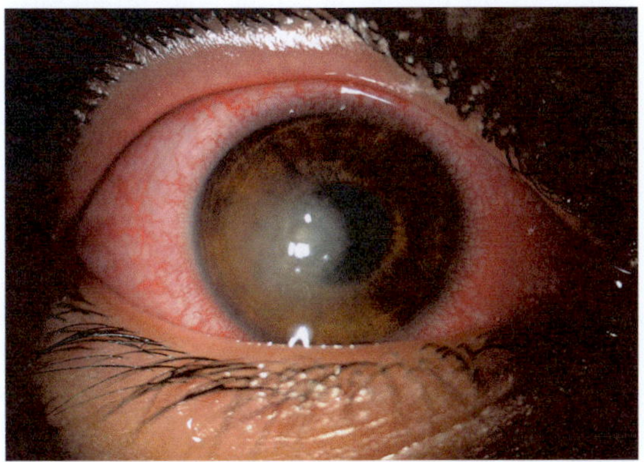

Fig. 8.13 Infectious keratitis. The cornea is hazy secondary to an infectious process. Corneal infections may be secondary to bacteria, viral, fungal, or parasitic etiology, and treatment should be adjusted accordingly to minimize corneal scarring

Glaucoma

While glaucoma is usually a chronic and painless condition, acute angle-closure glaucoma is painful and associated with a red "hot" eye. Patients experiencing a narrow-angle glaucoma attack usually present with deep boring pain, blurred vision, halos around lights, and nausea or vomiting. Anterior chamber aqueous fluid normally drains through the trabecular meshwork in the angle of the eye; if the meshwork becomes obstructed (usually by apposition of the iris due to anatomic configuration), a precipitous rise in intraocular pressure (IOP) may occur as fluid fails to drain. On exam, patients typically have perilimbal injection (ciliary flush), a hazy cornea, and a shallow anterior chamber. Initial treatment is targeted at rapidly lowering eye pressure.

Topical glaucoma therapies are often employed first, but oral (e.g., acetazolamide) or intravenous medications (e.g., mannitol) are often necessary to bring down the pressure. For primary angle-closure glaucoma, a peripheral iridotomy (or hole in the iris to allow drainage of fluid) can prevent further attacks. Treatment is time-sensitive, and prolonged, elevated IOP can damage the optic nerve and lead to permanent vision loss. Angle-closure glaucoma is discussed further in Chap. 15.

Conjunctival Tumors and Lesions

Benign growths of the conjunctiva are quite common and may give the appearance of a red eye directly (e.g., pterygia and inflamed pingueculae appear pinkish) or by irritation of the surrounding tissue (e.g., a conjunctival cyst). While less common, malignant growths of the conjunctiva can also give the appearance of a red eye and must therefore always be considered, as these lesions can be sight and health-threatening.

Conjunctival cysts are inclusion cysts of the conjunctival epithelium. They are typically asymmetric. They can be congenital or acquired and consist of a central cavity, lined by nonkeratinized conjunctival epithelium, filled with clear fluid (Fig. 8.14). Patients usually complain of foreign body sensation, especially with eye movement. Conjunctival cysts may occur after trauma or surgery. The surface irregularity may cause conjunctival injection. These benign cysts often reform after simple incision and drainage; if the patient is symptomatic, complete excision is usually necessary to prevent recurrence.

Granulomas are subconjunctival lesions which are benign inflammatory vascular tumors composed of fibroblasts and proliferating capillaries. They most commonly follow surgery (e.g., suture granuloma following strabismus surgery) or minor trauma. They are bright red and pedunculated and bleed easily. They often resolve with topical or intralesional steroids but can be excised and cauterized if they are recalcitrant (Fig. 8.15).

Pingueculae (singular pingueculum) and pterygia (singular pterygium) are benign lesions at the corneal limbus caused by UV exposure. Pingueculum are small and yellow in appearance. They are generally well tolerated, and do not cross the limbus onto the cornea, but can be associated with surface irritation and resultant thickening and hyperemia. Pterygia often arise from pingueculae. They are wing-shaped and highly vascular, giving a bright red appearance (Fig. 8.16). Pterygia cross the limbus and can encroach on the cornea and induce an irregular corneal curvature (astigmatism). If they advance far enough onto the cornea, they can also occlude vision. Patients complain of cosmetic issues, irritation, fluctuating injection, and progressive blurring of vision. While a pterygium outside the visual axis can be watched and treated with sur-

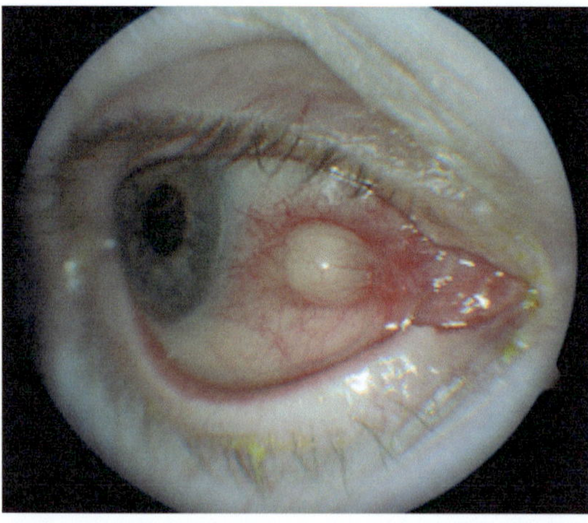

Fig. 8.14 Conjunctival cysts can cause surrounding irritation. They are benign and can be congenital or acquired. They can be treated conservatively with lubrication or occasionally a weak steroid. If they persist and cause substantial discomfort, they can be surgically removed

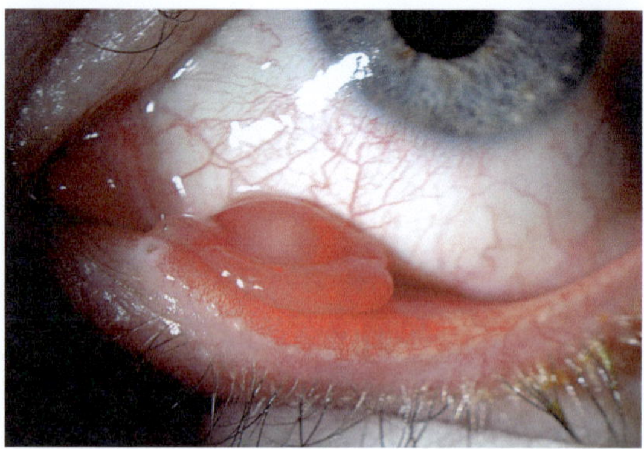

Fig. 8.15 A conjunctival pyogenic granuloma located in the medial canthal region

face lubrication, it should be excised if vision becomes compromised. Occasionally, pterygia may exhibit squamous metaplasia, so excised specimens should always be sent to pathology.

Conjunctival papillomas are benign (or pre-malignant) squamous neoplasias, associated with the human papillomavirus. They may be pedunculated or sessile and appear red with a fibrovascular core. On close inspection, they are smooth with numerous underlying corkscrew vessels

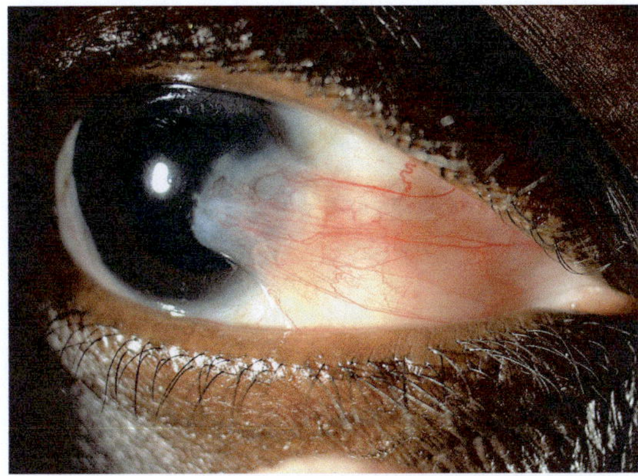

Fig. 8.16 Pterygia are benign lesions at the limbus secondary to elastotic degeneration of the conjunctiva and Tenon's layer, most commonly as a result of sun exposure. They can interfere with vision if they extend onto the cornea, both by occluding the central axis and also by producing corneal astigmatism

(Fig. 8.17a, b). They are often asymmetric and produce minimal foreign body sensation. They can become dysplastic. More worrisome findings include keratinization of the surface (leukoplakia), symblepharon (Fig. 8.4), and inflammation. Excised specimens must be sent to pathology to rule out squamous cell cancer.

Ocular surface squamous neoplasia (OSSN) is a broad term for dysplastic squamous cell lesions of the conjunctiva and cornea. These lesions are typically slow-growing and near the corneal limbus. Patients may have noted the lesion for many years. They may complain of slight foreign body sensation. OSSN is associated with UV exposure and may arise from a pre-existing pterygium or pingueculum. On examination, they may demonstrate gelatinous change, leukoplakia, and abnormal vasculature, including feeder vessels (Fig. 8.18). Treatment includes primary excision with cryotherapy and/or topical chemotherapeutic agents (e.g., interferon, mitomycin, or 5-fluorocuracil).

Conjunctival melanomas make up less than 1% of ocular malignancies, and amelanotic melanomas account for 25% of conjunctival melanomas. Conjunctival melanomas are heavily vascularized, thereby giving the eye a red appearance, and can bleed easily. They most commonly arise from areas of previous pigmentation (primary acquired melanosis). Conjunctival

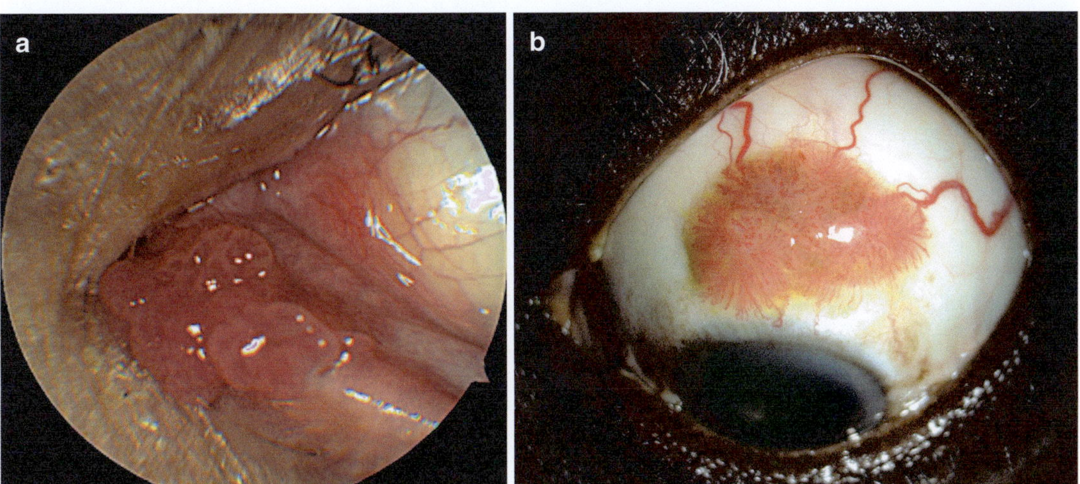

Fig. 8.17 (**a**, **b**) In these two examples of conjunctival papillomas, one can appreciate the characteristic corkscrew vessels. The lesions are well circumscribed. They are pre-malignant, and diagnosis usually involves conjunctival biopsy

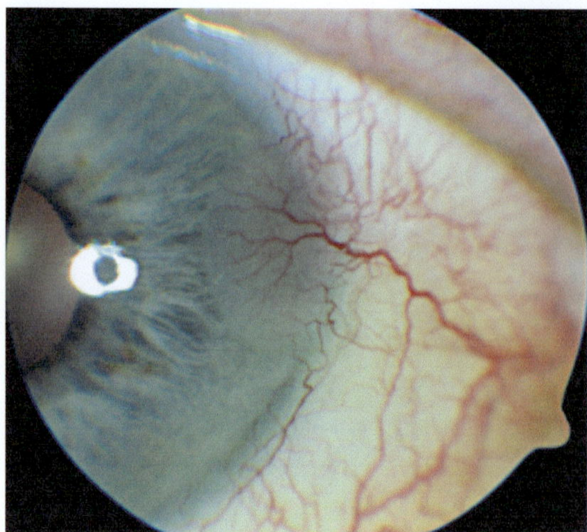

Fig. 8.18 This patient with ocular surface squamous neoplasia (OSSN) has a leukoplakic plaque of irregular tissue at the corneal limbus. Also seen here is a prominent feeder vessel. These lesions can be treated with excision and/or topical chemotherapeutic agents

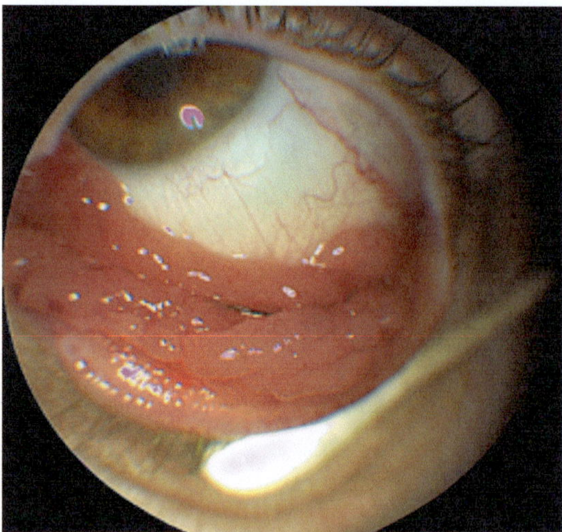

Fig. 8.19 Conjunctival lymphoma often presents as a smooth salmon-pink mass of the conjunctiva. In this patient, the lesion can be seen on simple lid eversion and is quite diffuse

malignant melanomas are potentially deadly tumors, and when possible, these patients should be referred to an ocular oncologist for further management.

Conjunctival lymphoma usually presents as a mobile, salmon-pink mass in the conjunctiva. When diffuse, it may present as a chronic conjunctivitis (Fig. 8.19). These lesions are painless and usually asymptomatic. Conjunctival lymphomas are usually non-Hodgkin B-cell lymphomas and are often treated by external beam radiation therapy in coordination with an oncologist.

Conclusion

The red eye is a common complaint and can be associated with many diverse etiologies. Most of these conditions are benign and self-limited; however, a few are sight- or health-threatening. The complaint of a red eye should always be taken seriously. A careful history and exam can narrow this vast differential and allow for targeted and appropriate treatment.

Suggested Reading

Blondeau P, Rousseau JA. Allergic reactions to brimonidine in patients treated for glaucoma. Can J Ophthalmol. 2002;37(1):21–6.

Channa R, Zafar SN, Canner JK, Haring RS, Schneider EB, Friedman DS. Epidemiology of eye-related emergency department visits. JAMA Ophthalmol. 2016;134(3):312–8.

Gritz DC, Wong IG. Incidence and prevalence of uveitis in Northern California; the Northern California Epidemiology of Uveitis Study. Ophthalmology. 2004;111(3):491–500.

Kumar NL, Black D, McClellan K. Daytime presentations to a metropolitan ophthalmic emergency department. Clin Exp Ophthalmol. 2005;33(6):586–92.

Blepharitis and Conjunctivitis

James Auran and Daniel S. Casper

Blepharitis

Blepharitis is a descriptive term meaning inflamed eyelids. It is a common condition, akin in some respects to chapped lips, in which moisture from the mouth irritates the skin of the lips, and also to acne, in which oil glands in the skin malfunction (Fig. 9.1). The lid margin area is packed with slightly modified sebaceous glands – the Meibomian glands – which add oil to the tear film (see Figs. 10.2 and 10.3). This oil creates a lipid bilayer on the tear film surface, lubricating the ocular surface and inhibiting tear evaporation. Along with mucous from conjunctival goblet cells and the aqueous tears, oil from the Meibomian

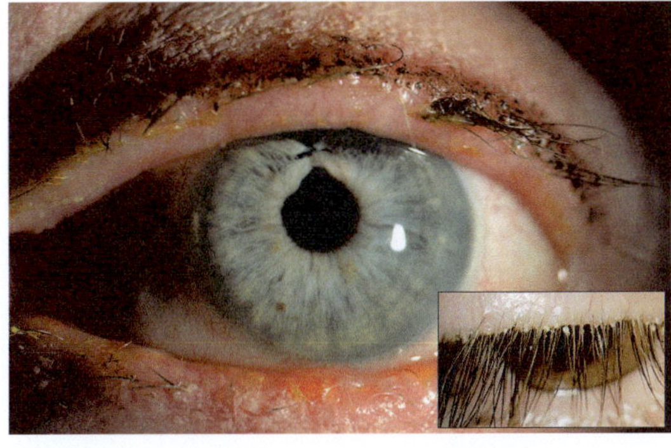

Fig. 9.1 Upper and lower lid blepharitis with associated lash loss, matting and misdirection, marginal lid crusting with fissures, and flaking of eyelid skin. Incidentally noted here is a surgical superior iridectomy with resultant mild superior pupillary distortion. Inset shows scurf and collarettes at lash bases

glands creates a breeding ground for bacteria, which can result in a low-grade superficial infection of the lid skin. This chronic condition, referred to as blepharitis, is managed rather than cured and, when mild to moderate, is treated to the extent that it bothers the patient. Blepharitis can have a significant adverse impact on people's lives, leading, for example, to difficulty reading for long periods and to contact lens intolerance. In more severe cases, treatment is aimed at preventing lash loss, scarring of the Meibomian glands and lid margins, and damage to the cornea. Blepharitis appears in several overlapping forms and is associated with dry eye, multiple systemic diseases, and chronic use of certain eye drops.

J. Auran, MD
Columbia University Irving Medical Center,
New York, NY, USA

Department of Ophthalmology, Edward S. Harkness
Eye Institute, Columbia University Vagelos College
of Physicians and Surgeons, New York, NY, USA

D. S. Casper, MD, PhD (⊠)
Columbia University Irving Medical Center, New York,
NY, USA

Department of Ophthalmology, Edward S. Harkness
Eye Institute, New York, NY, USA

Naomi Berrie Diabetes Center, Columbia University
Vagelos College of Physicians and Surgeons,
New York, NY, USA
e-mail: dsc5@cumc.columbia.edu

© Springer Nature Switzerland AG 2019
D. S. Casper, G. A. Cioffi (eds.), *The Columbia Guide to Basic Elements of Eye Care*,
https://doi.org/10.1007/978-3-030-10886-1_9

A common form of blepharitis is due to bacterial (typically staphylococcus) overgrowth. Staphylococcal blepharitis is characterized by symptoms worse on awakening (due to the buildup of irritants in the stagnant tear film overnight) and also worse after periods of visual effort, such as reading (due to increased evaporative dryness secondary to the decreased blinking associated with visual effort). Patients describe awakening with their lids glued together; crusting; mucus discharge, more than the minimal whitish collection of morning mucus in the inner corner of the eye (aka "sleep") that many people normally experience; burning; and blurred vision. There may be lid swelling, itching, burning, foreign body sensation, and tearing. The lid margins are thickened and erythematous, with crusting (scurf), lash loss, and irregular margins. Microscopic soap bubbles may be present on the lid margin due to saponification of tear lipids by bacterial lipases. With more severe cases, there is eyelash loss, conjunctivitis, corneal irritation, vascularization, and ulceration.

Approximately one third of blepharitis cases are classified as seborrheic, which is typically characterized by a greasy and flaky eyelid skin margin and is usually associated with seborrheic dermatitis elsewhere on the body.

Another category of blepharitis is that of Meibomian gland dysfunction, when the source of the pathology is within the lid margin oil glands. This may be associated with dermatologic conditions affecting the oil glands, such as rosacea. In blepharitis associated with Meibomian gland dysfunction, the glands are congested, and the oil (meibum) that is normally a golden, clear, low-viscosity liquid becomes thickened, even to a cheese-like in consistency, with an elevated melting point temperature.

Demodex is a mite which lives in the eyelash follicles; although often it may be part of the normal lid flora, it has been implicated as a relatively common contributing factor in some cases of blepharitis. It is unclear whether the mites exert a direct pathologic effect on the Meibomian glands or whether the mite or its by-products produce a secondary inflammatory reaction. Characteristic cylindrical dandruff-like sleeves (collarettes) are noted around the base of eyelashes during the ophthalmic examination. As the demodex tend to migrate downward along the lash shaft, eradication can be difficult, and a variety of treatments have been proposed. Treatment with hypochlorous acid disinfectant and tea tree oil has been found to be beneficial in some cases.

Superimposed on these conditions is the dry eye state caused by increased tear evaporation due to disruption of the oil layer. As tear glands are located just below the conjunctival surface, inflammation can shut down these glands, creating additional dryness due to tear production deficiency. Dry eye treatments (see

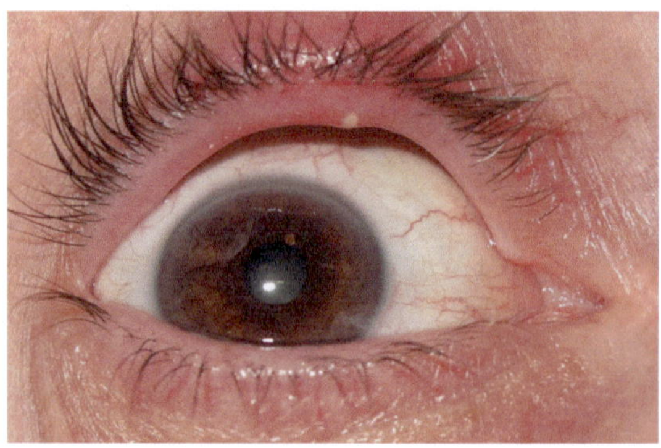

Fig. 9.2 A stye at the Meibomian gland orifice may be quite tender with symptoms of foreign body sensation in the eye

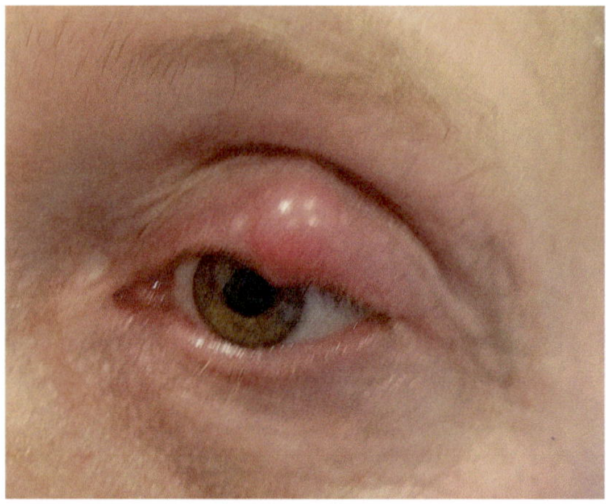

Fig. 9.3 An externally pointing chalazion with surrounding lid inflammation. Such surrounding lid inflammation may be mistaken for bacterial cellulitis. Large chalazia like these may persist for months, often requiring either intralesional injection of corticosteroids or surgical excision

Chap. 10) supplement and overlap with blepharitis therapy.

Styes and chalazia (Figs. 9.2 and 9.3) may develop secondary to blepharitis, appearing as a focal mass within the eyelid and often erythematous and tender. They usually are adjacent to the lid margin but may be up to a centimeter away, occurring anywhere along the length of the Meibomian glands. Styes (hordeola) are acute infections (microabscesses) within the lid; chalazia are chronic cystic lesions that develop from plugged Meibomian or Zeiss oil-producing glands; they may result from a prior stye. Styes are treated with hot compresses; antibiotic/steroid ointments (applied to the lid skin) or topical antibiotic solutions, typically macrolide (azithromycin) drops instilled into the eye and wiped onto the lid margin, with or without additional peri-lesional corticosteroid injections; and incision/drainage in severe cases. Chalazia are sterile and therefore are usually treated with hot compresses and, if necessary, corticosteroid injection or incision and drainage.

Blepharitis, and especially chalazia, may mask or be confused with eyelid tumors, most commonly basal cell carcinomas, and less likely with squamous cell or sebaceous cell carcinoma. New, non-inflamed, or persistent (and especially growing) eyelid masses and marked, chronic blepharitis resistant to treatment should be referred for ophthalmologic evaluation (e.g., via biopsy) for the presence of occult neoplasia (See Chap. 30).

Thyroid eye disease can present with complaints and findings related to ocular surface disease (dry eye, chronic conjunctivitis, blepharitis). Evaluation for thyroid eye disease should be a part of every workup for ocular surface disease (See Chap. 29).

Diagnosis of blepharitis is usually based on history and clinical examination. Tear osmolarity, matrix metalloproteinase-9 (MMP-9) immunoassay, tear breakup time, and new technologies to image the Meibomian glands and tear lipid layers are available. Culturing is useful for persistent, recalcitrant blepharitis, once neoplasia has been ruled out.

Treatment of mild-to-moderate blepharitis is first aimed at reassurance that this is almost always an uncomfortable nuisance rather than a sight-threatening condition. The goal of treatment is to maximize patient comfort and visual function, which is initially achieved by removing debris and controlling the local bacterial population. Treatment regimens include short- and long-term lid cleansing regimens (including lid scrubs, hypochlorous acid skin disinfectant, topical antibiotic drops, and ointments), hot compresses (hot enough to melt the thickened, abnormal meibum), lubricants (artificial tears, gels, and ointments), anti-inflammatory agents (topical corticosteroids, T-cell modulators cyclosporine and lifitegrast, oral omega-3 fatty acid supplementation, oral tetracyclines, and oral macrolides), debridement of the Meibomian gland orifices, intense pulsed light therapy, and mechanical devices to mechanically open or flush out the Meibomian glands using probing, heat, and pulsating pressure. The pulsed light and mechanical devices are not reimbursed by insurance and are often quite costly to the patient and are thus reserved for severe, recalcitrant cases.

Conjunctivitis

Patients often call to report that they have either conjunctivitis or "pink eye" and need a prescription for antibiotics; frequently, their diagnosis is incorrect, and even in those cases where it is correct, antibiotics may not be indicated. As shown in Chap. 8, "pink eye," or a red eye, is a nonspecific descriptive that may or may not represent an infectious process. The causes for pink, red, irritated, or tearing eyes are many, however, and infection is just one of the possibilities. Even so, a significant number of infections will be of viral etiology, for which antibiotics will not prove helpful. A small corneal abrasion, an inturned eyelash, a minute foreign body, or chronic dry eye, for example, may all produce "pink eye," but none of these conditions is a true conjunctivitis. Proper diagnosis will dictate treatment.

For the ophthalmologist, conjunctivitis, or "pink eye," refers to an inflammation of the mucous membrane covering the globe (bulbar conjunctiva) and the inside of the eyelid (palpebral conjunctiva). Although conjunctivitis has many etiologies, history and examination alone are often sufficient to diagnose the cause. Presentation may be acute (as with many allergic and infectious etiologies) or chronic. A typical presentation of acute conjunctivitis is a patient who complains of symptom onset over the course of hours in one or both eyes. It may be more difficult to ascribe a causative factor in chronic conjunctivitis, requiring culturing or other tests.

Allergic Conjunctivitis

The hallmark of allergic conjunctivitis (Fig. 9.4a–d) is itching, although patients may also present with complaints of tearing, dryness, burning, or foreign body sensation (at least in part induced by eye rubbing). There may be edema of the conjunctiva (chemosis), with patients describing the onset of a "drop of water" over the white of the eye which is actually edematous conjunctiva. The edema is often pallid, although redness (hyperemia) may also occur. Patients with allergic conjunctivitis often present with a history of seasonal or perennial allergy, facilitating diagnosis. Treatment includes artificial tears, cold compresses, avoidance of rubbing the eyes, avoidance of the inciting antigen, topical and systemic antihistamines, topical mast cell stabilizers, and short-term topical corticosteroids.

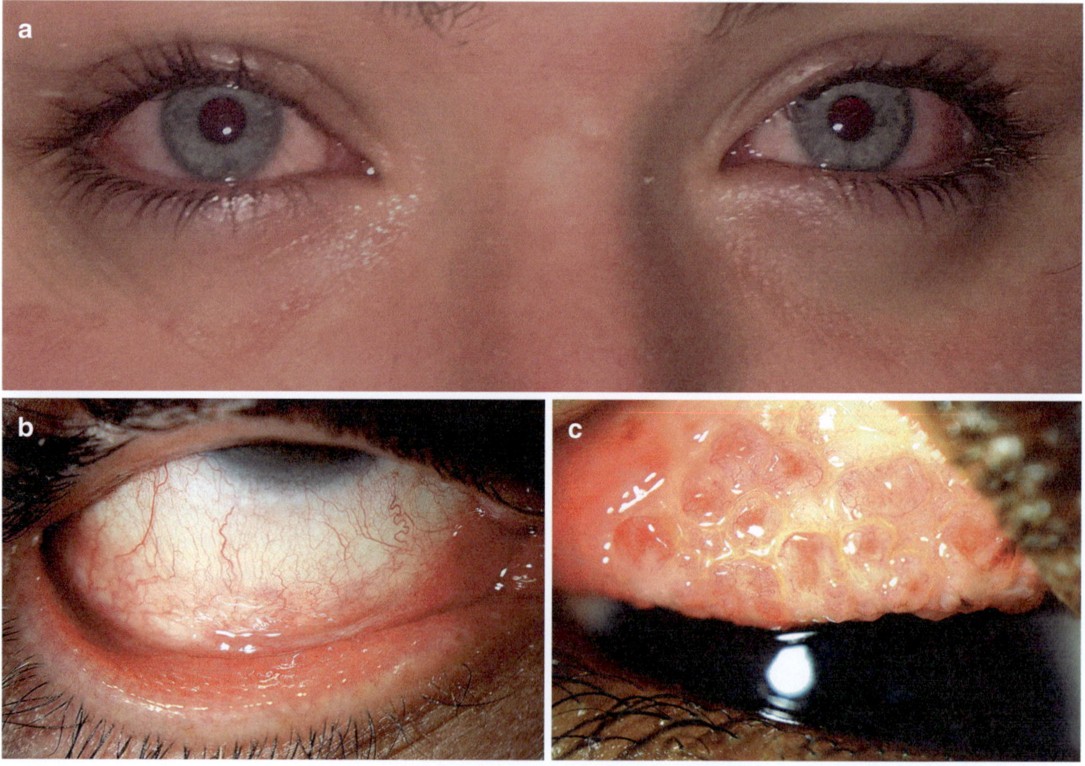

Fig. 9.4 (**a–d**) Allergic conjunctivitis may present with pallid or erythematous conjunctival edema, along with diffuse led swelling. (**a**) Allergic conjunctivitis with erythematous appearance. Note the associated mild erythema seen on the upper cheeks. (**b**) The inferior lid conjunctiva shows typical allergic papillae, resulting in a dimpled appearance to the normally smooth inner lid surface. (**c**) An everted lid shows the giant papillae classically associated with vernal (atopic) conjunctivitis. (**d**) Severe allergic conjunctivitis (a reaction to a topical eye drop) with chemosis, erythema, and periorbital lid edema

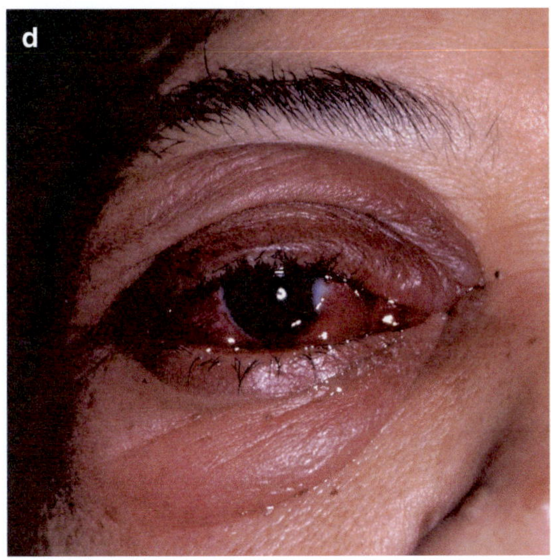

Fig. 9.4 (continued)

Viral Conjunctivitis

Viral (often adenoviral) conjunctivitis (Fig. 9.5a–c) is very common, with conjunctival involvement occurring frequently with any respiratory tract infection (e.g., the common cold or influenza). Conjunctival involvement can be subclinical or may manifest itself with mild symptoms such as tearing. However, multiple strains of viruses, particularly adenovirus, have a predilection for affecting the conjunctiva and can present with a very unpleasant course of conjunctivitis lasting days to weeks (see Fig. 8.3). Adenoviral conjunctivitis may start with one eye, migrating to the second eye (typically with a less intense course) a few days later. Conjunctival injection is diffuse, although typically worse inferiorly. There may be preauricular and

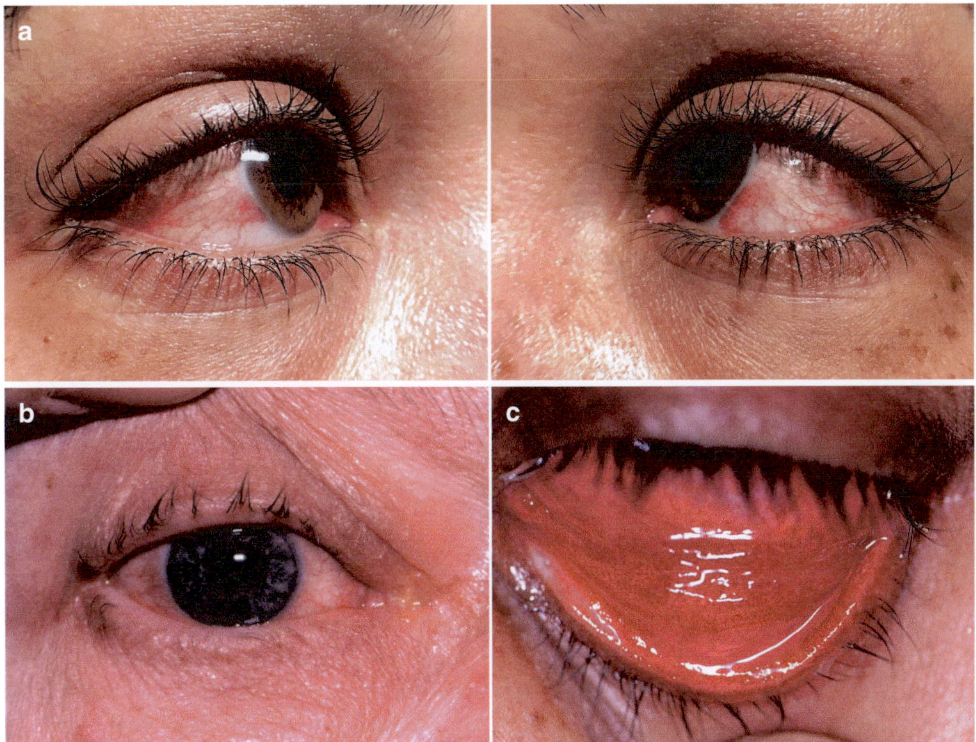

Fig. 9.5 (**a–c**) Viral conjunctivitis usually presents with a thin, watery discharge, conjunctival erythema, and edema. (**a**) Bilateral viral conjunctivitis with predominantly temporal erythema. (**b**) A patient with acute viral conjunctivitis. Discharge is typically scanty. The bulbar conjunctiva is diffusely red, typically more so inferiorly than superiorly, and subconjunctival hemorrhages may occur. (**c**). Epidemic keratoconjunctivitis (EKC), showing the typical inferior conjunctival follicular reaction. This is usually caused by an adenovirus, is highly contagious, and may be associated with preauricular adenopathy and systemic malaise. Fine corneal subepithelial infiltrates may persist for months and reduce visual acuity (see Fig. 12.11)

submandibular adenopathy (as the lymphatics from the superior/temporal conjunctiva drain into the preauricular nodes and the inferior/nasal conjunctival lymphatics drain into the submandibular nodes). Viral conjunctivitis stimulates lymphocytosis, and the lower lid (tarsal) conjunctiva, fornix, and even the lower bulbar conjunctiva may develop true lymphoid follicles manifesting as velvety nodules. Tearing may be profuse, with white to yellow discharge. Corneal involvement can be absent but can occur, leading to blurred vision and sensitivity to light (photophobia). If blurred vision or photophobia occur, referral to an ophthalmologist is very important because it may be a sign of corneal inflammation or iritis.

Treatment of adenoviral conjunctivitis is supportive. Treatment measures consist of warm or cool compresses, artificial tears, gels, or ointments, hygiene measures to remove discharge and other debris from the eyes, and oral or topical antihistamines for itching. Eyes with conjunctivitis are particularly sensitive to surface toxicity from eye-drop medications and their preservatives (typically benzalkonium chloride). If possible, preservative-free topical ophthalmic medication should be considered. It is very important to prevent the spread of adenoviral conjunctivitis. Patients with active adenoviral conjunctivitis should take all hand hygiene measures. Patients with adenoviral conjunctivitis should alert their families and coworkers, who should take extra hand hygiene precautions and refrain from touching their eyes. Healthcare personnel with active conjunctivitis should refrain from patient contact. As with any respiratory tract infection, consideration should be taken to keep infected individuals out of the school and workplace. Healthcare workers who examine a patient with adenovirus should wear gloves and disinfect all surfaces that have had contact with the patient, including waiting room pens and magazines.

Primary herpes can present as unilateral and occasionally bilateral conjunctivitis. Herpes simplex reactivation can occur secondary to trauma or to conjunctivitis caused by bacteria or a different virus. Herpes conjunctivitis is usually not

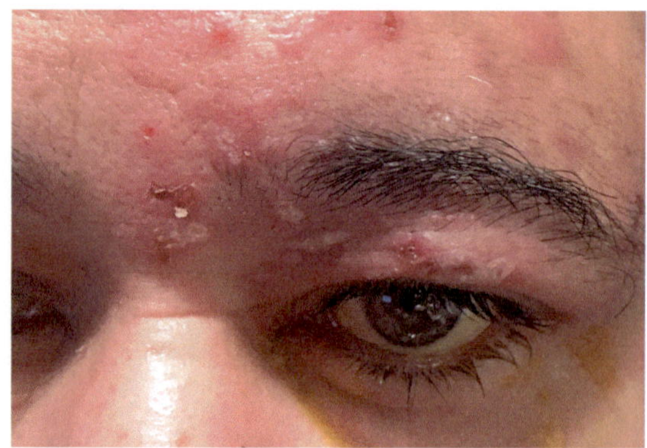

Fig. 9.6 Herpes zoster lesions on the lid margin can cause diffuse conjunctivitis, often most pronounced near the focal zoster eyelid margin lesion. This is not the same as ocular herpetic zoster, associated with involvement of the nasociliary branch of the trigeminal nerve, which is not a superficial conjunctival reaction and requires more aggressive treatment

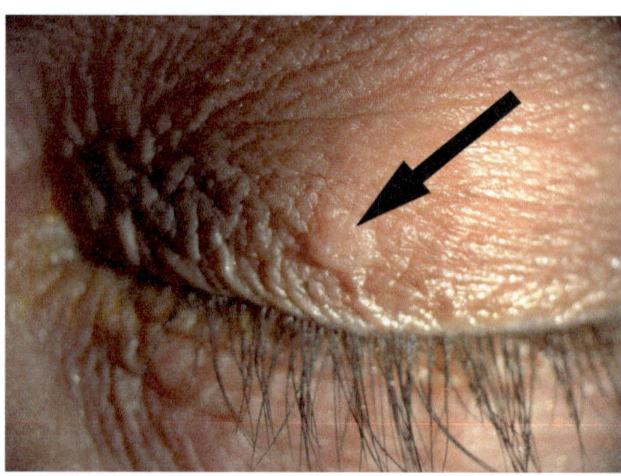

Fig. 9.7 Molluscum contagiosum near the eyes may cause a chronic conjunctivitis. The arrow shows a single molluscum lesion on the upper lid, which can easily be overlooked on examination, particularly when attention is focused on the red eye

detected unless there are focal skin, conjunctival and/or corneal lesions. If herpes simplex conjunctivitis is suspected, treatment with oral and/or topical antiviral medication is appropriate.

Herpes zoster ophthalmicus (HZO) can include conjunctivitis (Fig. 9.6). Any ocular redness in the setting of HZO should be referred to an ophthalmologist to investigate the possibility of keratitis, scleritis, and iritis. Treatment of HZO conjunctivitis consists of systemic antivirals, and lubricating drops.

Molluscum contagiosum skin infection of the forehead, brows, or eyelids (Fig. 9.7) is a rare cause of chronic conjunctivitis. Unless the lesions are numerous or large, they are easily missed on initial examinations.

Bacterial Conjunctivitis

Bacterial conjunctivitis (Fig. 9.8a–c) tends to have a more rapid onset, with a yellow-greenish discharge and no adenopathy or follicle formation. Due to a honeycomb-like attachment of the conjunctiva to the tarsus, there may be tiny clear bleb-like nodules (papillae) along the inferior tarsus. Typical bacterial conjunctivitis responds well to topical antibiotics and hot compresses. If a suspected bacterial conjunctivitis worsens on antibiotic treatment, referral to an eye specialist is necessary.

Unfortunately, the clinical signs used to differentiate viral from bacterial conjunctivitis are unreliable. Bacterial conjunctivitis is generally self-limited, and an eye with conjunctivitis is particularly susceptible to eye-drop toxicity. Nevertheless, it is often reasonable to initiate short-term (e.g., 5 days) treatment with antibiotic drops or ointments (in addition to warm or hot compresses) if bacterial infection (or superinfection) is suspected. Topical corticosteroids can reduce discomfort but should only be used if herpes simplex virus has been ruled out as a possible

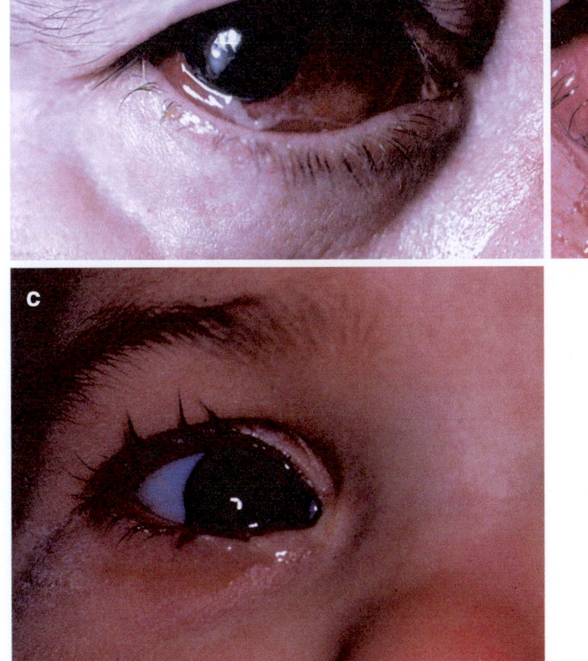

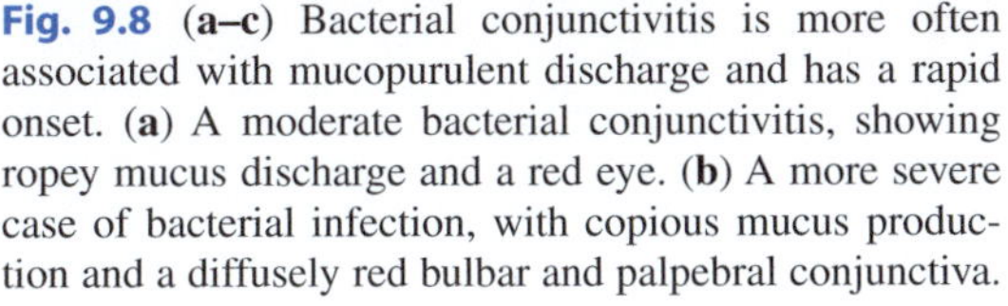

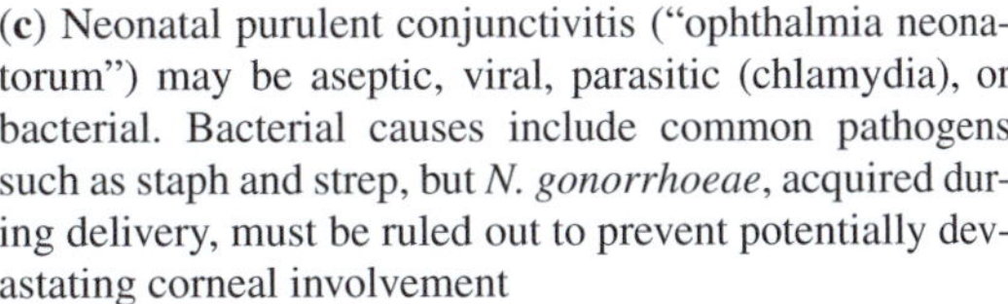

Fig. 9.8 (**a–c**) Bacterial conjunctivitis is more often associated with mucopurulent discharge and has a rapid onset. (**a**) A moderate bacterial conjunctivitis, showing ropey mucus discharge and a red eye. (**b**) A more severe case of bacterial infection, with copious mucus production and a diffusely red bulbar and palpebral conjunctiva. (**c**) Neonatal purulent conjunctivitis ("ophthalmia neonatorum") may be aseptic, viral, parasitic (chlamydia), or bacterial. Bacterial causes include common pathogens such as staph and strep, but *N. gonorrhoeae*, acquired during delivery, must be ruled out to prevent potentially devastating corneal involvement

etiology (which cannot be done without formal ophthalmologic examination) and should only be prescribed under the supervision of an ophthalmologist. As with viral conjunctivitis, bacterial conjunctivitis may have an allergic component manifesting itself as symptomatic itch. This may be treated with topical or oral antihistamines or topical mast cell stabilizers.

Contact Lens-Induced

Chronic giant papillary conjunctivitis may develop in contact lens wearers, in particular in reusable soft contact lens wearers who use chemical-based (multipurpose) contact lens disinfection systems (see Fig. 8.1). This syndrome is characterized by worsening intolerance of contact lenses, ocular irritation (sometimes worse when the contact lenses are not in the eye), and ocular redness. Treatment consists of switching to 1-day single-use contact lenses or discontinuance of contact lens wear. More severe cases may benefit from topical antihistamines, mast cell stabilizers, and corticosteroids.

Conclusion

It should be emphasized that the use of topical corticosteroids should only be used with extreme caution in the treatment of conjunctivitis. They should only be employed after it has been determined that herpes simplex infection is not present, as corticosteroids can cause an explosive worsening of corneal epithelial herpetic disease. Corticosteroids can also cause elevation of intraocular pressure after a few weeks of use, so intraocular pressure must be monitored.

Conjunctivitis of any etiology should be differentiated from other causes of red eye (see Chap. 8). Conjunctivitis of more than 1 or 2 weeks' duration warrants evaluation by an eye specialist. Chronic conjunctivitis or remitting conjunctivitis may indicate a resistant organism, systemic infection (e.g., chlamydia), or a secondary source of infection (e.g., an obstructed lacrimal drainage system.

Suggested Reading

Azari AA, Barney NP. Conjunctivitis: a systemic review or diagnosis and treatment. JAMA. 2013;310:1721–9.

Duncan K, Jeng BH. Medical management of blepharitis. Curr Opin Ophthalmol. 2015;26:289–94.

Patel DS, et al. Allergic eye disease. BMJ. 2017;359:j4706. https://doi.org/10.1136/bmj.j4706.

Pflugfelder SC, KArpecki PM, Perez VL. Treatment of blepharitis: recent clinical trials. Ocul Surf. 2014;12:273–84.

Dry Eye Syndrome

Danielle Trief

Dry eye syndrome (DES, also referred to as keratoconjunctivitis sicca, or KCS) is very common, affecting between 5% and 30% of the population. Symptoms range from occasional irritation to debilitating pain and visual compromise. Numerous studies have found that DES significantly affects patients' quality of life. In 2015 alone, the sale of dry eye medications and devices accounted for $3.2 billion, and this is expected to grow to $4.5 billion by 2020. While it is easy to identify the symptoms associated with dry eye (foreign body sensation, grittiness, epiphora, burning, etc.), it is much more challenging to define the syndrome itself. "Dry eye" is a multifactorial and complicated condition, dependent on tear production and evaporation, inflammation of the ocular surface, and patient symptomatology.

Dry eye syndrome is more prevalent in the aging population as a result of a decrease in tear production and can be accelerated in autoimmune conditions such as Sjögren's syndrome, rheumatoid arthritis, thyroid disease, etc. Other causes of dry eye include increased exposure of the ocular surface due to incomplete lid closure. Dry eye syndrome is also associated with the use of some medications, contact lens wear, prolonged usage of computer or personal devices, a history of prior corneal surgery like LASIK, and low-humidity work environments. Conditions that affect the composition of the normal tear film, which has layers of aqueous, oil, and mucin, such as inflammation of the eyelids called blepharitis, can also cause dry eye.

In 2007, the Dry Eye Workshop (DEWS) group defined DES as "a multifactorial disease of tears and ocular surface that results in symptoms of discomfort, visual disturbance and tear film instability with potential damage to the ocular surface. It is accompanied by increased osmolarity of the tear film and inflammation of the ocular surface." Thus, a DES diagnosis mandates that both symptoms and clinical findings be present. The more recent DEWS II (2017) defines dry eye as "a multifactorial disease of the ocular surface characterized by a loss of homeostasis of the tear film, and accompanied by ocular symptons, in which tear film instability and hyperosmoloarity, ocular surface inflammation and damage and neurosensory abnormalities play etiological roles." Both the more recent DEWS II and older definition of DES recognize that DES is a multifactorial disease, characterized both by signs and symptoms.

D. Trief, MD, MSc (✉)
Columbia University Irving Medical Center,
New York, NY, USA

Department of Ophthalmology, Edward S. Harkness
Eye Institute, Columbia University Vagelos College
of Physicians and Surgeons,
New York, NY, USA
e-mail: dft2102@cumc.columbia.edu

D. S. Casper, G. A. Cioffi (eds.), *The Columbia Guide to Basic Elements of Eye Care*,
https://doi.org/10.1007/978-3-030-10886-1_10

Anatomy

The tear film is critical in its lubricating, antimicrobial, and nutritional roles to the eye. A healthy tear film maintains ocular surface health, ensuring corneal transparency and visual quality and supporting surface stem cells. The health of the tear film is determined by the lacrimal functional unit (LFU), which consists of the ocular surface, eyelids, tear secreting glands, and sensory and autonomic nerves that control them. The LFU regulates tear film components and responds to environmental and physiological changes. Dysfunction in any of these LFU components can affect ocular surface homeostasis.

The healthy tear film consists of three components: an inner mucin layer derived from conjunctival goblet cells, a central aqueous layer derived from the lacrimal gland and accessory lacrimal glands (and not related to the aqueous fluid of the anterior chamber), and an outer, superficial oily layer derived from the meibomian glands at the lid margin. Disruption of any of these layers leads to instability of this trilaminar tear film. Lacrimal and accessory glands, meibomian glands, and conjunctival goblet cells are all innervated by autonomic nerve fibers. Our natural blink, which is controlled by motor fibers from the facial nerve, distributes tears over the ocular surface, and tears then drain through the punctae of the lids to exit the eye.

While the oily top layer of the tear film inhibits evaporation, tear stability also depends on proper positioning of the eyelids and punctae. A full blink is critical to properly redistribute the tear film evenly across the cornea, and disruptions in lid anatomy and lid closure can result in evaporative dry eye.

DES can be broadly characterized into (1) aqueous-deficient dry eye, or a failure of the lacrimal and accessory glands to produce adequate aqueous (the major component of the tear film), or (2) increased tear evaporation (evaporative dry eye), caused by meibomian gland dysfunction, disorders of the lid aperture, or extrinsic factors leading to increased evaporation. DES can also present as a mixed picture of both aqueous deficient and evaporative dry eye.

Signs and Symptoms

The cornea is one of the most densely innervated tissues in the human body. Thousands of nerve endings make it possible to feel, and be made quite uncomfortable by, the presence of a grain of sand, a fine eyelash, or a microscopic epithelial defect on the eye's surface. We can also sense irregularities in our tear film, and the associated dryness, precipitates (filaments), and mucus production can be quite bothersome.

Generally, people with dry eye complain about irritation. Patients typically state that they feel that something is present in their eye (so-called foreign body sensation). They may also experience burning, stinging, or a sensation of grittiness. A careful slit lamp exam is always necessary; not every patient with foreign body sensation has dry eye, and it is prudent to look at both the visible ocular surface and under the eyelids, as an unsuspected foreign body may actually be present.

Another common symptom is tearing or epiphora. Epiphora is an overflow of tears from the eye onto the face. It is commonly confusing to patients why dry eye would be associated with epiphora. The explanation for this apparent paradox is that this tearing is a reflex secondary to irritation, and reflex tears, in contrast to the nor-

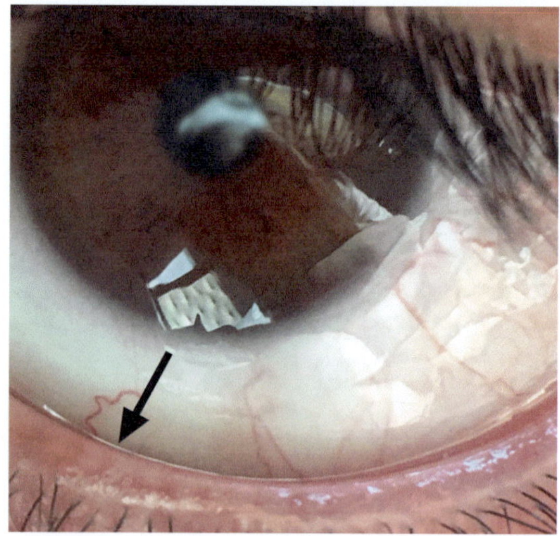

Fig. 10.1 A healthy tear lake or tear meniscus. The tear meniscus should measure approximately 1 mm in height; less than 0.3 mm is abnormal

mal trilaminar tear film, are essentially only lacrimal gland aqueous, which is not sufficient to provide the same lubricating role as the natural tear film does. Until this reflex loop is interrupted, epiphora will persist.

The tear lake, or meniscus (Fig. 10.1), should be observed. A decreased tear lake may be seen in dry eye, whereas an increased tear lake may point to an outflow obstruction. The eyelids also should be well apposed to the globe. If the eyelids turn inward (entropion) or outward (ectropion), tears will not properly drain (see Chap. 31).

Patients with DES may also complain of red eyes. Ocular injection seen with DES is generally diffuse, bilateral, and chronic. A focal area of injection or marked asymmetry between the two eyes is unlikely secondary to dryness. See Chap. 9 for further discussion of red eye.

As with foreign body sensation, not every patient with epiphora has "dry eye." A careful work-up for both epiphora and dry eye should be undertaken to uncover the etiology. In patients complaining of epiphora, the punctae must be carefully inspected. In healthy eyelids, the punctae abut the ocular surface. If they turn outward (punctal ectropion or eversion), they will not be able to adequately drain the tear film (Fig. 10.2). The four punctae should be patent. Nasolacrimal system patency can be tested by gentle probing the punctum and irrigating with fluid. The patient should normally feel fluid drain into the nose and mouth after irrigation. Obstruction anywhere along the nasolacrimal system can result in a reflux of tears or mucus through either punctum or failure of fluid passage. If nasolacrimal obstruction is suspected as the underlying cause of epiphora, the patient should be referred to an oculoplastic surgeon for further evaluation.

Dry Eye Testing

Surveying Patients

The ocular surface disease index (OSDI) is a questionnaire which patients can take to distinguish between normal, mild-to-moderate, and severe dry eye symptoms. Patients are asked about symptomatology, exacerbating conditions, and how DES affects activities of daily living. The answers are tallied, and patients are given a disease severity score from 0 to 100. The index has been found to correlate significantly with other dry eye indices as well as patient perceptions of symptoms and artificial tear usage.

Inspection

Patients often exhibit easily noticeable signs of DES even before formal examination. These may include conjunctival injection, crusting or scaling around the eyes, or associated signs of ocular surface disease (blepharospasm, lid ptosis). The patient's face should be examined for signs of rosacea (telangiectatic vessels and eyelid margin hyperemia), as many rosacea patients have concomitant dry eye.

At the slit lamp, the tear meniscus is measured. There should be a tear lake at the lower eyelid measuring approximately 1.0 mm in height (a meniscus <0.3 mm is abnormal). The quality of the tear film is closely observed, as there may be mucus or filaments present in the tear film. Careful inspection of the lids is paramount.

The tiny meibomian gland orifices at the lid margin should be examined. With gentle pres-

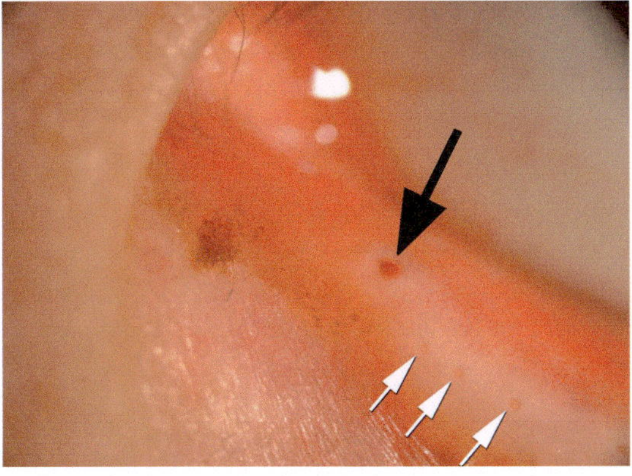

Fig. 10.2 The left lower punctum (black arrow), seen to be patent and the openings of adjacent meibomian gland orifices (white arrows). These glands contribute to the oily top layer of the tear film. The oil prevents tear evaporation

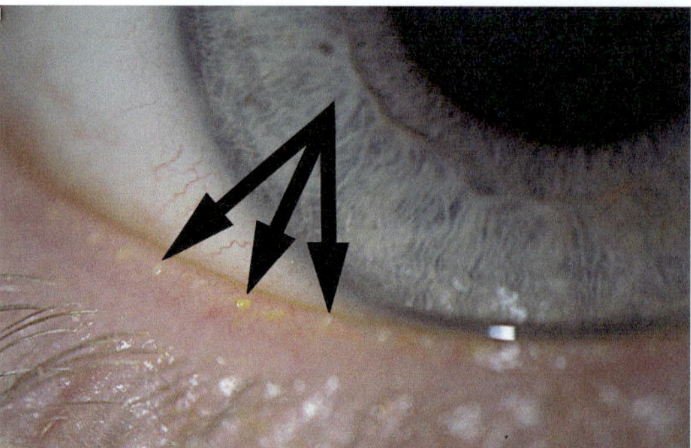

Fig. 10.3 Meibomian gland dysfunction. The small glands on the lid margin are clogged with keratin deposits and solid oils (arrows), which contribute to tear film instability. One can also appreciate fine telangiectatic vessels at the margin, which can be seen in chronic inflammation

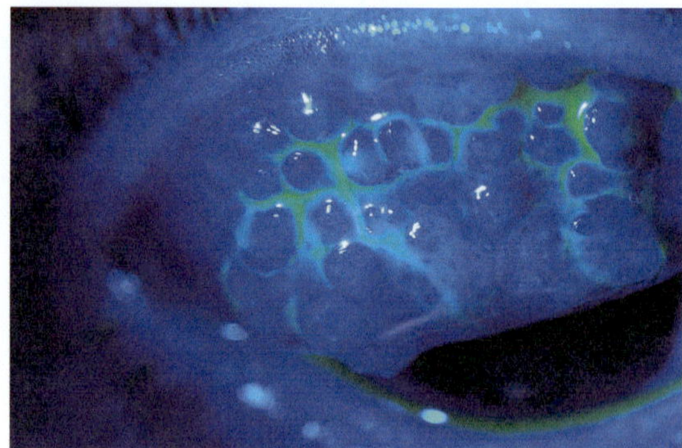

Fig. 10.4 Giant papillae. The topical fluorescein dye in this figure pools around the papillae, which can be seen here as "bumps" on the inner lid surface. Papillae are the result of vascular changes, spoke-like capillaries that are surrounded by edema, on the palpebral conjunctiva in the setting of inflammation or allergy

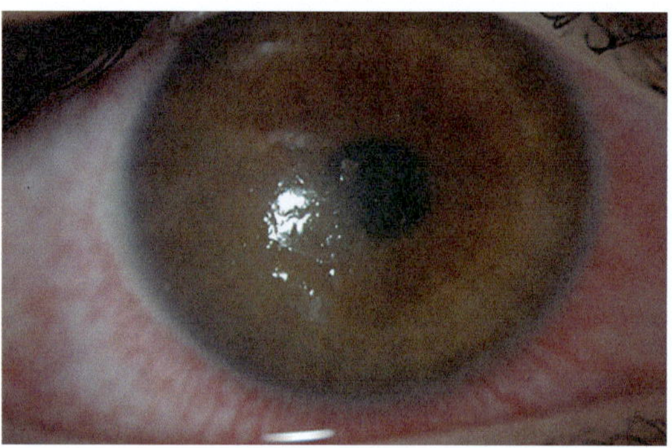

Fig. 10.5 Corneal punctate epithelial erosions in the setting of severe dry eye. One can appreciate the dull light reflex secondary to poor epithelium. The irregular epithelium seen here causes the surface to appear rough

sure, these glands should release a smooth oil. They are often clogged with solid oils and keratin in the setting of meibomian gland dysfunction (Fig. 10.3). Telangiectatic vessels can also be seen at the lid margin in the setting of rosacea. Punctae are assessed as above. The eyelids are everted and inspected for foreign bodies, concretions (yellow subconjunctival deposits seen in chronic irritation), scarring, or signs of ocular allergy like papillae (Fig. 10.4).

The lids are inspected, and particular attention is paid to movement and closure. Failure of the eyelids to close completely (lagophthalmos) can result in a chronic loss of the tear film and resultant exposure keratopathy. Eyelid laxity can be tested by a simple snap back test: the lower lid is pulled away from the globe for several seconds and then released. A healthy eyelid returns to the globe immediately ("snaps back"); a delay indicates eyelid laxity, which is often seen in ectropion and floppy eyelid syndrome and can contribute to dry eye.

The cornea is carefully examined. It should be smooth with a uniform sheen. Punctate epithelial erosions, which are discrete disruptions of the epithelial surface known as superficial punctate keratopathy (SPK), and/or a dull reflex, can be seen in dry eye disease (Fig. 10.5). Larger abrasions or corneal infiltrates should be treated appropriately. The conjunctiva is also carefully examined. In addition to conjunctival injection, areas of redundant conjunctiva (conjunctivochalasis) are noted. This redundant conjunctival tissue can result in epiphora through obstruction of the punctal openings.

The lacrimal gland, located superotemporally, can be seen by asking the patient to look down and toward their nose (see Fig. 2.2). The gland should appear pink and smooth. Occasionally, fibrosis or inflammation of the gland may be noted.

Tear Breakup Time (TBUT)

TBUT is a functional measure of tear film stability. It is determined by instilling fluorescein solution onto the eye and then observing the amount of time it takes for the tear film to become discontinuous without blinking.

Fluorescein is a water-soluble, vital dye that is most commonly used to determine areas of corneal epithelial irregularity and in applanation tonometry to check intraocular pressure. In this test, it is used instead to visualize the tear film coating the corneal surface. After fluorescein is placed in the patient's lower fornix, the time from last blink to the appearance of the first dry spot (i.e., exposed epithelium) on the cornea is recorded as the tear breakup time. A TBUT less than 10 s suggests tear film instability, and less than 5 s suggests definitive dry eye.

Schirmer Testing

The Schirmer test is one of the most well-known dry eye tests. It assesses the aqueous component of tear production. There are multiple variations of Schirmer testing, but all involve placing a thin strip of filter paper in the inferior cul-de-sac of the eye, waiting 5 min, and then recording the amount of filter paper wet by the tear film.

- Basic secretion test: topical anesthetic is instilled, and the amount of filter paper wetting is measured. A normal value is greater than 10 mm. Less than 5 mm is highly suggestive of aqueous deficiency, and 5–10 mm is equivocal.
- Schirmer I test: the test is performed like the basal secretion test but without the use of topical anesthetic. It therefore tests both basal and reflex tearing. Wetting of the filter paper less than 10 mm is diagnostic for aqueous tear deficiency.
- Schirmer II test: like the Schirmer I test, the Schirmer II test is performed without anesthetic. Additionally, a cotton tip applicator is used to irritate the nasal mucosa. This measures reflex secretion. Wetting of less than 15 mm after 5 mm suggests a problem in reflex secretion.

Tear Composition Assay

The Dry Eye Workshop defined as a key feature of dry eye disease an increase in tear osmolarity. Increased tear osmolarity is thought to cause

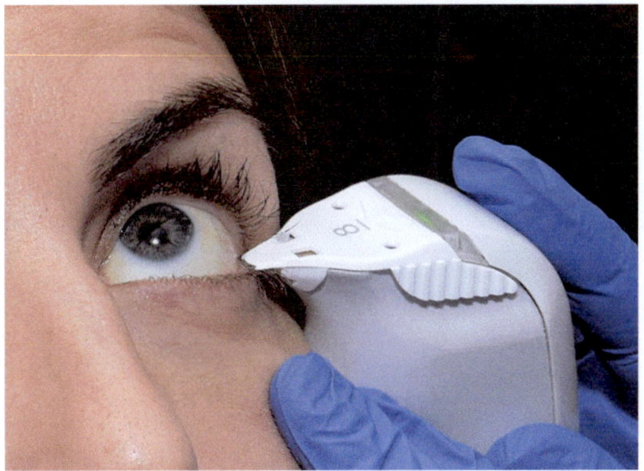

Fig. 10.6 Tear osmolarity testing. Tears are collected in the inferior temporal fornix with a device, and the osmolarity, or concentration of solute particles in the tears, can be tested. The normal tear osmolarity is around 300 mOsm/L and is elevated in patients with dry eye disease

damage to the ocular surface by activating a cascade of inflammatory events and inflammatory mediators in tears. This can, in turn, lead to further damage to conjunctival goblet cells and aqueous producing tear glands, perpetuating the cycle of dry eye.

- Tear osmolarity
  Clinicians can collect and measure tear osmolarity (Fig. 10.6). In one study, a cutoff of more than 308 mOsms/L achieved a 91% rate of correct diagnosis of severe dry eye patients and a true negative rate of 81%.
- Tear inflammatory markers
  Commercially available point of care tests are available which measure matrix metalloproteinase 9 (MMP-9) levels in the tear film. MMP-9 has been found to be significantly elevated in patients with blepharitis, dry eye disease, and allergic eye disease.

Vital Dye Staining

- Fluorescein (see above, TBUT testing) is very useful in assessing ocular surface disease, as it collects in corneal epithelial defects (Fig. 10.7). With a cobalt blue filter, fluorescein will stain punctate and macro epithelial defects green (positive staining). It can also

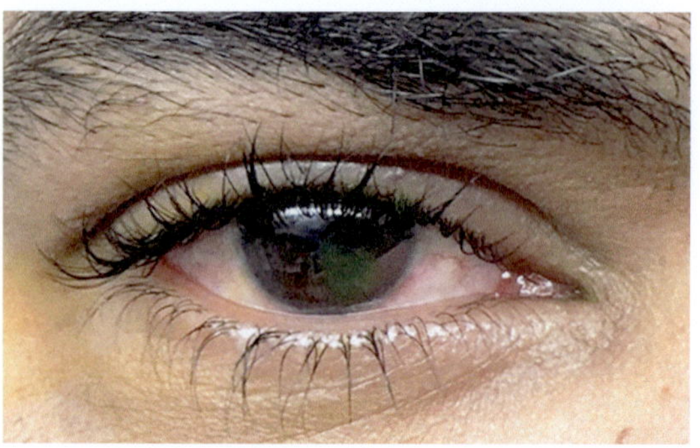

Fig. 10.7 Fluorescein stains an epithelial defect, also known as a corneal abrasion. The area with the damaged epithelium appears green and is even more apparent with a cobalt blue light filter

highlight nonstaining raised areas that project through the tear film (negative staining).

- Rose Bengal is another water-soluble dye used in anterior segment evaluation. Rose Bengal stains any part of the ocular surface that is not covered by mucin. It therefore stains areas without an adequate tear film. It is toxic to epithelial cells, and patients complain of stinging on administration.
- Lysamine green is a synthetic organic acid dye that, like Rose Bengal, stains areas where there is a disruption in the mucous coating but is better tolerated with fewer toxic effects to the epithelial cells.

Impression Cytology

In impression cytology, nitrocellulose filter paper is applied to the ocular surface, which removes the superficial two to three layers of cells. This can then be sent for histological, immunohisto-chemical, and molecular testing and provides information about the composition of cells on the ocular surface and helps in the diagnosis of limbal stem cell disease or ocular surface neoplasia.

Esthesiometry

Normal cornea sensation is critical in the functioning of the LFU. It can be tested crudely with the wisp of a cotton swab, lightly touched to the non-anesthetized cornea. It can also be measured with esthesiometers. Pictured here (Fig. 10.8) is the Cochet-Bonnet esthesiometer, which has a fine nylon filament whose length can be adjusted to apply different intensities of stimuli. Sensation can be graded depending on the stiffness of the testing filament.

Classification

DES can be broadly classified into (1) aqueous tear deficiency (ATD) and (2) evaporative tear dysfunction (ETD). The hallmark of ATD, by definition, is decreased aqueous tear production, as measured by Schirmer testing. ATD can be further categorized as Sjögren's syndrome or non-Sjögren's syndrome dry eye. Non-Sjögren's syndrome ATD can result from damage to the lacrimal gland or reduced tear production secondary to systemic disease or medications. ETD, by contrast, is the result of tear film instability and increased evaporation. It can be further defined as *intrinsic*, secondary to disorders of the lid or meibomian glands, or *extrinsic*, secondary to ocular surface disease, medications, or contact lens wear (Fig. 10.9). With advanced DES, ATD and ETD commonly coexist.

Aqueous Tear Deficiency (ATD)

ATD conditions affect the lacrimal gland and accessory lacrimal glands, thereby causing decreased tear production and ATD. Sjögren's syndrome is a common cause for ATD. Sjögren's is an autoimmune condition characterized by dry eye, dry mouth, and immune dysfunction. While the clinical presentation is variable, to be diagnosed with primary Sjögren's syndrome, patients must have the presence of four out of six of the criteria below or the presence of three of four objective criteria (items 3–6):

Sjögren's syndrome criteria:

1. Ocular symptoms
2. Oral symptoms

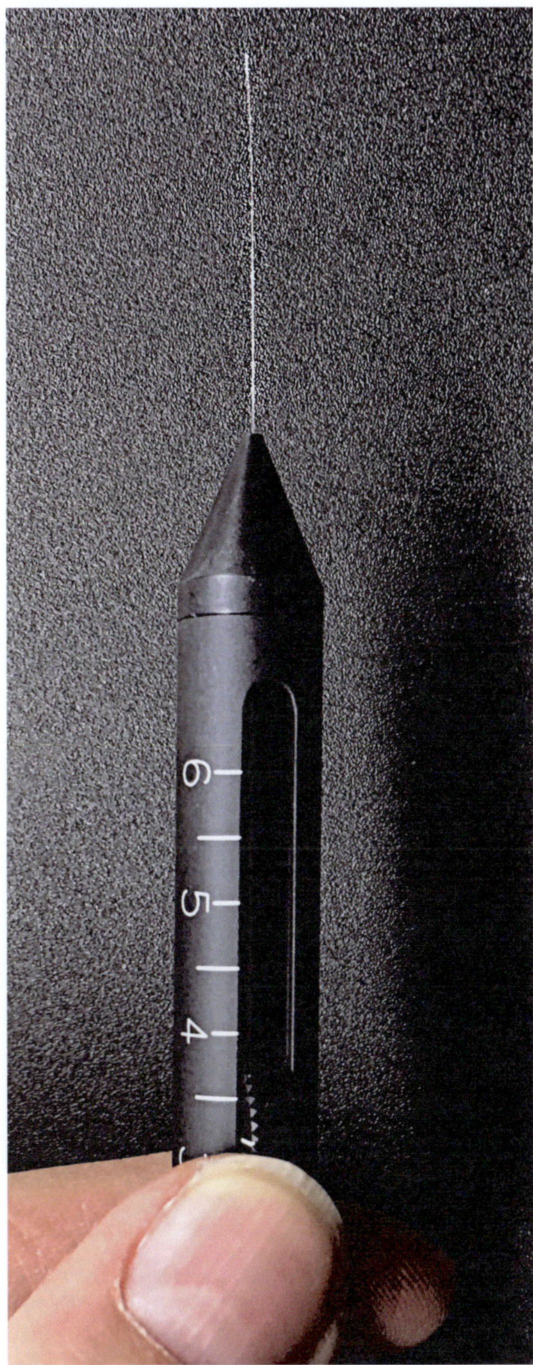

Fig. 10.8 Esthesiometers can be used to measure corneal sensation. Pictured here is a Cochet-Bonnet esthesiometer. It has a fine filament, whose height can be adjusted. The shorter the filament, the stiffer it becomes, and the easier it is to sense when it is touched to the cornea. By adjusting the length of the filament, corneal sensation can be graded

3. Ocular signs
4. Histopathologic features
5. Salivary gland involvement
6. Autoantibodies

Secondary Sjögren's syndrome occurs in patients with a well-defined connective tissue disease, most commonly rheumatoid arthritis. Histopathologic changes seen in the lacrimal and salivary glands in patients with Sjögren's syndrome are similar. There is marked diffuse lymphocytic infiltration, resulting in glandular destruction.

Lacrimal gland dysfunction can also be seen in other systemic conditions like HIV, sarcoidosis, or graft-versus-host disease (GVHD). Rarely, there is congenital absence of the lacrimal gland from birth (alacrima) or dysfunction secondary to other congenital conditions (Riley-Day syndrome or Shy-Drager syndrome). Lacrimal gland outflow can also be obstructed secondary to scarring from chemical burns, cicatrizing conjunctivitis, trauma, or surgical damage. Certain systemic medications can also cause decreased aqueous production.

Evaporative Tear Dysfunction (ETD)

The most common etiology of ETD is meibomian gland dysfunction (MGD) (Fig. 10.3). Meibomian glands produce the oily layer of the tear film, which diminishes aqueous evaporation; consequently, dysfunction of these glands will result in tear film instability and a shortened tear breakup time. Patients with MGD typically exhibit increased inflammation at the lid margin and are prone to develop chalazia and the chronic lid inflammation known as blepharitis (see Chap. 9). The gland orifices may be plugged with keratin and solid oils and ultimately scar or "drop out." MGD is commonly found in patients with rosacea.

An abnormal blink or lagophthalmos can also result in ETD. The normal blink restores and evenly redistributes the tear film. In lagophthalmos, the eyelid does not close completely, and

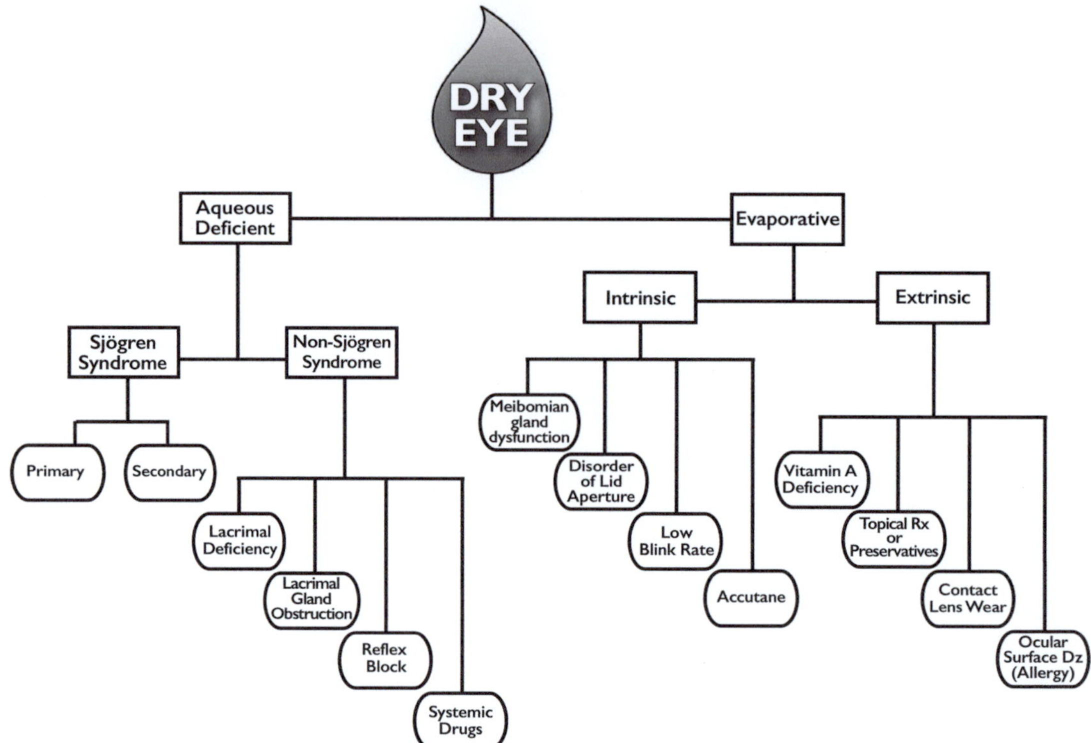

Fig. 10.9 Schematic showing the classification of dry eye syndrome. Dry eye can be broadly defined by a problem in aqueous production (aqueous deficiency) or a problem in tear film stability (evaporative disease) (Adapted from BCSC External Disease and Cornea)

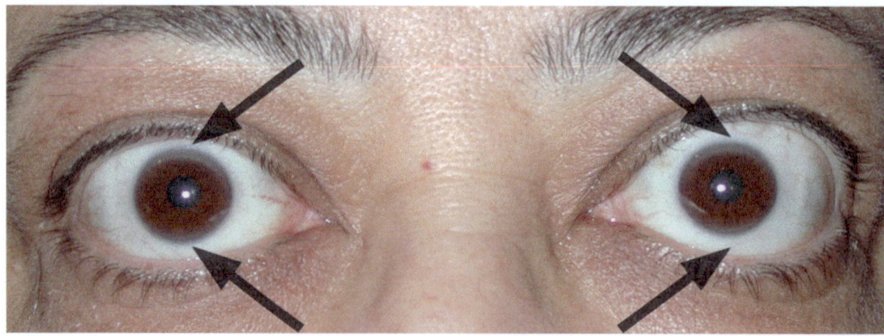

Fig. 10.10 Scleral show in the setting of thyroid orbitopathy. The lids should normally slightly cover the superior and approximate the inferior limbus. Here there is a wide palpebral fissure, and one can appreciate the exposed sclera above and below the cornea (arrows), which contributes to evaporative dry eye

surface irritation and dryness are especially apparent inferiorly.

Accelerated evaporative loss is frequently seen with abnormally large interpalpebral fissures, often demonstrating scleral "show" above and/or below the limbus (as is often present in thyroid disease or with orbital masses) with increased corneal and conjunctival area exposed and resultant greater tear evaporation (Fig. 10.10).

Topical and systemic medications can affect the tear film. Damage to the mucin layer of the tear film can be caused by drops containing the preservative benzalkonium chloride (BAK), which is found in many glaucoma medications, as well as other eye drops. Prolonged contact lens wear can also alter the tear film and lead to ETD.

Vitamin A deficiency can lead to a loss of mucus production by goblet cells and ETD. Internationally, vitamin A deficiency causes blindness in 20,000–100,000 people each year. Patients with vitamin A deficiency may show a Bitot spot, a superficial foamy triangular area of the bulbar conjunctiva with keratinized epithelium. Ultimately, vitamin A deficiency can cause ulceration and melting of the cornea as well as retinal pathology. This treatable condition has a high morbidity and mortality and is important to recognize.

Treatment

Environmental Changes

DES can be exacerbated in environments with low humidity or wind. Room humidifiers can be helpful in dry environments. Patients should avoid air conditioning drafts and may benefit from protective glasses outside. When possible, patients should avoid medications with anticholinergic side effects (e.g., antihistamines and certain antidepressants) that can contribute to dry eye. Some patients find relief with moisture chamber eyeglasses (wraparound, goggle-type spectacles which seal off the eyes, to minimize evaporative loss). Patients with nocturnal lagophthalmos should maintain lubrication through either a tear gel or closing of the lid (by nightly lid taping or lateral tarsorrhaphy).

Several studies have found benefits in diets rich in omega-3 fatty acids. Foods that are rich in omega-3 fatty acids include cold-water fish, flax seed, and walnuts. There are also numerous commercial supplements that contain omega-3 fatty acids.

Artificial Tears

Topical artificial tears can provide symptomatic relief for DES. They come in a variety of preparations and consistencies including drops, gels, and ointment. If patients are using tears more than four times a day, they should be encouraged to use preservative-free preparations. Some preparations contain electrolytes and buffers, which may temporarily normalize the tear film and osmolarity. They will not, however, permanently reverse damage to the ocular surface.

Punctal Plugs

Punctal occlusion is considered in patients where artificial tears and lubrication is not sufficient. By closing the punctae, naturally produced tears or instilled artificial tears will remain on the ocular surface longer. Punctal plugs come in many forms. There are dissolvable collagen rods that can be inserted directly into the punctae. There are semipermanent plugs made of silicone that last months to years (Fig. 10.11), with a mushroom-shaped plug head that sits at the punctal opening. Permanent

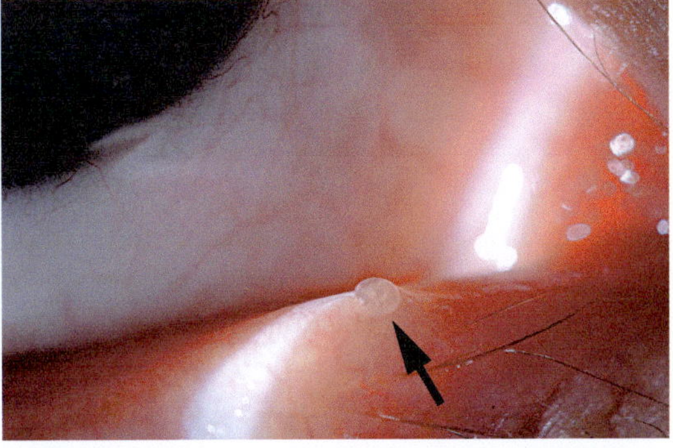

Fig. 10.11 The punctual plug seen here is made of silicone. It is located in the inferior punctum, where tears normally drain. It consists of a cap and a stem and can be removed if necessary. Punctal occlusion retards normal tear loss, thereby decreasing the symptoms of dry eye disease

punctal occlusion can also be achieved with cautery or a radio-frequency probe, which scars the punctal tissue to result in aperture constriction and closure.

Anti-inflammatory Therapy

Ocular surface inflammation is a hallmark of DES, and multiple studies have shown that anti-inflammatory therapy can significantly improve the signs and symptoms of dry eye.

- Topical cyclosporine A is a fungal-derived peptide that prevents activation of factors required for T-cell activation and inflammatory cytokine production. Topical cyclosporine 0.05% (Restasis™) is available by prescription and has been proven to decrease fluorescein staining, improve blurred vision symptoms, and reduce dependence on artificial tears in patients with moderate-to-severe DES.
- Lifitegrast inhibits lymphocyte function-associated antigen 1 (LFA-1), which also downregulates inflammation caused by T lymphocytes. Lifitegrast ophthalmic solution 5% (Xiidra™) is also available by prescription and has been found to improve patient-reported symptoms of dry eye.
- Topical corticosteroids decrease ocular surface irritation, but long-term use can be associated with significant side effects (elevated intraocular pressure, cataract development, and periocular dermal atrophy). Topical corticosteroids come in different strengths and often a low-dose steroid such as fluorometholone or loteprednol etabonate is enough to get a patient through a DES exacerbation. Steroids for DES treatment are most appropriately used in short courses as pulse therapy.

Autologous serum tears can be formulated with the help of an eye bank. Serum tears have growth factors and trophic function similar to natural tears and can be helpful in refractory dry eye. Serum tears require special storage and are often costly to prepare.

Warm compresses to the eyelid margins can liquefy thickened meibomian gland secretions and also soften eyelid incrustations at the lid margin, resulting in easier removal. Some practitioners recommend an eyelid massage following warm compresses. Newer technologies like LipiFlow™ automate this process by providing heat and pressure to the inner eyelid by machine. Treatments may be costly.

Tetracyclines have anti-inflammatory properties, including the inhibition of production of inflammatory cytokines and MMP. Systemic use of tetracyclines has been found to improve symptoms, increase tear film stability, and improve ocular surface disease and rosacea. Doxycyline is frequently used as a first-line treatment because it does not need to be taken on an empty stomach and can be dosed BID and then tapered to daily. Patients are often treated for 3–4 weeks and then tapered to daily dosing.

Specialty contact lenses and tarsorrhaphy are occasionally employed for refractory DES and severe corneal epithelial disease. Specialty contact lenses provide an additional barrier to the fragile cornea and help with epithelial healing: bandage contact lenses can be used for short durations to improve corneal defects, and long-term scleral lenses or the PROSE lens™ can be used in patients for severe ocular surface diseases. These lenses bathe the cornea in a continuous aqueous reservoir. Tarsorrhaphy, or eyelid closure, can be used in patients with poor lid closure, blink abnormalities, or neurotrophic disease.

Suggested Reading

American Academy of Ophthalmology. Ocular surface disease: diagnostic approach. Basic and clinical science course, section 8, 2011–2012. San Francisco: American Academy of Ophthalmology; 2011. p. 51.

Barabino S, Labetoulle M, Rolando M, Messmer EM. Understanding symptoms and quality of life in patients with dry eye syndrome. Ocul Surf. 2016;14(3):365–76.

Craig JP, Nichols KK, Akpek EK, Caffery B, Dua HS, Joo CK, Liu Z, Nelson JD, Nichols JJ, Tsubota K, Stapleton F. TFOS DEWS II definition and classification report. Ocul Surf. 2017;15(3):276–83.

Lemp MA. Advances in understanding and managing dry eye disease. Am J Ophthalmol. 2008;146(3): 350–6.

Lemp MA, Bron AJ, Baudouin C, Benítez Del Castillo JM, Geffen D, Tauber J, Foulks GN, Pepose JS, Sullivan BD. Tear osmolarity in the diagnosis and management of dry eye disease. Am J Ophthalmol. 2011;151(5):792–8.

Schiffman RM, Christianson MD, Jacobsen G, Hirsch JD, Reis BL. Reliability and validity of the ocular surface disease index. Arch Ophthalmol. 2000;118(5):615–21.

The definition and classification of dry eye disease: report of the definition and classification subcommittee of the international dry eye workshop (2007). No authors listed. Ocul Surf. 2007;5(2):75–92.

Vitali C, Bombardieri S, Jonsson R, Moutsopoulos HM, Alexander EL, Carsons SE, Daniels TE, Fox PC, Fox RI, Kassan SS, Pillemer SR, Talal N, Weisman MH, European Study Group on Classification Criteria for Sjögren's Syndrome. Classification criteria for Sjögren's syndrome: a revised version of the European criteria proposed by the American-European Consensus Group. Ann Rheum Dis. 2002;61(6):554–8.

Cataract

Leejee H. Suh and Steven A. Kane

Cataracts are a leading cause of blindness in the world, contributing to approximately 51% of world blindness, which represents about 20 million people (WHO 2010). The most significant and discouraging aspect of this fact is that while cataract blindness is reversible, the number of people blind from cataracts increases each year due to a shortage of healthcare providers. In the United States, cataract surgery is the most commonly performed surgical procedure in the Medicare-aged population. Cataracts affect more than 24.4 million Americans age 40 or older, and by age 75, approximately half of all Americans have cataracts. Cataracts affect a much smaller population of children but with significant socioeconomic impact. In 2015, about 3 million cataract procedures were performed in the United States with an estimated $6.8 billion in direct costs. Because of the magnitude of both the number of individuals affected and the associated healthcare costs, considerable effort has been spent to ensure the highest quality care is delivered using the most cost-effective techniques.

Cataract is defined as an opacification of the crystalline lens of the eye. There is a functional impairment produced by the cataract, as opacities within the lens diminish or impede the passage of light into the eye and focusing of an image on the macula. Development of these opacities is found in almost all individuals as the result of normal aging. Surgical intervention is warranted when there is a "visually significant cataract," whereby the degree of opacification affects the individual's vision to the extent that it affects his/her daily activities of living.

The crystalline lens of the human eye is a biconvex structure and is made up of three main parts (Fig. 11.1). A thin capsule makes up the outer coat of the lens and is comprised of basement membrane material. The next layer is a soft cortical layer and at the center is the nucleus. The central nucleus is harder and denser than the cortex. The lens is approximately 65% water and 35% crystalline and albuminoid proteins, and is supported by hundreds of fibers known as zonules which attach to the equator of the lens and muscular ciliary body within the wall of the eye. The lens, in conjunction with the cornea, focuses light onto the retina. In youth, the crystalline lens is pliable, and its shape can be changed by altering the tension of the zonules, altering the curvature of the front and back surface of the lens. This change of shape allows for a variable focus and the clear

L. H. Suh, MD
Columbia University Irving Medical Center,
New York, NY, USA

Department of Ophthalmology, Edward S. Harkness
Eye Institute, Columbia University Vagelos College
of Physicians and Surgeons, New York, NY, USA
e-mail: lhs2118@cumc.columbia.edu

S. A. Kane, MD, PhD (✉)
Department of Ophthalmology, Edward S. Harkness
Eye Institute, Columbia University Vagelos College
of Physicians and Surgeons, New York, NY, USA
e-mail: sak6@cumc.columbia.edu

© Springer Nature Switzerland AG 2019
D. S. Casper, G. A. Cioffi (eds.), *The Columbia Guide to Basic Elements of Eye Care*,
https://doi.org/10.1007/978-3-030-10886-1_11

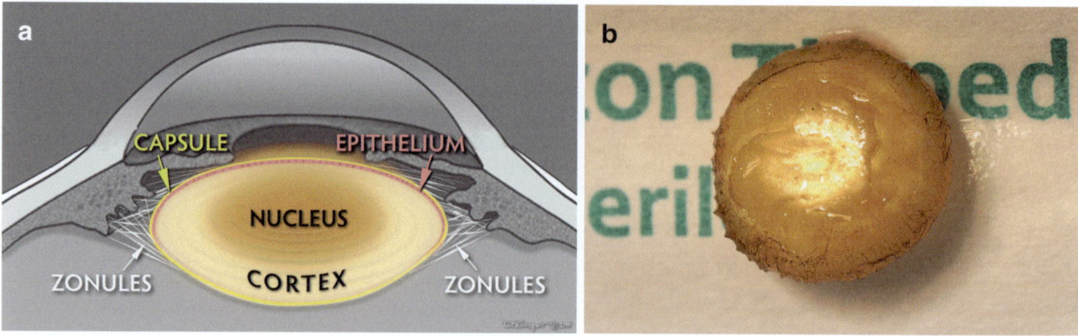

Fig. 11.1 (**a**) Lens diagram. (**b**) Photograph of brunescent cataract removed during cadaver dissection, showing dense opacity which prevents viewing lettering behind it

Table 11.1 The prevalence of lens opacities and visually significant cataracts depends on age

Study	45–54	55–64	65–74	75–84	>84
Framingham					
Lens opacities	–	41.7	73.2	91.1	
Cataract	–	4.5	18.0	45.9	
NHANES					
Lens opacities	11.2	27.6	57.6	–	
Cataract	2.6	10.0	28.5	–	
Watermen					
Lens opacities	5.7	37.0	72.1	94.2	100
Cataract	–	5.0	25.0	59.0	

viewing of objects both close and distant. With aging, the composition of the lens changes, and so the lens becomes more rigid, limiting its ability to focus on close objects (accommodation). The normal loss of accommodation is called presbyopia and affects all individuals in their middle age. These changes in the internal composition of the lens also may lead to loss of clarity and cataract formation (Fig. 11.1b).

The prevalence of both lens opacities and visually significant cataracts depends largely on age (Table 11.1). Between 18% and 28.5% of patients over the age of 65 experience significant cataracts and as many as 12% of patients over the age of 45 have some degree of lens opacification.

Adult Cataract

Clinical Manifestations

Cataracts can be classified by the extent, characteristics, and location of the lens opacification.

The most common types of age-related cataracts are nuclear, cortical, and posterior subcapsular (PSC), although there are many other types of cataract which occur. Usually, there is no identifiable cause for which type of cataract occurs, although some are frequently related to antecedent medications or medical conditions. For instance, PSC cataracts are often associated with prior use of corticosteroids, coronary cataracts are seen with diabetes, and Christmas tree (also called crystalline or polychromatic) cataracts are noted in myotonic dystrophy (Figs. 11.2 and 11.3f).

Nuclear sclerotic cataract (NSC) is the most common type of cataract in which the lenticular nucleus becomes harder, less clear, and more pigmented. This change to the lens initially allows for greater magnification for individuals and an enhanced ability to see at close range, a phenomenon known as "second sight." With time, however, the sclerotic changes (brownish coloring or brunescence and hardening) of the nucleus lead to a decrease in vision. Cortical cataracts (CO) appear as spokes or radial opacities within the cortical material of the lens and are soft in density. Posterior subcapsular cataracts (PSC) occur in younger individuals and are characterized by focal opacities just anterior to the posterior capsule and usually in the central visual axis and are often associated with uncontrolled diabetes mellitus, systemic corticosteroid use, and previous trauma. They often progress more rapidly than other types of cataracts. In addition, because they are often located centrally, directly in the visual axis, they can cause more vision loss in earlier states of cataract.

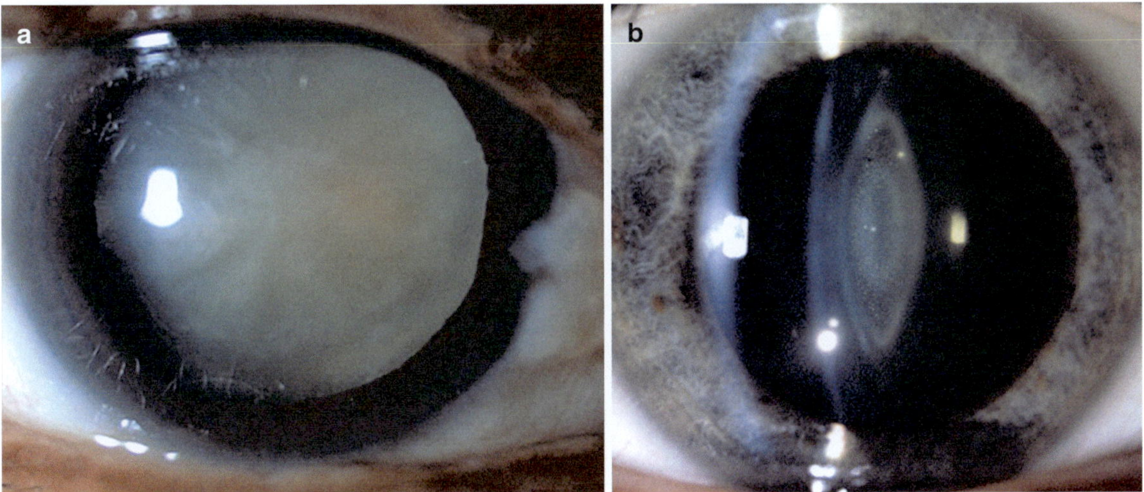

Fig. 11.2 (**a**, **b**) Nuclear sclerotic cataract, slit lamp views

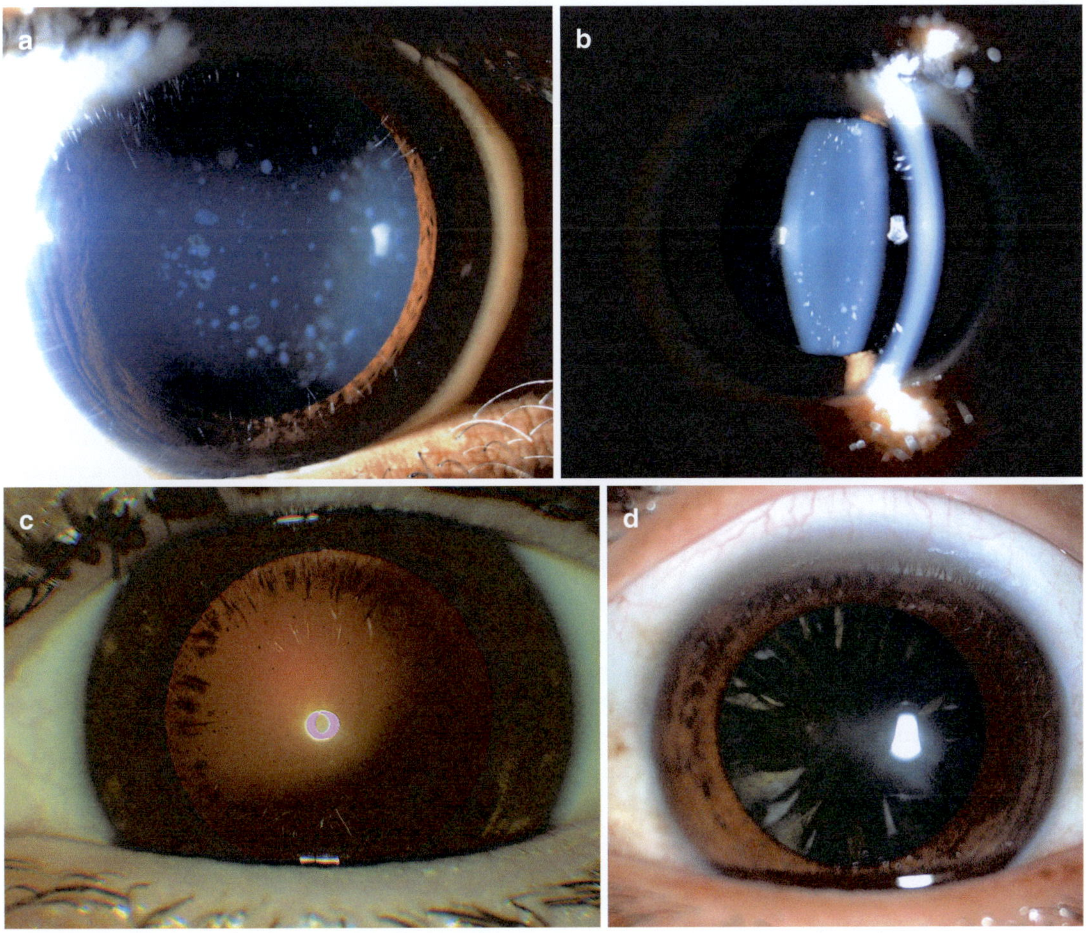

Fig. 11.3 (**a–h**): Examples of cataract types: (**a**, **b**) cortical specks; (**c**) diabetic coronary; (**d**) cortical spokes; (**e**) PSC; (**f**), Christmas tree/polychromatic; (**g**, **h**) bilateral congenital

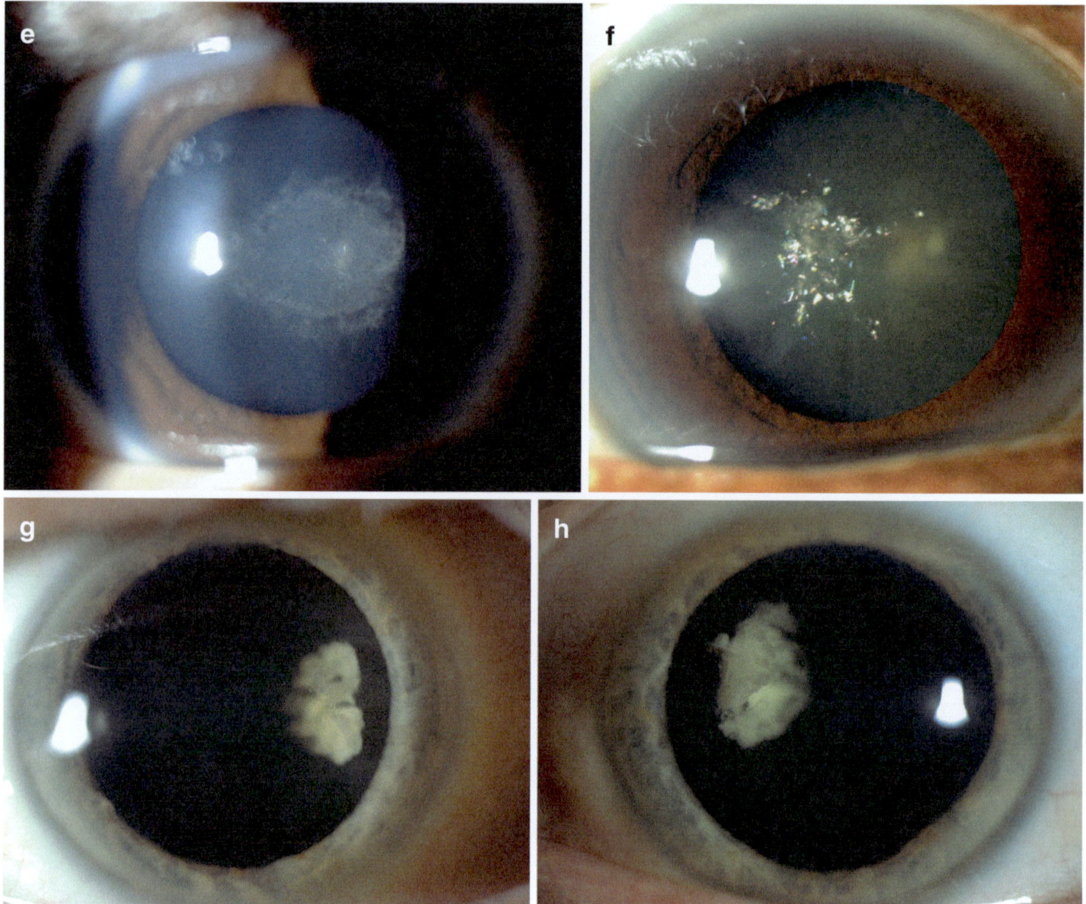

Fig. 11.3 (continued)

Functional impairment from cataracts varies. Patients with early cataracts often have nonspecific complaints of generalized visual disturbances in daily activities of living, such as driving (particularly night driving from glare), reading, and near work such as computer or small handheld device usage. As cataracts progress, the ability to perform activities of daily living becomes more and more difficult. Snellen visual acuity is not a good predictor of visual disturbance as someone with 20/40 vision may be more functional than someone with 20/25 vision. For example, someone with a posterior subcapsular cataract may have better than 20/40 Snellen visual acuity but cannot drive at night due to intense glare. As such, the ophthalmic exam not only includes an assessment of the cataract but also a history of the patient's visual functionality. Over time, eyeglass or contact lens prescriptions may change due to worsening of the cataract, in which case an updated prescription would be dispensed. Cataract surgery is recommended when an updated refractive correction is not optimal and/or when the patient reports difficulty with daily activities. For most patients, cataract surgery is initially discussed at visual acuities of 20/40 or worse.

Differential Diagnosis

The diagnosis of cataracts is made by clinical examination of the eye using the slit lamp biomicroscope. The functional significance of a cataract is made by interviewing the patient and determining his/her visual needs. Since cataract surgery is almost always an elective procedure, the functional impairment of the patient far outweighs the anatomic appearance of the cataract on clinical examination. A complete eye examination is always necessary to rule out other reasons for gradual visual decline. Particular attention is paid to the presence of other opacities in the visual axis, such as corneal scarring or vitreous opacities, as well as the health of the neurosensory retina and optic nerve. Removing a cataract in the setting of other media opacities or retinal or optic nerve pathologies would provide no real functional benefit.

Prevention and Risk Factors

Many studies have shown a higher prevalence of cataracts in geographic regions with high ultraviolet B (UVB) radiation levels. This data suggests there is potential benefit in wearing sunglasses to reduce ocular exposure to UV rays. Diabetes mellitus is another risk factor associated with cataract formation. Many drugs are cataractogenic, such as corticosteroids, certain tranquilizers (i.e., phenothiazines), and possibly diuretics. Cigarette smoking and heavy alcohol consumption are also risk factors for cataract development. Although many attempts have been made to identify cataractogenic or preventative vitamin supplements, no single supplement has been identified.

Treatment

Surgical Indications

The decision to perform cataract surgery is made after assessing visual function and the degree of cataract formation. Nonsurgical interventions include providing the most updated refractive correction with eyeglasses and/or contact lenses. As the cataracts progress, however, these interventions become inadequate. Visual acuity less than 20/40 is often accepted as sufficient visual loss to justify cataract extrac-

tion. 20/40 or better vision in at least one eye is needed to obtain a driver's license in most states. In those with better than 20/40 vision, visual disturbances such as glare, monocular double vision, or visual disparity between the eyes may warrant surgical intervention. Much less common reasons for surgery include lens-induced diseases such as uveitis or glaucoma from the cataract and the need to visualize the fundus for adequate diagnosis and treatment of disorders in the posterior pole, such as diabetic retinopathy or macular degeneration.

Preoperative Ophthalmic Testing

As discussed, the most critical preoperative ophthalmic assessment is to rule out the presence of concurrent ocular disease. Glare testing may be performed in an office setting to simulate bright light situations such as oncoming headlights or bright sunny environments. In some individuals, it is difficult to assess the relative amount of visual loss due to cataract and to predict the potential for visual rehabilitation following cataract extraction. This is especially true for an eye with concomitant eye disease such as glaucoma, diabetic retinopathy, or macular degeneration. In these cases, potential acuity meter (PAM) measurements, which assess retinal visual potential, can be performed prior to surgery.

For the most part, cataract surgery involves extraction of the crystalline lens and replacement with an artificial intraocular lens implant (IOL). The power of the IOL is determined by utilizing various formulas that take into account the axial length of the eye, specific characteristics of the particular intraocular lens to be used, and the corneal power, related to curvature of the cornea. Optical biometry is a highly accurate, noninvasive, and automated method of measuring these parameters of the eye and is most often utilized; a more traditional method of measuring the ocular axial length utilizes an A-scan ophthalmic ultrasound. Often, mature, dense cataracts require A-scan ultrasound measurement, as optical biometry readings may not be accurate due to the cataract density. Finally, the keratometry readings, which determine corneal curvature, can be influenced by recent wearing of contact lenses. In these cases, patients are usually asked to refrain from contact lens use for at least a week to normalize corneal readings for IOL measurement.

Preoperative Medical Examination

A preoperative medical examination should be performed for all individuals undergoing cataract surgery, whether in the hospital or ambulatory surgical facility and regardless of the type of anesthesia administered. Preoperative medical assessment is guided by the patient's age and medical condition.

Anesthesia

Anesthesia for cataract surgery can be either local or general. Local anesthesia is usually preferred to general by both the patient and surgeon. In most settings, local anesthesia is administered with concurrent oral or intravenous sedation. Local anesthesia includes a regional block to the retrobulbar space which provides akinesia and anesthesia to the eye. An additional block of the facial nerve may be performed to prevent eyelid squeezing during surgery. More commonly, however, topical anesthesia with anesthetic eye drops and intracameral anesthetics has become the preferred modality, especially in cooperative patients. General anesthesia is used for those who cannot cooperate fully, due to behavioral issues, hearing loss, neurologic or neurodegenerative conditions, or in pediatric cases.

Surgical Techniques

Microsurgical techniques used for cataract surgery have undergone tremendous technological advancements in the past few decades. In the 1970s, there was a transition from traditional intracapsular cataract extraction (ICCE, a technique which involved whole lens removal, including the surrounding capsule) to extracapsular cataract extraction (ECCE, in which the lens nucleus and cortex are removed but the capsule is left behind). In extracapsular cataract extraction, a 10–14 mm incision is made near the corneoscleral junction, the anterior capsule of the lens is opened, and the lens nucleus is removed intact. The lenticular cortex is then aspirated, leaving the lens capsule to support the placement of an artificial intraocular lens implant. Unlike the older method of intracapsular surgical technique, in which the whole lens and capsule were removed, extracapsular cataract surgery prompted development of improved artificial intraocular lenses, eliminating the need for thick cataract glasses or contacts, both of which had severe limitations for the typical elderly patient.

In the 1980s, a new surgical technique called phacoemulsification cataract extraction was developed and has become the mainstay of modern cataract surgery (Fig. 11.4a, b). In phacoemulsification, a smaller, self-sealing incision is made in the cornea, the anterior capsule is opened with a circular incision (capsulorrhexis) (Fig. 11.5), a probe producing sound energy is used to fracture (emulsify) the lens (= phaco) nucleus into

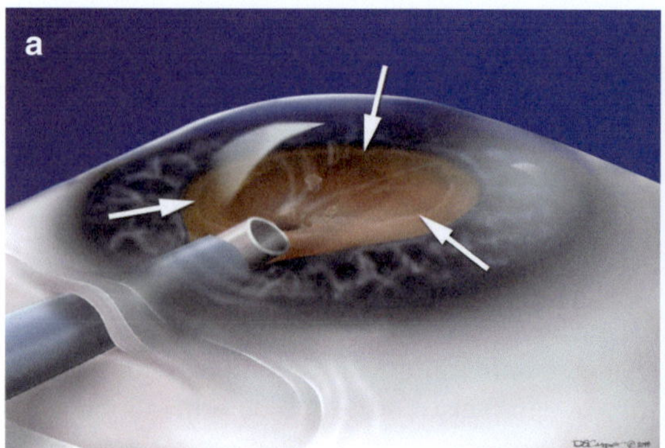
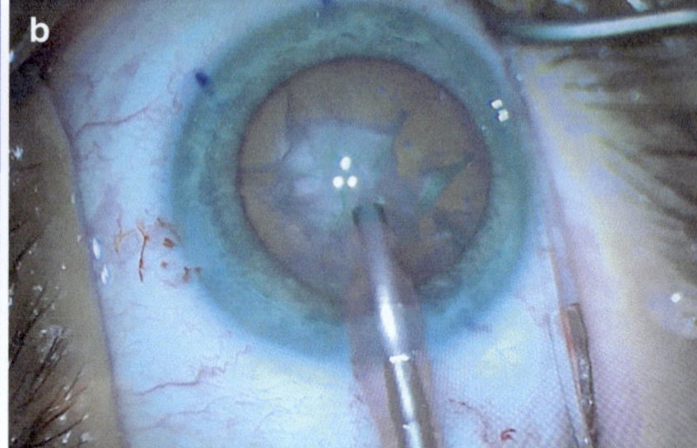

Fig. 11.4 (**a**) Phacoemulsification illustration showing the anterior capsulotomy (white arrows) and lens fragments, and (**b**) intraoperative photograph taken during phacoemulsification

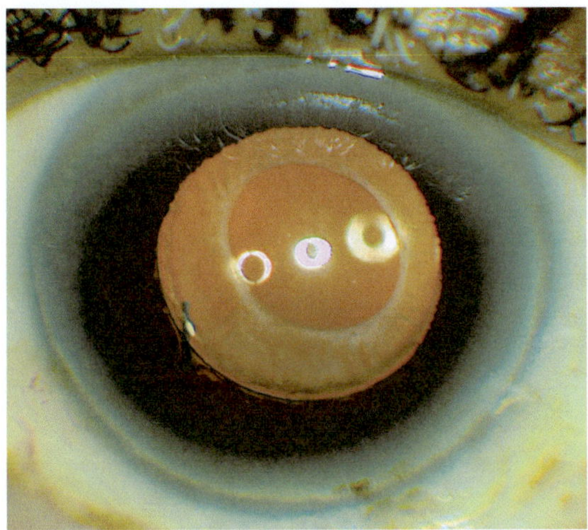

Fig. 11.5 Anterior capsulorhexis

fragments which are vacuumed out, and a separate aspiration instrument is used to remove the cortex. A foldable IOL is then injected and in the capsular bag, where it unfurls to replace the removed crystalline lens. The capsular bag must have an intact posterior capsule for the stability of intraocular lens implantation. The use of a smaller incision allows for a safer, more controlled cataract extraction with quicker postoperative visual rehabilitation. Currently, the older extracapsular technique is utilized for mature or hypermature cataracts, in which removal of the nucleus in toto is safer than attempts to fracture the nucleus with phacoemulsification. Phacoemulsification cataract extraction with IOL implantation has become the most commonly performed surgical technique for cataract surgery.

More recently, the initial steps of the phacoemulsification procedure have been modified with laser-assisted instrumentation. This technique, called femtosecond laser-assisted cataract surgery (FLACS) (Fig. 11.6a, b), utilizes a femtosecond laser to make custom incisions on the cornea for the wound and any necessary astigmatic correction, then the central circular anterior capsulotomy, and finally softens the nucleus with a grid-like pattern of laser sculpting. The surgeon is assisted in this laser-enhanced technique by the guidance of a simultaneous, real-time, cross-sectional lens image (anterior segment optical coherence tomography). The remaining nucleus and cortex removal and insertion of the intraocular lens are performed manually by the surgeon as is done with traditional phacoemulsification. FLACS became FDA approved in the United States in 2010. The option of FLACS has not, however, become a covered service under insurance, and so there are added costs for patients who elect to undergo this procedure. Studies have shown its efficacy in reproducible corneal incisions and the reduction for phacoemulsification power usage (and hence less potential damage to the corneal endothelium) for lens removal. More outcome studies are needed, however, to show improved results in uncorrected vision with FLACS compared to those found with more traditional phacoemulsification techniques, which are generally covered by most insurances.

Intraocular lenses are routinely placed at the time of cataract extraction to replace the removed crystalline lens. Over the past several decades, a variety of synthetic materials have been developed to manufacture intraocular lenses, including plastics such as polymethylmethacrylate (PMMA), silicone, and acrylic. Intraocular lenses are well tolerated in the eye and are used in most surgeries to enhance the visual outcome. In select cases, intraocular lens placement at the time of surgery is avoided, e.g., in eyes with concurrent severe inflammation (uveitis), in infants where contact lens correction is preferred, and in certain combined cataract-retinal surgeries. In addition, in eyes where the posterior capsule is not intact, placement of the intraocular lens may be more difficult or unsuitable. Recent surgical techniques have been developed which allow placement of an intraocular lens even in the absence of a posterior capsule; this delayed IOL placement may be performed years after the original cataract removal.

The choice of intraocular lenses has also expanded over recent years. Traditional monofocal intraocular lenses (Fig. 11.7) leave the patient either farsighted (hyperopic) or nearsighted (myopic) (see Chap. 7). With the development of "presbyopia-correcting" IOLs, patients can potentially perceive a full range of vision (both distance and near vision) without additional spectacle overcorrection. There are two main types of presbyopia-correcting lenses: accom-

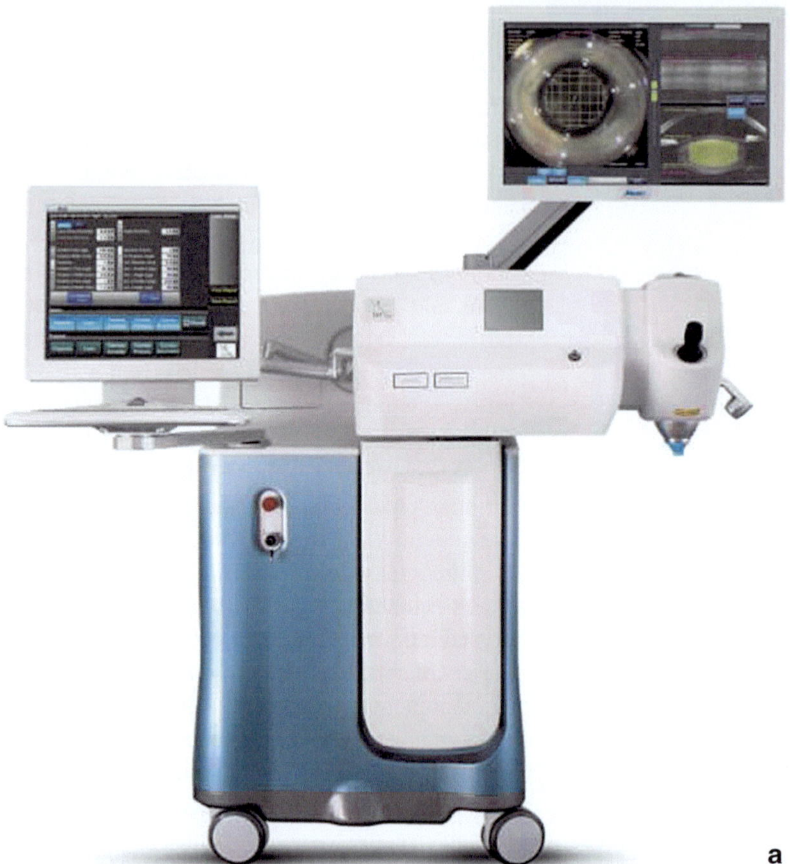

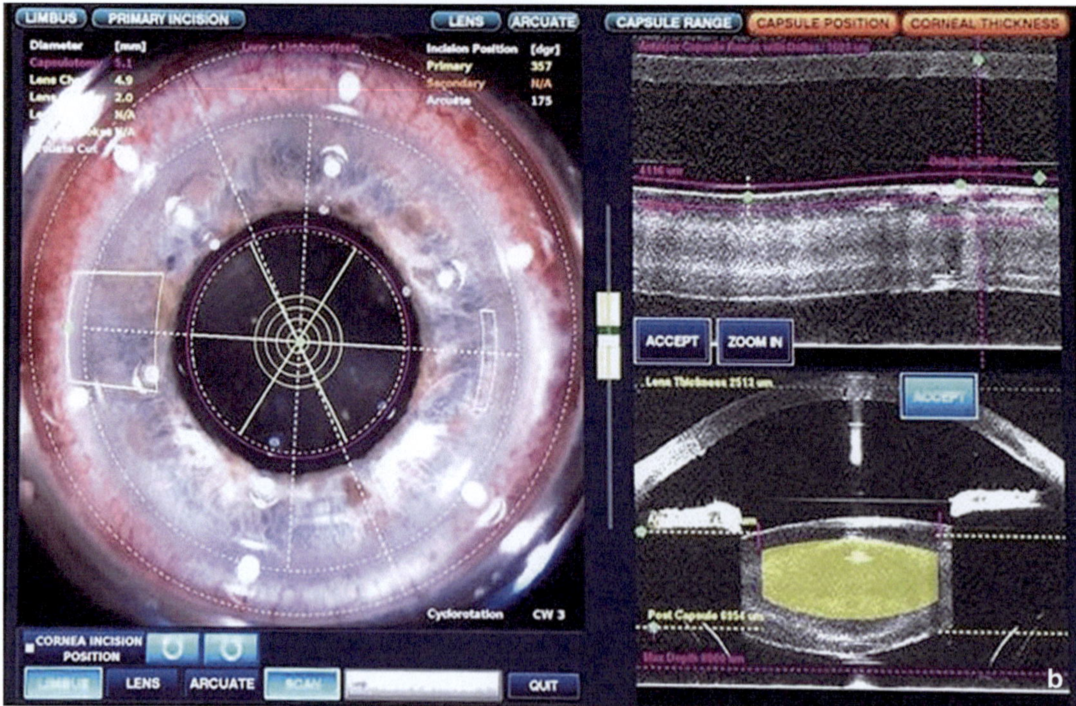

Fig. 11.6 (**a**) LenSx femtosecond laser console. (Courtesy of Alcon). (**b**) Femtosecond console readout

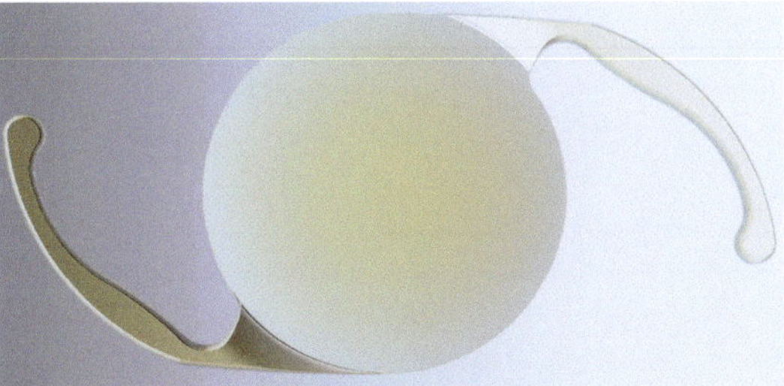

Fig. 11.7 Acrylic monofocal AcrySof intraocular lens. (Courtesy of Alcon)

modating lenses and multifocal lenses (Fig. 11.8). These lenses are usually not a covered service under insurance but are an option for patients who want an extended focal range that enables vision at multiple distances. While there are several benefits with these lenses, they are not well tolerated in patients with other ophthalmic comorbidities such as corneal disease, glaucoma, and macular degeneration. Some side effects experienced with multifocal lenses that usually diminish over time include halos and glare around light sources and reduced contrast sensitivity. Toric intraocular lenses are another option for patients; these are monofocal lenses that provide corneal astigmatic correction and are an option for patients with significant corneal astigmatism.

With several options of surgical techniques (manual phacoemulsification and FLACS) and intraocular lenses (standard monofocal, toric monofocal, accommodating, and multifocal) now available, the patient must have a thorough discussion with their surgeon to best assess the appropriate combination, weighing the risks and benefits of each option.

Visual Outcomes Following Cataract Surgery

Cataract surgery is one of the safest surgical procedures performed. Most patients can expect recovery of excellent vision with well over 90% achieving a final postoperative visual acuity of 20/15 to 20/40, short of any other ophthalmic conditions. The majority of patients postoperatively need some spectacle correction.

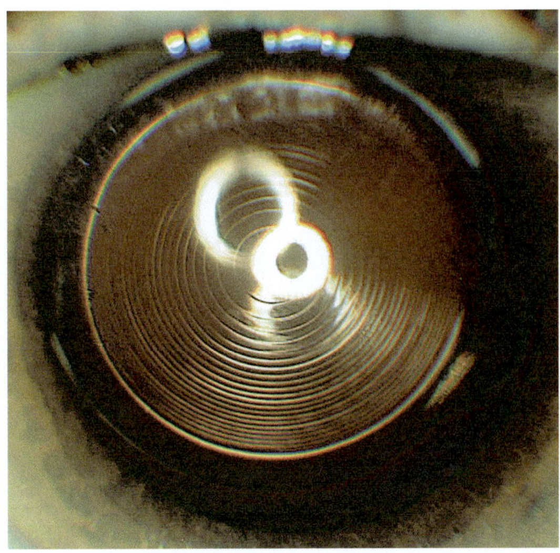

Fig. 11.8 Intraocular acrylic multifocal intraocular lens seen through a dilated pupil

Patients often wonder if their cataract can recur. This is not the case, as the actual nucleus and cortex are removed during surgery. Posterior capsular opacification (PCO), also known as "secondary cataract," can diminish the patient's vision over time, however, and is a common occurrence after cataract surgery (Fig. 11.9a). As described, the posterior capsule of the crystalline lens is purposely preserved at the time of cataract surgery in both extracapsular and phacoemulsification cataract extraction to support the implanted IOL and prevent vitreous humor from entering the anterior segment of the eye and surgical wound. Rupture of the posterior capsule at the time of cataract extraction is considered an undesirable complication that may prevent immediate intraocular lens implantation and limit visual outcome. However, long-term vision is largely dependent on maintaining clarity of the posterior capsule. Opacification of the posterior capsule occurs in 15–20% of eyes within the first postoperative year and in as many as 50% of patients by the fifth postoperative year. If the PCO becomes visually significant, a small posterior capsulotomy can be performed with an in-office neodymium-YAG laser that is minimally invasive, requires no sedation, and is a low-risk procedure. The capsulotomy procedure produces a small central opening in the hazy posterior capsule, which usually results in a rapid and dramatic improvement in visual acuity (Fig. 11.9b).

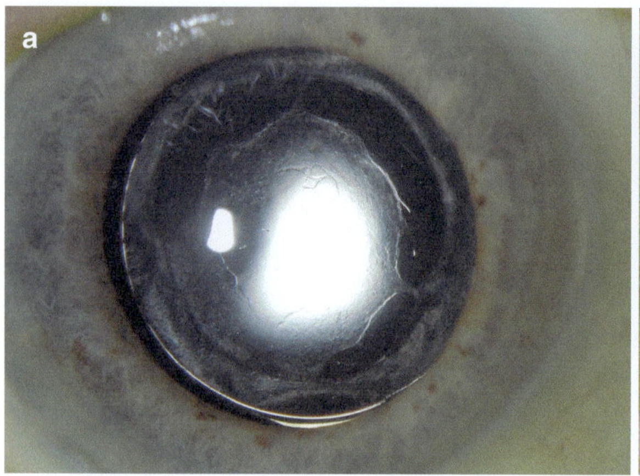
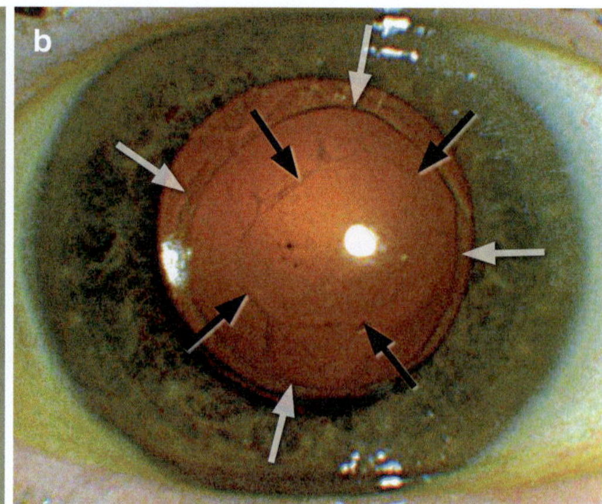

Fig. 11.9 (**a**, **b**): (**a**) Dense central posterior capsular opacification (PCO). (**b**) YAG capsulotomy (black arrows) performed postoperatively for PCO. White arrows show the anterior capsulorrhexis performed intraoperatively for cataract removal

Table 11.2 The most common complications following cataract surgery

Complication	Rate (%)
Bullous keratopathy	<0.3
Intraocular lens malposition	<1.0
Endophthalmitis	<0.3
Retinal detachment	<1.0
Significant macular edema	<3.0

Complications of Cataract Surgery

As with any surgical procedure, complications and adverse outcomes can occur. Table 11.2 lists the most common complications seen following cataract surgery. Elevated intraocular pressure, corneal edema, ptosis, and small hemorrhages on the conjunctiva may all occur following otherwise uncomplicated cataract surgery. Usually these are self-limited and respond to medical therapies. In rare cases, the IOL may shift position, sometimes resulting in partial pupil occlusion ("IOL capture") or dislocation out of the visual axis (Fig. 11.10a, b). Endophthalmitis (intraocular infection), retinal detachment, and bullous keratopathy (significant corneal decompensation and persistent edema) are of greater concern because of the likelihood of permanent visual impairment. Fortunately, these complications are rare and can often be addressed with additional surgery or other interventions to reduce long-term vision loss. Significant edema of the central macula can occur 4–12 weeks after uncomplicated surgery; this complication is thought to be related to postoperative intraocular inflammation causing leakage of fluid into the macular region from breakdown of the blood-retinal barrier (Fig. 11.11). Fortunately, most cases of macular edema can be treated with topical, nonsteroidal and/or topical corticosteroid eye drops. Intraoperative expulsive choroidal hemorrhage is a very rare complication (1/10,000 cases) which can result in complete vision loss. It can be largely avoided by maintaining normal blood pressure and vascular status preoperatively and intraoperatively. All patients should be informed of the possibilities of these complications preoperatively to allow them to weigh the relative risks against the expected benefits of cataract surgery.

Preoperative and Postoperative Care

Preoperative assessment of a patient with cataracts should include a complete ophthalmic examination, measurement of the eyes for intraocular lens selection, a discussion of the preferred surgical technique and type of intraocular lens, and a discussion of the risks and benefits of the procedure. Withholding systemic anticoagulation should be discussed with the patient's internist. For most cataract surgeries where anesthesia is largely topical, anticoagulation cessation is not necessary, but the

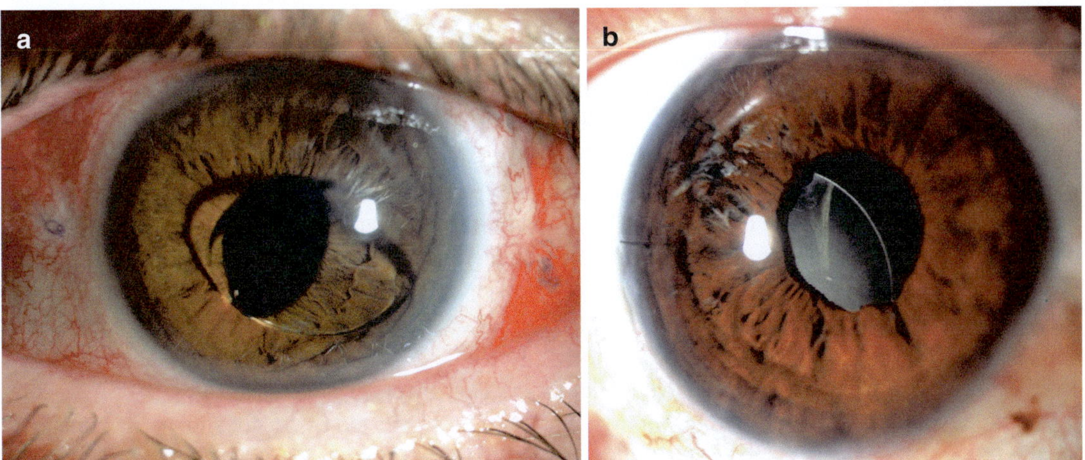

Fig. 11.10 (**a**, **b**): (**a**) Recent postoperative photos showing lens capture within the pupil and (**b**) IOL inferior dislocation. Post-surgical iris atrophy is seen from 9:00 to 10:30

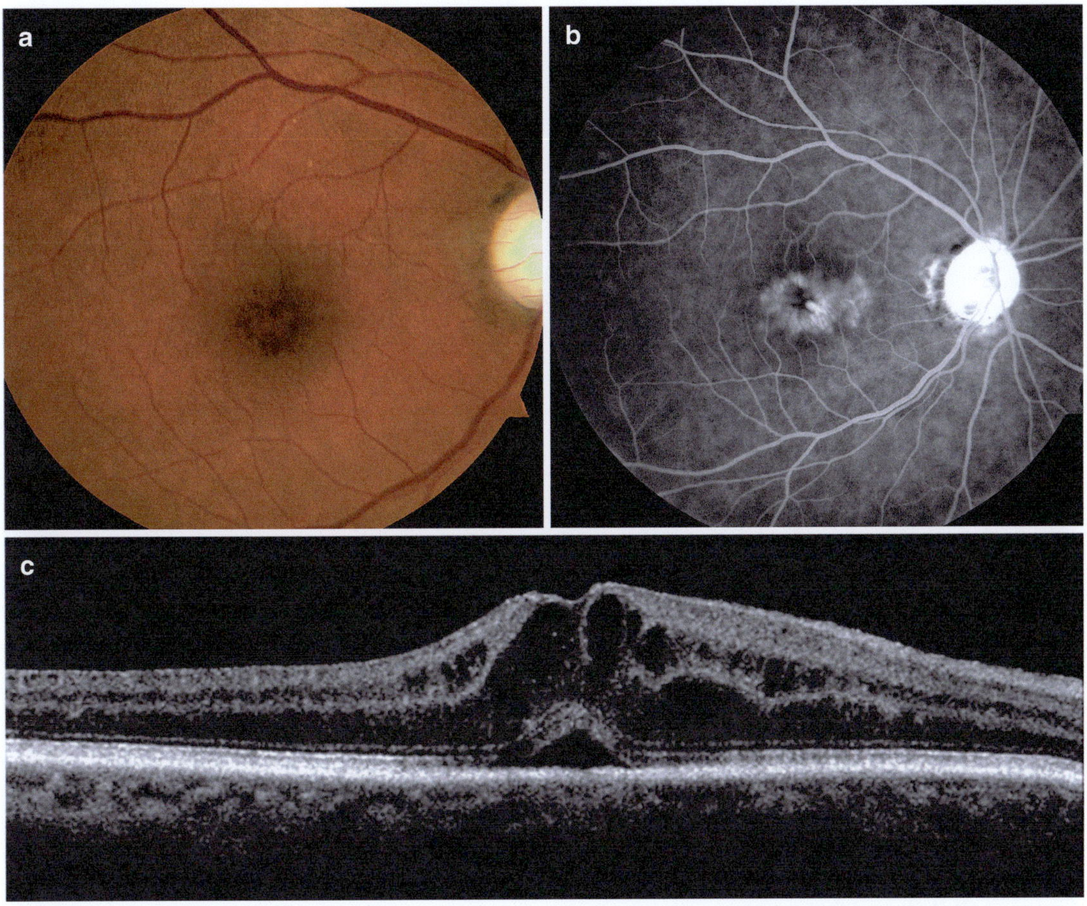

Fig. 11.11 Case of 84 years old woman, 5-week post-uncomplicated cataract removal, with cystoid macular edema. (**a**) Fundus image; (**b**) fluorescein angiography showing classic petalloid leakage of dye into the central macula; (**c**) optical coherence tomography showing cystic foveal edema and distortion

decision should be made on a case-by-case basis. Following cataract extraction, the patient's eye is protected with a plastic shield and may be briefly patched if the patient received deeper ocular anesthesia. Topical antibiotic and corticosteroid therapy is often initiated right after surgery and usually maintained for a period of 1–4 weeks. Some patients are also placed on topical nonsteroidal therapy if there is a higher risk of macular edema. Patients are usually seen the first postoperative day, when the shield and/or patch are removed and then again 1 and 4 weeks after surgery. Visual rehabilitation with a new corrective lens prescription, if required, is usually achieved 4–6 weeks following surgery. Variations in the timing of the final refractive correction depend largely on the healing response of the individual patient.

Pediatric Cataract

Considerations Peculiar to the Child with Cataract

Pediatric cataracts are a treatable cause of potentially lifelong visual impairment. In contrast to the more common adult cataracts, pediatric cataracts can profoundly affect neurodevelopment, education, and economic security in young adulthood and beyond. The projected lifetime risk of vision loss in the non-amblyopic eye for an individual with amblyopia is at least 1.2% (Rahi et al. 2002), so a significant number of adults with untreated pediatric cataract can be expected to experience a decline in quality of life and independence later in life.

Between 1 and 15 per 10,000 children are affected by pediatric cataract worldwide, a range reflecting population heterogeneity and varying definitions. Between 1 and 3 per 10,000 children are affected in more developed countries where communities tend to be less insular and public health interventions such as the rubella vaccination program are successfully implemented.

Types of Childhood Cataracts

A classification of childhood cataracts is presented in Table 11.3. The number and diversity of associated conditions is noted. Primary cataracts are genetic or developmental in origin; many are associated with a metabolic disorder or syndrome. They may be present during infancy or appear later in childhood. At the time of this writing, more than 70 genes have been associated with childhood cataract, and many can be efficiently screened with gene chips. Secondary cataracts are acquired and indicate an external process that interfered with early development of the crystalline lens or later damaged a normal lens.

The onset of cataract development in a child may be suggested by the location and appearance of the lens opacity. Blemishes affecting posterior lens fibers and capsule can be transparent upon delivery and remain undetected until opacification develops. After birth, the crystalline lens continues to enlarge and gradually, over decades, acquires features of the adult lens. Common adult cataracts – nuclear, subcapsular, and cortical – typically reflect aging and toxic or metabolic influences on lens fibers rather than delayed effects of early lens maldevelopment.

Associated Ocular Pathologies

Congenital cataract may be the most conspicuous feature of a more generalized ocular malformation. When cataract is present in only one eye at birth, the affected eye is often smaller than the unaffected eye. Asymmetries of iris stroma and musculature may range in severity and result in asymmetries of eye color, stromal texture and color, and pupil characteristics. If the posterior segment is also involved and the retina or optic disc is severely malformed, the visual potential of the affected eye may be limited.

Congenital cataracts are often associated with nystagmus, and visual acuity in eyes with nystagmus is typically worse than in eyes without nystagmus. Risk factors for nystagmus include visually significant bilateral cataract, eyes that are small, and eyes with concurrent anatomic abnormalities such as foveal or optic nerve dysplasia. Nystagmus associated with congenital cataracts typically appears by 2–3 months of age and is not necessarily prevented by early cataract surgery. It rarely occurs in children who develop cataracts at older ages.

Table 11.3 Abbreviated table for primary and secondary childhood cataracts

I. Primary (genetic) cataracts
  A. Inherited without systemic abnormalities
    1. Autosomal dominant (various types)
    2. X-linked
    3. Autosomal recessive (rare)
  B. Chromosomal abnormalities (examples)
    1. Trisomy 21 (Down's syndrome)
    2. Trisomy 13 (Patau's syndrome)
  C. Metabolic disorders (examples)
    1. Galactosemia
      a. Transferase deficiency
      b. Kinase deficiency
    2. Hypocalcemia
    3. Hypoglycemia
    4. Diabetes mellitus
    5. Fabry's disease
    6. Mannosidosis
    7. Zellweger's syndrome
  D. Systemic syndromes/diseases (examples)
    1. Skeletal
      a. Albright's disease
      b. Chondrodysplasia punctata
      c. Majewski's syndrome
      d. Myotonic dystrophy
      e. Osteogenesis imperfecta
    2. Dermatological
      a. Atopic dermatitis
      b. Cockayne syndrome
      c. Congenital ichthyosis
      d. Incontinentia pigmenti
      e. Rothmund-Thomson syndrome
      f. Ectodermal dysplasia of Marshall
    3. Central nervous system
      a. Laurence-Moon-Bardet-Biedl
      b. Marinesco-Sjögren
      c. Sjögren-Larsen syndrome
      d. Neurofibromatosis type 2
    4. Craniofacial
      a. Hallermann-Streiff syndrome
      b. Pierre Robin syndrome
      c. Alport's syndrome
      d. Crouzon's syndrome
      e. Smith-Lemli-Opitz
    5. Multisystem
      a. Noonan's syndrome
      b. Werner's syndrome
      c. Lowe's syndrome
      d. LEOPARD syndrome
  E. Ocular diseases
    1. Persistent fetal vasculature
    2. Posterior lenticonus
    3. Retrolental fibroplasia
    4. Uveitis, especially JIA
    5. Aniridia
    6. Retinal degeneration syndromes
    7. Wagner's vitreoretinal degeneration
    8. Gyrate atrophy
    9. Endophthalmitis
    10. Retinoblastoma
    11. Phthisis bulbi (Norrie disease)
    12. Acute glaucoma
    13. Intraocular foreign body
    14. Associated with ectopia lentis
      1. Marfan syndrome
      2. Homocystinuria
      3. Weill-Marchesani syndrome
      4. Hyperlysinemia
      5. Ectopia lentis et pupillae

II. Secondary (acquired) cataracts
  A. Intrauterine infections
    1. Maternal rubella syndrome
    2. Severe toxoplasmosis
    3. HSV infection
    4. Maternal varicella syndrome
    5. CMV
  B. Trauma
    1. Cesarean section
    2. Child abuse
    3. Cataracts of prematurity
      a. Transient
      b. Laser for ROP complication
    4. Blunt or penetrating trauma
    5. Electrical injury
    6. Radiation induced
    7. Chronic head banging
    8. Glaucoma surgery
      1. Cyclocryotherapy
      2. Trabeculectomy
      3. Goniotomy
      4. Tube shunt
    9. Vitrectomy
  C. Drug induced
    1. Steroids (topical or systemic)
    2. ACTH

Early Detection

Detection of congenital cataract largely occurs in the nursery or primary care setting by inspection (Fig. 11.12) or an abnormal red pupillary light reflex (Fig. 11.13). The red reflex is assessed with a direct ophthalmoscope, and comparison is made between eyes. The clinician's past experiences observing red reflexes, visual behaviors and measured acuities, other observations, and

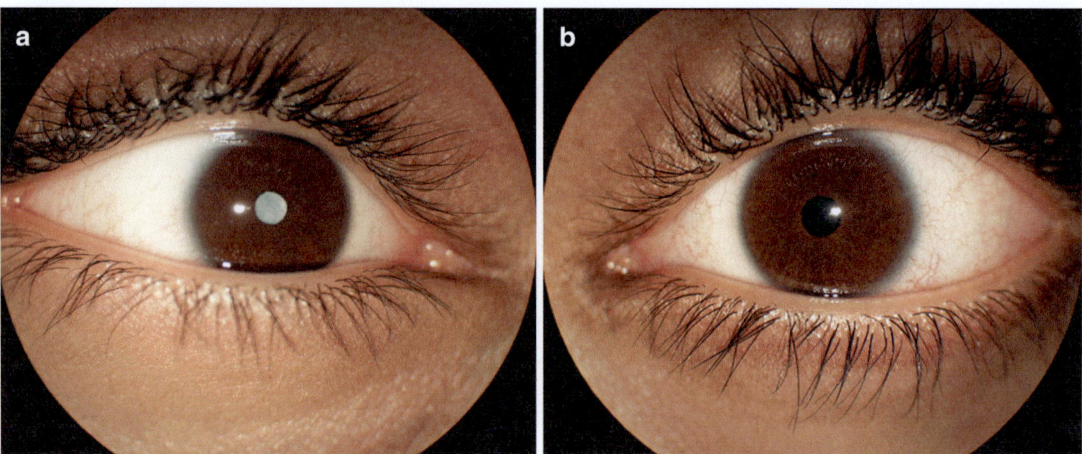

Fig. 11.12 Opacification of the anterior crystalline lens is often visible by inspection. (**a**) Right eye cataract. (**b**) Clear left pupil

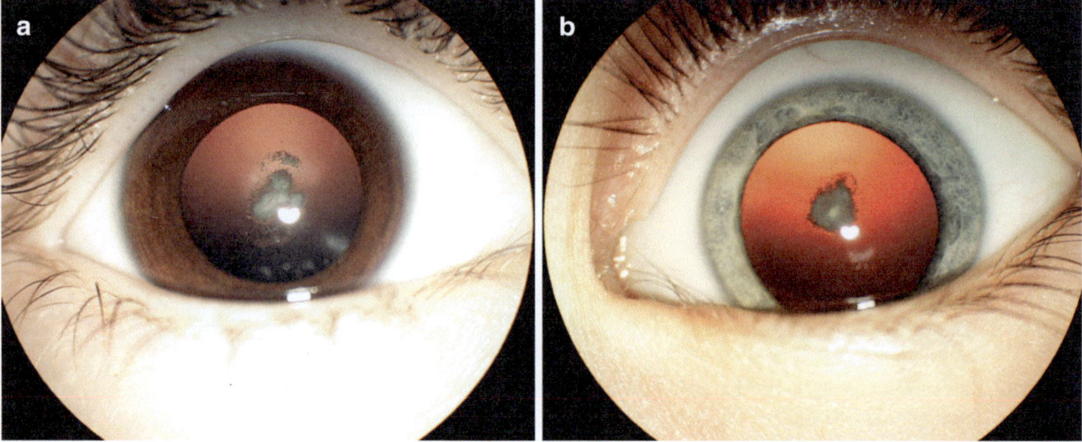

Fig. 11.13 Some central and posterior lens opacities are more clearly appreciated against the red pupillary light reflex as in this case of bilateral posterior lenticonus. (**a**) Right eye. (**b**) Left eye

parental concerns aid interpretation. If a red reflex is obscured by miosis despite dim ambient light, a subsequent attempt may be more successful later during the visit. Occasionally a parent will bring a photograph that documents a pupillary abnormality on one or both sides (Fig. 11.14). Suspicion of pathology should be heightened if other anomalies are present, such as strabismus, a smaller-than-normal cornea or pupil, a displaced or distorted pupil, unusual iris color, nystagmus, or if there is family history of childhood cataract. Leukocoria (Table 11.4) has many causes in addition to cataract, some ominous, and many with posterior segment pathology. Because early detection is vitally important for successful treatment of conditions such as retinoblastoma and cataract, immediate referral and prompt ophthalmic examination are warranted if any of these conditions is suspected.

Assessment of Vision in Children with Lens Opacities

When a cataract is found, careful ophthalmic examination is required to assess visual significance. This determination in a preverbal child is based on visual behavior and the size, density,

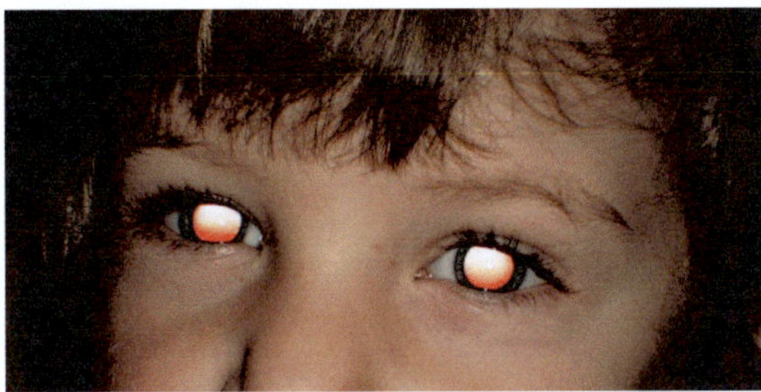

Fig. 11.14 Cameras with closely spaced flash and aperture can produce red eye that can detect abnormality of the ocular media. Not all abnormal red reflexes indicate cataract; this child has bilateral leukocoria due to large colobomas of each ocular fundus. In this case the large area of exposed white sclera around each optic disc is magnified by the eye's optics to create these pupillary appearances

Table 11.4 Common leukocoria causes

Cataract
Retinoblastoma
Coats disease
Persistent fetal vasculature
Ocular toxocariasis
Familial exudative vitreoretinopathy
Retinopathy of prematurity
Astrocytic hamartoma
Vitreous hemorrhage
Coloboma
Endogenous endophthalmitis
Rhegmatogenous retinal detachment

and location of the lens opacity. Strabismus, resistance to occlusion of preferred eye, asymmetric visual behaviors, visual acuity in one or both eyes that lags behind the normal range for age, and inability to visualize the fundus with a direct ophthalmoscope through an undilated pupil all strongly suggest visual impairment. Opacities that are 3 mm across or larger are almost always visually significant; smaller opacities may also be visually significant, particularly if in sensitive locations or if surrounding lens tissue is clear but distorted, effectively enlarging the opacity (Fig. 11.15a). Axial opacities are the most significant, particularly when the nucleus, posterior lens fibers, or posterior capsule are involved. When cataract precludes visualization of the ocular fundus, sonography is indicated to look for potentially occult posterior segment pathology. Depending on these assessments, the child may be initially observed, treated with spectacles or patching, or offered early surgery.

Amblyopia (see Chap. 39)

Amblyopia compounds visual loss from ocular disease during childhood. Without concurrent amblyopia treatment, benefits from the best med-

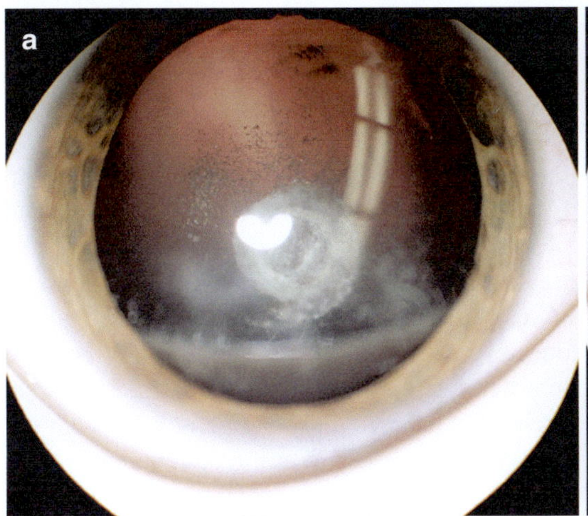
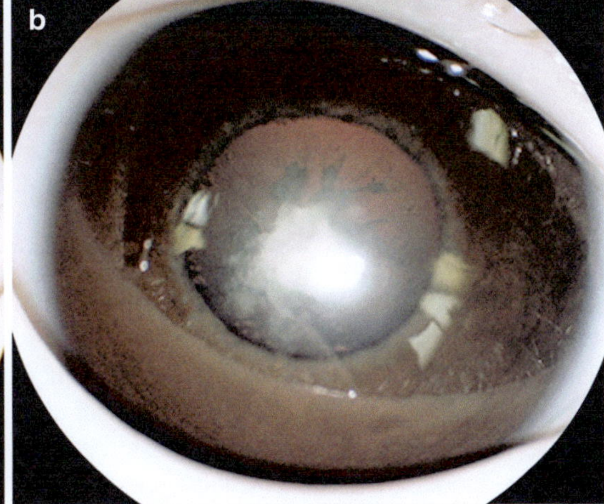

Fig. 11.15 (**a**) This child with unilateral posterior lentiglobus was found to have 20/800 visual acuity on the left at 2.5 years. The opacity is paraxial with adjacent distortion of the most central lens tissue. Central lens tissue must have been clearer and permitted good visual devel- opment during infancy since she had 20/40 at the conclusion of amblyopia therapy. (**b**) This boy with bilateral axial membranous cataract due to Lowe's syndrome would not have the opportunity to develop good visual acuity without early lensectomies

ical and surgical therapies may not result in visual improvement. Deprivation amblyopia, a particularly profound amblyopia, is commonly associated with congenital cataracts.

For useful vision to be obtained, the window of opportunity to recognize and begin treatment for unilateral congenital cataract is brief, typically spanning only the first few months of life. Deprivation-related ocular dominance changes in the visual cortex can become permanent if allowed to establish without challenge (Wiesel and Hubel, 1965). The window of opportunity to recognize and treat bilateral congenital cataract is longer, typically spanning a few to several months or more, depending on cataract characteristics. Nuclear and large axial posterior lens opacities often require earlier surgery (Fig. 11.15b). Small anterior polar and lamellar cataracts can permit surprisingly good visual development and may only require observation until cataract growth begins to degrade acuity, sometimes years later or never.

Virtually all children with visually significant unilateral cataract develop strabismus and impaired stereopsis. Strabismus typically persists despite early lensectomy and dedicated optical rehabilitation. Most children with visually significant bilateral cataract also develop strabismus and amblyopia.

Surgery

With rare exception, such as early cataract due to galactosemia, cataract in children is not reversible, and surgery may be needed. Biomechanical properties of the eye differ between child and adult. In children, eyes are small, growing, and the ocular coats and intraocular tissues are elastic and soft. In adults, eyes are large, fully grown, and ocular coats and intraocular tissues are less distensible. Relatively large incisions in an adult's eye can self-seal and not require suturing, whereas smaller incisions in a child's eye may leak without suturing. Increased tissue elasticity and wound instability can make control of fluid dynamics significantly more challenging in a child's eye.

The lens epithelium typically has a soft, liquid consistency in childhood, despite the optical density of the opacity, in contrast to the firm, sclerotic consistency in adulthood. Surgical approaches thereby vary according to age. In a child's eye, the elastic lens capsule can be opened, and the lens nucleus and cortex aspirated through a 1 mm incision with a suction-cutting instrument (vitrector), whereas in an older adult's eye, the nucleus must first be emulsified with ultrasound (phacoemulsification) or laser energy through a 2–3 mm incision before it can be aspirated.

Surgery for pediatric cataract, like most ophthalmic surgical procedures in children, is performed under general anesthesia. A patch and shield may be applied at the conclusion of surgery and either a protective shield or spectacles worn after the patch is removed. Postoperative care typically includes application of a topical antibiotic, a topical steroid, and a mydriatic for several days. Occasionally systemic anti-inflammatory medications are also given.

Optical Rehabilitation of Pediatric Aphakia

The eye of a child grows and changes rapidly during the first 2–3 years, particularly in the first several months, whereas the eye of an adult changes little in axial length and corneal curvature, the major determinants of refraction. If the third determinant of refraction, the crystalline lens (see Chap. 7), is removed, compensation or optical rehabilitation is needed for images to focus properly on the retina. In adulthood and older children, a permanent intraocular lens implant is almost always placed. In infants, a static intraocular lens implant may not be placed during this period of rapid eye growth because long-term refractive goals may be impossible to accurately achieve and may be at odds with the more pressing needs of amblyopia therapy.

Spectacles or contact lenses can well compensate bilateral aphakia, and a single contact lens can well compensate unilateral aphakia in young children. The powers of these devices can be easily adjusted according to eye growth and the child's expanding visual world. Bifocals, either traditional or progressive, are often added around the time a child begins to walk to enable clearer vision of both near and far stimuli. If the prescription of an intraocular lens implant is chosen for emmetropia at a young age, significant myopia will develop by adulthood (McClatchey and Parks 1997). Accurately predicting how much an eye will grow, and choosing a lens implant for a very young child to accurately achieve emmetropia in adulthood, are not currently possible and may not be optimal for amblyopia therapy.

Pediatric ophthalmologists have debated whether visual outcome would be better with an intraocular lens implant than with a contact lens for infants with cataract. Some theoretical arguments predicting less aniseikonia and risk of aphakic glaucoma supported the use of lens implants. Success with more conservative methods of optical rehabilitation and the surgical difficulties of intraocular lens implantation argued against their use. The Infant Aphakia Treatment Study Group (2014) followed two groups of children who underwent unilateral cataract surgery during their first 6 months of life. One group received an intraocular lens implant and the other group a contact lens for optical rehabilitation. Both groups have been followed for years. Subsequent acuities, sensory outcomes, and incidences of strabismus and aphakic glaucoma were found equivalent, so the theoretical advantages of intraocular lens implantation were not realized. The group that received an intraocular lens implant had more postoperative complications and required significantly more additional surgeries. Because a clear benefit for primary intraocular lens implantation at the time of surgery for congenital cataract was not identified, most pediatric ophthalmologists now use contact lenses or spectacles after early lensectomy and avoid intraocular lens implantation until a child is at least 2–3 years old or if the initial method of optical rehabilitation fails.

Choices to minimize dependency on spectacles with techniques such as monovision, multifocal contact lens wear, refractive surgery, and toric and multifocal lens implants can sometimes be appropriate according to age and need.

Amblyopia Therapy

Recognition and treatment of amblyopia are discussed in Chap. 39. Care for the child with cataract is a subset of the treatment of amblyopia that often begins with optical rehabilitation as discussed above.

Amblyopia treatment for the child with bilateral cataract and superimposed strabismus can be challenging, particularly at older ages when patching can be refused. Since accommodation is not possible after cataract surgery, pharmacological penalization with atropine drops to paralyze accommodation and blur vision in the preferred eye is not an effective option. If bilateral contact lenses are or could be used, withholding the contact lens from the preferred eye for the desired amount of time each day may be an effective alternative to occlusive patching.

Amblyopia treatment for the child with unilateral cataract can be challenging for similar reasons and because the preferred eye can also accommodate, another reason to dominate the cataractous eye. Patching may be needed nearly throughout the child's first decade. Unfortunately, waiting to patch until a child is sufficiently old enough to understand its purpose is not possible if the best visual outcome is desired. The dominant eye is often patched for one hour per month of life and up to ½ or more of waking hours. Acuities are monitored to document improvement in amblyopia without the development of deprivation amblyopia in the dominant eye.

If a child frequently falls asleep, becomes reclusive, or fails to demonstrate improvement despite adequate amblyopia treatment, the amblyopia may be too deeply seated to justify continued patching.

Monitoring Visual Acuity After Cataract Surgery

Long-term ophthalmic follow-up is indicated following any intraocular surgery in children. The most useful method to test acuity in a child will vary according to age. Different acuity tests may not measure the same parameters of visual function and cannot be simply converted from one to another or easily compared. Furthermore, the range of normal responses may vary for the young child according to the type of test, age, and particular abilities. Frequent refraction and changes in spectacle or contact lens prescriptions may be necessary to optimize, and possibly determine, the best treatment program for a particular child. Acuities in infants and toddlers are typically assessed by visual behaviors, signs of binocularity, refractions, and general ocular health. Recognition acuities can typically be obtained beginning at 3 years and with Snellen line letters beginning at 5 years.

Late Complications of Pediatric Cataract Surgery

The lens capsule is typically used to support an intraocular lens implant, both at the time of cataract surgery in older children and adults and years after cataract surgery in very young children with aphakia. Because the lens and other ocular structures grow rapidly during early childhood, lens capsule and epithelium are more reactive in a child's eye than in an adult's eye. If the posterior capsule is left intact at the time of cataract surgery in a child, it virtually always thickens and opacifies within months to years, eventually becoming another source of visual deprivation and amblyopia. Because of this concern, the posterior capsule may be opened in the child's eye during cataract surgery (Fig. 11.16) with or without primary intraocular lens implantation but left intact in an adult's eye where it may remain clear and require no further management or may be easily opened with a YAG laser capsulotomy procedure in the office. Lens epithelial cells lining the anterior capsule actively divide during early childhood. Despite meticulous aspiration during pediatric cataract surgery, if anterior capsule is left, microscopic clusters of these cells remain and proliferate on the lens capsule, intraocular lens implant, and vitreous face. Globular excrescences called Elschnig pearls (Fig. 11.17) can form due to this epithelial proliferation and can be seen along the pupillary margin or within the

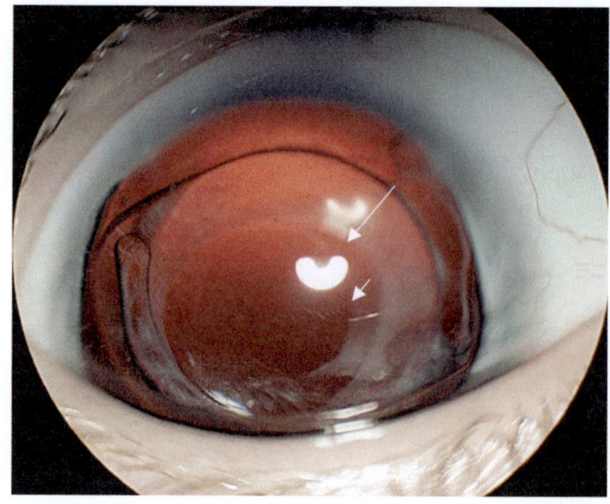

Fig. 11.16 An Alcon AcrySof lens implant can be seen in its entirety in a child with congenital absence of the iris (aniridia). The implant is located within the capsular bag. The anterior and posterior capsules are mildly hazy except where central apertures were created: anterior capsulotomy, long arrow, posterior capsulotomy, short arrow

pupil. This postoperative complication may be a risk factor for developing aphakic glaucoma and requires treatment such as additional vitrectomy or YAG laser ablation if the visual axis becomes obstructed. Alteration of the red reflex may signify this development and may initially be noted in the primary care setting.

Retinal detachment can develop after childhood cataract surgery, particularly in the presence of associated posterior segment disease such as persistent fetal vasculature, retinopathy of prematurity, and ocular trauma. As instrumentation has improved, the incidence of retinal detachment has decreased but not been eliminated. This complication may also alter the red reflex and be detected in the primary care setting.

Glaucoma is often associated with childhood cataract and its surgery. Topical steroids are commonly prescribed after ophthalmic surgery to reduce inflammation and increase patient comfort. A topical steroid, particularly if given with high frequency, can cause elevated eye pressure (steroid-induced glaucoma) as quickly as 2–3 days after the onset of treatment. Once the lens is removed, adhesions can develop between residual lens tissue and iris, resulting in alteration of the normal aqueous outflow

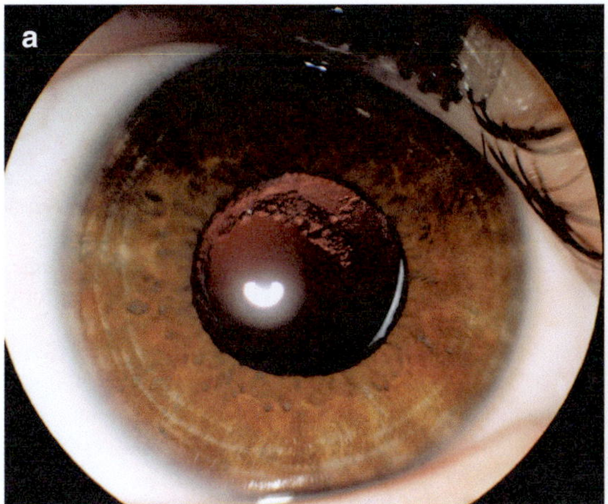

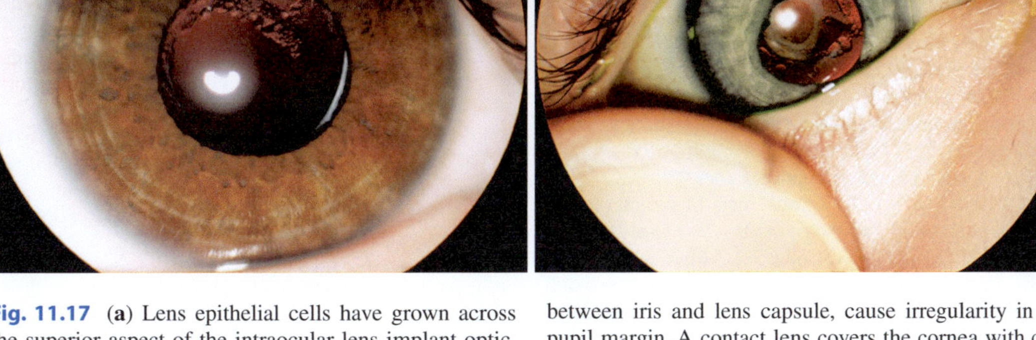

Fig. 11.17 (**a**) Lens epithelial cells have grown across the superior aspect of the intraocular lens implant optic. (**b**) Lens epithelial cells have proliferated within the capsular bag in this eye with aphakia and only a small central aperture surrounded by a white annulus due to lens capsule contraction remains. Posterior synechiae, adhesions between iris and lens capsule, cause irregularity in the pupil margin. A contact lens covers the cornea with central optical element. Despite the proliferation of lens epithelial cells and formation of partial opacities known as Elschnig pearls, neither eye has a visually significant secondary cataract that would require further surgery

pathway. Pupillary block by posterior synechia or vitreous can result in acute angle closure glaucoma soon after lensectomy or years later; this complication, which may present with headache, emesis, and abdominal pain, can be mistaken for migraine or a gastrointestinal disturbance, delaying diagnosis and leading to catastrophic visual loss. Symptoms of headache and vomiting should garner particular attention in the context of prior ophthalmic surgery, prompting immediate ophthalmic examination and, if indicated, urgent surgery to resolve a pupillary block. Prophylactic peripheral iridectomy at the time of cataract surgery can be protective (Fig. 11.18).

Aphakic or pseudophakic glaucoma may develop months to decades after surgery. The incidence of aphakic glaucoma varies widely across the literature; a 10–40% likelihood is typically quoted to parents. If children are followed well into adulthood, the total incidence of aphakic glaucoma becomes much higher. Children at greatest risk are those who are younger than 6 months at the time of cataract surgery. This glaucoma can have the typical signs and symptoms of primary congenital glaucoma if onset is within the first 2–3 years of life. When onset occurs at older ages, the child may be asymptom-

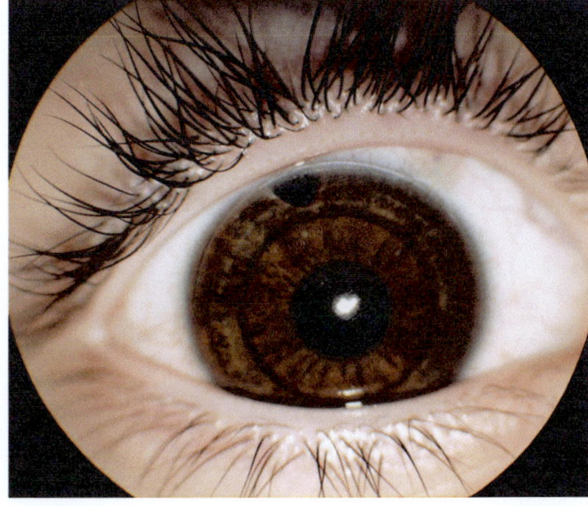

Fig. 11.18 This eye has aphakia following recent lensectomy. A peripheral iridectomy, a secondary opening in peripheral iris, is seen at 11:00. A contact lens covers the cornea with central optical element

atic until central vision declines because of glaucomatous optic atrophy. Aphakic glaucoma typically requires surgical intervention with trabeculectomy or a tube shunt to control eye pressure.

Given the scope of potential late complications, lifelong ophthalmic care for children with cataract is mandatory.

Suggested Reading

Adult Cataract

Cataract Management Guideline Panel. Clinical practice guidelines (4): cataracts in adults: management of functional impairment. AHCPR publication no. 93-0542. Rockville: US Department of Health & Human Services; 1993.

Grewal DS, Schultz T, Basti S, Dick HB. Femtosecond laser-assisted cataract surgery- current status and future directions. Surv Ophthalmol. 2016;61(2):103–31.

https://www.nei.nih.gov/eyedata/cataract

Lee CM, Afshari NA. The global state of cataract blindness. Curr Opin Ophthalmol. 2017;28(1):98–103.

Olson RJ, Braga-Mele R, Chen SH, Miller KM, Pineda R, Tweeten JP, Musch DC. Cataract in the adult eye preferred practice pattern. Ophthalmology. 2017;124(2):120–43.

Thompson J, Lakhani N. Cataracts. Prim Care. 2015; 42(3):409–23.

Pediatric Cataract

Infant Aphakia Treatment Study Group. Comparison of contact lens and intraocular lens correction of monocular aphakia during infancy: a randomized clinical trial of HOTV optotype acuity at age 4.5 years and clinical findings at age 5 years. JAMA Ophthalmol. 2014;132(6):676–82.

McClatchey SK, Parks MM. Theoretic refractive changes after lens implantation in childhood. Ophthalmology. 1997;104(11):1744–51.

Rahi JS, Logan S, Timms C, Russell-Iggitt I, Taylor D. Risks, causes, and outcomes of visual impairment after loss of vision in the non-amblyopic eye: a population-based study. Lancet. 2002;360(9333): 597–602.

WHO. 2010. https://www.who.int/blindness/causes/priority/en/index1.html

Wiesel T, Hubel D. Comparison of the effects of unilateral and bilateral eye closure on cortical unit responses in kittens. J Neurophysiol. 1965;28:1029–40.

Corneal Trauma, Infection, and Opacities

12

Jonathan Fay and Leejee H. Suh

Corneal Abrasion, Laceration, and Foreign Body

The cornea and conjunctiva comprise the surface structures of the eye. They are in direct contact with the outside world and, as such, are susceptible to a particular set of injuries from exposure or trauma. Indeed, approximately 2.4 million eye injuries occur in the United States each year resulting in approximately 630,000 emergency room visits. Nearly half of the injuries occur at home, and the majority occur in patients age 44 years and younger. Corneal abrasion, a foreign body in the eye, and blunt trauma are common types of eye injury.

Many features of the face and orbit protect the eye from injury. The bony orbit protrudes beyond the surface of the eye, protecting it from direct impact by large objects. The eye is also suspended within the orbit, cushioned by orbital fat. Eyelids and eyelashes act as physical barriers to the outside world and, along with the blink reflex, protect the globe from many oncoming threats. Tears bathe the ocular surface with nutrients and immune factors but also trap and sweep away small particles.

Understanding the anatomy of the surface of the eye is critical for the clinician to accurately assess the severity and prognosis of an ocular injury. The corneal stroma is comprised mostly of collagen, and the clarity of the cornea is in large part due to the highly organized structure of the collagen lamellae. Disruption of the corneal stroma caused by a laceration, for example, disrupts the lamellae, resulting in scar formation, opacification of the cornea, and potentially a loss of vision (Fig. 12.1a–f). Overlying the corneal stroma is Bowman's layer of condensed collagen and, finally, a layer of stratified squamous epithelium. The epithelium is adherent to the stroma by hemidesmosomes. Even minor trauma to the corneal surface, especially with accompanying shearing force, causes epithelial cells to separate from their underlying attachments. Epithelial disruption is known as a corneal abrasion. Fortunately, if underlying the corneal stroma is not damaged, the epithelium will regenerate without scar formation and normal visual acuity will be restored.

Clinical Signs and Findings

A corneal abrasion is the loss of part or all of the corneal epithelium without injury to the underlying stroma; a corneal laceration occurs when the deeper corneal stroma is disrupted (Fig. 12.2). If the cause

J. Fay, MD
Klamath Eye Center, Klamath Falls, OR, USA

L. H. Suh, MD (✉)
Columbia University Irving Medical Center, New York, NY, USA

Department of Ophthalmology, Edward S. Harkness Eye Institute, Columbia University Vagelos College of Physicians and Surgeons, New York, NY, USA
e-mail: lhs2118@cumc.columbia.edu

© Springer Nature Switzerland AG 2019
D. S. Casper, G. A. Cioffi (eds.), *The Columbia Guide to Basic Elements of Eye Care*,
https://doi.org/10.1007/978-3-030-10886-1_12

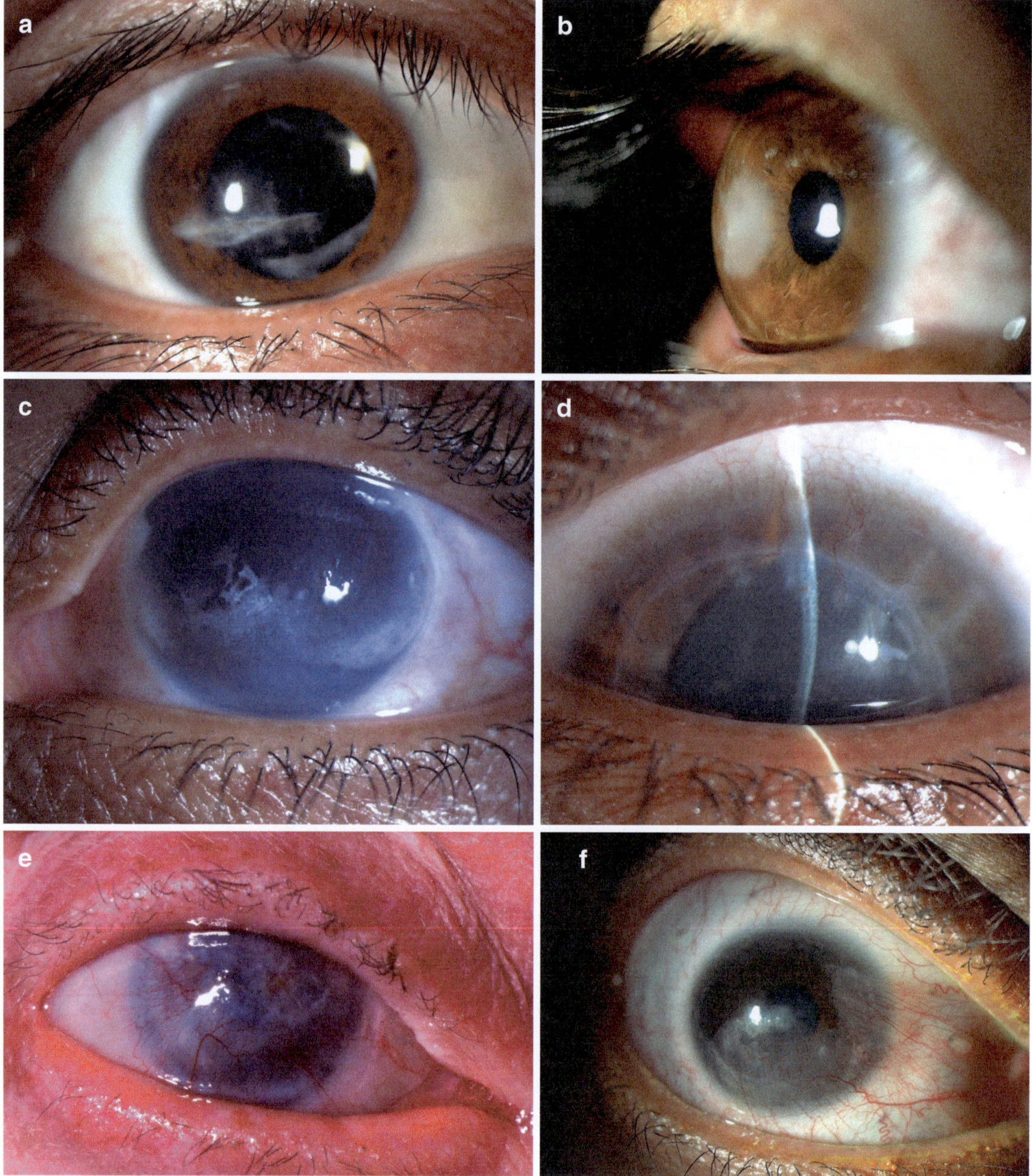

Fig. 12.1 (**a**) Scar formation after corneal laceration. (**b**) Corneal scar after ulcer formation of unclear etiology in a patient with inflammatory bowel disease. (**c**) Band keratopathy. (**d**) Post-corneal transplant (penetrating keratoplasty) with pannus and scarring at wound interface and suture lines. (**e**) Severe lid and corneal scarring with pannus after chemical burn. (**f**) Scleritis and scarring associated with rheumatoid arthritis. (**g**) A 61-year-old man who had bilateral radial keratotomies performed to correct myopia in 1990. The linear scars from the procedure are clearly visible. Radial keratotomy, introduced in the 1970s, has been almost entirely replaced with newer surgical refractive procedures

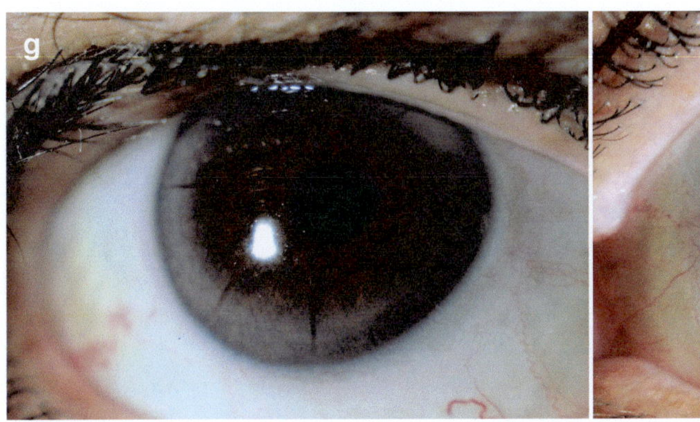
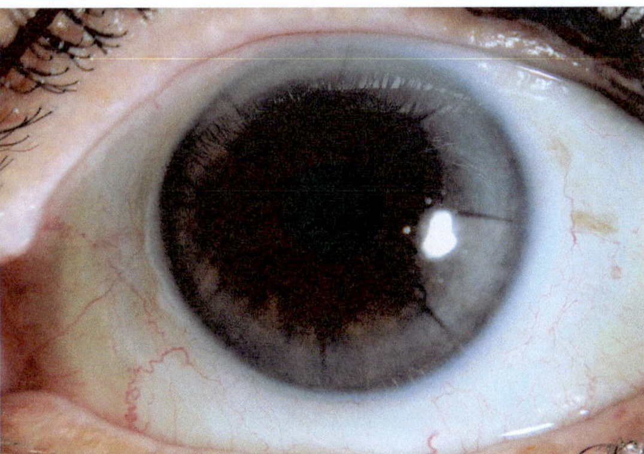

Fig. 12.1 (continued)

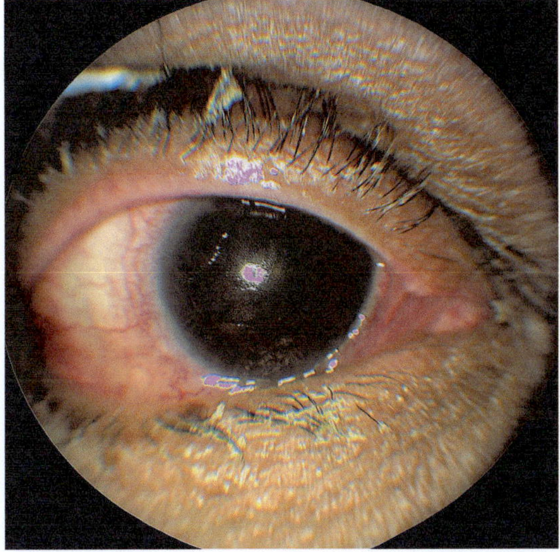

Fig. 12.2 An unstained, large, irregular central corneal abrasion

of injury is a foreign body, for example, a small fleck of metal, it may be retained within the corneal epithelium or stroma. Retained metallic foreign bodies within the cornea often exhibit "rust rings," consisting of oxidized ferrous materials, due to reaction with the overlying tear film, which leach into the surrounding tissue (Fig. 12.3a, b).

An appropriate history is essential to making the correct diagnosis. The patient should be able to report a specific place and time that an injury occurred. Common causes for corneal abrasion include fingernails, paper, makeup applicators, and plants. A retained corneal foreign body is often seen in patients who were grinding, hammering, or working with metal. If the patient is unable to identify a discrete injury, the physician should be concerned about other potentially serious causes for an epithelial defect.

The patient will typically complain of intense pain, photophobia, foreign body sensation, and tearing. They may have difficulty voluntarily opening the affected eye. The pain primarily results from stimulation of exposed nerve endings at the denuded corneal surface. For this reason, instillation of a topical anesthetic drop such as proparacaine or tetracaine can temporarily relieve the discomfort and facilitate carrying out the remainder of the exam.

On examination, the visual acuity of a patient with a corneal abrasion may be decreased if the abrasion disrupts the normally smooth contour of the central corneal surface. The presence of a corneal epithelial defect is best assessed using fluorescein stain and cobalt blue illumination. Ideally, the cornea is evaluated under magnification with the aid of a slit lamp. The examiner should note the extent of any abrasion and be particularly cognizant of any underlying tissue disturbance. Aside from what might be furled or folded edges of epithelium, the de-epithelialized corneal stroma should be smooth and clear. A cotton-

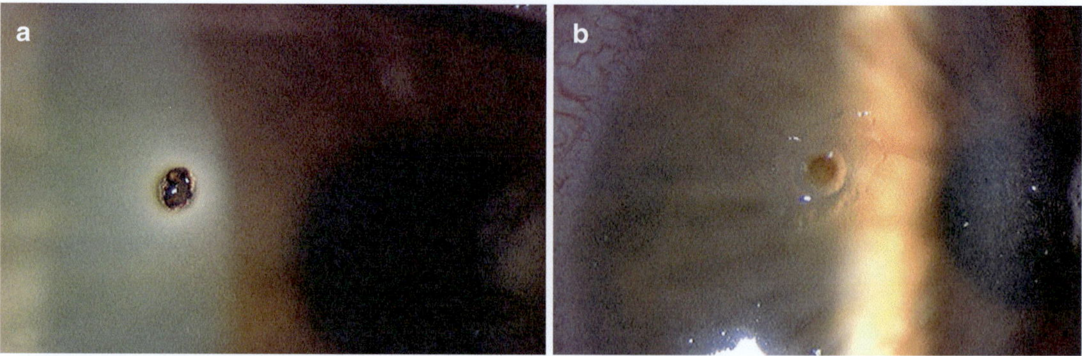

Fig. 12.3 (**a**) Metallic corneal foreign body. (**b**) After removal of the metallic foreign body, a residual rust ring can be seen in the superficial corneal stroma with a small overlying epithelial defect

tipped applicator soaked in topical anesthetic can be used to debride loose epithelium and aid in a careful evaluation. If the denuded area is not smooth, a deeper laceration or perforation of the cornea must be considered, and immediate referral to an ophthalmologist should be made. If the area is not clear, the examiner may assume that a cellular infiltrate has caused opacification of the underlying cornea, and infectious keratitis must be considered, and immediate referral to an ophthalmologist should be made. In evaluating the anterior chamber, the clinician should look for a normal chamber depth, a normal iris, and a round pupil; any disruption of these structures may indicate a perforating injury, with an occult intraocular foreign body presumed to be present. The upper and lower lid should also be everted and examined for presence of any foreign material. A foreign body embedded in the palpebral conjunctiva can result in a vertical corneal abrasion from blinking.

Differential Diagnosis

Corneal abrasions and foreign bodies are usually easily diagnosed in the primary care setting. Entities that present in a similar fashion include infectious keratitis (corneal ulcer), herpes simplex keratitis, recurrent erosion syndrome, ultraviolet keratitis (welder's "burn"), and severe dry eye syndrome. In any patient who wears contact lenses, particularly with overnight lens wear or poor lens hygiene, one must entertain a very high degree of suspicion for infectious keratitis.

Treatment

If a corneal foreign body is present and it is safely determined that the cornea is not perforated, the foreign body should be removed. In general, this should be performed under slit lamp magnification. A superficially embedded foreign body can sometimes be removed with a cotton-tipped applicator alone. However, it is often necessary to use a 25-gauge needle to gently remove the corneal foreign body. If a metallic foreign body has been retained for 12–24 h, a rust ring may form (see above, Fig. 12.3). This can be gently abraded away with a corneal burr while carefully avoiding excessive disruption of the corneal stroma.

A primary concern in the treatment of corneal abrasion and corneal foreign body is the potential for secondary infectious keratitis as this carries a risk of irreversible vision loss. A break in the corneal epithelium from any cause disrupts the normal defense mechanisms against infection. Furthermore, the object that caused the corneal abrasion may introduce infectious microbes directly to the eye, particularly in the case of corneal abrasions caused by fingernails or vegetable matter. For this reason, all patients with a corneal abrasion are started on prophylactic topical antibiotics. In the case of abrasions from organic matter (e.g., tree branches), it is important to monitor the patient for delayed-onset fungal infection.

Proper topical antibiotic selection is important and may not be the same in all cases. For a non-contact lens wearer, topical erythromycin, bacitracin or bacitracin/polymyxin ointment, or polymyxin B/trimethoprim drops are all reasonable options which are commonly used. If the injury was from a fingernail or vegetable matter, a broader spectrum antibiotic, such as a fourth-generation fluoroquinolone, is usually the antibiotic of choice. Similarly, a contact lens wearer should be covered with a fourth-generation fluoroquinolone as well. Antibiotic treatment is typically continued for 5–7 days or until the epithelial defect has resolved.

For large abrasions, a cycloplegic agent (i.e., cyclopentolate 1%) is often used to reduce pain and photophobia secondary to ciliary body spasm. Patching the eye is rarely necessary and is not done if the injury involves fingernails, vegetable matter, or if the patient wears contact lenses, as, in these cases, proliferation of anaerobic infection is a serious consideration, and patching may enhance bacterial growth. Under no circumstance should a patient be sent home with topical anesthetic, as this may cause toxicity to the ocular surface, with delayed epithelial healing. With any abrasion, topical corticosteroids or antibiotic-steroid combinations should also be avoided, due to an associated increased risk of infection and delayed healing.

Follow-up should occur every 1–2 days to assure appropriate healing and resolution and to confirm that no secondary keratitis is present. Contact lens wearers should forgo any contact lens wear for at least 1 week beyond full recovery and the completion of a complete antibiotic course.

Corneal Infection and Ulceration

Corneal ulceration, or ulcerative keratitis, refers to a wide array of conditions which cause damage to the corneal stroma, resulting in loss of tissue and corneal thinning. Most commonly, a corneal ulcer is caused by an infectious agent such as bacteria, fungus, virus, or parasite and is usually associated with an overlying epithelial defect. Noninfectious ulcers can also occur from autoimmune, neurotrophic, toxic, allergic, iatrogenic, and a host of other etiologies. In all cases, ulcerative keratitis is a potentially sight-threatening emergency, and timely diagnosis and management is critical. If left untreated, ulcerative keratitis can not only cause irreversible vision loss but can even result in corneal perforation and loss of the eye. For the primary care physician, early recognition of the signs and findings of ulcerative keratitis is the first step to making an appropriate referral and getting the patient timely, urgent treatment.

Background

An estimated 30,000 cases of microbial keratitis occur in the United States annually. Although the incidence and etiology vary by region, more than half are due to bacterial infection with the remainder being due to fungal, viral, and parasitic infection. Due to the robust natural defense mechanisms of the eye, infectious keratitis rarely occurs in a normal healthy eye with the exception of viral keratitis. Natural defense mechanisms include protection by the eyelids, flushing by the tear film, a barrier to invasion by the corneal epithelium, and immune defenses present in the tear film and cornea. A careful assessment of a patient's risk for infection is therefore a critical step in correctly diagnosing infectious keratitis.

Risk factors for infectious keratitis include any disruption of the normal ocular defenses caused by external factors, ocular surface disease, and systemic disease. Likely the most common risk factor for infectious keratitis is contact lens wear. Contact lenses of all types predispose the cornea to infection especially when associated with overnight wear, overwear, and poor contact lens hygiene. The clinician should entertain a high degree of suspicion for infectious keratitis for any contact lens wearer who presents with eye redness or pain. Other ocular risk factors include trauma to the ocular surface especially when involving vegetable matter or fingernails, ocular medication use, dry eye disease, prior eye surgery including LASIK or corneal transplant, prior eyelid surgery, improper closure of the eyelids (e.g., in Bell's palsy or ectropion of the eyelid), and neurotrophic keratopathy (Fig. 12.4). Systemic risk factors include Stevens-Johnson syndrome, ocular mucous membrane pemphigoid, diabetes mellitus, immunocompromised status, graft versus host disease, and chronic assisted ventilation status (Table 12.1).

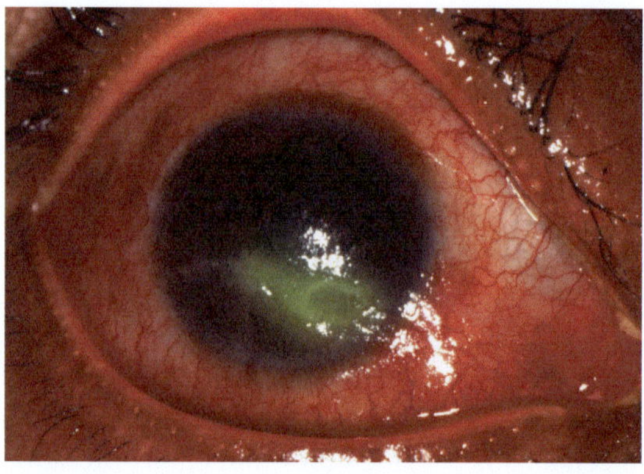

Fig. 12.4 Chronic neurotrophic corneal ulcer in patient with a history of previously excised cerebellopontine angle tumor and secondary trigeminal corneal sensory nerve damage

Table 12.1 Risk factors associated with ulcerative keratitis

Ocular risk factors	Contact lens wear
	Ocular surface trauma
	Ocular medication use
	Dry eye disease
	Prior eye surgery, i.e., corneal transplant
	Improper closure of eyelids
	History of eye infection
Systemic risk factors	Stevens-Johnson syndrome
	Ocular mucous membrane pemphigoid
	Diabetes mellitus
	Immunocompromised status
	Graft versus host disease
	Chronic assisted ventilation status

Presentation/Evaluation

Patients with infectious keratitis generally present with pain and redness, most commonly unilaterally. Photophobia and foreign body sensation are also common features. Decreased vision may occur when an infection involves the central portion of the cornea. Discharge is less common in infection keratitis than in conjunctivitis. Noninfectious ulcerative keratitis may be asymptomatic or minimally symptomatic as in neurotrophic keratitis.

Evaluation begins with a careful history including onset and duration of symptoms. The evaluation should include a careful assessment of risk as mentioned above, including a history of contact lens wear or other potential inciting factors. Past ocular history is also important, in particular a history of prior eye infections, a history of eye surgery especially penetrating keratoplasty or LASIK, and current ocular medications. Topical steroids are a notable risk factor for infectious keratitis. Topical anesthetics or NSAIDs are associated with sterile corneal infiltrates.

An examination for ulcerative keratitis begins with visual acuity and intraocular pressure. Next, an external examination should focus on the face, periorbital skin, and the eyelids. Any defect in eyelid apposition on gentle closure or when blinking should be noted. Next, evaluation of the ocular surface should be performed at the slit lamp for proper magnification and illumination. The examiner should note any injection of the conjunctiva or sclera, and the eyelids can be flipped to exclude an embedded foreign body. Evaluation of the cornea itself should include a careful search for any infiltrate (whiteness or loss of transparency) of the cornea at any level. Evaluation for corneal sensation using the fine strands of a cotton-tipped applicator may be indicated. A topical anesthetic and fluorescein should then be applied to the ocular surface which, under cobalt blue illumination, will highlight a defect in the epithelium, a dendritic ulcer, a foreign body, or a loose suture. Under high magnification, the anterior chamber should be evaluated for cell, flare, or hypopyon (a layered collection of inflammatory cells).

Herpetic keratitis may present with a pathognomonic dendritic ulcer of the epithelium which appears as a branching lesion highlighted by fluorescein stain (Fig. 12.5a, b). Alternatively, herpetic keratitis can present with opacification of the corneal stroma without an epithelial defect or as an endotheliitis resulting in overlying corneal edema and loss of clarity. The appearance of bacterial keratitis is variable; it may present as a discrete circular infiltrate with an overlying epithelial defect or as a highly suppurative lesion with extensive thinning of the cornea (Fig. 12.6). By comparison, fungal keratitis classically presents with feathered edges and satellite lesions (Fig. 12.7). *Acanthamoeba*, a parasite found in tap water, classically presents with a ring-shaped infiltrate and pain out of proportion to the clinical findings. Early Acanthamoeba infections can mimic herpetic keratitis, so a high index of suspicion is necessary. Thinning and ulceration of the

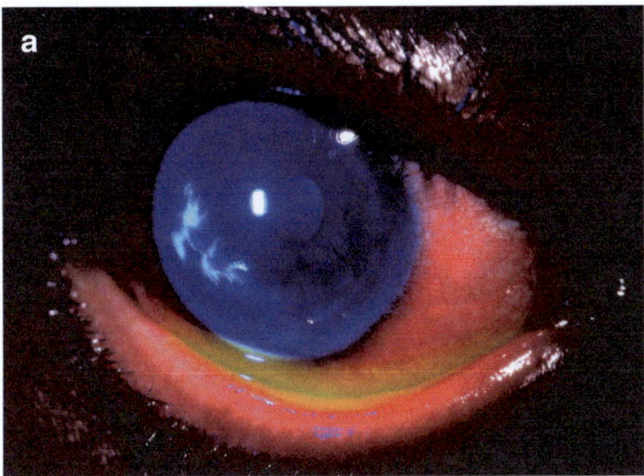

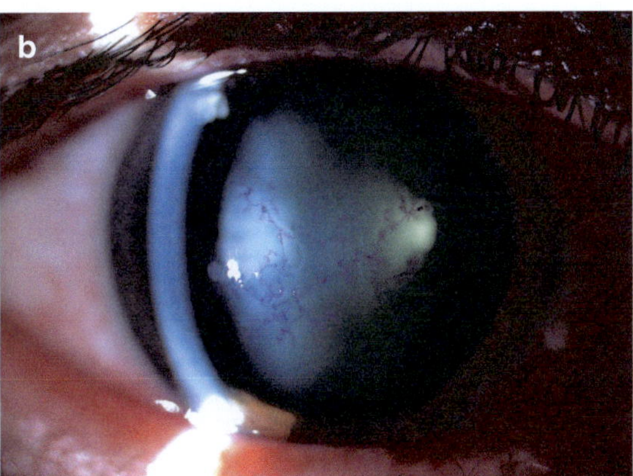

Fig. 12.5 (**a**) Herpes simplex epithelial keratitis, typical dendritic de-epithelialization pattern visualized using fluorescein and a cobalt light. (**b**) Another case of HSV keratitis, with the dendritic pattern revealed using a different vital dye, rose bengal stain

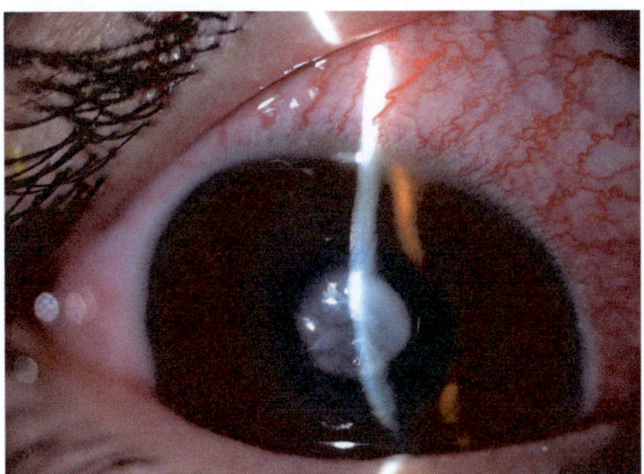

Fig. 12.6 Central corneal ulcer in a diabetic patient with chronic contact lens overwear. Cultures grew out Pseudomonas

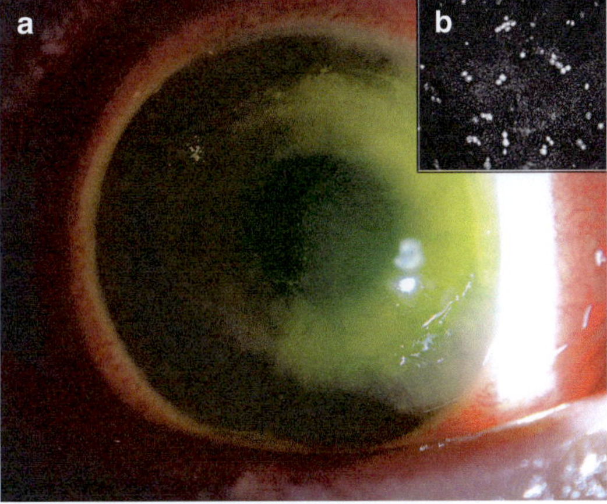

Fig. 12.7 (**a**) A corneal ulcer, suspected of being Acanthamoeba, showing a large central ring ulcer. (**b**) In vivo confocal microscopy of the cornea, seen in inset, revealed Acanthamoeba cysts, confirming the diagnosis; Acanthamoeba eventually grew out in the laboratory

peripheral cornea is seen in peripheral ulcerative keratitis associated with systemic rheumatologic disease.

The differential diagnosis for ulcerative keratitis includes any ocular condition presenting with pain, redness, and photophobia. This includes conjunctivitis (bacterial, allergic, or viral), contact lens-associated keratopathy, corneal abrasion, iritis, chemical injury, corneal foreign body, pterygium, blepharitis, and dry eye syndrome.

Diagnostic Testing

In the appropriate setting, small peripheral ulcers that appear bacterial in nature are often treated empirically with a topical broad-spectrum antibiotic, such as a topical fourth-generation fluoroquinolone. If the infiltrate is central, large, or atypical, however, several diagnostic tests are indicated to aid in diagnosis and management.

Most commonly, gram stain, cultures, and sensitivity testing are performed. Due to the small sample size and specialized techniques, corneal cultures are usually collected and plated by the ophthalmologist directly. The ophthalmologist will use a sterile blade or swab to collect pathologic corneal material which is then inoculated onto a series of culture media including thioglycolate, chocolate agar, blood agar, and Sabouraud agar. After incubation, the cultures may identify the causative organism, and sensitivity testing can guide appropriate therapy. Other diagnostic tests include various smears and stains, corneal biopsy, in vivo confocal microscopy imaging, and PCR.

In the case of noninfectious or inflammatory ulcerative keratitis such as peripheral ulcerative keratitis, systemic testing is mandatory to rule out potentially life-threatening disease. These patients should be evaluated for rheumatoid arthritis, systemic lupus erythematosus, Wegener's granulomatosis (granulomatosis with polyangiitis), polyarteritis nodosa, and sarcoidosis according to clinical judgment.

Etiology

A plethora of microorganisms are implicated in infectious keratitis (Table 12.2). Among bacterial causes, *Pseudomonas* and *Staphylococcus* are the most common in the United States, accounting for approximately 30% of cases each. Fungal keratitis is caused by yeasts, including *Candida*, and filamentous fungi including *Fusarium* and *Aspergillus*. Herpes simplex and herpes zoster are the most common viral etiologies. Acanthamoeba is the most common parasitic keratitis to occur in the United States. Worldwide, Onchocerciasis (river blindness) is a major cause of blindness.

Management/Prevention

As variable as the etiologies of infectious and noninfectious keratitis are, the treatment modalities are numerous. In all cases, however, prompt recognition of the problem and expeditious referral is absolutely critical to treatment success.

Topical antibiotic therapy is generally successful in the treatment of bacterial keratitis. For small peripheral ulcers, the treatment may be a topical fourth-generation fluoroquinolone. For larger or unresponsive bacterial infections, specialty compounded fortified antibiotics including vancomycin, tobramycin, gentamicin, and clindamycin are frequently employed. Dosing

Table 12.2 Common infectious organisms associated with ulcerative keratitis

Bacterial	*Staphylococcus aureus*
	Staphylococcus epidermidis
	Streptococcus pneumoniae
	Pseudomonas aeruginosa
	Enterobacteriaceae
	Serratia marcescens
	Mycobacterium species
Fungal	*Candida* species
	Aspergillus species
	Fusarium species
Viral (more commonly type 1 than type 2)	Herpes simplex (more commonly type 1 than type 2)
	Herpes zoster
Parasitic	*Acanthamoeba*

may be as frequent as every 30 minutes to 1 hour initially and is adjusted according to clinical response. Fungal infections are frequently slower to respond to therapy, but effective antifungals do exist, and fungal keratitis is often successfully treated with topical therapy such as with topical natamycin, voriconazole, and amphotericin. Acanthamoeba is the most difficult to treat, and the available drugs are often associated with significant ocular surface toxicity. In all cases, difficult to treat infectious keratitis has the potential to progress to corneal perforation, endophthalmitis, or extension to the sclera. In these cases, appropriate management may include emergent penetrating corneal transplantation to excise the offending agent, yet even this option is met with significant intraoperative and postoperative complications and morbidity. Systemic and or topical antiviral agents are the mainstay treatment for active herpes viral keratitis. Corticosteroids, topical or systemic, may be used cautiously in select types of ulcerative keratitis.

Risk reduction is another important consideration in the management of ulcerative keratitis. Patients with a history of improper contact lens use or contact lens-related infections should be carefully instructed on proper contact lens use. Patients with eyelid disease should undergo proper protective measures whether it be protection of the ocular surface with lubrication or a bandage contact lens or surgical correction of an eyelid malposition. Patients with systemic rheumatic disease should know to seek medical attention for the signs and symptoms of ulcerative keratitis.

A Final Note

Ulcerative keratitis includes a wide array of disease processes including infectious and noninfectious causes. Risk factor evaluation is important to making the correct diagnosis. Patients suspected to have ulcerative keratitis should be referred to an ophthalmologist promptly as definitive diagnosis and treatment could save the patient's vision or even eye.

Corneal Opacities

Opacities in the corneal and/or conjunctival surface can stem from a variety of etiologies and often cause the chief complaint of foreign body sensation. Patients often feel that "something is in my eye." The cornea, and to a lesser extent, the conjunctiva, is the most highly innervated surface in the body. The cornea contains a vast, dense network of nerve endings within the superficial epithelium. For this reason, drying of the epithelial surface, opacities on and of the cornea, and imbedded particles can all cause foreign body sensation.

Dry eye syndrome is one of the most common ophthalmic conditions seen by eye care specialists. Approximately, 30 million Americans have reported symptoms of dry eye, which include stinging, burning, grittiness, occasional blurry vision, and overall eye discomfort. Dry eye syndrome is more prevalent in the aging population as a result of a decrease in tear production and can be accelerated in autoimmune conditions such as Sjögren's syndrome, rheumatoid arthritis, thyroid disease, etc. Other causes of dry eye include increased exposure of the ocular surface due to incomplete lid closure. Dry eye syndrome is also associated with the use of some medications, contact lens wear, prolonged usage of computer or personal devices, a history of prior corneal surgery like LASIK, and low-humidity work environments. Conditions that affect the composition of the normal tear film, which has layers of aqueous, oil, and mucin, such as inflammation of the eyelids called blepharitis, can also cause dry eye. On examination, there are discrete disruptions of the epithelial surface, also known as superficial punctate keratopathy (SPK) (see Fig. 10.5). Patients with dry eye often undergo a validated symptom questionnaire and special testing in the ophthalmic exam. Rose bengal, lissamine green, and fluorescein staining are used to evaluate epithelial changes. Schirmer testing is used to aqueous tear production by placement of filter paper strips in the lower lid cul-de-sac to measure the amount of tear production. More recently, other assays of tear function, such as tear osmolarity, are being used. Primary therapy includes the use of supplemental topical

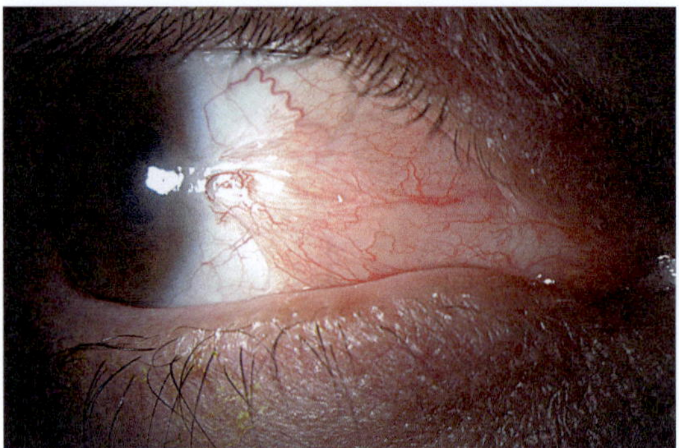

Fig. 12.8 Pingueculum. Note that the conjunctival overgrowth does not cross the limbus and encroach on the cornea, as occurs with pterygia

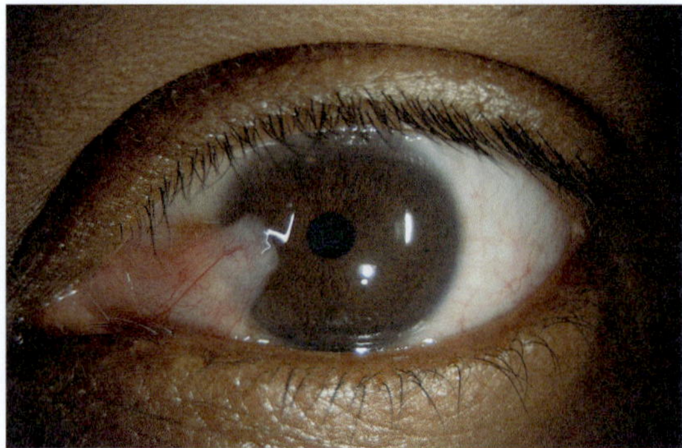

Fig. 12.9 Fleshy, elevated pterygium seen crossing the nasal limbus and approaching the central visual axis

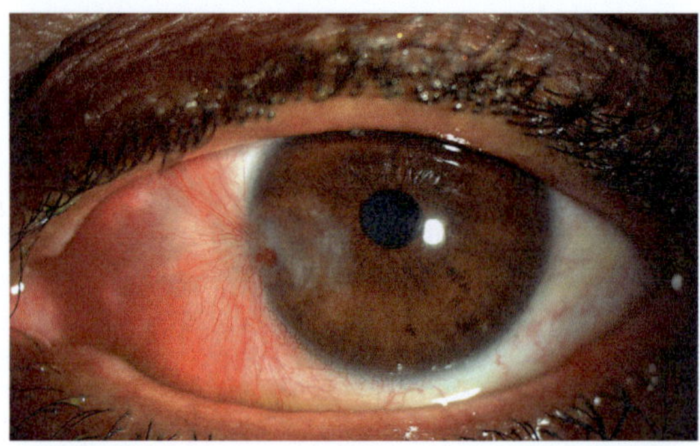

Fig. 12.10 Recurrent pterygium growth after previous excision, with residual corneal scar noted at the head of the advancing regrowth

lubricants or artificial tears, placement of punctal plugs, and anti-inflammatory eye drops.

Pinguecula and pterygium are benign, fleshy growths on the conjunctiva that are associated with chronic UV light exposure (from sun), dry eyes, and irritants like dust/wind (Figs. 12.8, 12.9, and 12.10). Commonly called "surfer's eye," the chronic sun and wind exposure with concomitant dry eye can cause these growths. Pinguecula are elevated growths that are limited to the conjunctiva, while pterygia cross the border of the conjunctiva and cornea and grow onto the corneal surface. Both lesions are slowly progressive and can cause ocular irritation, dry eye symptoms, and inflammation. Pterygia often start out as pinguecula and, with progression and growth onto the cornea, can cause blurred vision by inducing corneal astigmatism. In the early stages, use of UV protection sunglasses and lubricants like artificial tears can help with symptoms. If the growth interferes with the vision or comfort, surgical excision may be recommended.

Infections of the cornea can cause permanent opacities with resulting corneal scars (see section "Corneal Infections"). A common infection of the eye, acute conjunctivitis is also known as "pink eye." Acute conjunctivitis can result from either bacterial or viral etiologies. Adenoviral infections are the most common cause of acute conjunctivitis, also termed "epidemic keratoconjunctivitis (EKC)" as they are highly contagious. Acute redness, tearing, light sensitivity, and

watery discharge with development of membranes on the conjunctiva are hallmarks of EKC. The presence of enlarged preauricular lymph nodes is also common. Unique to EKC is the presence of corneal subepithelial infiltrates (Fig. 12.11a, b) that develop about 10 days after the onset of symptoms. These corneal opacities can often impair vision for weeks to months. Management of these opacities includes the use of topical steroids in a long, tapering fashion, topical antiviral medications, and other anti-inflammatories such as topical cyclosporine drops.

Foreign bodies of the cornea can often be picked up on examination. The patient often has a clear history of exposure to something in his/her environment. If the foreign body causes a breakdown of the corneal or conjunctival epithelial surface, significant pain and tearing will be

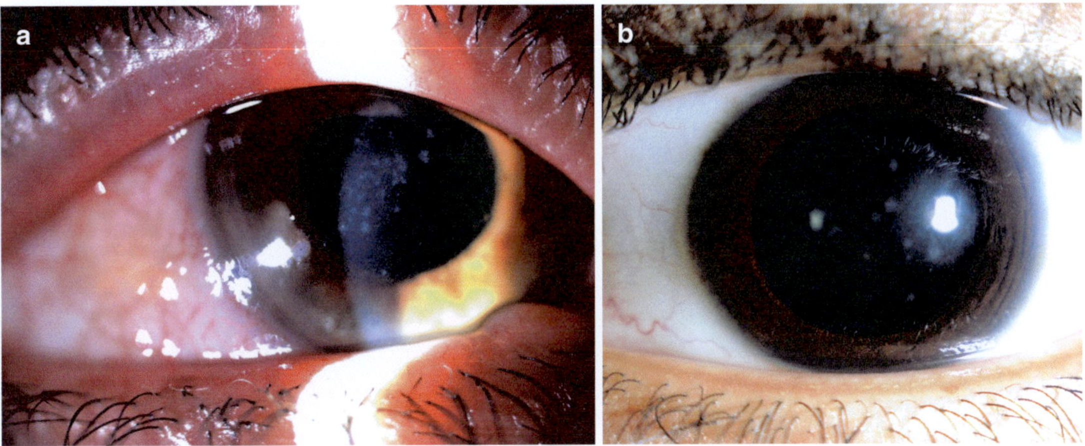

Fig. 12.11 EKC. (**a**) Acute infection showing subepithelial deposits and ocular injection. (**b**) Chronic epithelial deposits after resolution of infection are seen in a quiet eye

present. Most conjunctival foreign bodies wash away with tearing, but corneal foreign bodies remain embedded. As mentioned in the section on corneal trauma, all foreign bodies in the cornea should be removed with prompt referral to an eye care specialist.

Suggested Reading

Trauma

http://www.preventblindness.org/sites/default/files/national/documents/fact_sheets/FS93_Scope EyeInjury_0.pdf

Owens PL, Mutter R. Emergency department visits related to eye injuries, 2008. Healthcare cost and utilization project. Statistical brief #112. May 2011.

Infection and Ulcer

American Academy of Ophthalmology Cornea/External Disease Panel. Preferred practice patterns – bacterial keratitis. San Francisco: American Academy of Ophthalmology; 2013.

Krachmer J, Mannis M, Holland E. Cornea: fundamentals, diagnosis and management. 3rd ed. St. Louis: Mosby Elsevier; 2011. p. 119–1023.

Sarah A, Collier SA, Gronostaj MP, MacGurn AK, et al. Estimated burden of keratitis – United States, 2010. MMWR Morb Mortal Wkly Rep. 2014;63(45):1027–30.

Weisenthal RW. Basic and clinical science course. Section 8: External disease and cornea, 2013–2014. San Francisco: American Academy of Ophthalmology; 2014.

Opacities

Jhanji V, Chan TC, Li EY, Agarwal K, Vajpayee RB. Adenoviral keratoconjunctivitis. Surv Ophthalmol. 2015;60(5):435–43.

Paulsen AJ, Cruickshanks KJ, Fischer ME, et al. Dry eye in the beaver dam offspring study: prevalence, risk factors, and health-related quality of life. Am J Ophthalmol. 2014;157(4):799–806.

Corneal Dystrophies

Joaquin O. De Rojas and George J. Florakis

Dystrophies of the cornea are progressive, inherited genetic disorders that lead to bilateral deposits in one or more corneal layers. Most corneal dystrophies tend to begin early in life, with the notable exception of Fuchs' endothelial dystrophy, and are usually inherited in an autosomal dominant fashion. Dystrophies are generally not associated with systemic diseases or corneal inflammation. Corneal neovascularization is usually absent.

As a general rule, symptoms of a corneal dystrophy tend to correlate with the corneal layer(s) involved. For example, epithelial basement membrane dystrophy (EBMD) and other Transforming Growth Factor Beta Induced (TGFBI) mutation dystrophies affect the anterior layers of the cornea, which house sensory nerves that are closest to the ocular surface. They tend to present with recurrent, painful erosions and glare due to early scattering of light. On the other hand, dystrophies that affect the endothelial layer of the cornea, such as Fuchs' endothelial dystrophy, may lead

J. O. De Rojas, MD
Department of Ophthalmology, Johns Hopkins Medicine, Baltimore, MD, USA

Department of Ophthalmology, Edward S. Harkness Eye Institute, Columbia University Vagelos College of Physicians and Surgeons, New York, NY, USA

G. J. Florakis, MD (✉)
Department of Ophthalmology, Edward S. Harkness Eye Institute, Columbia University Vagelos College of Physicians and Surgeons, New York, NY, USA
e-mail: gjf2@cumc.columbia.edu

to corneal edema resulting in blurred vision and, if the edema progresses sufficiently, painful bullous keratopathy.

Anterior Corneal Dystrophies

Epithelial Basement Membrane Dystrophy (EBMD; Formerly Called Map-Dot-Fingerprint Dystrophy)

This is the most common of the anterior corneal dystrophies occurring in 6–18% of the population and results from deficient epithelial cell adhesions to the epithelial basement membrane, which in turn leads to excessive compensatory subepithelial production of collagen and duplication of the epithelial basement membrane (Fig. 13.1).

Affected patients will often present with recurrent corneal erosion syndrome, which is characterized by recurring bouts of eye pain cause by partial or complete detachment of the epithelium from the basement membrane. Other symptoms include double vision, tearing, and decreased visual acuity. On slit lamp exam, EBMD presents with diffuse gray or white patches, cysts, and lines in the subepithelial space that may look like whorled patterns reminiscent of "geographic maps, dots, or fingerprints." The most common treatment options for this dystrophy are hypertonic saline drops and/or ointment for treatment of the recurrent erosions, bandage

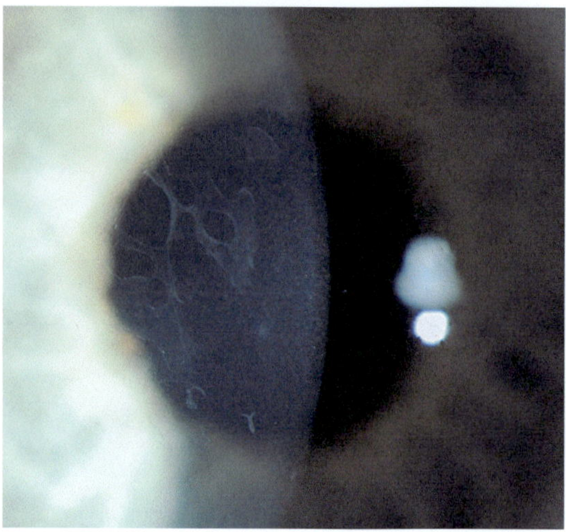

Fig. 13.1 Epithelial basement membrane dystrophy on slit lamp

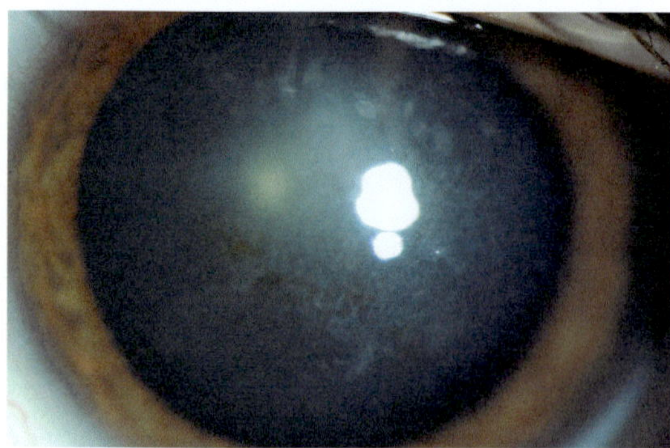

Fig. 13.2 Reis-Buckler corneal dystrophy with opacification of Bowman's layer on slit lamp examination

contact lenses, as well as superficial lamellar keratectomy (SLK) and phototherapeutic keratectomy (PTK) to ablate the epithelium and superficial Bowman's layer to promote better adhesion. Other treatment options include topical steroids and doxycycline, micropuncture with a needle, or Neodymium:YAG (Nd:YAG) laser.

Corneal Dystrophies of Bowman's Layer

Bowman's layer of the cornea is a thin (10 μ), acellular layer of collagen fibrils that underlie the epithelium and sit just above the stroma or "body" of the cornea. Dystrophies of this layer include "Reis-Buckler" and "Thiel-Behnke" dystrophies, both of which arise from mutations of the TGFBI gene. Similar to epithelial basement membrane dystrophy, Bowman's layer dystrophies may present with recurrent corneal erosions and blurry vision. Slit lamp examination shows a honeycomb-like appearance in Theil-Behnke and geographic-like opacities in Reis-Buckler, although phenotypically they may appear similar (Fig. 13.2). Treatment options for symptomatic cases include SLK or PTK or, less frequently, corneal transplantation surgery such as deep anterior lamellar keratoplasty (DALK) or penetrating keratoplasty (PK) when vision is significantly affected.

Corneal Stromal Dystrophies

The stromal dystrophies are a set of disorders caused by the progressive accumulation of intrastromal deposits. Classically they are classified by their phenotypic appearance on slit lamp examination. More recently, the genetic basis of the dystrophies is taken into account in a new classification defined by International Committee for Classification of Corneal Dystrophies (IC3D; http://www.corneasociety.org/sites/default/files/publications/ic3d_class_cornealdystrophies.pdf). This classification differentiates between phenotypically similar conditions, which are different genotypically, and genotypically similar conditions, which are different phenotypically.

Lattice Dystrophy

Lattice dystrophy is characterized by refractile, linear lesions within the stroma. Genetically, lattice dystrophy is caused by a transforming growth factor beta 1 (TGF-beta 1) cytokine mutation. On histopathology, there is amyloid deposition within the stroma that stains with Congo red. Patients may present with decreased visual acuity or recurrent, painful erosions sometimes as early as the first decade of life (Fig. 13.3). PTK, DALK, or PK are treatment options in severe cases, although a 40% recurrence rate 3–5 years after transplant has also been reported.

A rare variant of amyloid corneal deposits, "gelsolin type" or "familial amyloidosis," presents with

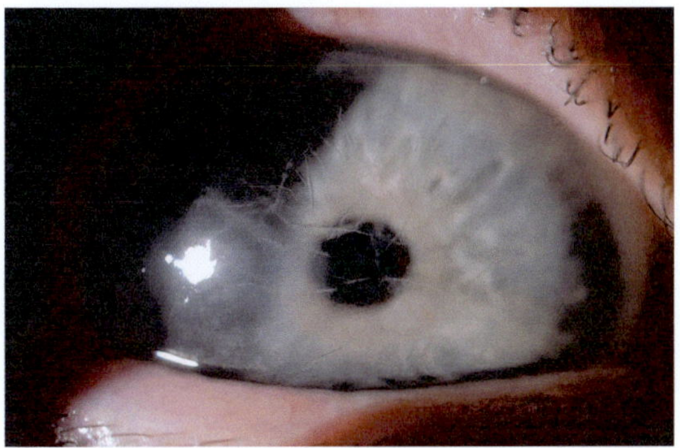

Fig. 13.3 Lattice corneal dystrophy showing refractile lesions in the stroma

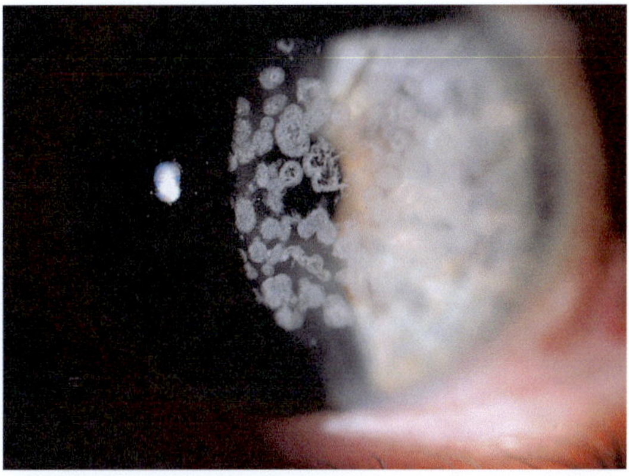

Fig. 13.4 Granular corneal dystrophy with "bread crumb-like" opacities in the stroma

systemic amyloidosis in addition to lattice changes of the cornea that do not stain with Congo red. This condition is not a true corneal dystrophy, however, as it is a consequence of a systemic problem.

Granular Dystrophy

The most common of the stromal dystrophies, granular dystrophy is characterized by hyaline deposition which produces "bread crumb-like" opacities within the stroma (Fig. 13.4). On histopathology, these deposits are best visualized with Mason's trichrome stain.

This disease is also caused by a TGFBI mutation and, like other such dystrophies, is autosomal dominant and often presents with recurrent, painful erosions. As the disease progresses, the crumb-like opacities can become confluent and lead to glare, photophobia, and visual impairment. When symptoms or decreased visual acuity interfere with the patients' daily activities, PTK, DALK, or PK are treatment options.

Granular-Lattice Dystrophy ("Avellino Dystrophy")

True to its name, this dystrophy presents as a combination of the two aforementioned dystrophies and is characterize by stromal deposition of both hyaline and amyloid elements. The deposits look like icicles in the anterior stroma (Fig. 13.5). Avellino dystrophy is caused by a TGFBI mutation and leads to signs and symptoms similar to

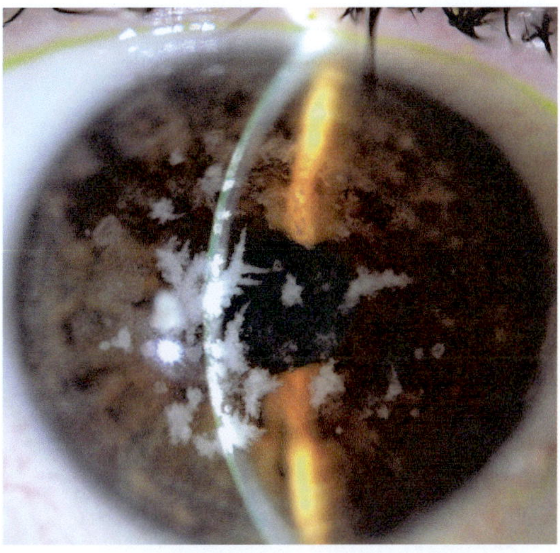

Fig. 13.5 Granular-lattice dystrophy ("Avellino dystrophy") with slit lamp examination showing stromal deposits composed of both hyaline and amyloid elements

both granular and lattice dystrophy. Treatment options for this condition are the same as for other stromal dystrophies when they become visually significant, namely PTK with excimer laser, DALK, or full thickness PK.

Macular Dystrophy

Unlike the other stromal dystrophies, macular dystrophy is autosomal-recessive and is not linked to a TGFBI mutation. This dystrophy is characterized by gray-white stromal opacities with poorly defined edges. Also, unlike other

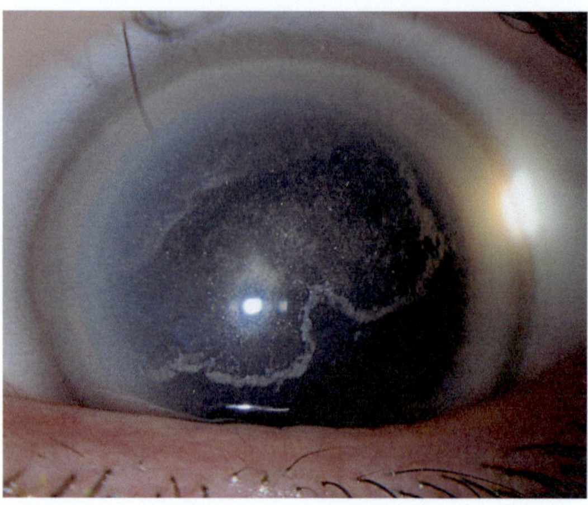

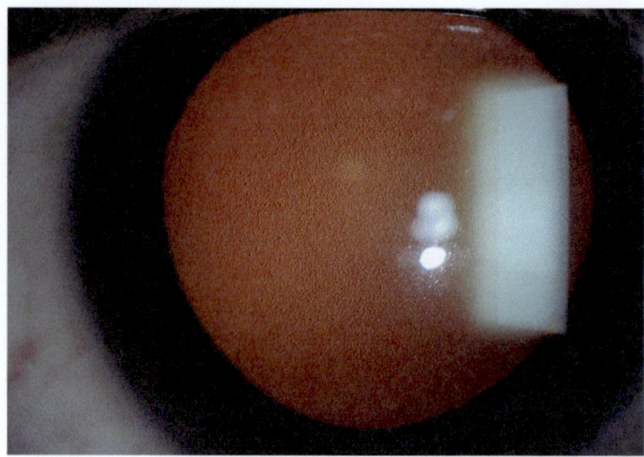

Fig. 13.7 Fuchs dystrophy with guttata at the level of the endothelium visualized with slit lamp retroillumination

Fig. 13.6 Schnyder dystrophy with cholesterol crystals in the cornea

dystrophies, the entire corneal surface from periphery to periphery and the entire depth of the cornea are affected by the deposits of macular dystrophy. Histologically, the lesions arise from deposition of mucopolysaccharides that stain with Alcian blue or Colloidal iron.

The most common presentation is blurred vision and glare symptoms in the first or second decade of life. Recurrent erosions can also occur but are less common. Since all layers of the cornea are involved, definitive treatment is with full thickness corneal transplantation.

Central Crystalline Corneal Dystrophy ("Schnyder Corneal Dystrophy")

A rare disorder that is infrequently visually significant, central crystalline corneal dystrophy can be diagnosed by the presence of yellow to white superficial stromal and epithelial crystals composed of cholesterol that migrate deeper into the cornea over time (Fig. 13.6). This dystrophy can be associated with systemic lipid abnormalities and, thus, requires an appropriate workup.

Corneal Endothelial Dystrophies

Fuchs' Dystrophy

Fuchs' dystrophy is one of the most common dystrophies and is the most common indication for endothelial corneal transplantation. Symptoms include blurred vision from corneal edema and associated "endothelial folds" visualized on slit lamp (Fig. 13.7). Also, with slit lamp, and more definitively with specular microscopy which images the endothelial cell layer, one can identify faults or defects in this layer associated with bumps or excrescences of Descemet's membrane termed "guttata." Specular microscopy is diagnostic and will also show polymegathism and pleomorphism or high variability in size and shape of the endothelial cells, respectively. The disease is bilateral, but may present asymmetrically, and tends to present more in women than men and in patients older than 50 years. In the differential diagnosis, a clinician must consider other causes of corneal edema that includes other endothelial dystrophies as well as "pseudophakic bullous keratopathy," which is an acquired condition characterized by endothelial cell loss and decompensation that leads to corneal edema after cataract or other intraocular surgery. PK has historically been the standard of care but is now only reserved for the most severe cases, such as when there is stromal scarring. Endothelial keratoplasty, such as Descemet stripping automated endothelial keratoplasty (DSAEK) or Descemet membrane endothelial keratoplasty (DMEK), is now more commonly performed and has better visual results and less chance of rejection.

Posterior Polymorphous Corneal Dystrophy

Posterior polymorphous corneal dystrophy (PPMD, PPCD) is autosomal dominant in inheritance and may present with mild bilateral corneal edema, irregularity of the pupils ("corectopia"), and possible adhesions from the iris to the cornea. Slit lamp examination is notable for grouped vesicles, discrete gray lesions, and broad bands with scalloped edges comprised of Descemet's membrane endothelium (Fig. 13.8). Histopathology reveals an abnormal endothelial layer composed of multiple layers of cells that resemble and behave like epithelial cells. Most patients are asymptomatic, although PPCD can lead to significant corneal opacification and edema that may necessitate a corneal transplant. Broad iris adhesions may be discovered on exam and are associated with glaucoma. If these signs and symptoms are present unilaterally, one must consider the alternate diagnosis of iridocorneal endothelial syndrome (ICE), a sporadic, acquired corneal disorder.

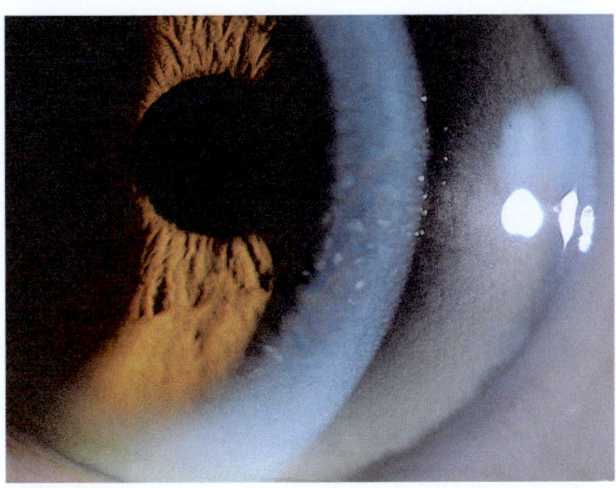

Fig. 13.8 Posterior polymorphous corneal dystrophy showing grouped vesicles and endothelial guttata

Congenital Hereditary Endothelial Dystrophy

Congenital hereditary endothelial dystrophy (CHED) presents with bilateral corneal edema in an infant or toddler in the absence of guttata. There are two distinct forms: an autosomal dominant form (CHED 1) that presents in childhood (ages 1–2 years) with pain, tearing, and photophobia, as well as a more severe autosomal recessive form (CHED 2) that presents at infancy with nystagmus secondary to visual deprivation. Unlike CHED 1, CHED 2 does not worsen throughout life.

Recently, CHED 1 has been reclassified as a subtype of posterior polymorphous corneal dystrophy, and CHED 2 has been renamed simply to "congenital hereditary endothelial dystrophy."

The above discussion represents descriptions of the most common corneal dystrophies of which the primary care doctor and general ophthalmologist should be aware of. As the genetic mutations of each dystrophy are further identified, the International Committee for Classification of Corneal Dystrophies (IC3D) classifications will be further reorganized and classified, and gene modification therapy may be developed to target specific gene mutations before they are expressed in the cornea.

Suggested Reading

Weisenthal RW, editor. 2015–2016 basic and Clinical Science Course (BCSC): sect. 8: external disease and cornea. San Francisco: American Academy of Ophthalmology; 2015. https://store.aao.org/2018-2019-basic-and-clinical-science-course-section-08-external-disease-and-cornea.html.

Weiss JS, Møller HU, Aldave AJ, et al. IC3D classification of corneal dystrophies – edition 2. Cornea 2015;34(2):117–59.

Cornea Transplantation

14

Jonathan Fay and George J. Florakis

Overview

The cornea is the transparent tissue at the front of the eye that covers the anterior chamber, iris, and pupil. It serves as a barrier to the outside world and is an important refractive component in the optical system of the eye. Without a clear, healthy cornea, good vision is not possible.

The cornea is composed of five layers: epithelium, Bowman's layer, stroma, Descemet's membrane, and endothelium (Fig. 14.1). At the surface lies the epithelium, a regenerative stratified squamous epithelium that plays an important role in host defense against pathogens. Next, Bowman's layer is a thin layer of condensed collagen located between the epithelial basement membrane and corneal stroma. The stroma is the thick middle layer of the cornea consisting of regularly arranged collagen fibers and sparsely distributed cells. Descemet's membrane is a modified basement membrane to the endothelium on the inner surface of the cornea. The endothelium (which is not related to a vascular endothelium, but shares the same name) is a single layer of non-regenerative cells that are responsible for regulating fluid and solute transport between the aqueous humor and corneal stroma; without proper endothelial function, the cornea becomes edematous and cloudy. Altogether, the cornea is approximately half a millimeter thick. As an avascular structure, the cornea receives oxygen from the air and nutrients from the aqueous humor; any disruption of this avascular nutritional system can have severe effects on corneal transparency and even viability. In addition, the avascular nature also contributes to the cornea's status as a relatively immune-privileged tissue.

A multitude of disease processes and injuries can alter the contour or clarity of the cornea, resulting in loss of visual acuity. If the loss of visual acuity is severe enough and corneal clarity cannot be restored, a surgical procedure, such as a corneal transplant, may be indicated. Based on recently published data, the most common indications for corneal transplantation include Fuchs' hereditary endothelial dystrophy, corneal swelling after cataract surgery (pseudophakic bullous keratopathy), keratoconus (an asymmetric, bulging contour of the cornea), and repeat corneal transplantation. Other indications include microbial infection, trauma, other corneal dystrophies, congenital opacity, corneal changes after refractive surgery, pterygium, and other causes for corneal scarring. Overall, approximately 44,000 corneal transplants are performed in the United States annually. All corneal transplantations require a donor corneal graft, obtained from

J. Fay, MD
Klamath Eye Center, Klamath Falls, OR, USA

G. J. Florakis, MD (✉)
Department of Ophthalmology, Edward S. Harkness Eye Institute, Columbia University Vagelos College of Physicians and Surgeons, New York, NY, USA
e-mail: gjf2@cumc.columbia.edu

© Springer Nature Switzerland AG 2019
D. S. Casper, G. A. Cioffi (eds.), *The Columbia Guide to Basic Elements of Eye Care*,
https://doi.org/10.1007/978-3-030-10886-1_14

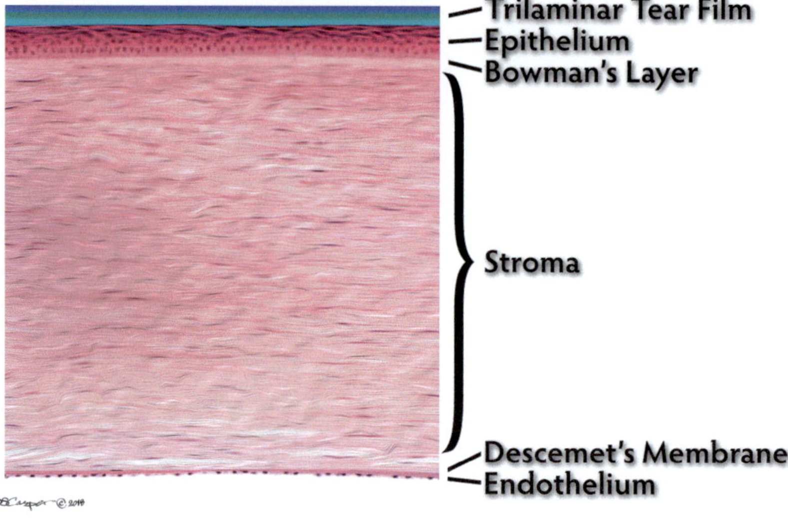

Fig. 14.1 The five layers of the human cornea: epithelium, Bowman's layer, stroma, Descemet's membrane, and endothelium

cadaveric donor eyes. In recent years, a variety of new procedures have been introduced in an attempt to improve the outcomes of corneal transplant surgery.

Corneal Transplantation

Corneal transplantation, also known as keratoplasty, is a fairly young surgery from a historical perspective. Tales of eye transplantation first appeared in ancient and medieval texts; however, true scientific advances did not begin until the early nineteenth century when experimentation in rabbits and chickens was met with limited success. Soon thereafter in 1837, a successful corneal transplantation was reported in a gazelle, and in 1838 a corneal xenograft with pig tissue on a human was attempted but was unsuccessful. A period of limited progress in corneal transplantation ensued, until 1905 when Eduard Zirm performed the first successful human allograft corneal transplantation in Europe, which remained clear for approximately 6.5 months.

Over the decades that followed, increasing knowledge of antiseptic technique, anesthesia, and immunology improved. The use of cadaver corneas became a new source of corneal transplant material, and Dr. R. Townley Paton established the world's first eye bank, located in New York City, USA. Another notable ophthalmologist, Dr. Ramon Castroviejo, performed the first corneal transplant of the modern era in the United States at the Edward S. Harkness Eye Institute of Columbia University Medical Center in 1933. He also made major contributions to techniques and instrumentation in corneal transplantation, popularizing a technique for full-thickness corneal transplantation (also known as penetrating keratoplasty, or PK) in the United States and around the world. Dr. Castroviejo's early full-thickness transplants utilized a square-shaped donor graft (Fig. 14.2). In modern full-thickness corneal transplantation, a circular button of tissue is removed from the patient's cornea, and a matching button of tissue from the cadaveric donor is sewn in its place (Figs. 14.3 and 14.4).

Another concept in corneal transplantation is the use of partial-thickness, or lamellar, transplantation, rather than a full-thickness tissue replacement (Fig. 14.5). First conceived of in the early 1900s, various techniques have been developed to transplant just the anterior portion or just the posterior portion of the cornea. Anterior

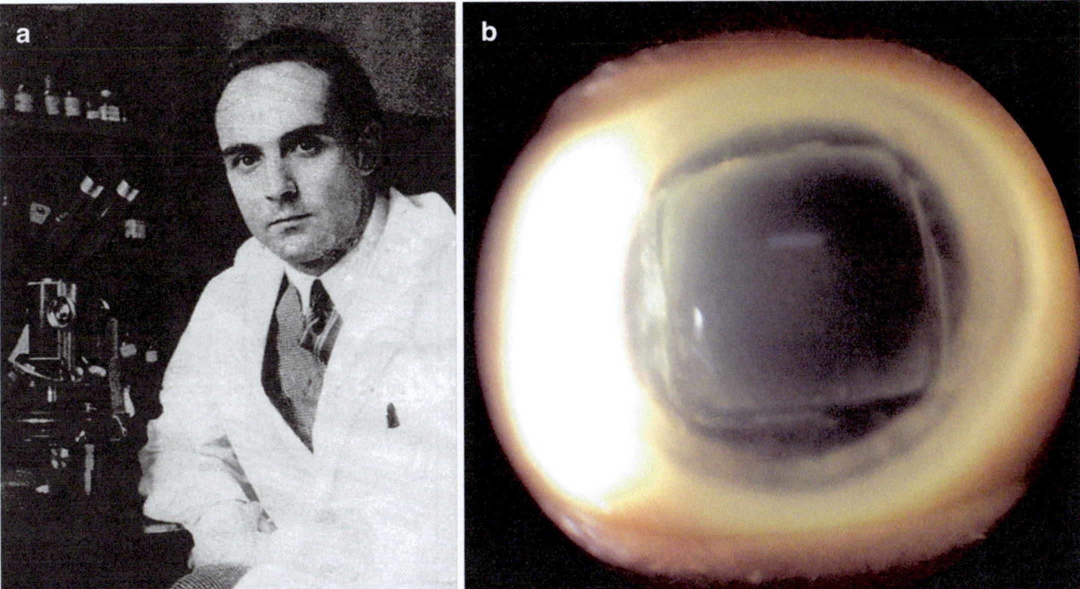

Fig. 14.2 (**a**) Photograph of Ramon Castroviejo. (**b**) The healed result of a square corneal graft typical of Dr. Ramon Castroviejo's early corneal transplants from the 1930s

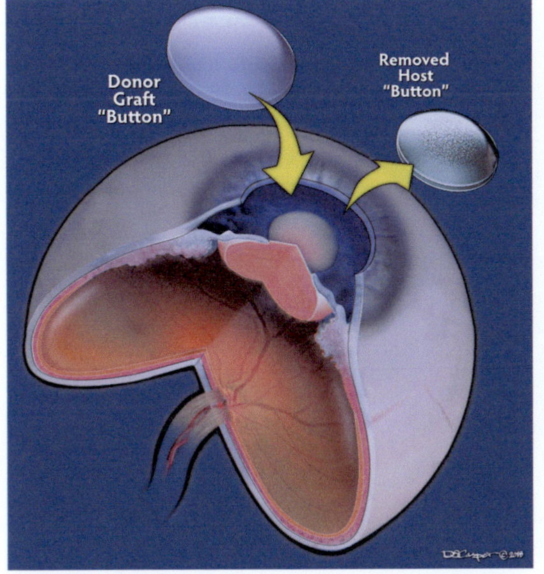

Fig. 14.3 Schematic representation of a full-thickness corneal transplantation (penetrating keratoplasty). A circular button of tissue is excised from the host cornea, and a circular button of tissue harvested from a cadaver cornea is sewn in its place

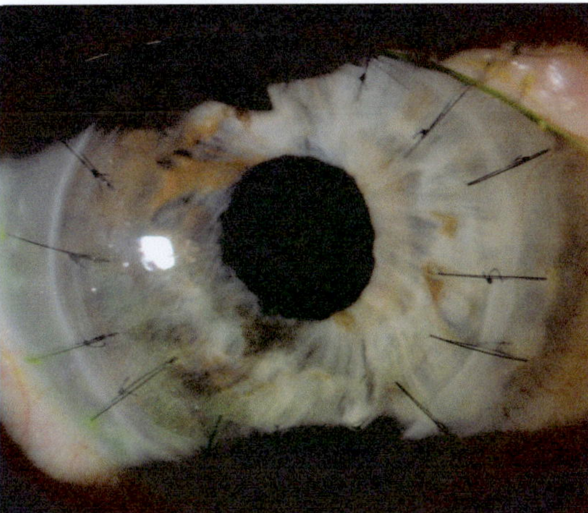

Fig. 14.4 This photograph demonstrates the appearance of a full-thickness transplant (penetrating keratoplasty); sutures are often removed many months after surgery

lamellar keratoplasty (ALK) and deep anterior lamellar keratoplasty (DALK) are techniques currently employed to replace only the anterior layers of the cornea. This technique can be used for anterior stromal scars, keratoconus, or other conditions where the patient's native endothelium at the inner layer of the cornea is healthy.

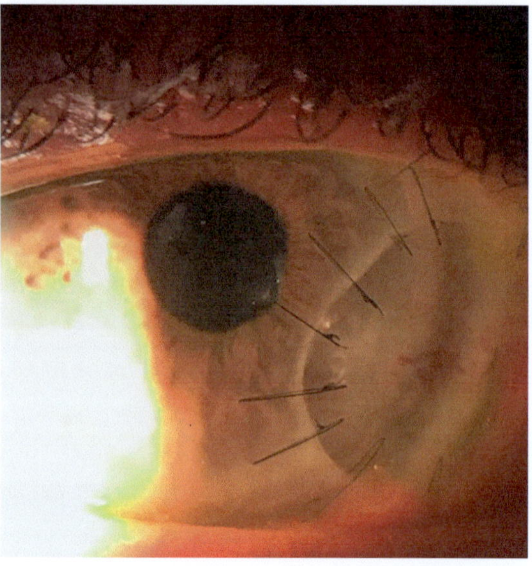

Fig. 14.5 This photograph demonstrates a lamellar patch graft which was placed over an area of thinned cornea and impending perforation

Anterior lamellar keratoplasty is also used to patch an area of damaged tissue or to repair a perforation or impending perforation in the cornea. In contrast, endothelial keratoplasty (EK) is a term that encompasses several techniques for replacing just inner corneal layers, which can successfully treat conditions affecting only the endothelium, such as Fuchs' endothelial dystrophy, or corneal edema occurring after cataract surgery (pseudophakic bullous keratopathy, PBK). Descemet's stripping (automated) endothelial keratoplasty (DSEK or DSAEK) is a technique developed and popularized in the beginning of this century which transplants a thin multilayered disc, consisting of donor stroma, Descemet's membrane and endothelium (approximately 1/10th of a millimeter thick) to the posterior aspect of a host cornea which has been stripped of the patient's Descemet's membrane and endothelium. Descemet's membrane endothelial keratoplasty (DMEK) is the newest technique in endothelial corneal transplantation, developed in 2006. In this technique, Descemet's membrane and adjacent endothelial cells, a layer of tissue as thin as 1/100th of a millimeter, are peeled from the posterior surface of a donor cornea and placed on the posterior surface of the host cornea through a small, 2.4 mm incision (Fig. 14.6). Much as

Fig. 14.6 Schematic comparison of the most common types of corneal transplantation: penetrating keratoplasty (PK), deep anterior lamellar keratoplasty (DALK), Descemet's stripping (automated) endothelial keratoplasty (DSEK or DSAEK), and Descemet's membrane endothelial keratoplasty (DMEK)

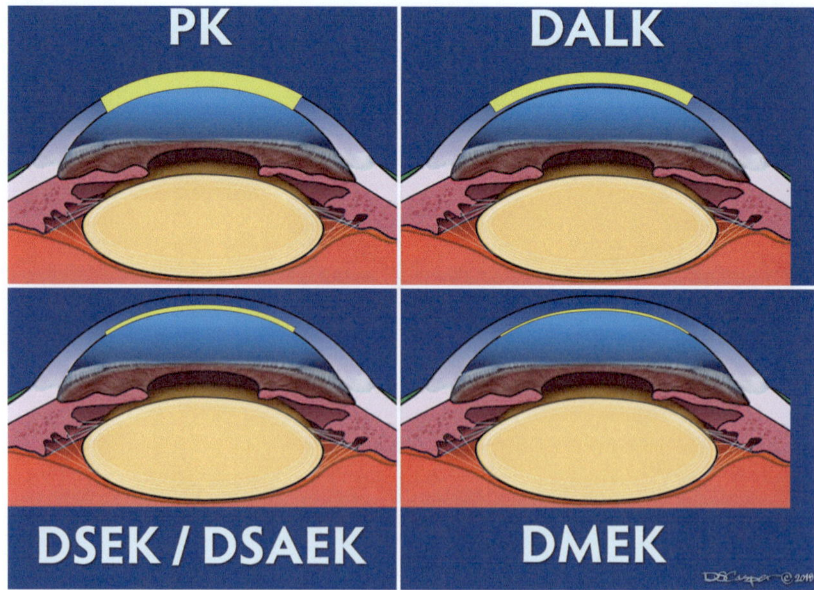

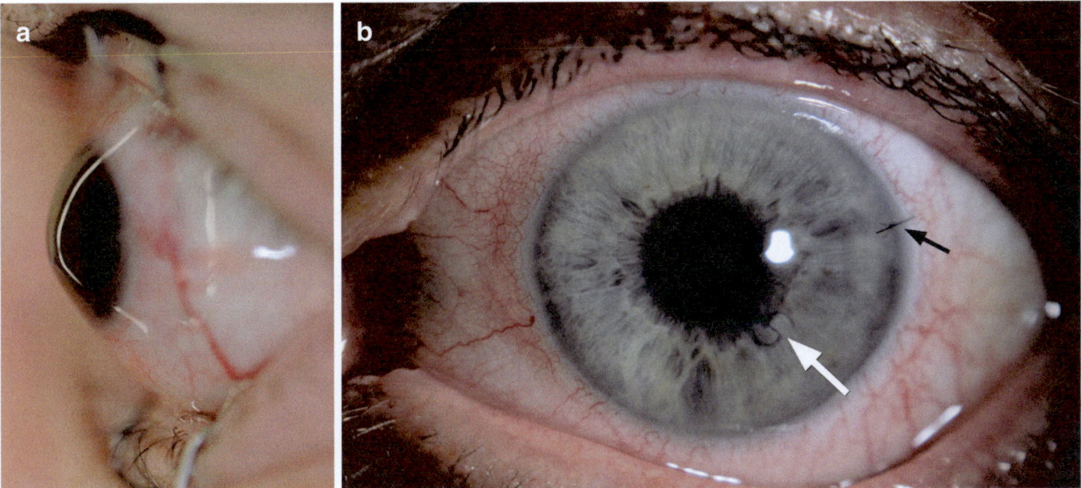

Fig. 14.7 (**a**) A distorted corneal curvature (a "cone") is clearly seen in this example of a keratoconic cornea. (**b**) The healed result of a DMEK transplant case. Note the excellent clarity of the cornea and the single suture (black arrow) which seals the small incision required in this type of endothelial transplantation. An "S" shaped stamp (white arrow) is used to confirm the correct orientation of the thin donor graft tissue after it is positioned in the recipient's eye. This "S" stamp fades with time and is typically unnoticeable to the naked eye

with general surgery and the use of laparoscopic procedures, one of the major advances in ophthalmic surgery has been the development of "small incision" techniques that employ remarkably small incisions, thus greatly reducing complications and accelerating healing. Modern surgical techniques in endothelial keratoplasty generally include the placement of a bubble of air or sulfur hexafluoride (SF-6) gas in the anterior chamber of the eye to hold the graft tissue in place during initial stages of healing. This bubble is naturally resorbed within 1–5 days after surgery (Fig. 14.7a, b).

Preoperative and Postoperative Considerations

In general, the decision to proceed with corneal transplantation entails a lifelong commitment to the care and management of the transplanted cornea, the eye, and the patient as a whole. This is in part due to the fact that the transplanted cornea, which is foreign to the host's immune system, carries a lifelong risk of rejection. Because of the privileged immune status of the cornea, most patients only require modification of the immune rejection mechanism (usually with topical steroids) in the early postoperative period. The majority of corneal transplant patients do not require lifelong use of immunomodulating medications, as is typical for other transplant procedures. In some cases, however, either acutely after surgery or later, sometimes years after transplantation, immune reactions may arise. Corneal graft rejection occurs when the host immune system attacks the epithelium, stroma, or endothelium of the transplanted cornea. In many cases, if recognized quickly, an episode of rejection can be treated, and the success of the cornea transplant can be maintained. However, sometimes an episode of rejection or recurrent episodes of rejection can result in a loss of clarity of the transplanted cornea and a loss of vision. In this case, a repeat corneal transplant may be indicated.

Although corneal transplantation is the most successful tissue transplantation procedure performed in humans relating to the cornea status as an "immune-privileged tissue," rejection is reported to occur in 20% of penetrating keratoplasties, 2.6–10% of DSAEK procedures and 1% of DMEK procedures. The lower risk of rejection after endothelial keratoplasty versus penetrating keratoplasty is one of the driving factors for the increasing popularity of endothelial transplantation when indicated. Potential risk factors for rejection include active inflammation or infection, corneal vascularization, younger age of the host, trauma, history of prior episodes of rejection, and prior ocular surgery.

Symptoms of rejection in all types of corneal transplantation include decreased vision, redness of the eye, light sensitivity, or pain that lasts longer than a few hours. Patients should be educated to recognize these symptoms and should understand that seeking prompt evaluation by their ophthalmologist could mean the difference between saving the cornea and irreversible failure of the transplant. Up to 70% of episodes of rejection are recognized by the patient based on symptoms, while 30% may be recognized on routine examination by the physician, highlighting the fact that regular follow-up with an ophthalmologist is another critical aspect of postoperative care.

If an episode of rejection occurs, it is typically treated with frequent application of topical steroid drops and sometimes an oral or intravenous steroid which reduces the immune response against the transplant. As an episode of rejection becomes controlled, the ophthalmologist will taper the dose of steroids to a lower maintenance dose. To reduce the risk of rejection, particularly after one has already occurred, many ophthalmologists keep their patients on a low dose of topical steroid drops for many years or, occasionally, indefinitely.

Expectations for visual recovery after corneal transplantation are another important consideration. With modern techniques in corneal transplantation, our goal is excellent visual acuity; however, in some cases excellent visual acuity is not a given, and in many cases improvement in visual acuity is not immediate. For penetrating keratoplasty (PK), visual acuity may be in the range of 20/400 initially, which will often improve significantly over the first 3 months after surgery. For these patients, vision usually will continue to improve for up to 1 year after surgery as the surgeon systematically removes sutures in a way that optimizes a regular curvature of the surface of the cornea, assuming the cornea remains transparent and without edema. At times, the use of glasses, a contact lens, or additional procedures may be required to optimize vision. For DSEK or DSAEK, visual recovery is much quicker and more predictable, with patients frequently achieving vision in the range of 20/25 within 1–3 months of surgery. For DMEK, recovery of visual acuity can occur as quickly as 2–4 weeks and with excellent visual acuity results. In all types of endothelial keratoplasty, fewer sutures are required and therefore an irregularity of the corneal surface, known as astigmatism, is much less concerning.

For patients who have undergone penetrating keratoplasty in particular, it is also important to note that even years after surgery, the eye can be more fragile than an eye that has not undergone surgery. With trauma to the post-transplant eye, it is possible for the scar between the graft and host tissue to break open (a wound dehiscence), which could result in catastrophic damage to the structures inside the eye. For this reason it is recommended that these patients always wear protective eyewear during any activities that might put them at risk of injury to the eye.

The Surgical Experience

Corneal transplantation is most commonly performed under monitored sedation anesthesia, although general anesthesia is considered for some cases. The duration of the surgery may range from 1 to 2 h, and it is performed on an outpatient basis with patients returning to their home on the same day. Patients usually wear a patch and shield over the operated eye for 12–24 h post-surgery, after which they wear a protective shield when sleeping during the post-op period. They are asked to prevent any water or other potential source of infection from getting into the eye and to avoid bending, lifting more than 10 lbs, or engaging in any strenuous activity for some time after surgery. Patients who undergo endothelial keratoplasty are asked to maintain face-up positioning with the eye looking toward the ceiling for 2–4 days after surgery with short breaks. This allows the intraocular gas bubble placed during surgery to anchor the transplanted tissue up against the inner surface of the cornea, until the tissue begins to heal in place.

A Final Note

Corneal transplantation would not be possible without the generous gift offered by registered tissue and organ donors and their families. Eye tissue donation is managed and processed by the many eye banks around the country and is regulated by the Eye Bank Association of America. After death, a donor is screened for various eye and systemic conditions by a local eye bank. As appropriate, the eye tissue may undergo a strict set of tests and processing to determine its safety and eligibility for use in corneal transplantation or use in other areas of ophthalmic surgery. If found appropriate for use in corneal transplantation, the tissue will be offered to the eye surgeon and transported to the site of surgery in a highly efficient and orchestrated process.

Suggested Reading

Crawford AZ, Patel DV, McGhee CN. A brief history of corneal transplantation: from ancient to modern. Oman J Ophthalmol. 2013;6(Suppl 1):S12–7. https://doi.org/10.4103/0974-620X.122289.

Eye Bank of Association of America. http://restoresight.org.

Park CY, Lee JK, Gore PK, Lim CY, Chuck RS. Keratoplasty in the United States: a 10-year review from 2005 through 2014. Ophthalmology. 2015;122:2432–42. https://doi.org/10.1016/j.ophtha.2014.08.017.

Part III

Glaucoma

George A. Cioffi

Prior to the 1980s, glaucoma was defined as a disease involving progressive visual loss due to elevated intraocular pressure (IOP). Although elevated IOP is now considered one of the major risk factors for glaucomatous damage, glaucoma is defined as a primary optic neuropathy; visual loss results from characteristic, progressive deterioration of the optic nerve due to loss of retinal ganglion cells and their axons, leading to irreversible loss of visual function. At least three million Americans suffer from glaucoma and many more have risk factors that require monitoring or treatment. In addition, 50% of Americans with glaucoma are unaware they have the disease.

Glaucoma is the leading cause of irreversible adult blindness, and it is also a leading cause of preventable blindness. Many glaucoma patients are already blind in at least one eye at the time of original detection, pointing to the need for better early diagnosis. Because glaucoma may not manifest any symptoms unless it is bilateral or severe, it is often likened to the "sneak thief of sight." Unlike the majority of eye diseases, most varieties of glaucoma are chronic, virtually "lifelong" disorders that can be controlled, but not cured.

Like diabetes mellitus, systemic hypertension, reactive airway disease, or arthritis, glaucoma requires some lifestyle modification, such as adherence to medical treatment regimens, regular physician visits, and acknowledgment of the disease, to achieve successful treatment.

Three areas of ocular anatomy are key to understanding the group of disorders known as glaucoma. These include the anterior optic nerve (referred to as the optic nerve head, the optic disc, or the optic papilla), the ciliary body, and the anterior chamber angle. Anterior optic nerve anatomy is described in detail below. The ciliary body is the midportion of the uveal tract lying just behind the iris and is the site of aqueous humor production (Fig. 15.1). The anterior chamber angle refers to the region between the cornea and the iris, which contains the trabecular meshwork, the principal site of outflow of aqueous humor from the

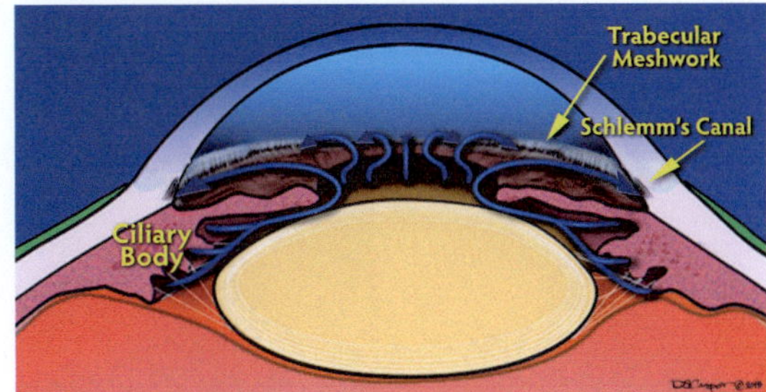

Fig. 15.1 Illustration shows production of aqueous humor within ciliary body, with flow through the pupil, draining via the trabecular meshwork to Schlemm's canal

G. A. Cioffi, MD (✉)
Columbia University Irving Medical Center, New York, NY, USA

Edward S. Harkness Eye Institute, Columbia University Vagelos College of Physicians and Surgeons, New York, NY, USA
e-mail: gac2126@cumc.columbia.edu

© Springer Nature Switzerland AG 2019
D. S. Casper, G. A. Cioffi (eds.), *The Columbia Guide to Basic Elements of Eye Care*,
https://doi.org/10.1007/978-3-030-10886-1_15

eye. Aqueous humor bathes the anterior segment of the eye, providing oxygen and nutrition to the region. Aqueous production is affected by diurnal and nocturnal variation, with greater production during waking hours. The trabecular meshwork acts as a sieve of tissue that connects, via the collector system and Schlemm's canal, to the venous system, where aqueous humor is returned to the bloodstream. Aqueous also leaves the eye via the uveoscleral (or nontraditional) pathway through the root of the iris ciliary muscle and into the suprachoroidal space (Fig. 15.2). Intraocular pressure (eye pressure) is therefore dependent on aqueous humor production and the resistance to aqueous humor outflow through the trabecular meshwork and the uveoscleral pathway. The trabecular and uveoscleral pathways are also known as the pressure-dependent and pressure-independent pathways, respectively.

The most important risk factor for glaucoma onset and progression is the pressure within the eye, the intraocular pressure. The majority of glaucoma cases in North America and Europe are associated with elevation of the intraocular pressure, although 50% of patients with glaucoma may have a statistically normal IOP (usually defined as approximately 10–21 mmHg) at the time of diagnosis. In theory, elevated IOP could result from either an excessive production of aqueous humor from the ciliary body or an obstruction of aqueous outflow through the chamber angle (trabecular meshwork). In reality, virtually all elevation of intraocular pressure arises from some form of decreased aqueous outflow through the trabecular meshwork and/or uveoscleral pathways. This blockage occurs either at the trabecular cellular level or from gross blockade of the tissue by fibrosis, iris tissue, or other material in the anterior chamber angle.

As mentioned above, many patients exhibit progressive glaucomatous optic neuropathy, but seldom, or never, manifest increased IOP. Controversy exists about whether these individuals have exquisitely pressure-sensitive optic nerves or whether other damaging factors such as compromised microcirculation cause the optic neuropathy. It is now generally accepted that other intraocular pressure-independent factors, including ocular perfusion pressure, genetic predisposition, and lamina cribrosa integrity, contribute to glaucomatous optic neuropathy, regardless of intraocular pressure. Glaucomatous optic nerve damage without elevated intraocular pressure is sometimes referred to as "low-tension glaucoma" or "normal pressure glaucoma," although the appearance of glaucomatous optic neuropathy across the range of intraocular pressures is similar. Conversely, in the condition known as "ocular hypertension," IOP may be elevated without the development of typical glaucomatous optic nerve damage.

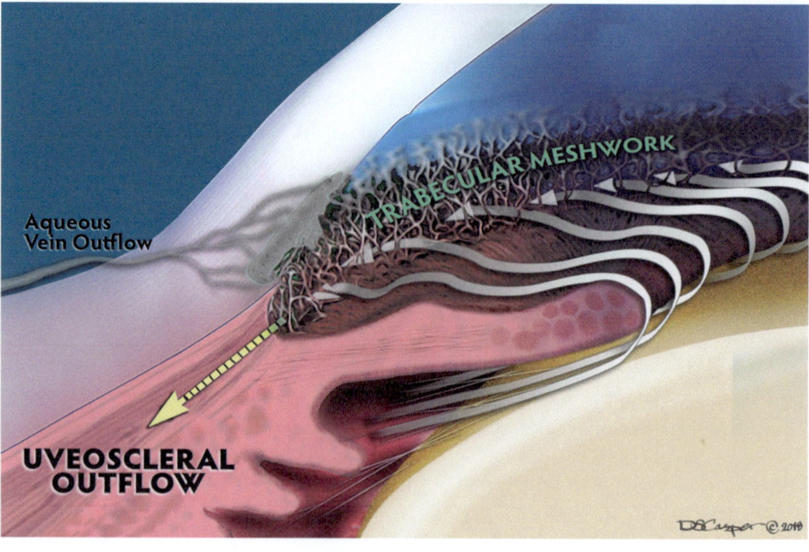

Fig. 15.2 Illustration of aqueous outflow through trabecular meshwork (conventional) and through uveoscleral (unconventional) pathways

Glaucoma Classifications

The glaucomas are often subdivided into two main groups: open-angle glaucoma and angle-closure glaucomas (see Chap. 16). Angle-closure glaucomas are characterized by iridotrabecular contact that limits aqueous access to the outflow system, whereas in open-angle glaucoma, aqueous humor has access to the outflow pathway, but the outflow pathway itself is dysfunctional. These two broad categories can be further broken down into primary (idiopathic) and secondary (associated with some other ocular or systemic conditions) mechanisms. The vast majority of glaucomas are chronic, although acute elevations of intraocular pressure can occur through a variety of open-angle and angle-closure mechanisms.

Although the majority of glaucoma patients in Western Europe and the United States have the primary open-angle type with no easily discernable underlying cause, some 50 different varieties of secondary glaucoma have been described, the most common of which are listed in Table 15.1. Worldwide, the prevalence of open-angle and angle-closure glaucoma is

Table 15.1 Common types of secondary glaucoma

Category	Factor	Prevalence	Incidence	Progression
State of the individual	Age	+	+	?
	Sex	0	0	0
	Ethnicity	Black +, Indian +, Hispanic +	Black +	?
	Family history	+		0
Ocular anatomy and physiology	Increased IOP	+	+	+
	Increased diurnal IOP variation	+	+	+
	Exfoliation syndrome	+	+	+
	Pigment dispersion	+		
	Myopia	+	0	0
	Decreased corneal thickness		+	
	Increased disc diameter	+		
	Disc crescent	+		+
Signs of damage	Increased CDR	+	+	
	Disc hemorrhage			+
	Decreased choroidal thickness	+		
Systemic disease	Hypertension	?	0	
	Diabetes	?	?	
	Thyroid	+	?	
	Cardiovascular disease	0		
	Migraine	+		
	Sleep apnea	+		
	Raynaud's		0	
Non-glaucoma medications	Corticosteroids	+	0	
	Cholesterol lowering	−		
	Calcium channel blockers	0		−
Personal behaviors	Exercise	Decreases IOP		
	Smoking	0	0	0
	BMI	0		
	Alcohol	0	0	
	Caffeine	0		
	Fat intake	?		
	Increased venous pressure	?		
	Acceptance of therapy			
	Persistence with therapy			

From Boland M, Quigley HA. Risk factors and open-angle glaucoma: classification and application. J Glaucoma. 2007;16(4):406–18, with permission approximately equal. In general, secondary open-angle glaucomas are not specifically attributable to endogenous dysfunction of the trabecular meshwork but rather to some other ocular or systemic disorders, such as inflammation, intraocular neovascularization, congenital anomalies, ocular trauma, or tumors. Although appropriate diagnosis of an unusual secondary glaucoma can make the difference between sight preservation and blindness, some secondary glaucomas are sufficiently uncommon to fall exclusively within the ken of the glaucoma subspecialist. A few are relatively common or afflict a specific group of patients, necessitating some familiarity by the primary care physician.

Glaucoma itself refers to a group of eye diseases, most of which are chronic and, when unrecognized, produce insidious irreversible visual loss. Blindness from glaucoma can be prevented or greatly reduced by appropriate screening, particularly by eliciting a family history of glaucoma and detecting the presence of glaucomatous optic neuropathy by ophthalmoscopy or the use of computerized imaging technologies. Glaucoma, like other chronic diseases, requires establishment of a strong physician-patient relationship, ongoing therapeutic regimen, and regular physician office visits. Patients in whom glaucoma is recognized in the early stages usually learn to cope with their disease and retain good functional vision throughout their life. Patients whose diagnosis is delayed until advanced visual field loss develops, who cannot cope with the rigors of chronic disease therapy, or who suffer from nonpressure risk factors have a much worse prognosis for retention of useful vision.

older age, family history, and African ancestry are most relevant for open-angle glaucoma. Other ocular and systemic risk factors remain debatable.

Two large, randomized clinical trials helped physicians better understand the main risk factors for glaucoma onset among subjects with statistically high intraocular pressure but no signs of glaucomatous damage: the Ocular Hypertension Treatment Study and the European Glaucoma Prevention Study. Both studies confirmed the significant role of intraocular pressure as the only proven, modifiable risk factor for the development of open-angle glaucoma. Each 1 mmHg higher pressure increased that risk by approximately 10%. In addition, older age, decreased corneal thickness, large cup-to-disc ratio, and abnormal results on visual field testing were significant and independent predictors for conversion to glaucoma.

Regarding progression among patients with established glaucoma, elevated intraocular pressure was also the most important predictor of future vision loss. In the Early Manifest Glaucoma Trial, for example, in which newly diagnosed, open-angle glaucoma patients were randomized to treatment or observation, there was a 12–13% average increase in risk for each mmHg higher pressure. Similar to the aforementioned studies on the risk of glaucoma onset, older age, worse disease status, decreased corneal thickness, and lower blood pressure significantly increased the risk of vision loss. Of note, the detection of small hemorrhages on the surface of the optic nerve (see Figs. 15.5 and 18.3c) was significantly associated with a greater risk of glaucoma onset and progression.

Risk Factors

Population-based studies, randomized clinical trials, and longitudinal observational studies have helped elucidate the main risk factors for glaucoma prevalence, onset, and progression. These studies have focused mainly on the open-angle glaucomas. Regarding risk factors for glaucoma prevalence, population-based studies have, in general, shown that elevated intraocular pressure,

Clinical Manifestations

Glaucomatous Optic Neuropathy

A characteristic deterioration of the optic nerve is the common denominator of all forms of glaucoma (primary or secondary, open or closed angle, chronic or acute). Glaucomatous optic neuropathy is the primary cause of permanent visual loss in glaucoma. Because of the visibility of the anterior optic nerve with any ophthalmoscope, recognition of the early signs of glaucomatous optic neuropathy becomes the single most useful clinical tool for glaucoma screening. With ophthalmoscopic visualization of the optic nerve head, recognition of glaucomatous optic neuropathy is not difficult. The circular optic disc border is visualized as the junction between the nerve head and the surrounding retina (Fig. 15.3). The optic nerve is composed primarily of axons

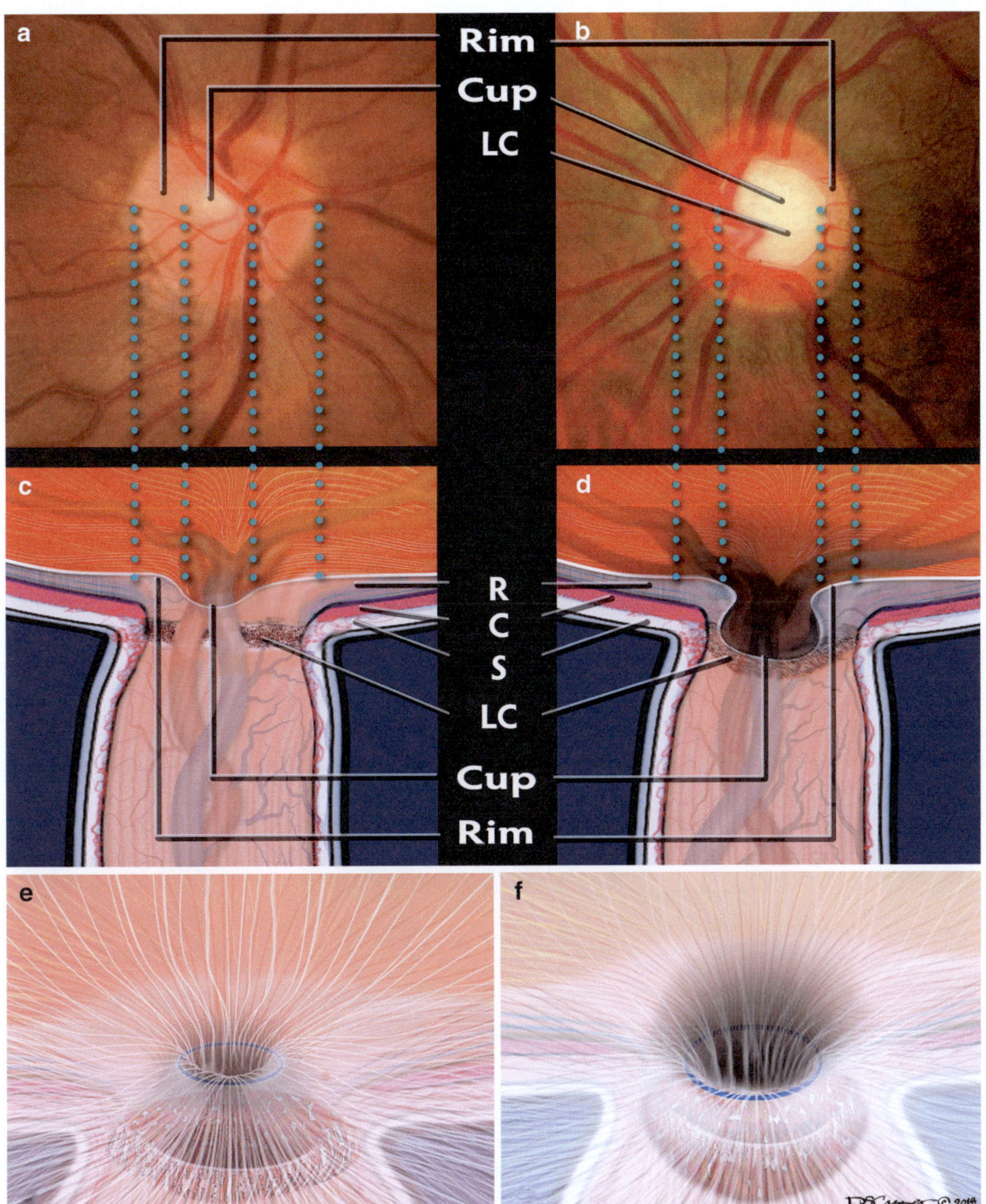

Fig. 15.3 Left panels (**a**, **c**, **e**) illustrate a normal optic nerve with a small central "cup" and a cup-to-disc ratio of approximately 0.2. Right panels (**b**, **d**, **f**) demonstrate an enlarged cup-to-disc ratio (approximately 0.7) with posterior displacement of the lamina cribrosa (LC). Thinning of the neuroretinal rim: Panels (**e**, **f**) show nerve fibers that make up the neural component of the optic nerve (*LC* lamina cribrosa, *R* retina, *C* choroid, *S* sclera)

(the retinal nerve fibers) from the retinal ganglion cells and acts as the neural connection between the neurosensory retina and brain. The optic nerve head represents the perpendicular transition of the retinal nerve fibers from the surface of the retina to the optic nerve as they exit the eye. The normal, healthy optic nerve is composed of approximately 1.2–1.5 million neurons or fibers, each originating from a retinal ganglion cell. With advancing age, there is often some atrophy of tissue surrounding the optic nerve that gives a pale halo around the disc edge and provides an obvious visual separation of the retina from optic disc tissue. Normal neural tissue of the disc has an orange-pinkish hue and a full, slightly elevated appearance, with a relatively distinct border at the disc edge. Centrally, the orange-pink neural tissue gradually gives way to a yellow-whitish central zone, the optic disc "cup," that is slightly more excavated than surrounding neural tissue. This renders a bagel-like or doughnutlike appearance to the nerve head, with neural tissue, or the "rim," surrounding the central physiologic cup. Retinal arteries and veins enter and exit the globe through the optic nerve in the area of the optic cup. In glaucoma, as neural tissue atrophies, the central cup appears to enlarge due to surrounding tissue loss. The normal ratio of the cup diameter

to the total diameter of the disc (cup-disc ratio) is usually 0.3 or less; a ratio greater than 0.6 should raise suspicion of glaucoma (Fig. 15.4). This is the most characteristic finding of glaucomatous neural change and is referred to as "cupping." This produces not only enlargement of the cup but also anterior-posterior elongation with retro-displacement of the supporting tissue. This posterior displacement causes a backward bowing of the tissue at the base of the central cup portion of the disc.

Most individuals have similar, symmetric optic discs and cups in each eye. An asymmetry of the cup-disc ratio of 0.2 or greater between the two eyes (not explained by differences in disc size) is easy to recognize and a useful sign of early glaucomatous optic neuropathy.

In addition to the diffuse enlargement of the physiologic cup, focal thinning of the optic nerve rim is also very characteristic of glaucoma. Typically, the lower pole of the nerve head shows a focal defect of the neural rim earlier than the superior pole of the optic nerve. This results in a concomitant, spatially consistent defect in the superior visual field. Small, "flame-shaped" hemorrhages at the disc edge are also often harbingers of advancing neural damage and visual field loss and are quite char-

Fig. 15.4 A comparison of fundus photos and visual field loss in progressive glaucoma

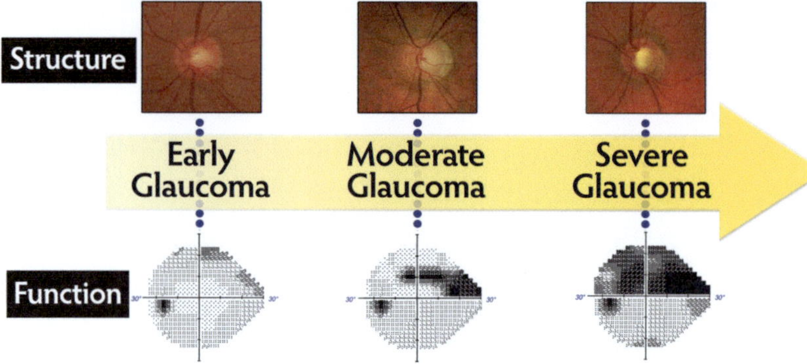

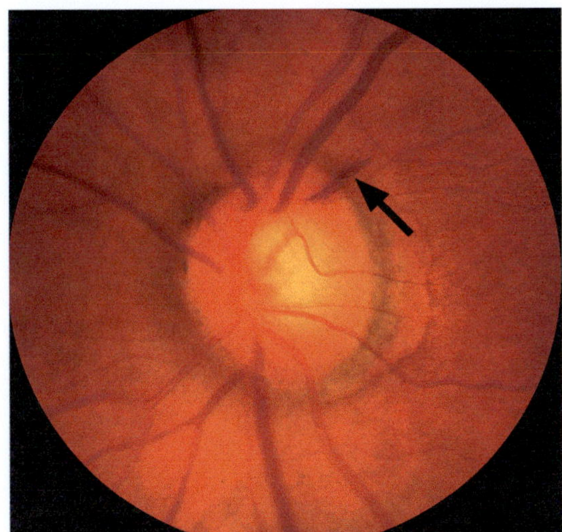

Fig. 15.5 Photograph demonstrating an optic nerve hemorrhage (arrow) which is often a sign of progressive glaucomatous damage. Note that the hemorrhages are easily confused with normal optic nerve vessels

acteristic of glaucomatous optic neuropathy (Fig. 15.5).

As the central cup enlarges and neural tissue of the optic nerve recedes, support for retinal vessels traversing the disc disappears, and vessels are displaced to the nasal aspect of the nerve. By the same token, because of the excavation of optic nerve tissue, displacement of the vessels may cause apparent abrupt changes in the course of vessels that suddenly veer in a new direction to accommodate topographic irregularities of the surrounding neural tissue (Fig. 15.6).

The vascular anatomy of the anterior optic nerve has been extensively studied. Its complex three-dimensional microanatomy and small vessel caliber, similar to that of the brain, have proven difficult to analyze until recently, with the advancement of novel in vivo imaging and post-mortem analysis. The arterial supply of the anterior optic nerve is derived almost entirely from branches of the ophthalmic artery. These branches (posterior ciliary arteries) divide from the oph-

thalmic artery itself, a branch of the internal carotid artery. The posterior ciliary arteries further divide just behind the globe, providing arterial supply to the surrounding choroid, the anterior optic nerve, and dural layers surrounding the optic nerve, beginning at the posterior aspect of the globe. The anterior optic nerve vasculature is almost entirely made up of capillaries that surround bundles of neurons (axons of the retinal ganglion cells) that comprise the neural elements of the optic nerve. Although the central retinal artery (also a branch of the ophthalmic artery) penetrates the optic nerve 10–15 mm behind the globe, it provides few arterial branches to the nerve itself. Instead, it terminates within the eye and provides arterial supply to superficial retina layers. Venous drainage of the optic nerve is almost entirely via tributaries to the central retinal vein, which parallels the central retinal artery and transits through the optic nerve (Fig. 15.7). It is believed that the unique vascular anatomy of the optic nerve may contribute to the development of glaucomatous optic neuropathy, either through insufficiencies in regional supply or alterations in tissue perfusion.

Visual Field Loss Resulting From Glaucomatous Optic Neuropathy

Progressive loss of optic neural fibers eventually leads to progressive loss of visual field and, ultimately, to complete loss of functional vision or blindness. However, in most forms of glaucoma, the individual patient will not experience any symptoms until late in the disease. Early peripheral visual field loss is undetectable to the patient, and its slow progression makes its recognition nearly impossible without special testing. In its normal physiologic state, greater than one million fibers of the optic nerve carry visual information from retinal ganglion cells through the nerve fiber layer of the retina, the optic nerve, and

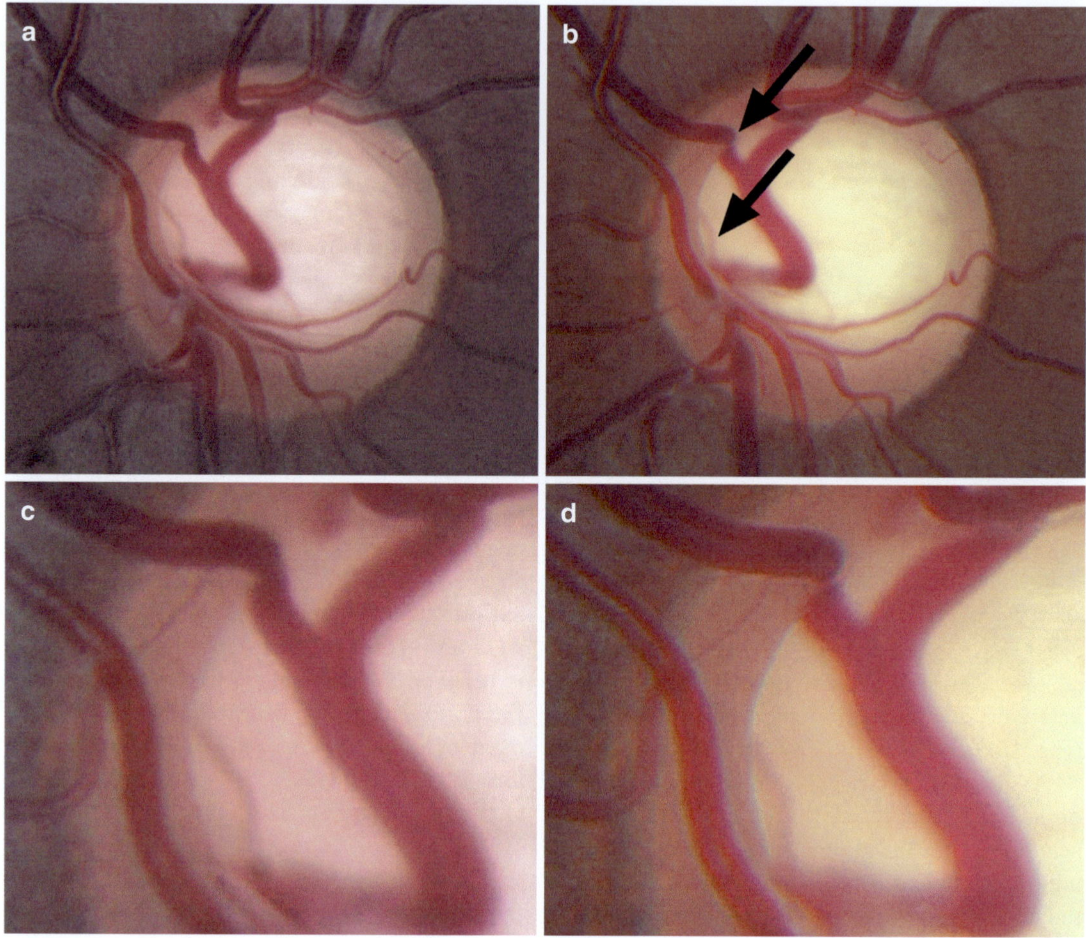

Fig. 15.6 Images (**a, c**) are taken 3 years before images (**b, d**) in an individual with progressive glaucomatous optic neuropathy. Note the enlarging cup with nasalization of the vessels (arrows) seen in (**b, d**)

to the lateral geniculate body of the brain. Fortunately, there is a certain amount of functional reserve (neural redundancy) in the optic nerve so that a considerable portion, perhaps even half, of the nerve fibers can be lost before significant visual field loss occurs. This offers the opportunity for early diagnosis of optic nerve changes before significant impending visual loss transpires, leading to timely therapeutic intervention. The functional status of the optic nerve can be assessed by specialized testing of the peripheral vision, called perimetry (Fig. 15.8).

The anatomy of the retinal nerve fiber layer produces visual field defects from glaucoma that follow a characteristic pattern. Nerve fiber layer loss in glaucoma usually arches from the physiologic blind spot of the optic disc, curving around the central region and ending abruptly along the horizontal axis temporally, corresponding to the temporal raphe of the retinal nerve fiber layer (Fig. 15.9). These arc-shaped defects are known by the eponym of "Bjerrum," or arcuate, scotomas (Fig. 15.10). Loss of the peripheral nasal visual field and/or paracentral region may occur

Fig. 15.7 Illustration of anterior optic nerve (ON) vascular supply and drainage. The central retinal artery penetrates the ON approximately 1–2 cm posterior to the globe and predominantly supplies the retina, while the central retinal vein is the major drainage site of the ON vasculature. The optic nerve vasculature is mainly composed of capillaries supplied by the short posterior arteries and pial vessels

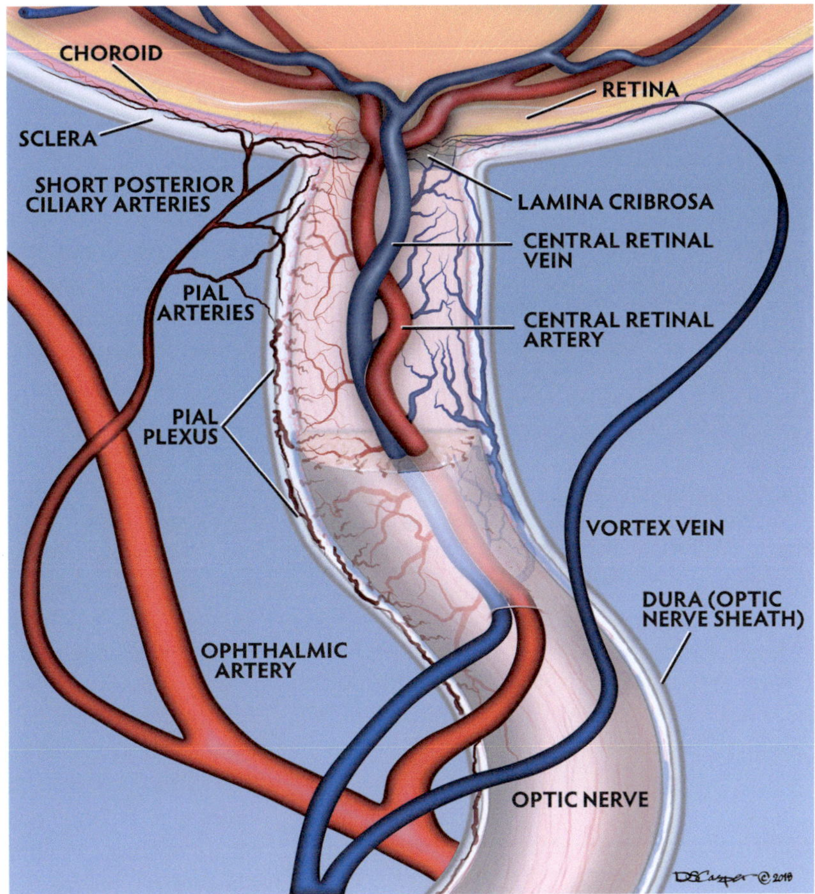

Fig. 15.8 Typical course of progression of retinal nerve fiber layer (RNFL) and visual field (VF) damage seen in progressive glaucoma

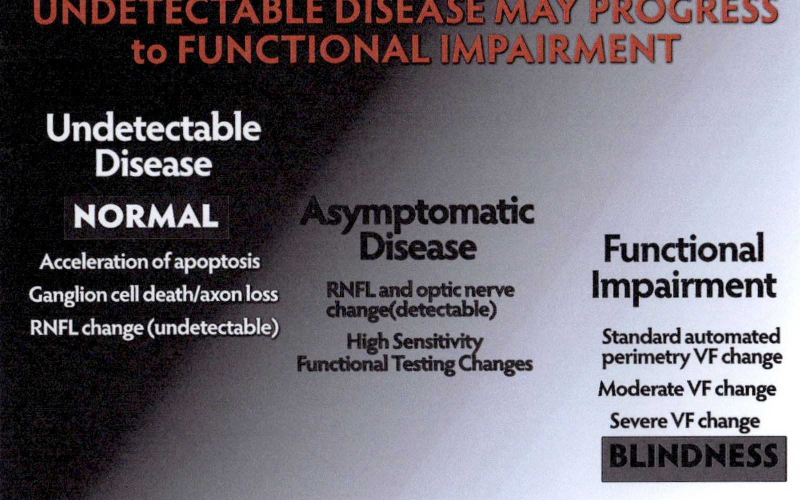

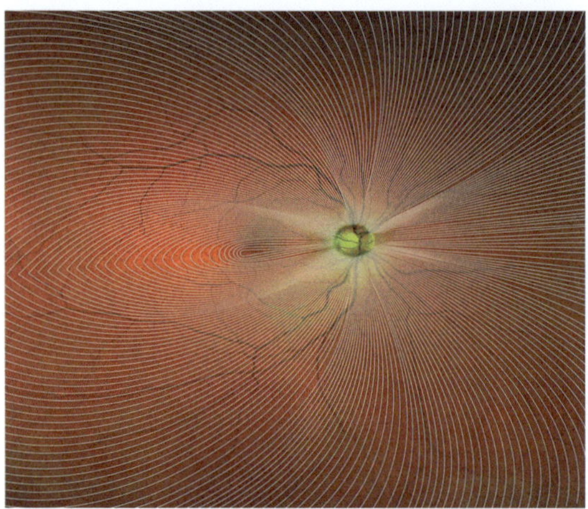

Fig. 15.9 Retinal photograph with a superimposed diagram of the pathways of retinal ganglion cell axons, converging to form the optic nerve, the neural component that transmits visual information to the brain

first in glaucoma. Following the progressive change and course of these visual field defects becomes the most critical aspect of managing the glaucoma patient.

Ophthalmic Examination for Glaucoma

In addition to the complete medical and ocular history and examination, particular emphasis on examination of the anterior chamber angle (gonioscopy), the optic nerve, and the visual field are essential in the ophthalmic examination for glaucoma. Because the anterior chamber angle structures cannot be seen without special optical prism or mirrored devices, gonioscopy becomes a crucial aspect of the glaucoma examination. Using one of a variety of specialized contact lenses, the peripheral iris, cornea, and trabecular meshwork can be directly visualized to determine the presence of angle closure, adhesions,

inflammatory foci, traumatic injury, masses, or other lesions. Gonioscopy is the most important test for the diagnosis of angle-closure glaucoma or the secondary glaucomas discussed earlier (see Figs. 16.1, 17.2, and 20.1).

Since glaucoma consists primarily of chronic progressive optic nerve deterioration, once the specific glaucoma diagnosis is confirmed, glaucoma is followed primarily with periodic assessment of optic nerve anatomy (ophthalmoscopy and/or computerized imaging), function (visual field assessment), and assessment of the most important modifiable risk factor, intraocular pressure. Glaucomatous optic neuropathy in moderate stages is easily recognized ophthalmoscopically by the presence of cupping, enlargement of the physiologic cup, or erosion of the neural rim tissue, especially if the erosion is focal within the nerve or asymmetrical between the two eyes. Anatomic changes in the optic nerve head are readily visualized by ophthalmoscopy but require sophisticated photographic or digital imaging techniques to record for prospective documentation of progressive change. Such documentation of change is done across the disease spectrum but is of utmost importance in earlier stages of glaucoma before extensive loss occurs. Ophthalmologists typically examine the optic nerve stereoscopically using the slit-lamp biomicroscope and specialized, hand-held condensing lenses. Documentation is also aided by fundus photography and modern imaging devices, such as optical coherence tomography. The latter provides objective, numeric values that can help differentiate patients from a database of normal subjects and help track progression over the course of follow-up. Modern visual field testing employs automated computer-generated light detection threshold measurements at multiple locations throughout the field of vision.

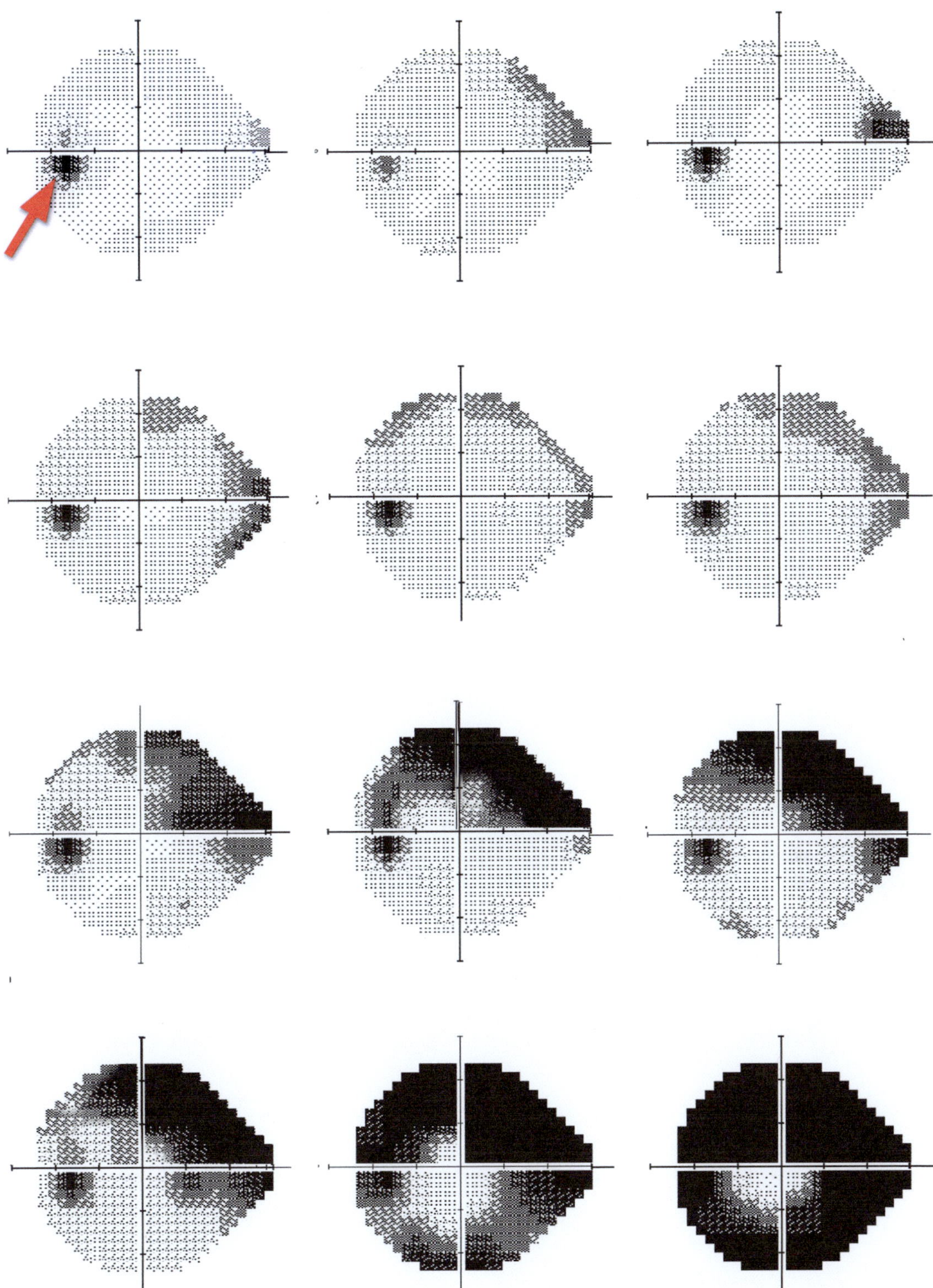

Fig. 15.10 A series of visual fields (all left eyes) demonstrating progressive loss of peripheral vision in glaucoma. The loss in this individual is initially in the superior nasal region and extends over time, to include superior and inferior field loss (arrow denotes the normal blind spot, where the optic nerve exits the eye)

Suggested Reading

Boland M, Quigley HA. Risk factors and open-angle glaucoma: classification and application. J Glaucoma. 2007;16(4):406–18.

Cioffi GA. Optic nerve: anatomy and physiology. In: Gross R, editor. Clinical glaucoma management: critical signs in diagnosis and therapy. Philadelphia: WB Saunders Co.; 2000. p. 34–47.

Van Buskirk EM, Cioffi GA. Glaucomatous optic neuropathy. Am J Ophthalmol. 1992;113(4):447–52.

Van Buskirk EM, Cioffi GA. Predicted outcome from hypotensive therapy for glaucomatous optic neuropathy. Am J Ophthalmol. 1993;116(5):636–40.

Carlos Gustavo De Moraes, Jeffrey Liebmann, and George A. Cioffi

Primary Open-Angle Glaucoma

Patients with open-angle glaucoma manifest a chronic, idiopathic disease associated with progressive degeneration of the anterior optic nerve, known as glaucomatous optic neuropathy. Although elevated intraocular pressure is an important causative risk factor, only about half of the three million North Americans with glaucoma will manifest elevated intraocular pressure at a single measurement. Therefore, measurement of intraocular pressure alone is a poor screening technique for glaucoma. Like most biologic parameters, eye pressure fluctuates diurnally and with other endogenous and exogenous influences, including hydration, sleep, blood pressure, and body position. With multiple measurements at different testing sessions, many, but not all of these glaucoma subjects, will eventually exhibit elevated intraocular pressure at least part of the time. The rise in intraocular pressure associated with primary open-angle glaucoma derives not from a clinically visible obstruction of the trabecular meshwork but rather from cellular dysfunction of the trabecular meshwork tissue leading to reduced permeability and increased aqueous humor outflow resistance. This outflow obstruction probably is associated with a progressive deterioration and loss of trabecular cells and a concomitant accumulation and reduced turnover of extracellular matrix within this complex tissue. Risk factors for primary open-angle glaucoma include family history, corticosteroid sensitivity, myopia, African ancestry, systemic hypertension, ocular hypertension (eye pressure >21 mmHg), diabetes mellitus, and age. In addition to these risk factors, early age of onset of disease and poor compliance with a medical regimen and physician visits are associated with a guarded prognosis. A series of gene defects have been associated with some forms of the disease. As mentioned earlier, some patients with progressive optic nerve damage characteristic of glaucoma never manifest intraocular pressures above the statistically normal range. These patients are commonly diagnosed with "low-pressure," "low-tension," or

C. G. De Moraes, MD, MPH
Columbia University Irving Medical Center,
New York, NY, USA

J. Liebmann, MD
Columbia University Irving Medical Center,
New York, NY, USA

Department of Ophthalmology, Edward S. Harkness
Eye Institute, Columbia University Vagelos College
of Physicians and Surgeons, New York, NY, USA

G. A. Cioffi, MD (✉)
Columbia University Irving Medical Center, New York,
NY, USA

Edward S. Harkness Eye Institute, Columbia
University Vagelos College of Physicians and
Surgeons, New York, NY, USA
e-mail: gac2126@cumc.columbia.edu

© Springer Nature Switzerland AG 2019
D. S. Casper, G. A. Cioffi (eds.), *The Columbia Guide to Basic Elements of Eye Care*,
https://doi.org/10.1007/978-3-030-10886-1_16

"normal-pressure" glaucoma. While recognizing that pressure-independent risk factors may play a stronger role in these than in their high-pressure counterparts, normotensive patients are managed similarly to those with conventional primary open-angle glaucoma.

Primary Angle-Closure Glaucoma

All physicians need to be cognizant of another form of glaucoma, closed angle or angle-closure glaucoma, which may present acutely or may be silent and chronic. Angle-closure glaucoma is more common in individuals of East Asian ancestry but occurs in all populations. This disorder, unrelated to open-angle glaucoma, derives entirely from blockade of the trabecular meshwork by the peripheral iris, either by simple and reversible anatomical apposition of the two tissues or by generally irreversible fibrotic adhesion (Figs. 16.1 and 16.2). These irreversible fibrotic adhesions may occur after unrecognized long-standing appositional angle-closure (chronic angle-closure glaucoma) or from other ocular conditions such as uveitis or neovascularization (secondary angle-closure glaucomas) (see Fig. 27.8b).

Classically, an acute angle-closure glaucoma attack is the well-known but less common variety of glaucoma that presents suddenly with severe ocular pain, blurring of vision, colored halos around lights (rainbows), nausea, and vomiting. Angle closure usually occurs in the hyperopic (far-sighted) eye, which is smaller in diameter than the average eye, thus crowding the iris, cornea, lens, and anterior chamber angle into a smaller than

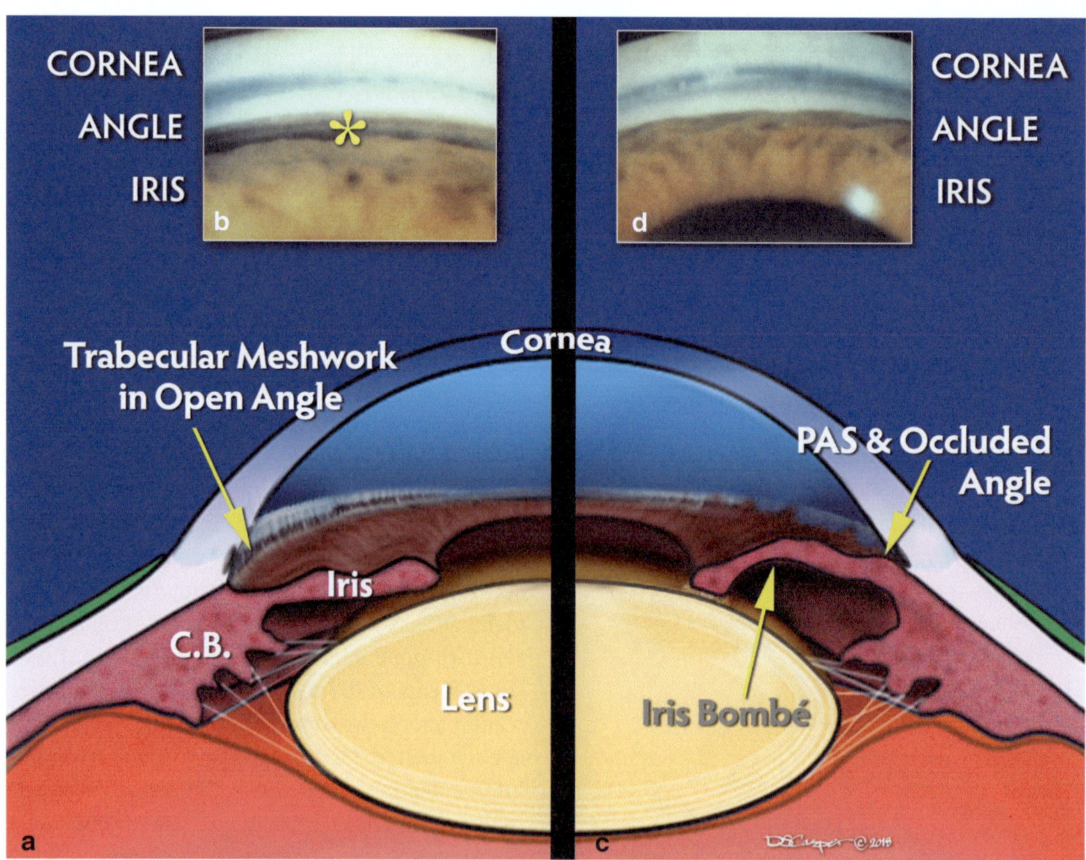

Fig. 16.1 (**a**) Normal anatomy of the anterior ocular structures. (**c**) Occlusion of the conventional outflow pathway as the peripheral iris blocks the trabecular meshwork. Insets (**b**) and (**d**) are gonioscopic photos of the same (*C.B.* ciliary body, *PAS* peripheral anterior synechiae)

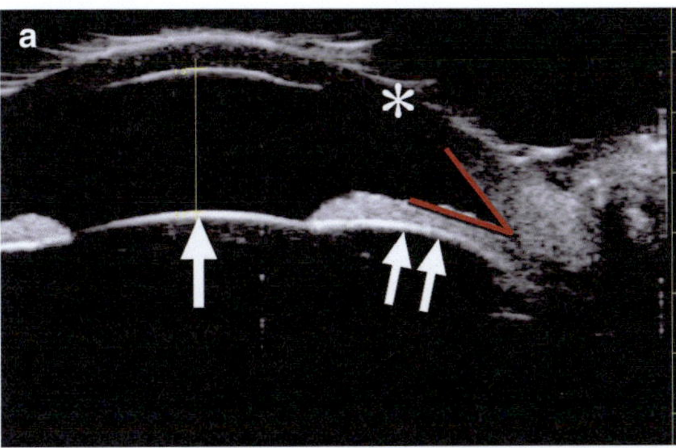
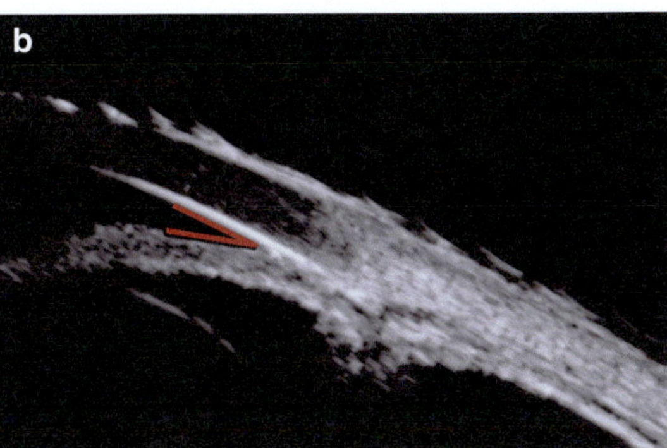

Fig. 16.2 Ultrasonic biomicroscopy of the normal eye (**a**) and eye with a narrow anterior chamber angle (**b**) (red lines indicate the angles). The angle between the periph- eral iris and cornea is nearly occluded in (**b**) (single arrow, anterior lens surface; double arrow, iris; asterisk, cornea). (Courtesy of Dr. Ronald Silverman)

average space. Eventually, as the crystalline lens gradually increases in size with aging (usually in the fifth to sixth decade of life), the lens-iris contact increases and limits the movement of aqueous from its site of production in the posterior chamber (ciliary body), through the pupillary aperture, to the anterior chamber. This partial obstruction of aqueous humor flow at the pupil, known as relative pupillary block, eventually becomes clinically significant and traps aqueous behind the pupil, raising the posterior chamber pressure above that in the anterior chamber and driving the iris anteriorly to lie against and block the trabecular meshwork. Trabecular meshwork blockade or angle-closure may lead to a sudden and dramatic rise of the intraocular pressure from its baseline normal level in the 10–20 mmHg range to 60 mmHg or more. This abrupt pressure elevation leads to corneal edema, with blurred vision, rainbow halos, and severe ocular pain from the corneal edema as well as iris ischemia. Pupillary block is typically maximal when the pupil is in the mid-dilated position, and partial dilation of the pupil by exposure to stress, darkness, or drugs (topically and systemically administered) may induce an acute attack of angle-closure glaucoma.

The immediate treatment of acute-angle closure is directed toward reversal of the pupillary block, usually by constriction of the pupil with various medications. Ultimately, however, the pupillary block can be reversed and prevented by creating a new aqueous channel with laser peripheral iridectomy (see Fig. 20.2).

Important Secondary Glaucomas

Glaucoma Associated with Ocular Trauma

Glaucoma may develop after ocular trauma. Penetrating injuries to the globe disrupt, or even destroy, intraocular contents and may lead to sustained elevation of intraocular pressure and glaucoma. A more subtle, insidious glaucoma may arise from blunt ocular injury or ocular contusion, as occurs when the globe is struck with a fist, ball, or other object. Blunt injury transiently deforms the globe causing shearing between its internal tissue layers. These shearing forces may tear the insertion of the iris (iridodialysis, Fig. 16.3) or ciliary body (cyclodialysis) from its attachment to the sclera. Most commonly, the fibers of the ciliary muscle that both control accommodation and modulate aqueous humor outflow are torn, leading to trabecular dysfunction and subsequent secondary glaucoma (angle recession glaucoma).

Acutely, the contused eye typically presents with intraocular hemorrhage (hyphema, see Fig. 2.12), and the intraocular pressure may be low, normal, or elevated. Angle recession glaucoma may not manifest for months or even years after the original injury. Thus, in any unilateral glaucoma, inquiry about a previous black eye, especially with hyphema, may help identify the underlying diagnosis. Gonioscopic examination

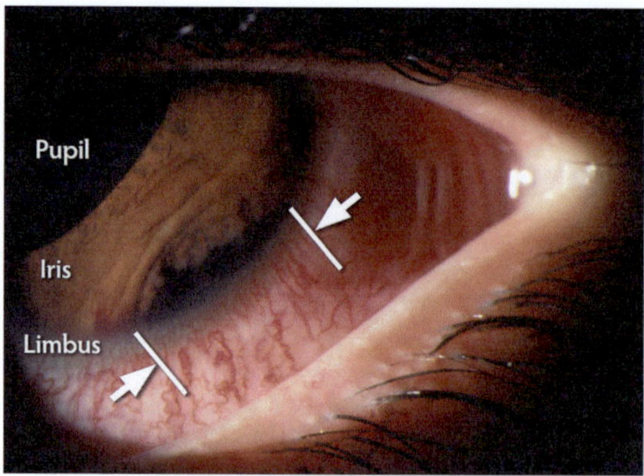

Fig. 16.3 Photograph of iris disinsertion (iridodialysis) secondary to blunt ocular trauma (arrows indicate extent of iridodialysis). (Modified with permission from Casper DS, Trokel SL, Chi TL. *Orbital disease: imaging and analysis.* New York: Thieme Medical Publishers Inc.; 1993.)

is also mandatory in these cases. Treatment of glaucoma from blunt ocular trauma follows a similar protocol for more common open-angle glaucomas. In addition, the trabecular meshwork is usually sufficiently damaged, so laser trabeculoplasty is similarly ineffective. Thus, when topical aqueous suppressant agents are ineffective, filtration surgery usually is required to reduce IOP.

Exfoliation Syndrome and Exfoliative Glaucoma

Exfoliation syndrome, also known as pseudoexfoliation syndrome, is the single most common identifiable cause of open-angle glaucoma worldwide and is associated with a defect in the LOXL1 gene. The disease is characterized by the production and deposition of white fibrillogranular material, visible during slit-lamp biomicroscopy, within the anterior segment, which results in trabecular dysfunction (Fig. 16.4). The condition may be bilateral, unilateral, or asymmetric and is notable for labile intraocular pressures. Treatment is similar to other open-angle glaucomas. Zonular laxity caused by exfoliation syndrome may cause anterior movement of the crystalline lens, pupillary block, and angle closure. Zonular laxity and the associated typical poor pupillary dilation lead

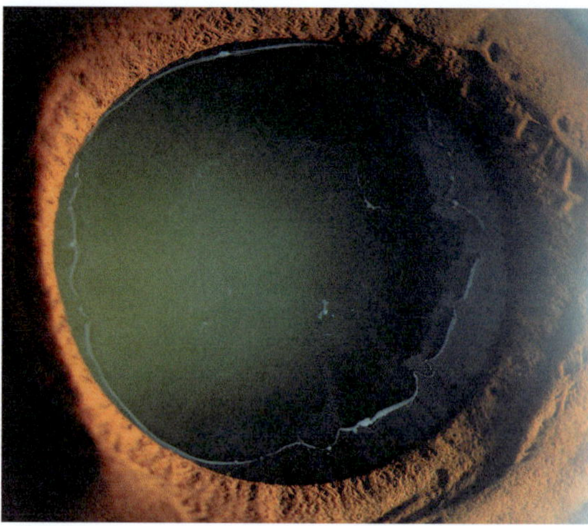

Fig. 16.4 Deposits of pseudoexfoliative material on the anterior lens surface. The protein appears as white "dusting" on many anterior segment structures

to an increased frequency of complications during cataract surgery.

Pigmentary Glaucoma

Pigmentary glaucoma is a relatively common secondary glaucoma in the young adult and appears to be exclusively an ocular disorder. This disease is significantly relevant because of the potentially severe consequences in young people in the presumed prime of life. Pigmentary glaucoma occurs primarily in young myopic (nearsighted) adults and is more common in males, usually manifesting between ages 20 and 40 years. Melanin pigment granules from the iris circulate freely in the aqueous humor and ultimately become deposited or entrapped in the surrounding tissues, including the cornea, iris, and lens and particularly within the interstices of the trabecular meshwork. This leads to obstruction of the meshwork and reduced aqueous outflow, elevation of intraocular pressure, and glaucoma. This condition may manifest with intermittent visual blurring or dull ocular pain but like other glaucomas may go unnoticed until severe visual loss occurs. Vigorous physical activity or pupillary dilation may induce a shower of pigment granules to be released acutely from the iris in these patients, resulting in a transient, acute rise in eye pressure, corneal edema, blurred vision, and ocular pain. Treatment of pigmentary glaucoma is similar to that for primary open-angle glaucoma, but some patients may respond to laser iridotomy to restore a more normal iris configuration.

Neovascular Glaucoma

Glaucoma is typically a disease of the middle aged and the elderly. Thus, its occurrence in children or young adults always raises the question of some associated condition, such as intraocular tumor, diabetes mellitus, and other vascular disorders which are frequently associated with neovascular glaucoma. The devastating consequences of diabetes upon the retinal vasculature and its associated diabetic retinopathy are well known. In addition to these problems, the diabetic patient may also develop glaucoma as a result of retinal ischemia, known as neovascular glaucoma. Neovascular glaucoma is one of the most devastating varieties of glaucoma. Just as retinal microangiopathy secondary to ischemia may result in retinal neovascularization and bleeding, retinal ischemia may also cause proliferation of fibrovascular tissue in the anterior segment of the eye. It is believed that angiogenic factors (such as VEGF) are produced by the ischemic retina which lead to new vessel formation inside the eye. Unfortunately, these vessels are aberrant and may cause a variety of vision-threatening sequelae, including secondary angle closure. Neovascular glaucoma derives from fibrovascular proliferation of friable new vessels on the iris (rubeosis iridis; see Figs. 16.5 and 22.13) and into the chamber angle. The trabecular meshwork provides a fertile template for neovascular growth, ultimately resulting in complete blockade of the aqueous humor outflow, marked elevation of intraocular pressure, and severe, often painful, blinding glaucoma. This process can also follow other vascular conditions associated with retinal ischemia, including occlusion of the central retinal vein, occlusion of the central retinal artery, and even carotid occlusive disease without manifest retinopathy. Treatment of neovascular

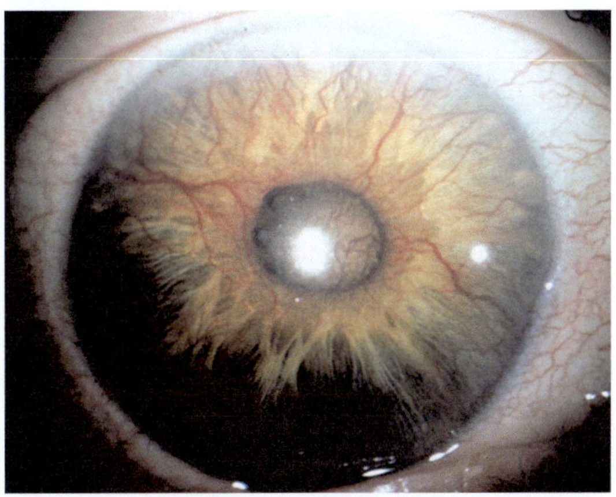

Fig. 16.5 Abnormal blood vessel growth on anterior surface of the iris (rubeosis iridis) secondary to ischemic eye disease in an individual with diabetes mellitus

glaucoma is multifaceted and involves diligent systemic management of related vascular disease, treatment of retinal ischemia, and lowering of the intraocular pressure with medical and, often, surgical therapy.

Glaucoma Associated with Increased Episcleral Venous Pressure

Another unusual form of glaucoma is that associated with increased episcleral venous pressure, typically derived from an intracranial arteriovenous shunt. Elevated episcleral venous pressure results in elevated intraocular pressure because the final step in the pathway of aqueous humor drainage is the episcleral venous system. Patients with elevated episcleral venous pressure present with a "red eye," sometimes with proptosis, chemosis, or even an orbital bruit. These findings are associated with an engorged venous system in the eye and orbit. The classic etiology is a carotid artery-cavernous sinus fistula with a high-flow shunt, often following trauma, and is more likely to present with the full spectrum of clinical findings. The fistulas most commonly referred to the ophthalmologist are low volume, low-flow shunts spontaneously occurring between dural arterial vessels and the venous system, often in elderly subjects. These present with less severe clinical signs – enlarged, dilated, tortuous episcleral veins that may mimic an inflamed, red eye from other causes such as conjunctivitis or thyroid ophthalmopathy. The absence of other clinical signs of inflammation, the identification of individual dilated, racemose vessels rather than generalized vascular engorgement, and the identification by the clinician or the patient of an orbital bruit help with diagnosis. Because the glaucoma derives from increased episcleral venous pressure, these eyes are usually resistant to medical therapy and require surgical intervention. Successful neuroradiologic intervention with closure of the fistula usually corrects the glaucoma.

Oculofacial hemangioma, associated with the Sturge-Weber syndrome (Fig. 16.6), classically presents with the facial port-wine stain and often ipsilateral glaucoma. All patients with Sturge-Weber syndrome should be evaluated for glaucoma. These glaucomas may occur in infancy or early childhood, or milder forms may be delayed until adulthood.

Congenital Glaucoma

Although glaucoma is commonly associated with adult and elderly patients, childhood or infantile glaucomas also exist (see Chap. 17). The most common primary congenital glaucoma occurs in children without other identifiable ocular or systemic abnormalities. Most cases become evident in the first year of life and often present in the newborn nursery or first few weeks of age. The exact cause of infantile glaucoma is unknown but appears related to a delay in development of aqueous humor outflow channels and is associated with a recessive gene (most often, CYP1B1).

Infants with congenital glaucoma present with photophobia (light sensitivity), epiphora (tearing), and blepharospasm. The principal clinical sign is an enlarged cornea, often bilateral. As the disorder advances, the cornea becomes edematous and appears cloudy. The appearance of an enlarged cloudy cornea in an infant is virtually pathognomonic for congenital glaucoma and can be obvious to causal penlight examination. Prompt referral to an ophthalmologist for intervention can make the difference between sight and permanent blindness.

Various forms of developmental glaucoma may also be associated with congenital malformations of the anterior chamber angle. Axenfeld-Rieger syndrome, associated with dental, facial, and other midline developmental abnormalities, adhesions between the cornea and iris, and glaucoma, is the most common. Aniridia is a bilateral congenital absence of the iris that may be inherited by autosomal dominant transmission or may occur spontaneously (see Fig. 1.22). These latter, spontaneous cases may be associated with Wilms' tumor or other anomalies of the genitourinary system. Glaucoma with aniridia usually occurs in early to mid-childhood and is not typically associated with megalocornea.

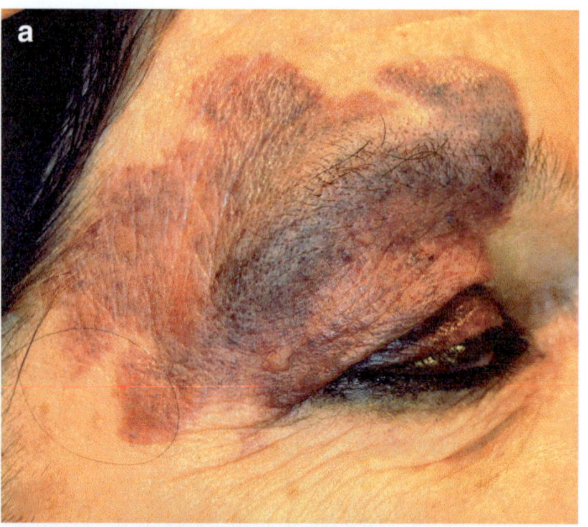
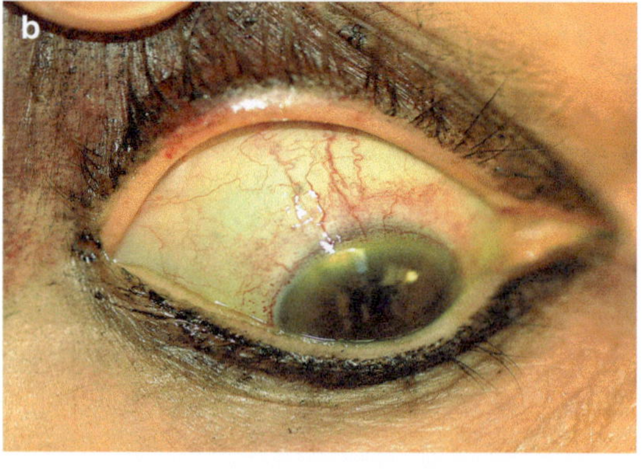

Fig. 16.6 (**a**) External photograph of "port-wine stain" in an individual with Sturge-Weber syndrome. Note the enlarged episcleral vessels on the surface of the eye (**b**)

Treatment

Although it is recognized that not all glaucoma patients manifest elevated intraocular pressure and not all glaucomatous optic nerve damage is attributable entirely to pressure damage per se, current standard glaucoma care is devoted almost exclusively to reduction of intraocular pressure (see Chaps. 19 and 20). Such pressure reduction, when substantial (to the normal or low normal range, 17 mmHg or less), can be expected to arrest progression or dramatically slow its course in the vast majority of cases. At the same time, it must be recognized that some unfortunate individuals, usually those diagnosed late with end-stage neural damage, those with an unusually vulnerable optic nerve, or those who are primarily sensitive to nonpressure factors, will continue to show unabated visual field loss despite significant pressure lowering. These are the individuals to whom future research regarding other pressure-independent causative factors and their treatment must be directed.

Three modalities for glaucoma hypotensive treatment are available – medicinal (usually topical eye drops), laser surgery, and incisional surgery – all of which are designed only to lower intraocular pressure. Since the threshold of pressure damage varies among patients, the only reliable indicator of glaucoma stabilization is stability of the visual field, arresting of visual field loss, and prevention of optic nerve damage. To date, reversal of glaucomatous damage is not possible. As with systemic hypertension, controversy exists about the appropriate time to institute hypotensive therapy and whether it should be medical or surgical. In the usual glaucoma therapy, intraocular pressure may be lowered by any or all of three methods (medical, laser, and surgery). In a normal, non-glaucomatous population, intraocular pressure averages approximately 16 mmHg, and most (95%) will fall between 10 and 21 mmHg, the most frequently cited normal range. In the untreated glaucomatous population, the mean intraocular pressure is somewhat higher, and the range much broader, even as high as 70 mmHg where arterial circulation to the eye begins to be compromised. Typically, however, the early, untreated open-angle glaucoma patient will manifest an eye pressure in the mid-20s. Measurement of intraocular pressure at different times of the day establishes the degree of pressure variability before hypotensive therapy is started. The experienced practitioner typically will determine a "target pressure" as a goal to achieve with hypotensive therapy, recognizing that the estimated target pressure may have to be revised based on further longitudinal assessment of the visual field and its progression.

Drugs placed on the ocular surface enter the systemic circulation by absorption through the mucosa of the nasolacrimal passages and the gut. Although systemic β-adrenergic blockade from topical β-adrenergic eye drops is the most common and best-known complication of topical glaucoma medication, all ocular drugs demonstrate some systemic absorption and can be associated with systemic effects. At the present time, most glaucoma patients are treated first with medical agents, then laser, and finally surgery. Immediate surgical therapy for early glaucoma may sometimes be required; however, the potential for surgical complications including cataract or devastating (and rare) intraocular hemorrhage may occur.

Frequency of Visits

After initial examination and diagnosis, glaucoma patients are managed much like patients with other chronic disease, requiring regular visits to assess disease severity and response to therapy. The primary criterion for disease status is the visual field, since it is the most accurate measure of visual function in this disorder. Typical open-angle glaucoma requires management much like other chronic disorders, with periodic medical examinations, diagnostic testing for progression or new findings, and titration of management with drugs or procedures as needed. Once the diagnosis and treatment regimen are established, the average patient needs to be seen two to four times yearly with one to two visual field tests per year (Table 16.1). Frequency of visits and testing depends upon risks for progressive damage and

Table 16.1 Average annual glaucoma care visits and tests adjusted for severity of illness

	Elevated IOP and normal VF	Early VF loss	Advanced VF loss	VF loss within central 5	Multirisk factors	"Low-tension glaucoma"
Number of annual visits	1–2	2–3	3–4	4	4–6	6
Visual fields per year	0.5–1	1	2	2	2–3	2–3
Dilated fundus examination per year	1	1	2	2	2	2–3
Optic nerve imaging	Initial exam	0.5–1	1–2	1–2	1–3	2–4

IOP intraocular pressure, *VF* visual field testing

severity of illness. It is generally recommended that patients undergo four to six visual field tests in the first 2 years, to increase the power to detect fast progression (see Chap. 18). Because subject performance of visual field testing shows some endogenous and exogenous variability, significant changes in management based upon apparent visual field deterioration require confirmatory retesting of the visual field.

Suggested Reading

Cioffi GA, Van Buskirk EM. What is glaucoma? In: Wright KW, editor. Textbook of ophthalmology. Baltimore: Williams and Wilkins; 1996. p. 563–8.

Killer HE, Pircher A. Normal tension glaucoma: review of current understanding and mechanisms of the pathogenesis. Eye (Lond). 2018;32(5):924–30.

Lascaratos G, Shah A, Garway-Heath DF. The genetics of pigment dispersion syndrome and pigmentary glaucoma. Surv Ophthalmol. 2013;58(2):164–75.

Marchini G, Chemello F, Berzaghi D, Zampieri A. New findings in the diagnosis and treatment of primary angle-closure glaucoma. Prog Brain Res. 2015;221:191–212.

Vesti E, Kivelä T. Exfoliation syndrome and exfoliation glaucoma. Prog Retin Eye Res. 2000;19(3):345–68.

Weinreb RN, Aung T, Medeiros FA. The pathophysiology and treatment of glaucoma: a review. JAMA. 2014;311(18):1901–11.

Pediatric Glaucoma

17

Steven A. Kane

In the primary care setting, an encounter with a child affected by glaucoma is unusual. When all pediatric glaucomas are considered, between 1 in 4000 and 1 in 6000 children are affected by these conditions. Though unusual, the pediatric glaucomas are treatable causes of permanent blindness, so timely recognition and treatment can have profound implications over a lifetime.

Pathophysiology

Glaucoma during childhood is the consequence of abnormal eye pressure, most commonly elevated pressure. Elevated eye pressure in children and adults damages ocular structures vital for the transduction of visual imagery and transmission of this visual information to the brain. Persistently elevated eye pressures are necessary to diagnose active pediatric glaucoma. The progressive glaucomatous visual loss seen in some adults with typically normal eye pressures (low-tension glaucoma, see Chap. 15) is not known to occur in children.

In a normal eye, aqueous humor is produced at the ciliary body and is drained at the filtration angle (Fig. 17.1). Nearly all aqueous humor drains across trabecular meshwork, into Schlemm's canal, and then along collector channels that end at the intravascular space in episcleral vessels. The pediatric glaucomas all share a common feature: derangement of aqueous humor circulation, typically due to obstruction around the pupil or angle or higher resistance along this drainage system. Understanding the nature of a pediatric glaucoma can often be enhanced when the filtration angle is visualized through a contact lens (Fig. 17.2a, b). Because the development of other ocular tissues occurs in concert with the development of the filtration angle, concomitant anomalies of other ocular tissues such as the iris stroma can often be seen. In infantile primary congenital glaucoma (PCG), the development of these drainage tissues is interrupted and the angle is anomalous (Fig. 17.2c). The trabecular meshwork is found compressed during histological analysis and is believed to be the primary site of increased resistance to aqueous humor drainage, a hypothesis supported by the highly successful results of goniotomy, a surgical procedure to incise the trabeculum.

Acquired disease processes can damage a normal eye in children and adults and secondarily impair aqueous humor circulation. Processes which can impair aqueous drainage include traumatic, inflammatory, neoplastic, surgical, toxic, vascular, developmental lens, and infectious conditions during childhood.

S. A. Kane, MD, PhD (✉)
Department of Ophthalmology, Edward S. Harkness
Eye Institute, Columbia University Vagelos College
of Physicians and Surgeons, New York, NY, USA
e-mail: sak6@cumc.columbia.edu

© Springer Nature Switzerland AG 2019
D. S. Casper, G. A. Cioffi (eds.), *The Columbia Guide to Basic Elements of Eye Care*,
https://doi.org/10.1007/978-3-030-10886-1_17

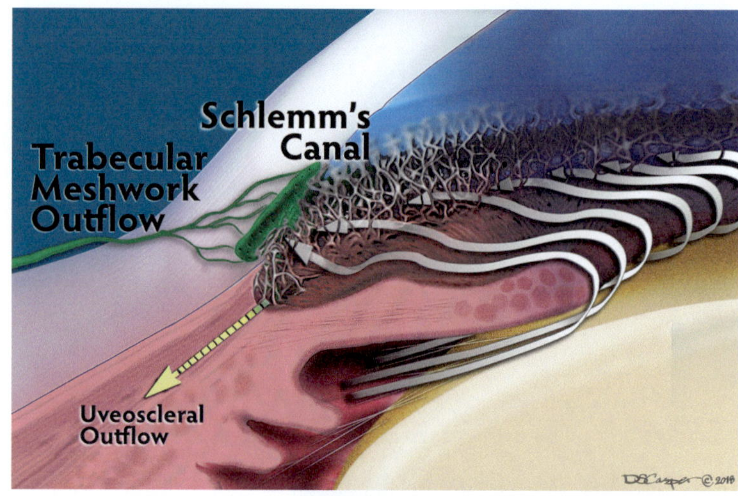

Fig. 17.1 Normal aqueous production at the ciliary body, flow through the pupil and toward the angle, and drainage primarily through Schlemm's canal to the aqueous venous system and the alternative uveoscleral outflow path

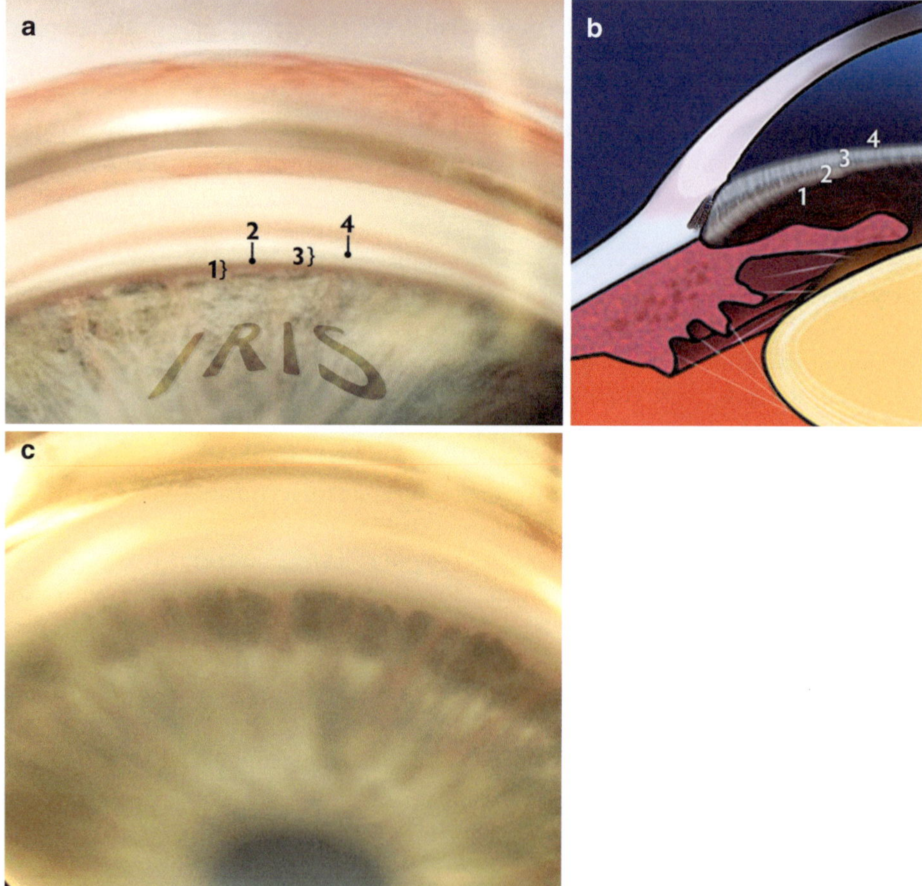

Fig. 17.2 (**a**, **b**) Normal angle structures seen through a contact lens. The textured iris extends from the pupil at the bottom of the image to its root. Just above the iris root is the brown ciliary body band. Trabecular meshwork is seen as a pale, tan band just above the ciliary body band. (1) Ciliary body, (2) scleral spur, (3) trabecular meshwork, (4) Schwalbe's line (not well visualized here). (**c**) The angle structures in an eye affected by PCG are anomalous. The iris root is anteriorly displaced with a palisading margin, ending at trabecular meshwork and obscuring the ciliary body band. ((**b**) Modified from Fig. 31.1: Al-Aswad LA, Casper DS. Laser trabeculoplasty. In: Albert DM, Lucarelli M, editors. Clinical atlas of procedures in ophthalmic and oculofacial surgery. New York: Oxford University Press; 2012. p. 308–312, with permission)

Classification

Table 17.1 contains a shortened list of the pediatric glaucomas organized according to primary and secondary etiologies. The diversity of these conditions is noted, and ophthalmic examination for any child affected by them is a consideration.

Primary glaucomas, listed along the left column, are genetically determined conditions which result in abnormal development of ocular

Table 17.1 Table for primary and secondary childhood glaucomas

I. Primary (developmental) glaucomas	II. Secondary glaucomas
A. Primary congenital glaucoma	A. Traumatic glaucoma
1. Newborn PCG	1. Acute glaucoma
2. Infantile PCG	(a) Hyphema
3. Late-recognized PCG	(b) Ghost cell glaucoma
B. Juvenile open-angle glaucoma	2. Angle recession glaucoma
C. Primary angle-closure glaucoma	B. Intraocular neoplasms
D. Associated with systemic disease	1. Retinoblastoma
1. Sturge-Weber syndrome	2. Juvenile xanthogranuloma
2. Neurofibromatosis type 1	3. Leukemia
3. Stickler syndrome	4. Mucogenic iris stromal cyst
4. Lowe syndrome	C. Chronic uveitis
5. Rieger syndrome	1. Open-angle glaucoma
6. Zellweger syndrome	2. Angle-blockage mechanisms
7. Marfan syndrome	(a) Synechial angle closure
8. Rubinstein-Taybi syndrome	(b) Iris bombe, pupillary block
9. Infantile glaucoma associated with mental retardation and paralysis	D. Lens-induced glaucoma
10. Oculodentodigital dysplasia	1. Subluxation with pupillary block
11. Glaucoma with microcornea and absent sinuses	(a) Marfan syndrome
12. Mucopolysaccharidosis	(b) Homocystinuria
13. Trisomy 13	2. Spherophakia with pupillary block
14. Cutis marmorata telangiectasia	3. Phacolytic glaucoma
15. Warburg syndrome	E. Glaucoma following lensectomy
16. Kniest syndrome	1. Pupillary block
17. Michel's syndrome	2. Aphakic glaucoma
18. Nonprogressive hemiatrophy	F. Steroid-induced glaucoma
19. PHACE syndrome	G. Secondary to rubeosis
20. Soto syndrome	1. Coats' disease
E. With profound ocular anomalies	2. Medulloepithelioma
1. Aniridia	3. Familial exudative vitreoretinopathy
(a) Congenital aniridic glaucoma	4. Subacute/chronic retinal detachment
(b) Acquired aniridic glaucoma	H. Angle closure glaucoma
2. Congenital ocular melanosis	1. Retinopathy of prematurity
3. Sclerocornea	2. Nanophthalmos
4. Iris ectropion uvea syndrome	3. Persistent fetal vasculature
5. Peters syndrome	4. Pupillary-iris-lens membrane syndrome
6. Posterior polymorphous dystrophy	5. Topiramate therapy
7. Idiopathic elevated episcleral venous pressure	I. Malignant glaucoma
8. Congenital anterior staphyloma	J. Increased episcleral venous pressure
9. Congenital microcoria	1. Sturge-Weber syndrome
10. Congenital hereditary endothelial dystrophy	2. Arteriovenous fistula
11. Axenfeld-Rieger anomaly	K. Intraocular infection
	1. Acute recurrent toxoplasmosis
	2. Acute herpes iritis
	3. Maternal rubella infection
	4. Endogenous endophthalmitis

From Yeung HH, Walton DS. Clinical classification of childhood glaucomas. Arch Ophthal. 2010;128(6):680–4 tissues variably associated with elevated eye pressure. They can be distinguished by genotype and phenotype, yet many share a common feature, a developmental abnormality of the filtration angle that is present at birth. By emphasizing the diverse genetic bases of these primary glaucomas, such a classification can promote understanding of ocular development at a molecular level as well as the differential effects of treatments. In newborn PCG, abnormal eye pressure is found at birth and accompanied by a more severe developmental anomaly or hypoplasia of the filtration angle than is seen in infantile PCG. The often disappointing results of goniotomy for newborn PCG support the involvement of tissues deep to the trabeculum as the primary site of increased resistance to aqueous humor drainage in this condition.

Secondary glaucomas are listed along the right column. These acquired conditions are distinguished by normal aqueous humor circulation at birth that becomes impaired by disease. They are highly variable and include blockage of aqueous humor at the pupil due to lens disorders, inflammatory conditions, and posterior masses and impairment of the filtration angle such as by blood or hyphema, chronic inflammation or uveitis, neovascularization, and infection.

Genetics

The primary or genetically determined pediatric glaucomas are notable for their diversity in genotype, phenotype, and inheritance. The most common group of primary glaucomas, primary congenital glaucoma (PCG), can occur sporadically or as an autosomal recessive trait. Consanguinity and a high carrier rate within a community are known to increase the incidence of PCG from 1 in 10,000 to 12,500 births in western countries to 1 in 1250 births in Slovak Roms. Mutations in two genes, CYP1B1 and LTBP2, are known to cause PCG. Mutations in the CYP1B1 gene are highly penetrant with variable expressivity. Variable gene expressivity explains how some affected children can have only a subtle anomaly

of the filtration angle with normal eye pressure, while others have a marked anomaly of the filtration angle and elevated pressure. Severity of PCG disease has been correlated with certain mutations in CYP1B1. The classification of pediatric glaucomas in Table 17.1 also finds conditions such as aniridia and the Sturge-Weber syndrome associated with glaucoma during early infancy, yet due to mutations in genes other than CYP1B1 and LTBP2. Clearly the genetics of ocular development are complex. Genetic counseling is often appropriate and can utilize individual family structure, biomolecular data, and available statistics to advise parents and caregivers.

Symptoms and Signs

Suspicion of pediatric glaucoma is developed by recognition of characteristic symptoms and signs, recognition of an associated systemic or ocular syndrome such as listed in Table 17.1, family history, or the presence of active or past intraocular disease.

The symptoms and signs of glaucoma in childhood listed in Table 17.2 are highly variable and influenced by age. Some, such as irritability, headache, epiphora, and vomiting, are frequently encountered in the primary care setting. For a child with significant active or past intraocular disease or with a family history of intraocular disease, the possibility that such frequently encountered and perhaps nonspecific symptoms and signs are due to an ocular problem is significantly increased. Examples illustrating the importance of such consideration of past ocular history could

Table 17.2 Symptoms and signs of childhood glaucoma

Pain
Irritability
Light sensitivity
Epiphora
Corneal enlargement
Cloudy cornea
Myopia
Unexplained vomiting
Vision loss
Optic disc cupping
Optic atrophy

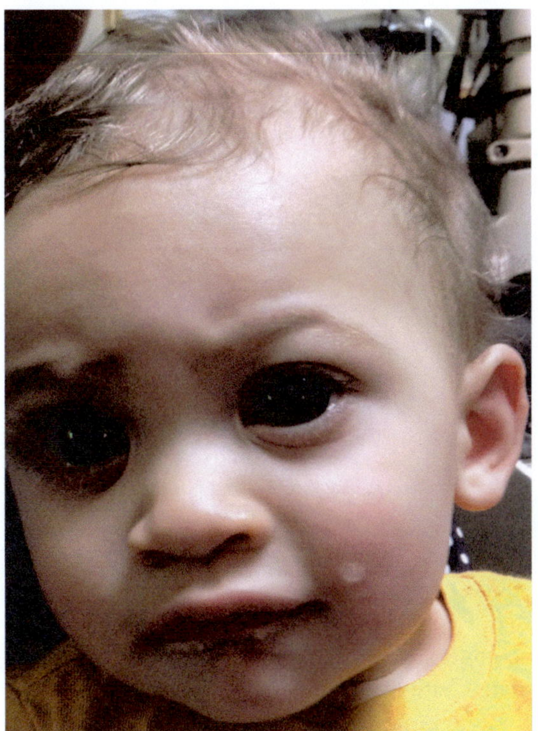

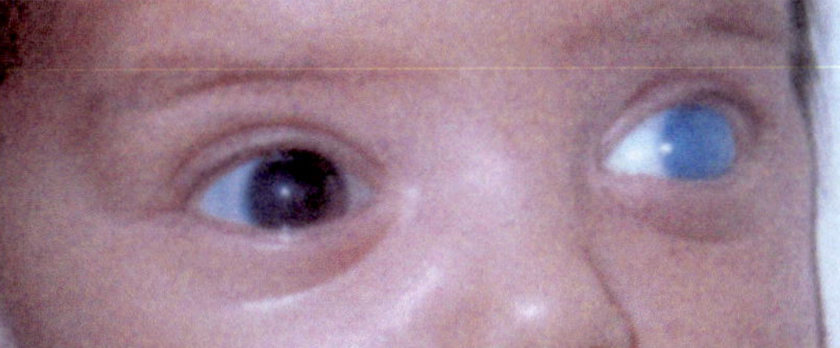

Fig. 17.4 This child developed striking and complete opacification of the left cornea within 10 min while at home. Examination revealed the presence of primary congenital glaucoma due to aniridia

Fig. 17.3 This child with infantile PCG has excessive light sensitivity, requiring drawn curtains at home and dim lighting during ophthalmic examination to open his eyes. He displays spontaneous tearing without crying and bilateral corneal enlargement. Before his symptoms progressed, he was thought to have beautifully large eyes

include a child of extreme prematurity with severe headache attributed to new onset migraine and a child with congenital cataract with recent onset recurrent vomiting and lethargy, attributed to atypical gastroenteritis. In both instances catastrophic visual loss could result if the possibility of acute glaucoma is not considered.

Other symptoms and signs such as extreme light sensitivity, blepharospasm, corneal haze, and corneal enlargement are infrequently encountered but more suggestive of glaucoma. The significance of the symptoms and signs displayed by the child in Fig. 17.3 is enhanced by the medical history and the results of careful physical examination.

A cloudy cornea is the most common first sign of childhood glaucoma recognized by a parent, physician, or nurse practitioner. The normal hydrostatic balance is altered by high eye pressure, and aqueous humor is driven into the cornea, lessening its clarity. If the eye pressure rises slowly or is only mildly elevated in both eyes, the corneas may be subtly hazy and impart or exaggerate a blue coloration that may initially appear pleasing. Recognition of the abnormality may be delayed until more significant corneal opacification develops. If only one eye is affected, heterochromia, asymmetric eye color, and pupil asymmetry typically gain attention promptly and, like any other ocular asymmetry, merit referral to a pediatric ophthalmologist.

Abnormal corneal enlargement is unique to children under 3 years of age. The ocular coats are elastic in early childhood, and eye growth accelerates in response to elevated eye pressure, similar to head growth acceleration due to elevated intracranial pressure. When bilateral, corneal enlargement can initially be interpreted as pleasingly large eyes. The abnormality can be recognized during a side-by-side comparison of cornea sizes between child and parent; no feature of a child should be larger than the corresponding feature of the parent. When unilateral or asymmetric, corneal enlargement is often detectable by inspection and careful consideration, even when the disparity between corneal diameters is as little as 0.25 mm. The onset of corneal clouding may be sudden (as seen in Fig. 17.4) if, as the cornea stretches, its posterior layer tears, resulting in a region of cornea overlying the tear, or sometimes the entire cornea, becoming opaque due to edema. Once the cornea recovers, opacification usually clears, and stretch marks called Haab stria can be visualized with a slit lamp (Fig. 17.5a) and sometimes as an anomaly of the red reflex (Fig. 17.5b). Haab stria remains as a

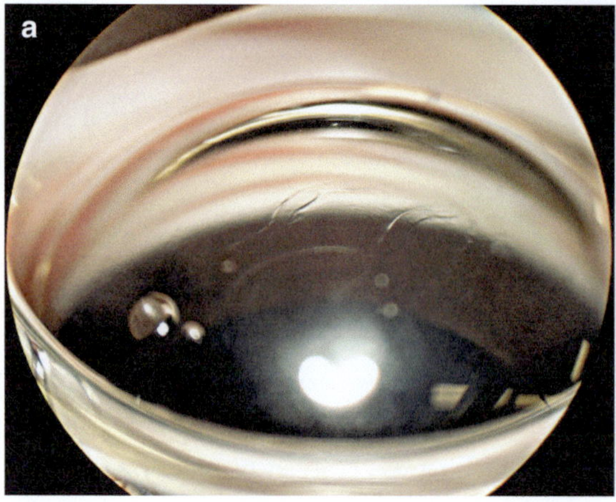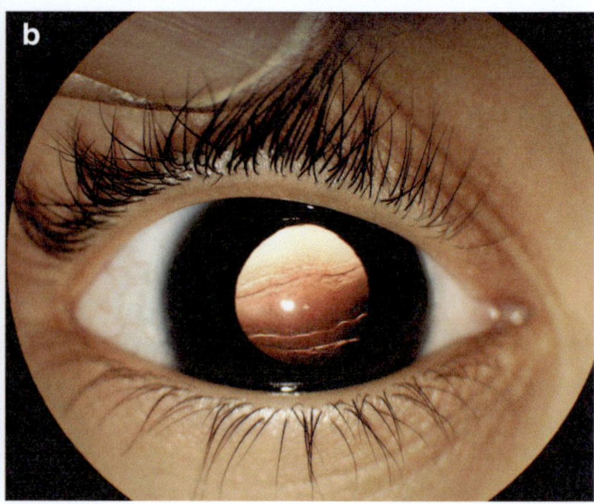

Fig. 17.5 The cornea of this child with infantile PCG was photographed through a (Koeppe) contact lens. (**a**) Two Haab striae are directed upward and rightward, each pair of curvilinear raised edges on the corneal endothe-lium representing the margins of a posterior corneal tear. (**b**) Central, horizontal Haab striae are seen as an abnormal red reflex

permanent sign of prior elevated eye pressure in the first 2–3 years.

Elasticity of the ocular coats lessens after 3 years, so glaucoma with later onset in childhood can develop and progress without these symptoms and signs and lead to occult visual loss. Children with juvenile open-angle glaucoma, a dominantly inherited condition that can develop sporadically, often do not have symptoms despite elevated intraocular pressure. They typically come to ophthalmic attention later in the first decade or in teenage years as a result of failed vision screening, not because of refractive error, amblyopia, or strabismus but because of loss of central fixation due to irreversible optic atrophy.

Differential Diagnosis

The symptoms and signs in Table 17.2 can be seen in the context of more common causes. As mentioned before, pain, irritability, and vomiting are frequently encountered in the primary care setting due to numerous conditions not associated with a syndrome, family history, or intraocular disease. Many normal children shy away from bright sunlight, enough so some parents may share concern that is distinct from the child who cannot even tolerate normal indoor room light. Uveitis and cataract can also be associated with light sensitivity and blepharospasm.

Epiphora due to obstruction along the lacrimal drainage system is much more common than due to pediatric glaucoma. Such obstruction is often accompanied by mucopurulent discharge due to bacterial stasis and typically resolves during the first several months. Epiphora due to PCG is typically not accompanied by ocular discharge. The two conditions, one common and the other rare, may coexist. Tearing with discharge is often followed in the primary care setting, presuming other signs of pediatric glaucoma are absent.

Myopia, optic disc cupping, and optic atrophy are difficult to determine for a child in the primary care setting. Myopia may be familial, common in some cultures, or due to an unrelated ocular syndrome rather than glaucoma. Pediatric ophthalmic examination can confirm glaucoma by measuring eye pressures, assessing ocular sizes through measurements of corneal diameter and biometry to assess axial length, and looking with magnification for other signs of tissue stretching and developmental anomalies. Myopia or relative myopia, detected by refraction, can also be a sign of globe elongation.

The possible presence of glaucoma can be better seen within a more typical framework used to determine ophthalmic referral for children (Table 17.3). Strabismus and amblyopia have

Table 17.3 Reasons to refer a child for ophthalmic examination

Strabismus
Abnormal red reflex
Nystagmus
Abnormally large or hazy cornea
Tearing
Premature birth
Torticollis
Acute eyelid swelling or proptosis
Unexplained abnormality; asymmetry
Family history of ophthalmic disease

Table 17.4 Pediatric glaucoma examination

History
General observations
Vision assessment
Anterior segment examination
Lens assessment
Funduscopy
Gonioscopy
Tonometry
Ultrasonography

Table 17.5 Instruments for glaucoma examination

Handheld slit beam
Binocular loupe
Portable and standard slit lamps
Handheld tonometer
Indirect ophthalmoscope
20 and 14 diopters condensing lenses
Scleral transilluminator
Koeppe lens
Handheld biomicroscope
Retinoscope
A- and B-scan sonography equipment

familial and refractive causes that are more common than induced anisometropia, corneal opacification or scarring, or optic atrophy due to glaucoma. An abnormal red reflex may suggest cataract or retinoblastoma but can also be caused by corneal opacification or haze, Haab stria, and high refractive error or anisometropia, all possibly due to pediatric glaucoma. Nystagmus, a disturbance of gaze-holding, can be due to sensory deprivation from congenital cataract or early retinal disease as well as central processes. Early glaucoma can cause sensory deprivation by corneal opacification and optic atrophy or be associated with another causative process such as foveal hypoplasia. Premature birth is associated with retinopathy, strabismus, amblyopia, and high refractive errors. Acute glaucoma can develop years later and can be anticipated based on careful serial observations of anterior chamber configuration. Torticollis can have ocular origins, typically in response to strabismus or nystagmus, but can also be a sign of light sensitivity due to pediatric glaucoma. Proptosis can be due to orbital tumor, unilateral high myopia or large globe, or a large eye due to glaucoma. Many anterior segment anomalies such as a decentered or irregular pupil, irregular iris color, iris defects, and heterochromia can be visualized in the primary care setting and suggest the presence of other hidden anomalies, some of which may be localized in the angle.

Examination

Physical examination can clarify the nature of the presenting signs and symptoms, contribute information about an associated systemic illness or syndrome, and help choose the most appropriate treatment. Elements of the pediatric glaucoma examination are listed in Table 17.4.

Instruments helpful in the primary care setting include a focused flashlight, magnifying glass, direct ophthalmoscope, and a selection of toys. Additional instruments helpful in the ophthalmic setting are listed in Table 17.5.

In the primary care setting, careful inspection of face and eyes can suggest abnormality and asymmetry such as ptosis, proptosis, asymmetry in corneal diameter or iris color, irregular shape and asymmetric size of pupils, and disturbance of the ocular media such as corneal haze and cataract. A magnifying glass can be used to further assess anterior segment structures, and a direct ophthalmoscope can be used to assess clarity and symmetry of the ocular media. General health and unusual physical features should be documented.

In the ophthalmic setting, a complete ophthalmic examination is performed after a detailed medical history. Though much can be done in an office setting, examination under anesthesia can sometimes be valuable to answer persistent questions.

Treatment of the Pediatric Glaucomas

Medical and surgical treatments are employed for pediatric glaucomas. The effectiveness of medicines (Table 17.6) is often disappointing, and surgery is frequently required to achieve eye pressure control. Systemic effects of drugs must be considered and parents instructed in their administration and potential complications.

A topical medication is typically employed first, such as a beta-blocker, prostaglandin analog, or combination preparation such as dorzolamide/timolol. Beta-blockers decrease the production of aqueous humor. Treatment with beta-blockers must be carefully monitored in infants and children with asthma because of potential cardiopulmonary complications. Prostaglandin analogs lower eye pressure by enhancing drainage through the alternate pathway. They have a good safety profile in children, but their effectiveness is often disappointing. Alpha adrenergic agonists often do not add much additional benefit over beta-blockers and are avoided in children before school age because of central nervous system depression. Miotics are not typical first-line medications except when treating aphakic or pseudophakic glaucoma, where they can sometimes be singularly effective.

The most effective medication for treating pediatric glaucoma remains oral acetazolamide, given up to 15 mg/kg/day in divided doses. Acetazolamide can be compounded into a flavored suspension such as 25 mg/ml and given with formula or juice. It is often prescribed for acute situations, to decrease eye pressure while awaiting surgery, and during postoperative care. It is rarely used as a long-term treatment. In infants, a supplementary base can help lessen induced metabolic acidosis.

Some of the surgeries performed for pediatric glaucoma are listed in Table 17.7. Sometimes pressure control is achieved with a single operation, although success is not easily won, and many surgeries, all with general anesthesia, are often required.

The operation that gives the best chance of success for controlling a particular pediatric glaucoma can be determined using evidence-based results from available treatment trials and case series. Only goniosurgeries are unique to the treatment of pediatric glaucoma. A technique for goniotomy is depicted in Fig. 17.6. After the trabeculum is incised, blood refluxes into the anterior chamber, a surgically induced hyphema that can sometimes produce high eye pressure and require surgical evacuation of hyphema. External trabeculotomy also incises the trabeculum, by utilizing an external approach. These surgeries work best when the site of increased resistance to aqueous drainage is at the trabeculum. When the angle abnormality involves the collector channels or episcleral vessels, surgery that bypasses the angle's filtration system may be needed. Trabeculectomy, often with adjunctive use of an antimetabolite, creates a guarded leak across angle and sclera. A tube shunt similarly bypasses the normal filtration system with a small silicone tube. Its tip connects the anterior or posterior chamber to a space around a plate anchored on the scleral surface from which

Table 17.6 Some medications used for pediatric glaucoma

Timolol 0.5 or 0.25%
Betaxolol 0.25% (cardioselective)
Latanaprost 0.005%
Bimatoprost
Travoprost
Dorzolamide 2%
Brimonidine 0.1, 0.15, or 2%
Apraclonidine 0.5%
Echothiophate 0.125%
Pilocarpine 1 or 4%
Acetazolamide 15 mg/kg/day, oral

Table 17.7 Surgeries for pediatric glaucomas

Goniosurgery
Goniotomy
Trabeculotomy
Trabeculectomy (filtration surgery)
Tube shunt (Ahmed, Baerveldt, Molteno)
Iridotomy and iridectomy
Cycloablation
Enucleation

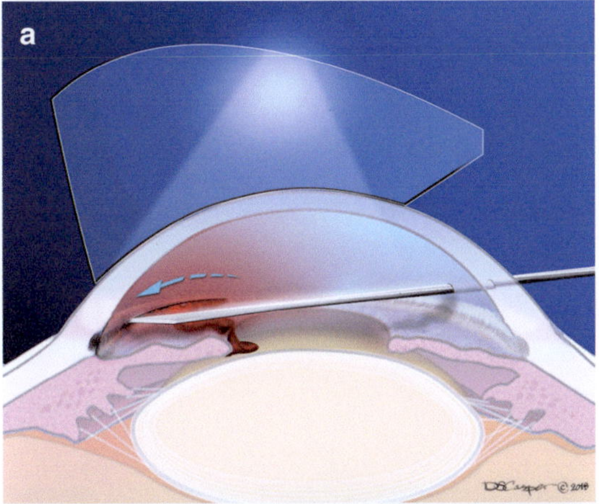

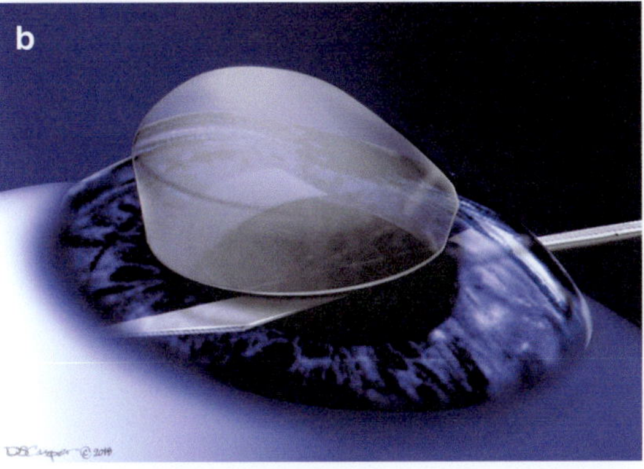

Fig. 17.6 (**a**) Goniotomy can be performed with a non-tapered knife inserted through limbal cornea, into and across the anterior chamber. Several clock hours of trabecular meshwork (trabeculum) can be incised as an assistant holds and rotates the eye. Blood refluxes into the anterior chamber from Schlemm's canal after the knife is withdrawn. (**b**) The surgeon uses a contact lens directly to view the angle during goniotomy

aqueous humor is absorbed by adjacent blood vessels (see Chap. 20). Cycloablative procedures utilize laser energy or localized freezing to produce permanent ciliary body injury to decrease production of aqueous humor. Complications are frequent and repeat procedures often required for children. Enucleation is indicated for deformed eyes that are painful, unsightly, and blind and represents an important treatment for some children. The goal of all these treatments is the prevention or treatment of amblyopia and the very best vision possible.

Summary

The pediatric glaucomas are infrequently encountered in the primary care setting. The recognition of this diverse group of disorders is enhanced by identification of characteristic symptoms and signs, an associated systemic or ocular syndrome, family history, or active or past intraocular disease. Prompt recognition and referral to a pediatric ophthalmologist for confirmation can have profound implications over an entire lifetime. The child may then be referred to a pediatric ophthalmologist experienced in the surgical treatment of the pediatric glaucomas for treatment.

Suggested Reading

Aponte EP, Diehl N, Mohney BG. Incidence and clinical characteristics of childhood glaucoma. Arch Ophthalmol. 2010;128(4):478–92.

Hollander DA, Sarfarazi M, Stoilov I, et al. Genotype and phenotype correlations in congenital glaucoma. Trans Am Ophthalmol Soc. 2006;104(12):183–95.

Suri F, Yazdani S, Narooie-Nejhad M, et al. Variable expressivity and high penetrance of CYP1B1 mutations associated with primary congenital glaucoma. Ophthalmology. 2009;116(11):2101–9.

Yeung HH, Walton DS. Clinical classification of childhood glaucomas. Arch Ophthalmol. 2010;128(6):680–4.

Visual Fields and Imaging in Glaucoma

Carlos Gustavo De Moraes

Background

Given that glaucoma is defined based upon the presence of characteristic structural abnormalities at the optic nerve and retinal nerve fiber layer which can be associated with corresponding loss of function, it is recommended that all patients with known or suspected glaucoma be followed with a combination of structural and functional tests.

Several ancillary tests are available to assist in diagnosing and managing patients with glaucoma. Their results allow an evaluation of the patient's visual function and the integrity of structures in the eye that may be affected by glaucoma. These tests are usually obtained at baseline and follow-up visits, to aide in the diagnosis of glaucoma and subsequent monitoring of glaucomatous progression. Here we discuss the three main tests most commonly employed in clinical practice for that purpose: visual field testing, optic disc photography, and optical coherence tomography (OCT).

Visual Field Testing

Visual field testing, often also called perimetry, is the subjective measurement of the patient's field of vision. The visual field is the total area in which objects can be seen in central and peripheral vision while the individual focuses on a given target. In daily life, peripheral vision allows individuals to be able to track what is happening in their surroundings while still focusing on a specific task with their central vision. Normally, the field of vision is more sensitive in the central part (corresponding to the macula and fovea) and decreases with eccentricity (as it approaches the periphery). Because there are no photoreceptors in the optic nerve, a physiologic "blind spot" is present in the field location corresponding to the optic nerve head.

Loss of visual field can occur for many reasons, such as glaucoma, cataract, retinal, and neurologic diseases. Glaucoma causes typical patterns of damage to the visual field that can be detected with this test. Therefore, perimetry is an important test to assess the status of patients' vision and determine if or how much of that vision has been lost. It is used to determine the severity of glaucoma and to monitor changes due to disease progression. The results of this test may influence treatment decisions, as well as help determine stratification for risk of future visual impairment and blindness.

C. G. De Moraes, MD, MPH (✉)
Columbia University Irving Medical Center,
New York, NY, USA
e-mail: cvd2109@cumc.columbia.edu

© Springer Nature Switzerland AG 2019
D. S. Casper, G. A. Cioffi (eds.), *The Columbia Guide to Basic Elements of Eye Care*,
https://doi.org/10.1007/978-3-030-10886-1_18

Originally, the visual field was tested using either a confrontational test, with the patient seated opposite to the examiner, who utilizes an outstretched hand to estimate peripheral field extent in each eye. A somewhat more rigorous format, the tangent screen test, employs a large, wall-mounted screen in a similar fashion. Both these tests are still used, but more easily quantifiable methods are routinely employed for glaucoma diagnosis and management. The older, Goldmann test (GVF) utilizes a large, hemispheric bowl in which the patient views varied illuminated targets presented by the examiner. Newer computerized systems, such as the Humphrey (HVF), are currently the most commonly used field testing modality.

There are different types of computerized perimeters, with different types of light stimulus, each measuring different features of vision. For glaucoma, the gold standard for functional evaluation is standard automated perimetry (SAP), which measures contrast sensitivity. In its most commonly used form, SAP employs a white stimulus of 4 mm^2 area of different intensities, ranging from very dim (0.08 apostilbs, asb) to very bright (10,000 asb). This stimulus, which lasts 200 ms, is projected at 54 locations of the field of vision on a dome-shaped hemisphere of 33 cm radius with a uniform white background illumination (31.5 asb). Because it employs a white stimulus on a white background, SAP is also called "white-on-white perimetry."

While testing one eye at a time, the patient is asked to fixate on a central target and click a button whenever they see the stimulus. At each location tested, the machine will alternate light stimuli of different intensities until it converges to the estimated threshold sensitivity of each location. Threshold sensitivity corresponds to the dimmest light stimulus that a can be seen at least 50% of the times it is presented. Because presenting a stimulus 100 times, at each of the 54 locations, would be very time-consuming and cause patient fatigue, the device employs an algorithm that converges to the estimated threshold sensitivity using a Bayesian approach. Such algorithms allow testing each eye of an individual in 5–10 min, on average. The most commonly used

SAP test evaluates the central 24° from fixation (fovea) – except for the nasal field, where it extends to 30° – and each tested location is 6° apart from each other. This strategy is called 24-2 testing.

Once the threshold sensitivity of each location is defined, the algorithm retests each location randomly with stimuli that are either dimmer or brighter than its threshold sensitivity. If the patient clicks the button when the stimulus is dimmer than the pre-defined threshold sensitivity, this is flagged as a false positive. On the contrary, if the patient does not click the button when the stimulus is brighter than the pre-defined threshold sensitivity, this is flagged as a false negative. In addition, an eye tracker helps determine if the patient moved their focus away from fixation during the test. Also, by retesting the location of the blind spot, the algorithm determines the number of fixation losses (remember that the patient should not be able to see any stimulus presented at the blind spot; if they do, it is probably because the eye moved and the stimulus now fell in an area outside the blind spot). These reliability indices (false positive, false negative, and fixation losses, along with the eye tracker output) help the clinician determine if the visual field is reliable.

As a subjective test that is dependent on patient's attention and cooperation, results of visual field tests may vary significantly from one test to the other. It is also common for there to be a definite learning curve associated with visual field testing, where the initial tests show decidedly abnormal results, with very poor reliability indices; for most patients, this initial difficulty with the test diminishes over time. Therefore, clinicians often request repeats if a test is deemed unreliable or in order to confirm if a visual field defect is truly present. In addition, repeated tests are obtained during follow-up to assess whether there is change over time caused by progressive disease. It is important to note that patients with glaucoma can sometimes have normal results on SAP. This usually happens when glaucomatous optic nerve damage has not yet reached a level of severity to affect the ability to detect the light stimulus on perimetry testing. It may also happen if the damage exists in an area of the field that the device did not test or if the test results were unreliable.

Figure 18.1 depicts the 24-2 SAP test printout of the right eye (OD) of a healthy individual (a) and a glaucomatous patient (b). Note in both cases the presence of the normal blind spot in the temporal field, indicating the location of the optic nerve. The main features of the printout discussed above are shown. Both patients had reliable tests, as described in the reliability indices section.

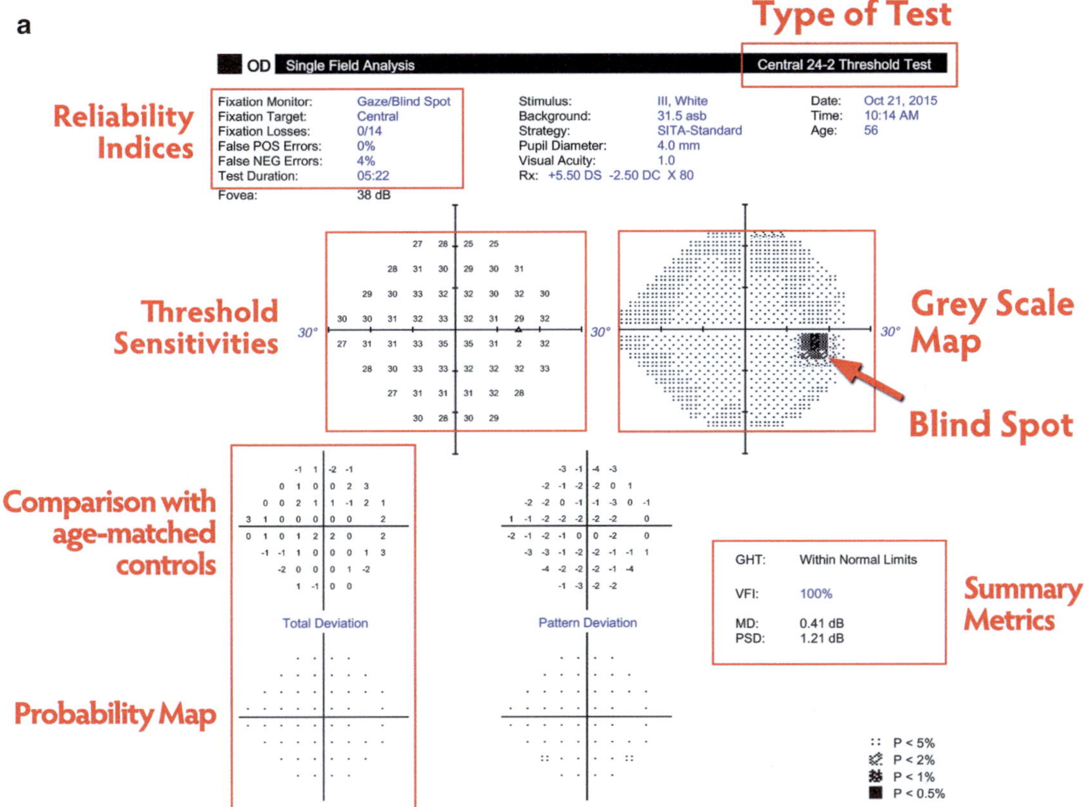

Fig. 18.1 (**a**) Standard automated ("white-on-white") perimetry result of the right eye (OD) of a healthy subject. The top panel describes the test and patient information at the time of the examination. The middle panel shows the threshold sensitivities (see text for definition) of each tested location of the 24-2 strategy (left) and the corresponding gray-scale map for illustration purposes. Note that the blind spot – corresponding to the optic nerve head location – is located inferiorly and temporally to the central field (corresponding to the fovea). The bottom panel shows the results when one subtracts the threshold sensitivity values from age-matched controls. Negative values represent values worse than the average of age-matched eye. Each point is assigned a probability that the difference could be found in normal subjects (i.e., the lower probability, the less likely that the value could be seen in healthy eyes and hence the more likely that it represents disease). In glaucoma, one would expect a cluster of three or more adjacent points with probabilities less than 5%, which did not happen in this case. The box on the right depicts the summary metrics which are based upon the weighted average of all points in the total deviation map [mean deviation (MD), in this case, the eye was 0.41 dB better than the average age-matched control]. The visual field index (VFI) summarizes what percentage of the visual field that is preserved. The other indices [pattern standard deviation (PSD) and glaucoma hemifield test (GHT)] summarize the level of variability and asymmetry, respectively, within the visual field. More variability and asymmetry are suggestive of glaucoma (as seen in **b**). (**b**) Results of the test of the right eye (OD) of a glaucomatous patient. Note the clusters of statistically abnormal points. As a result, the MD shows that the eye is 3.72 dB worse than the average age-matched control, and this difference was significant at $P < 1\%$. The VFI suggests that the eye has lost about 8% (100–92%) of its sensitivity. Similarly, the PSD and GHT depict high variability in the field (note the dispersion of normal and abnormal locations) and a significant degree of superior versus inferior asymmetry

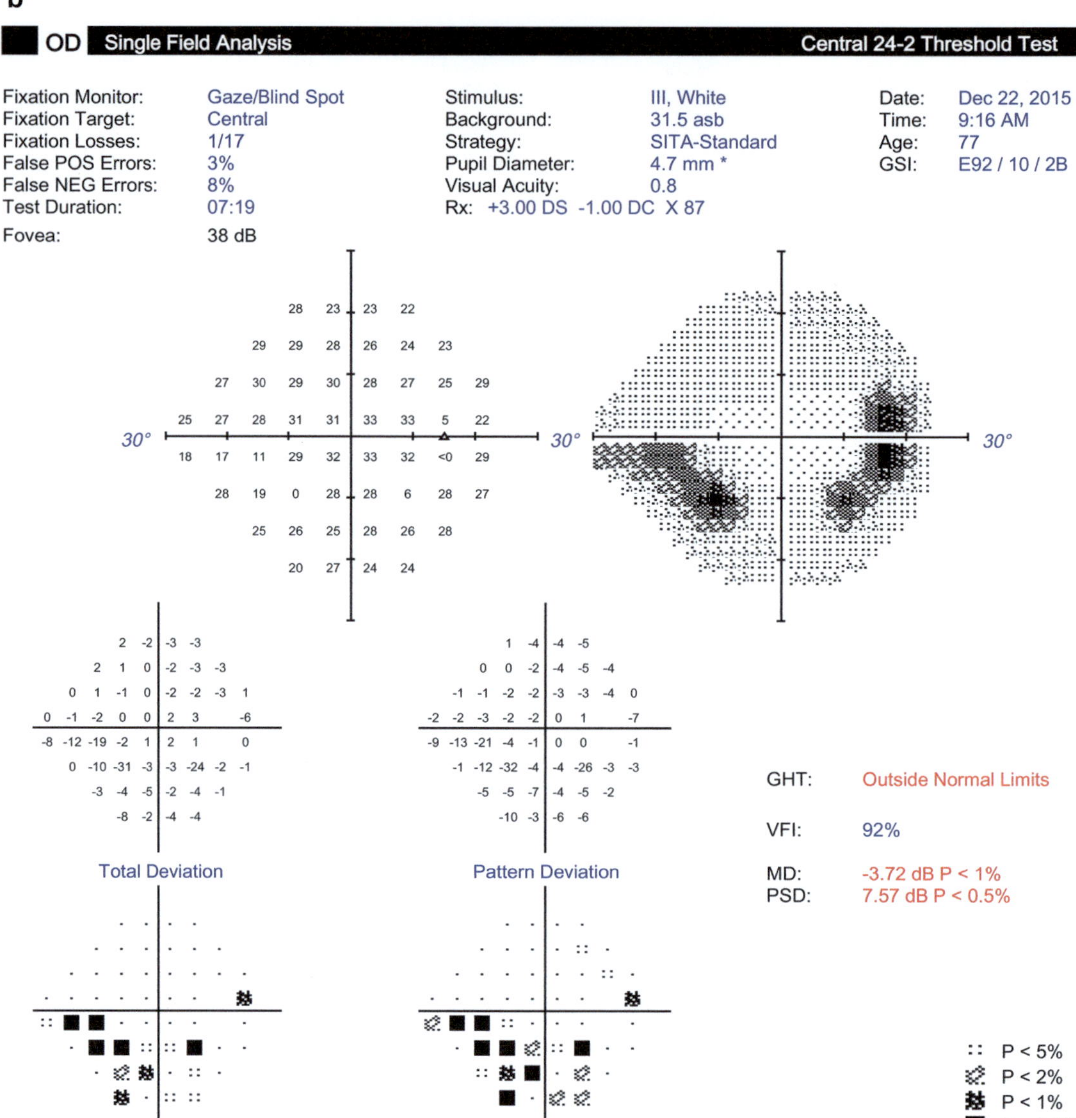

Fig. 18.1 (continued)

In the printout of the glaucomatous patient, note the inferior field defect ("scotoma") with a curved "arcuate"-like pattern. This pattern is characteristic of glaucoma, and the test result suggests that the patient has poor contrast sensitivity in the inferior field, which may affect their ability to perform daily tasks.

When looking for progression, clinicians monitor changes in depth (i.e., how depressed the threshold sensitivities are) and size of scotomas, as well as the development of new scotomas. Figure 18.2 shows an example of an eye of a glaucoma patient who experienced visual field loss progression. With the help of a computerized algorithm, the clinician selects two reliable baseline tests to which the last test (or test of interest) will be compared. The printout shows the rate of progression (in units per year) for the summary (average) metrics and projects the estimated loss in 5 years – assuming no changes in treatment are

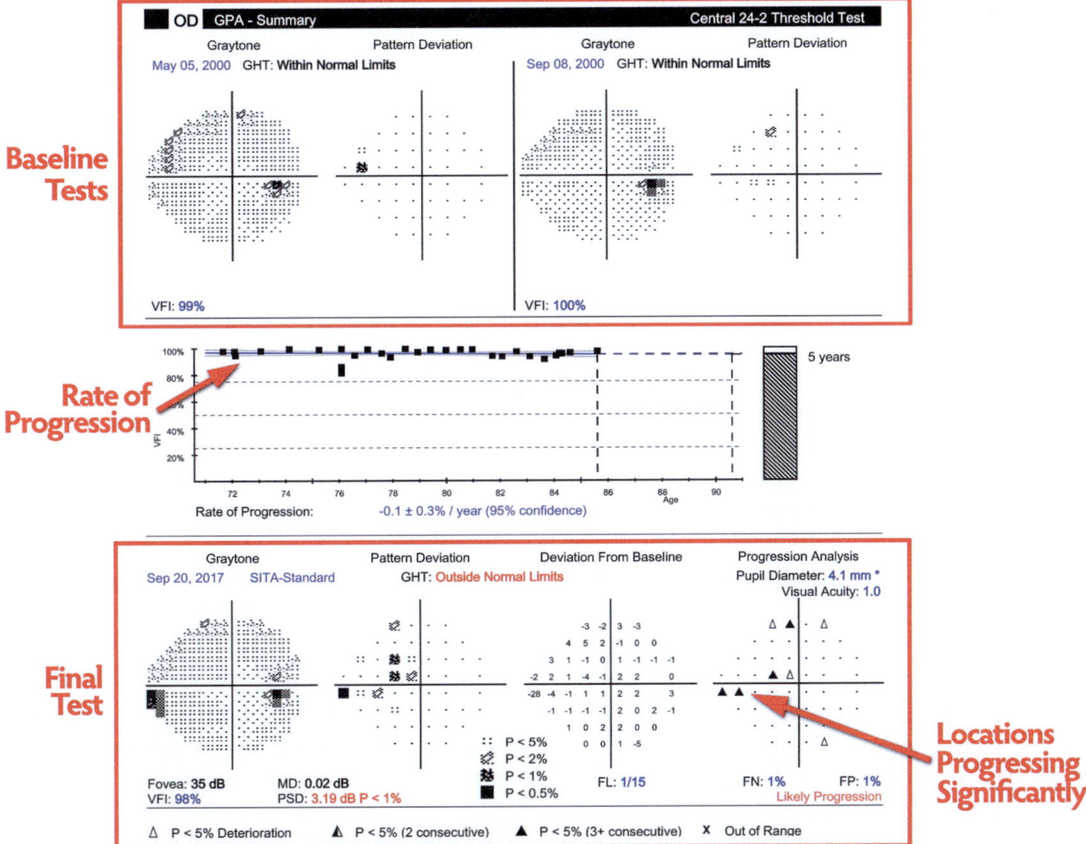

Fig. 18.2 Visual field progression analysis of the right eye (OD) of a glaucomatous patient. Top panel: note that the two baseline tests (performed about 4 months apart) are suggestive of a superior hemifield abnormality. Middle panel: the VFI is plotted over time (each black square is a different test on a different date) and shows the trend of change, i.e., the rate of progression in %/year ($-0.1 \pm 0.3\%$/year). Bottom panel: the final test performed about 17 years after the two baseline tests. The pattern deviation map shows an increase in the severity and number of abnormal points, which are depicted in the progression analysis as black triangles

implemented. It also shows which test locations progressed significantly relative to the average of two baseline tests.

Visual field testing with white-on-white perimetry (SAP) is the gold standard to measure visual function in glaucoma. It allows detection of damage, classification of severity, risk stratification, and monitoring progression. SAP results correlate with vision-related quality of life and have been used to define endpoints of glaucoma in randomized clinical trials. Due to its subjective nature, clinicians must pay attention to test reliability and may need to repeat a test numerous times to confirm damage and track progressive changes. Visual field test results should always be correlated with the results of structural tests (see further).

Optic Disc Photography

Optic disc photography is an examination in which a picture of the retina and optic nerve is taken with a customized camera. This technique was the first imaging modality available for optic disc structural evaluation. In fact, disc photography is the reference technique in many places where computerized technologies are not available. Photographs are usually acquired using a technique called stereophotography to produce a three-dimensional (3D) view of the optic nerve head (ONH), although plain (2D) photos can also be obtained and used in clinical practice. Serial optic disc imaging allows a qualitative evaluation of the structure of the optic nerve.

Since glaucoma is a disease characterized by damage to the optic nerve, disc photographs assist clinicians in diagnosing structural glaucomatous damage and detecting signs of disease progression. In some patients, glaucomatous damage can happen in the optic nerve before visual field abnormalities are manifest. Therefore, clinicians often obtain optic disc photographs to look for early signs of disc anatomic changes suggestive of glaucoma, which may help in deciding if treatment should be initiated, even in the absence of visual field loss. In addition, by acquiring serial optic disc photographs, clinicians can compare the relative appearances of the optic nerve over time in order to evaluate if glaucoma is progressing or is stable. One important advantage over direct or indirect ophthalmoscopy is that optic disc documentation with photos overcomes challenges related to patient examination, such as eye movement and the more obvious interviewer agreement discrepancies associated with optic disc drawings, and enables a more detailed evaluation of the disc at different time points, side by side.

During optic disc photography, patients are asked to look at a target while a technician takes a photo of the retina and ONH with a special fundus camera. Only light – no radiation or laser – is used. In most cases, pupil dilation is needed to obtain the high-quality images required for analysis. The photo is then saved to a computer or printed for subsequent clinical evaluation.

Figure 18.3a shows what the optic nerve looks like in a photograph of a person without glaucoma. The ONH looks like a "doughnut." The middle part, a depression in the nerve head ("doughnut hole"), is called the "cup" (dashed line). The ring around the cup (the "doughnut" itself) is composed of nerve tissue (the aggregated axons of the ~1.25 million retinal ganglion cells) and is called the "rim." In glaucoma, there is enlargement of the cup because of loss of nerve tissue (rim) (Fig. 18.3b). In addition to evaluating nerve tissue loss, optic disc photography may also help detect other signs of glaucomatous damage, such as the presence of a small area of bleeding, often "flame-shaped" in appearance, called an optic disc hemorrhage (Fig. 18.3c, arrow). This small hemorrhage usually disappears in a couple of months but is often indicative of uncontrolled disease. Disc photos are also important to help rule out other optic nerve diseases, such as compressive (e.g., tumors of the chiasm or meninges), ischemic (e.g., autoimmune or thromboembolic), or traumatic neuropathies.

Optic disc photography enables a structural evaluation of the optic nerve head and its surrounding tissues as a component of the investigation for the presence of, or progression of, glaucoma. Besides helping differentiate

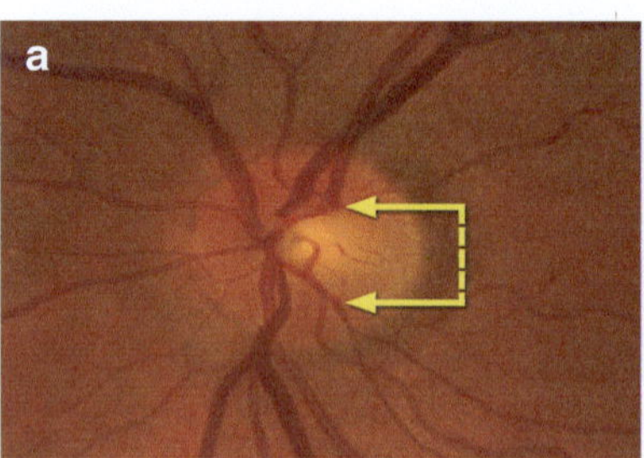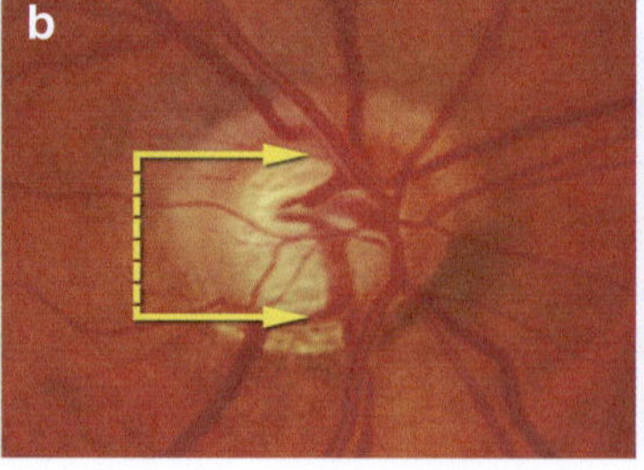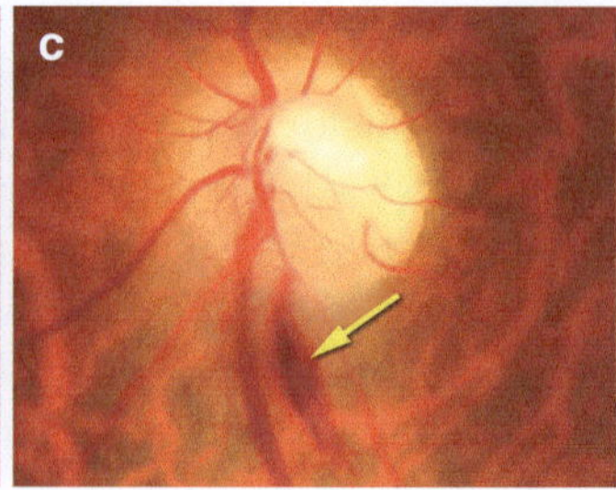

Fig. 18.3 Optic disc photography. (**a**) Optic nerve head of a healthy, non-glaucomatous eye. Note the blood vessels emerging from the center of the disc, which has a donut shape: the central, yellow part (dashed line connecting arrows) represents the cup, and the surrounding orange-red part represents the neural tissue (rim). (**b**) Note the enlarged cup of this glaucomatous eye, which led to almost complete loss of the neural rim tissue. (**c**) A cupped disc of a glaucomatous eye that experienced bleeding ("flame-shaped" disc hemorrhage, seen at yellow arrow), which is an important predictor of future progression if not treated adequately

glaucoma from other optic neuropathies, this technique is inexpensive and has remained relatively stable since its implementation, which helps the evaluation of progressive changes over long periods of time. Its main disadvantage is its subjective nature, which results in moderate to poor inter-rater agreement to detect glaucoma and monitor progression.

Optical Coherence Tomography

Optical coherence tomography (OCT) is a recently available, noninvasive, rapid ancillary test to evaluate structural damage caused by glaucoma. OCT provides high-definition microscopic images of the retina, macula, and ONH. Unlike photographs, OCT measures the thickness of the nerve fibers and neuronal layers of the retina and provides quantitative (numeric), objective measurements. These measurements are then compared with a database of subjects without glaucoma, which helps clinicians define whether retinal or optic nerve parameters are thinner or similar to those expected in healthy individuals with same age. If thinner (i.e., below the lower limits of variability of healthy eyes), it increases the probability of presence of glaucoma or other optic neuropathies. In addition, ONH measurements can directly measure both cup and rim size. Over time, increasing cup and decreasing rim size, combined with thinning of the retina, strongly suggest the presence of progressive glaucoma.

OCT is an objective test, that is, it is less dependent on the subjective interpretation of the clinician (which was discussed above as a limitation of visual field testing and optic disc photography). This can be helpful when clinicians disagree if photographic images of the ONH are suggestive of glaucoma or whether glaucoma is progressing. By quantifying the amount of nerve tissue loss over time, OCT can help the evaluation of disease progression. It is important to note that just like any other ancillary diagnostic test, the OCT result alone may not be able to confirm the diagnosis of glaucoma or whether the disease is progressing. Moreover, it cannot always differentiate glaucoma from other optic neuropathies (in which case, optic disc photographs may help). OCT results should be interpreted in conjunction with medical history, clinical examination, and other tests such as photographs and visual fields.

The OCT uses laser light to acquire high-resolution images of the structures in the posterior segment. It employs similar principles as ultrasound, but instead of soundwaves, it employs laser-emitted light waves. As the light travels from the OCT device through the eye and retinal layers, some light is back-reflected, the intensity of which depends on inherent tissue properties. The computer analyzes differences between the propagated and reflected light and generates an image of the layer in focus (optic nerve in Fig. 18.4a and macula in Fig. 18.5). Finally, an algorithm defines the boundaries between different layers and measures the distance between them (Fig. 18.4b). These measurements are compared with a normative database, and the output shows areas that fall within or outside the limits expected in healthy eyes (Fig. 18.4c, d). The laser used by OCT is safe for use in the eye, and the whole test can usually be performed in just a few minutes. After the images are acquired, the device produces a printout illustrating the results. Depending on the manufacturer of the device, these printouts may appear different.

Figure 18.4 shows an example of printouts obtained from an OCT examination of a patient with glaucoma. The OCT software provides a classification of normal (green), borderline (yellow), or abnormal (red) based on the thickness of the nerve fiber layer around the ONH compared to age-matched subjects without glaucoma. In addition to the optic nerve, the device also evaluates the thickness of the layer of neurons in the macula (Fig. 18.5). Such classification is shown for each eye tested. The presence and range of abnormal areas around the ONH and macula will help the doctor diagnose if glaucoma is present. Also, when the retinal thickness measurements decrease over time, this might indicate that glaucoma is progressing.

Due to its objective nature, high resolution, and highly reproducible results, OCT has gained

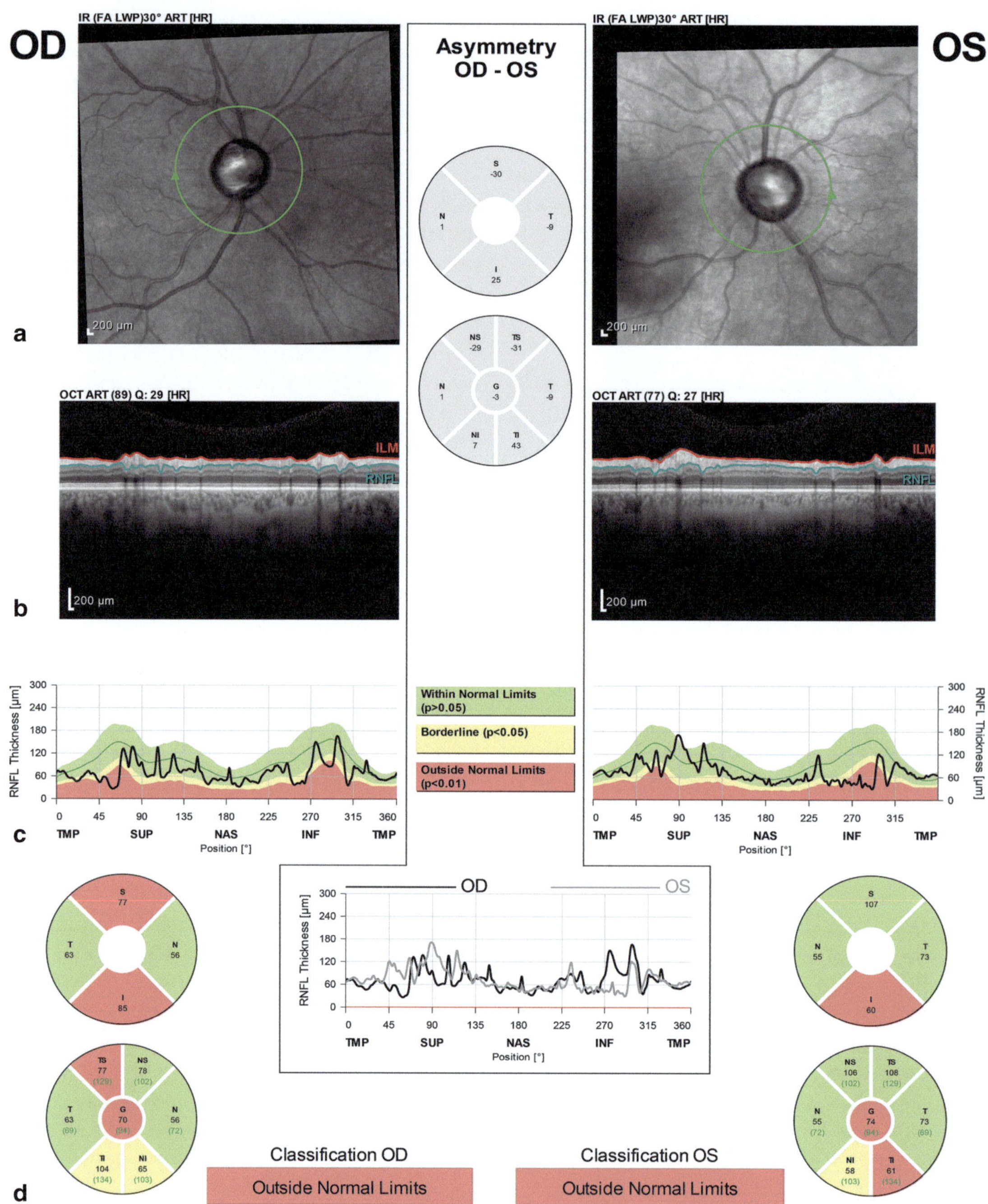

Fig. 18.4 Optical coherence tomography (OCT) analysis of the optic nerve head of the right eye (OD) and left eye (OS) of a glaucomatous patient. (**a**) The green circle shows where the scan was performed. In (**b**) the two-dimensional b-scan from the circle line in (**a**) is "stretched," so it can be seen as a straight line. The red line corresponds to where the algorithm detected the interface between the internal limiting membrane and the vitreous cavity. The blue line corresponds to the interface between the retinal nerve fiber layer (RNFL) and the retinal ganglion cell layer (RGCL). (**c**) Comparison between the eye's RNFL thickness and age-matched controls: red represents a probability less than 1% (abnormal); yellow between 1% and 5% (borderline); and green above 5% (normal). (**d**) The difference between the red and blue lines in (**b**), corresponding to the RNFL thickness, is plotted as a function of the different probabilities relative to healthy controls

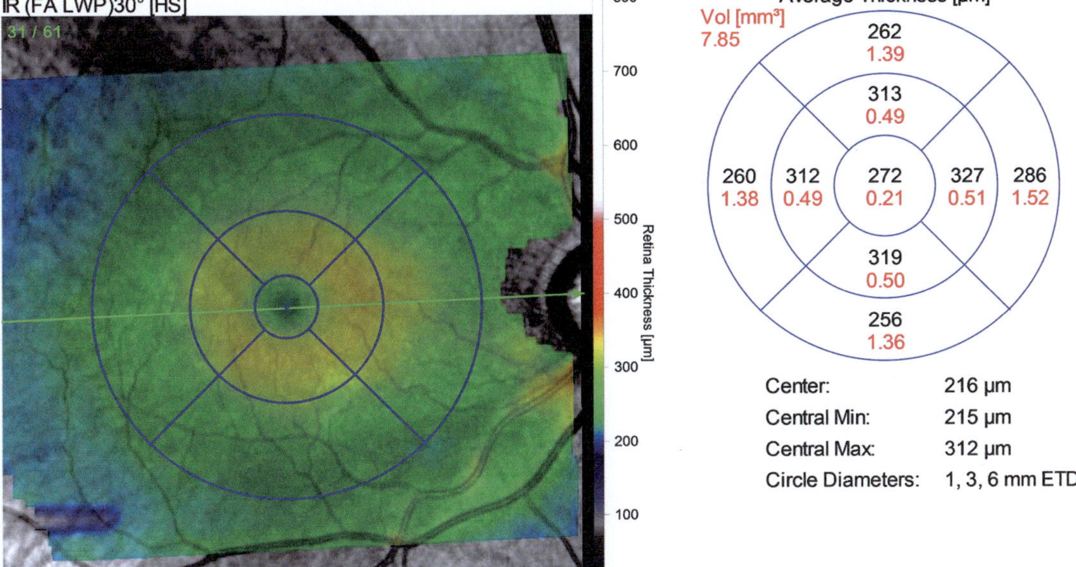

Fig. 18.5 Optical coherence tomography (OCT) analysis of the macula of the right eye (OD) of the same patient shown in Fig. 18.4. The left panel shows the fundus image with a pseudo-color map overlaid. Green corresponds to thinner and yellow thicker, full retinal thickness. Note that the retina is thicker around the fovea (macula) and surrounding the blood vessels emerging from the optic nerve head. In right panel, the macular region is divided into nine sectors, and their thickness and volume are shown in black and red, respectively

growing importance in glaucoma management. However, its interpretation should always take into account the results of clinical examination and visual field testing.

greatly to the ability to accurately diagnose glaucoma in its earliest stages and to adequately assess the patient's response to ongoing treatment.

Summary

In recent decades, glaucoma diagnosis has evolved. Once defined as a disease of high intraocular pressure, current definitions of glaucoma instead focus on the disease as a primary disorder of the optic nerve, often, but not always, accompanied by elevated pressures. This evolution in the understanding of glaucomatous optic nerve disease has been a motivating factor behind the shift in glaucoma identification and progression. Both visual field and fundus disc imaging, which have been used for many years, have seen technological improvements which have enhanced glaucoma management, and the addition of objective, noninvasive, and rapid OCT testing has added

Suggested Readings

Hood DC. Improving our understanding, and detection, of glaucomatous damage: an approach based upon optical coherence tomography (OCT). Prog Retin Eye Res. 2017;57:46–75.

Heijl A, Patella VM, Bengtsson B. The field analyzer primer: effective perimetry. 4th ed. Dublin, CA: Carl Zeiss Meditec; 2012.

Moustafa Y. Visual fields interpretation in glaucoma: a focus on static automated perimetry. Community Eye Health. 2012;25(79–80):1–8.

Sathyan P, Shilpa S, Anitha A. Optical coherence tomography in glaucoma. J Curr Glaucoma Pract. 2012;6(1):1–5.10008-1099

Susanna R Jr, Vessani RM. New findings in the evaluation of the optic disc in glaucoma diagnosis. Curr Opin Ophthalmol. 2007;18(2):122–8.

Medical Treatment of Glaucoma

19

Gene Kim and Dana Blumberg

Glaucoma is a group of diseases that exhibit a characteristic optic neuropathy which, untreated, initially causes loss of peripheral and ultimately central vision. It is a leading cause of blindness worldwide and is estimated to affect over three million people in the United States. Although vision loss due to glaucoma is irreversible, blindness can typically be prevented when it is detected and treated in its earlier stages.

Elevated intraocular pressure (IOP) plays a causative role in the progressive optic nerve damage seen in glaucoma and is the only known modifiable risk factor. As such, the goal of glaucoma treatment is to reduce IOP below a presumed "safe" target pressure that arrests disease progression and prevents further visual field loss. Current treatment methods for glaucoma are thus all aimed at lowering IOP and include topical and oral medications, laser therapy, and incisional surgery. The Collaborative Initial Glaucoma Treatment Study (CIGTS) showed that initial management with

medicine or surgery resulted in similar visual field outcomes after 5 years of follow-up. Given its relative safety and ease of use, medical therapy remains the preferred first choice of treatment for most forms of glaucoma in the United States.

A number of different medication classes are currently in use to treat glaucoma, including prostaglandin analogues, β-adrenergic antagonists, adrenergic agonists, carbonic anhydrase inhibitors, parasympathomimetics, and hyperosmotic agents. In general, these medications reduce IOP either by reducing aqueous humor secretion from the ciliary body or by increasing aqueous outflow from the eye (Figs. 19.1 and 19.2). To avoid potential adverse events due to patient difficulty in distinguishing between multiple topical medications, a uniform color-coding

G. Kim, MD
Department of Ophthalmology and Visual Sciences, Albert Einstein College of Medicine, Montefiore Medical Center, Bronx, NY, USA

D. Blumberg, MD (✉)
Columbia University Irving Medical Center, New York, NY, USA

Department of Ophthalmology, Edward S. Harkness Eye Institute, Columbia University Vagelos College of Physicians and Surgeons, New York, NY, USA
e-mail: dmb2196@cumc.columbia.edu

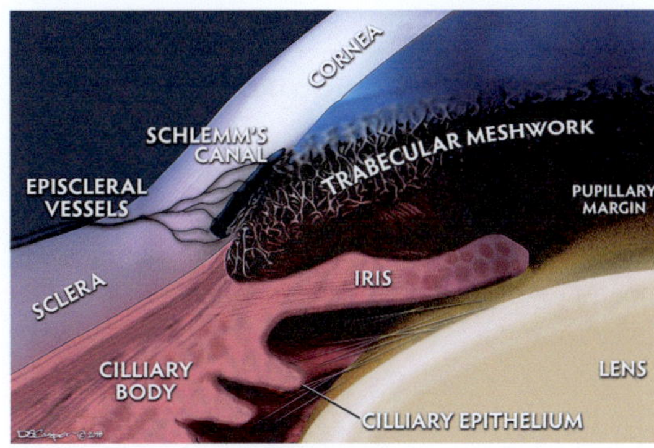

Fig. 19.1 Anatomy of the anterior chamber angle and surrounding area, location of the aqueous humor production and outflow systems

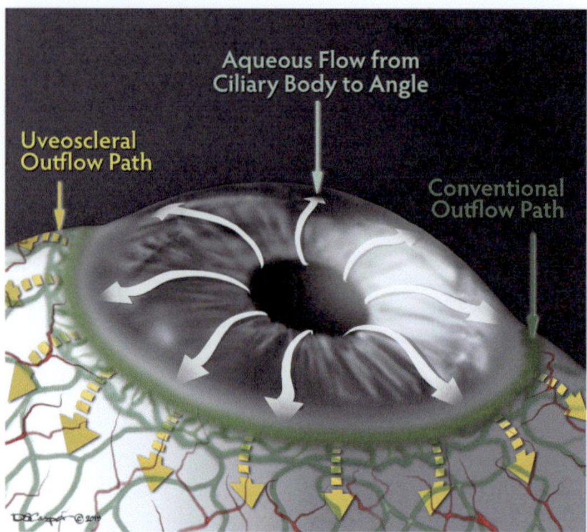

Fig. 19.2 Aqueous (white arrows) formed in the ciliary body flows through the pupil, over the iris, and toward the angle. In the conventional outflow system (shown in green), aqueous passes through the trabecular meshwork, into the canal of Schlemm (located 360° around the peripheral cornea) and drains via collector channels, and eventually into aqueous veins and the systemic venous system, much like lymphatic fluid. In the alternative uveoscleral outflow system (yellow arrows), clearly defined anatomic drainage structures are not utilized as in the conventional system. Rather, aqueous penetrates into the ciliary muscle and then passes into the supraciliary and suprachoroidal spaces, eventually draining into adjacent sclera and the lymphatic system

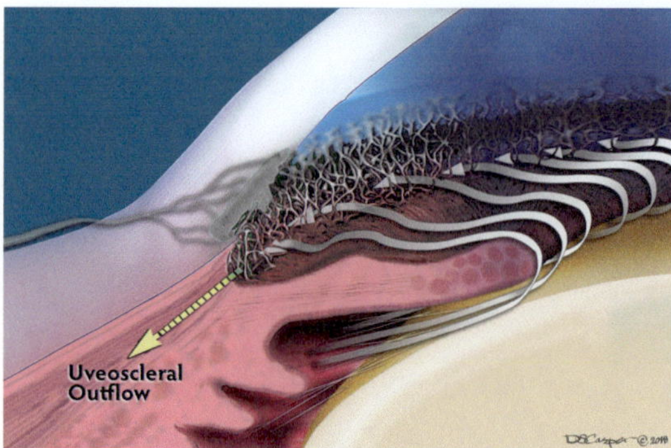

Fig. 19.3 A diagram of uveoscleral aqueous outflow

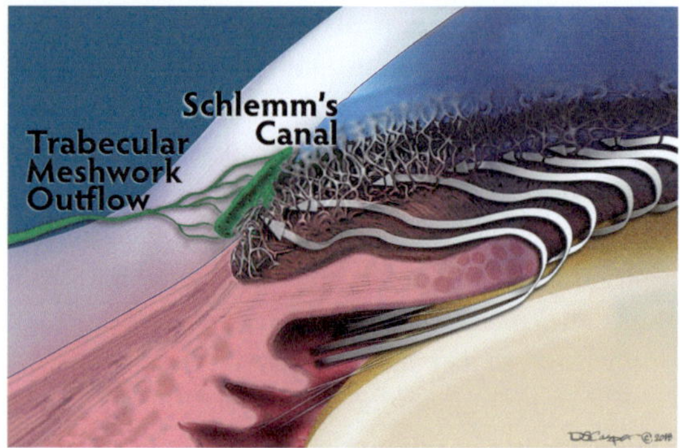

Fig. 19.4 A diagram of conventional aqueous outflow through trabecular meshwork

system has been developed in which a specific Pantone color is assigned to the bottle cap of each medication class, thereby reducing patient medication errors (see Appendix 4).

Prostaglandin Analogues

Although they are a relatively newer drug class, prostaglandin analogues are currently the most widely used first-line agent in the treatment of open-angle glaucoma. Medications in this class have a turquoise cap color and include latanoprost (Xalatan), travoprost (Travatan), bimatoprost (Lumigan), tafluprost (Zioptan), and unoprostone isopropyl (Rescula). Their mechanism of action is to increase aqueous outflow facility, primarily via the uveoscleral pathway, but with some effect on the trabecular meshwork as well (Figs. 19.3 and 19.4). Although the exact mechanism is not fully understood, it is thought that the increase in uveoscleral outflow is mediated by stimulation of the FP class of prostaglandin receptors at the iris root and ciliary body. Activation of these receptors leads to upregulation of matrix metalloproteinases, which promotes extracellular matrix remodeling and widening of intermuscular spaces in the ciliary body, and thus decreasing resistance to aqueous outflow. Increased aqueous outflow results in decreased IOP.

Prostaglandin analogues typically yield a 25–30% reduction in IOP. They are dosed once daily, typically at night, as they produce a relatively flat IOP curve over 24 h and reach peak effect approximately 10–14 h after administration. Maximum IOP reduction may take up to 6 weeks of use to occur. They are indicated in the treatment of both open-angle and angle-closure glaucoma and are generally considered safe and effective to use in the pediatric population as well.

Prostaglandins are generally well-tolerated, with very few systemic side effects. One potential ocular side effect that is unique to this class is increased iris pigmentation, which can occur in up to 33% of patients after 5 years of use. This color change is permanent but does not otherwise confer any risk to the patient. Other common side effects include eyelash growth, conjunctival hyperemia, and hyperpigmentation of the periocular skin. Although their effect on eyelash growth may be considered desirable in some patient populations, the potential cosmetic effects of these agents must be taken into consideration, particularly when used unilaterally. Prostaglandins have also been associated with increased risk of uveitis, cystoid macular edema, and, rarely, reactivation of herpes simplex virus (HSV) keratitis. For this reason, prostaglandin use is often suspended during the immediate postoperative period and avoided in patients with active inflammation or a history of HSV keratitis.

β-adrenergic Antagonists

Topical β-antagonists have a yellow cap color and are generally categorized as either nonselective (β1 and β2 blockade) or selective (β1 ≫ β2 blockade). The nonselective β-blockers include timolol (Timoptic), levobunolol (Betagan), metipranolol (OptiPranolol), and carteolol (Ocupress). Carteolol, although nonselective in β-blockade, is thought to have intrinsic sympathomimetic activity and consequently may have less effect on lipid profiles. Betaxolol (Betoptic) is the only commercially available selective β1 antagonist and is thus associated with fewer pulmonary side effects than its nonselective counterparts. β-blockers lower IOP by reducing aqueous humor production, which is thought to occur by inhibiting cyclic adenosine monophosphate (cAMP) production in the ciliary epithelium. They are indicated in the treatment of both open-angle and angle-closure glaucoma.

Medications in this class typically produce a 20–25% IOP reduction with peak effect within 2–6 h after administration, although betaxolol-may have slightly lower efficacy. Evidence suggests that β-blockers have little activity during the evening and nighttime hours. Therefore, although many are approved for twice-daily dosing, most of the benefit can be achieved by a single morning dose. Their efficacy may be reduced in patients already taking a systemic β-blocker, and approximately 10–20% of all patients fail to respond to treatment. Loss of efficacy can occur in some patients due to both the "short-term escape" and "long-term drift" phenomena, although both of these effects are controversial. Short-term escape occurs within 2–3 weeks of starting treatment and is thought to be due to an upregulation of β-receptors in response to initial complete blockade. Long-term drift, or tachyphylaxis, may also be seen over time due to downregulation of β-receptors. Additionally, unilateral administration of β-blockers may elicit a "crossover" response of IOP reduction in the fellow eye due to systemic absorption, which may limit the utility of monocular treatment trials.

β-blockers have few ocular side effects, most commonly dry eye syndrome and corneal anesthesia. Due to their relatively high systemic absorption, however, they are associated with several potentially serious systemic side effects including bronchospasm, bradycardia, and heart block. Other systemic side effects include lethargy, headache, depression, impotence, decreased exercise tolerance, and altered serum lipid profiles (decreased HDL and increased triglycerides). Importantly, nonselective β-blockers must be used with extreme caution in patients with asthma or obstructive pulmonary disease as well as those with a history of bradycardia or more than first-degree heart block. Cardio-selective β-blockers such as betaxolol, although somewhat less effective in reducing IOP, are associated with fewer pulmonary side effects and may be a safer alternative in this population. β-blockers may also mask the symptoms of hypoglycemia in diabetic patients and the symptoms of thyrotoxicosis in patients with thyroid disease, and abrupt cessation may exacerbate thyroid symptoms. Although they are often considered first-line therapy for glaucoma in children due to their long track record, they must be used with caution in children with underlying medical comorbidities given their high systemic absorption.

Adrenergic Agonists

Medications in this class have a purple cap color and can be categorized as nonselective adrenergic agonists or selective α2-adrenergic agonists. The older, nonselective agonists include epinephrine and dipivefrine (a prodrug of epinephrine) and function by activating both α- and β-receptors. They are no longer used in most countries and have largely been replaced in clinical practice by the α2-agonists. The α2-agonists include apraclonidine (Iopidine) and brimonidine (Alphagan) and have relatively selective activity at the α2-receptor which prevents the release of norepinephrine at presynaptic nerve terminals. Although the exact mechanism is unclear, they reduce IOP by decreasing aqueous production and may also have some effect on episcleral venous pressure and uveoscleral outflow.

The α2-agonists produce a 20–25% IOP reduction, with peak effect occurring within 2–3 h. Given their relatively rapid onset of action, they are often used in the laser surgery setting to block postoperative IOP rises. Although approved for three times daily dosing, they are commonly used twice daily, particularly when used as an adjunctive agent. In addition to their IOP-lowering effect, there is controversial evidence that α2-agonists may confer a neuroprotective effect for retinal ganglion cells. They are indicated in the treatment of both open-angle and angle-closure glaucoma. Brimonidine, due to its miotic effect, has been used off-label after refractive surgery to decrease symptomatic glare and halos.

The most common ocular side effect is a local allergic reaction which manifests as follicular conjunctivitis and periorbital blepharodermatitis (Fig. 19.5). The rate of allergy is significantly higher with apraclonidine (up to 40%) than brimonidine (10–20%), and long-term intolerance is common due to these local adverse effects. Possible systemic adverse

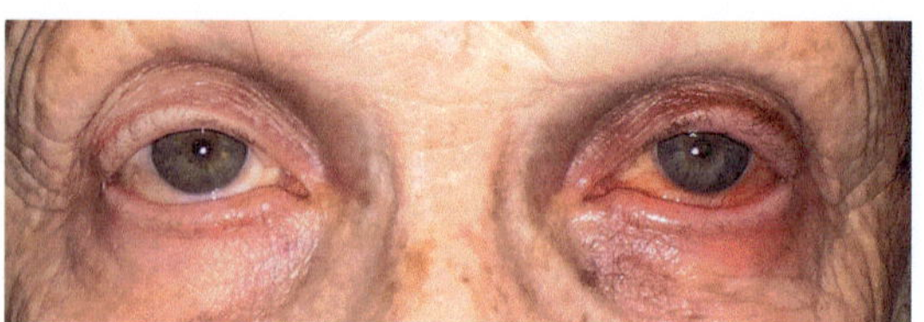

Fig. 19.5 Allergic periorbital blepharodermatitis OS. Also present is bilateral mild inferior lid ectropion

effects include hypotension, dry mouth and nose, lethargy, headache, anxiety, depression, and fatigue. Brimonidine is absolutely contraindicated in infants and young children as it crosses the blood-brain barrier and can lead to CNS depression, including somnolence, apnea, hypotension, bradycardia, and seizures. α2-agonists should also be used with caution in patients taking monoamine oxidase inhibitors (MAOIs) and tricyclic antidepressant medications, due to the respective risks of hypertensive crisis and CNS depression.

Carbonic Anhydrase Inhibitors (CAIs)

Medications in this class are available both as topical drops and systemic medications, which can be given orally or intravenously. Topical agents include dorzolamide (Trusopt) and brinzolamide (Azopt); these have an orange cap color and are generally used for long-term IOP management. Systemic agents include acetazolamide (Diamox) and methazolamide (Neptazane) and are typically reserved for acute situations. Their shared mechanism of action is to reduce aqueous production by inhibiting carbonic anhydrase in the ciliary body epithelium, which decreases bicarbonate formation and thus lowers sodium and fluid transport. More than 99% of the enzyme activity must be inhibited, however, to achieve successful aqueous suppression.

Topical carbonic anhydrase inhibitors produce approximately a 20% reduction in IOP, with peak effect occurring at 2–3 h after administration. Topical medications are approved for three times daily dosing, although they are generally used twice daily. In comparison, oral CAIs cause a more profound 25–30% reduction in IOP. They begin to act within 1 h of consumption, with maximal effect occurring in 2–6 h. Acetazolamide is available both as regular tablets (62.5, 125, and 250 mg) which are typically dosed QID and timed-release 500 mg tablets (or "Sequels") which are dosed BID. Methazolamide is available as either 25 or 50 mg tablets and is dosed two to three times daily. Patients who are already on an oral CAI do not receive any added IOP-lowering benefit from the addition of a topical CAI. Both topical and systemic CAIs are indicated in the treatment of open-angle and angle-closure glaucoma. Topical CAIs are considered excellent second-line agents in pediatric glaucoma, although systemic formulations are avoided in this population.

Common side effects of the topical CAIs include bitter taste, dry eye syndrome, and transient blurred vision or burning after administration. They can also lead to corneal decompensation and should be used with caution in eyes with compromised corneal endothelium. Systemic side effects are rare with topical CAIs but not uncommon with systemic agents and are generally dose-dependent. These include paresthesias, metallic taste, fatigue, malaise, anorexia, GI upset, depression, increased risk of kidney stones, electrolyte imbalances (metabolic acidosis, hypokalemia), and hematologic abnormalities, including rare cases of aplastic anemia. They are to be used with caution in patients with impaired renal function, who should have their electrolytes monitored regularly. Although CAIs are sulfonamide derivatives, they are generally tolerated in those with sulfa allergies as the level of cross-reactivity is low. In one retrospective study by Lee et al., 27 patients with documented sulfa allergies received acetazolamide, and none experienced a severe allergic cross-reaction. Nevertheless, given their numerous potential systemic side effects, systemic CAIs are typically reserved for situations in which topical options have been exhausted or an acute decrease in IOP is required.

Parasympathomimetics (Miotics)

Parasympathomimetic agents are one of the oldest medication classes and have been used in glaucoma treatment for over 100 years. They were traditionally categorized as either indirect-acting or direct-acting agents. Indirect-acting agents, which include echothiophate iodide (Phospholine Iodide) and demecarium bromide (Humorsol), enhance acetylcholine activity by blocking acetylcholinesterase. These agents fell out of use due to ocular and systemic side effects and are no longer commercially available in the United States. Direct-acting agents mimic the activity of acetylcholine on motor end plates of postganglionic parasympathetic junctions. Pilocarpine, a direct-acting agent, is the only miotic that is still in use as a glaucoma medication.

Pilocarpine reduces IOP by inducing contraction of the longitudinal ciliary muscle, which puts tension on the trabecular meshwork by pulling the scleral spur, thereby increasing aqueous outflow through the meshwork (Fig. 19.6). However, its action may coincidentally reduce aqueous outflow through the uveoscleral pathway. It produces a 15–25% IOP reduction, with peak effect at about 2 h. It is available in 1–4% concentrations and is typically dosed four times daily.

Pilocarpine has traditionally been utilized in the treatment of both open-angle and

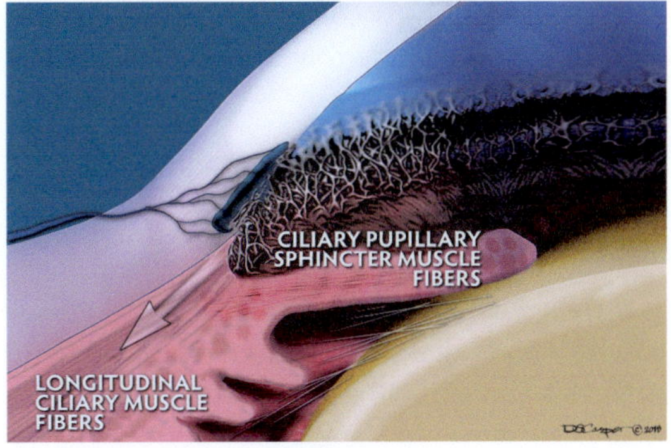

Fig. 19.6 Pilocarpine mechanism of action on the longitudinal ciliary muscle, resulting in opening of the drainage pathway

narrow-angle glaucomas. Currently it is often used prophylactically for angle-closure glaucoma prior to iridectomy and in patients with persistently occludable angles despite prior iridectomy. Despite its common use in narrow-angle glaucoma due to its miotic effect, pilocarpine does carry a small risk of inducing paradoxical angle closure via anterior shifting of the lens-iris diaphragm and subsequent exacerbation of pupillary block (a condition where the closely apposed anterior lens and posterior iris surfaces form a seal which prevents aqueous circulation through the pupil, thus blocking normal drainage via the angle).

In general, miotic agents are poorly tolerated due to their higher daily dosing requirement and numerous side effects and have been associated with poor compliance. These factors have limited their use in the management of primary open-angle glaucoma, and they are now typically spared for use as an adjunctive therapy when other medications have failed or are insufficient. Side effects include headache, brow ache, accommodative spasm, decreased vision (due to pupillary miosis as well as induced myopia), and chronic follicular conjunctivitis. They have also been associated with increased risk of retinal detachment, cataract development, and intraocular inflammation, particularly after surgery. They must be used with caution in patients with high myopia or other known risk factors for retinal detachment. As mentioned previously, they also carry a 1–2% risk of paradoxical angle closure and are thus relatively contraindicated in patients with phacomorphic narrow angles or malignant glaucoma (see Chap. 15).

Topical Combination Agents

It is estimated that 30–50% of glaucoma patients require more than one topical medication to achieve adequate IOP control. Compliance rates have been shown to significantly decrease as the number of medications increases, due in part to complex dosing schedules, financial cost considerations, and higher side effect rates. Combination products containing two agents in a single bottle have the potential benefit of improving convenience and compliance for such patients.

Prostaglandins are currently the most common choice for first-line therapy given their efficacy, once-daily dosing, and favorable side effect profile. β-blockers, α2-agonists, and CAIs have all been used as single medication adjunctive agents to prostaglandins, although they differ in their additive IOP reduction and dosing schedules. Although they are not available in the United States, combination products containing prostaglandin analogues and β-blockers are used in many other countries.

In the United States, numerous other fixed combination products are available or can be used both as sole therapies and as adjunctive agents. The most common of these include Cosopt (dorzolamide and timolol), Combigan (brimonidine and timolol), and Simbrinza (brimonidine and brinzolamide). In general, it is thought that the efficacy and side effect profiles of these fixed combinations are similar to that of each component given separately.

Hyperosmotics

Hyperosmotic agents are only used in acute situations to rapidly reduce IOP and never for chronic glaucoma management. When given systemically, they lower IOP by increasing serum osmolality and creating an osmotic gradient between the blood and the vitreous humor, which thereby draws fluid from the eye. The most commonly used hyperosmotic agents include intravenous mannitol, oral glycerin, and oral isosorbide.

Hyperosmotic agents are typically administered rapidly, as large doses to create a greater osmotic gradient, and are rarely administered for longer than a few hours. Their IOP-lowering effect is transient due to the rapid re-equilibration of the serum-vitreous osmotic gradient.

Hyperosmotic agents are associated with numerous systemic side effects, including headache, thirst, nausea/vomiting, diuresis, and mental status changes. The fluid shifts may precipitate or exacerbate congestive heart failure, and rare cases of subdural or subarachnoid hemorrhages have been reported. Due to their associated fluid and electrolyte disturbances, they are contraindicated in patients with renal failure or on dialysis. As oral glycerin may lead to hyperglycemia, it is often avoided in diabetic patients and substituted with oral isosorbide. In general, these medications are spared for use as a last resort in an emergency setting.

Recently Introduced Medical Treatment

The newest class of drugs is the rho-kinase, or ROCK, inhibitors. ROCKs mediate various important cellular functions such as cell shape, motility, secretion, proliferation, and gene expression. Inhibition of the ROCK pathway has been shown to contribute to the cardiovascular benefits of statin therapy. With regard to glaucoma, these drugs lower IOP by relaxing the trabecular meshwork. In December 2017 the FDA approved netarsudil for commercial use. The approval was based on results from three randomized trials which found that netarsudil was associated with a reduction in intraocular pressure of up to 5 mmHg. The most common side effect of netarsudil is conjunctival hyperemia, which has been reported to occur in approximately half of all users. Additional reactions, in approximately 20% of users, include corneal verticillata, instillation site pain, and conjunctival hemorrhage. There are minimal reported systemic adverse events and no contraindications, to date.

Preservative-Free Agents

Benzalkonium chloride (BAK) is the most commonly used preservative in topical medications. It is a quaternary ammonium compound and a cationic surfactant, and its biocidal properties prevent microbial contamination of medication bottles. It can also enhance corneal penetration of some drugs by acting as a detergent and disrupting corneal epithelial zonula occludens (tight junctions), increasing permeability to water-soluble substances.

BAK can also cause numerous adverse effects on various ocular tissues, and chronic BAK use in the glaucoma population can lead to significant toxicity. Most commonly, BAK can cause or exacerbate ocular surface disease, including compromised epithelial cell integrity, aqueous tear deficiency, Meibomian gland dysfunction, and blepharitis. It is a frequent and often underdiagnosed cause of eye discomfort and can lead to symptoms including redness, tearing, irritation, foreign body sensation, burning, and intermittent visual degradation. Although 8–15% of the general elderly population may experience some degree of ocular surface disease, the prevalence of symptoms increases to 40–58% in the glaucoma population. The severity of symptoms is directly related to the number of topical medications used.

Several alternative options exist for patients with severe BAK-related ocular surface disease or allergies. Available preservative-free preparations include timolol (Timoptic Ocudose), a dorzolamide/timolol fixed combination (preservative-free Cosopt), and tafluprost (Zioptan). Additionally, some gentler oxidizing preservatives have recently been introduced in topical glaucoma medications, including a stabilized oxychloro complex (Purite) and an ionic-buffered solution containing borate, zinc, and polyols (sofZia). These preservatives can be found in BAK-free formulations of brimonidine preserved with Purite (Alphagan-P) and Travatan preserved with sofZia (Travatan-Z). Minimizing BAK exposures in patients with symptomatic ocular surface disease can significantly improve quality of life and eyedrop tolerance, which in turn can lead to improved medication compliance.

Barriers to Successful Treatment

Inadequate medication compliance is highly correlated with treatment failure rates and is one of the major obstacles in long-term management of glaucoma. Nonadherence is often multifactorial in etiology, and patient education is critical in addressing its various underlying causes.

Simply remembering to take medications as prescribed can present a significant challenge to patients, particularly in the elderly population or those with neurological issues. Simplifying drug regimens to include the fewest number of medications given with the least frequency is optimal, and coordinating dosing schedules with meals or daily events can be a helpful memory aid. Newer technologies are also available such as the Travatan Dosing Aid (Alcon Laboratories, Ft Worth, TX), an electronic bottle-holder which reminds patients to take their eye drops, aids in dispensing medication, and records each instillation.

Improper administration of topical medications can also be a major source of non-compliance. As such, it is vital to teach patients the correct way to instill eye drops and to verify that the patient or someone else they live with can successfully administer them.

In some cases, patients may actively choose not to comply with their prescribed therapy. Willful negligence may be due to intolerance of side effects, financial cost, or various other social or environmental factors. Drug tolerance can often be improved by adjusting the medication regimen according to a patient's underlying medical comorbidities, which may be impacting their side effects. Optimizing the ocular surface with lubrication and the use of preservative-free medications can also improve tolerance and compliance. Switching medications to more affordable generic alternatives can significantly reduce the financial burden for patients in which cost is a prohibitive issue.

Regardless of the cause, patient education remains the first step in increasing medication compliance. Although it can prove difficult in a busy clinic setting, effective patient-provider communication is essential in order for patients to understand the nature of their disease, the risks and benefits of treatment, and the importance of regular follow-up. As glaucoma medications can only be effective when used properly, improving medication adherence is paramount to optimizing treatment outcomes and visual prognoses in the glaucoma population.

Suggested Reading

Camras CB, Alm A, Watson P, Stjernschantz J. Latanoprost, a prostaglandin analog, for glaucoma therapy efficacy and safety after 1 year of treatment in 198 patients. Latanoprost Study Group. Ophthalmology. 1996;103(11):1916–24.

Lee AG, Anderson R, Kardon RH, Wall M. Presumed "sulfa allergy" in patients with intracranial hypertension treated with acetazolamide or furosemide cross-reactivity, myth or reality? Am J Ophthalmol. 2004;138(1):114–8.

Liu JH, Kripke DF, Weinreb RN. Comparison of the nocturnal effects of once-daily timolol and latanoprost on intraocular pressure. Am J Ophthalmol. 2004;138(3):389–95.

Emre Göktas and Lama A. Al-Aswad

The goal of treating patients with glaucoma is the successful control of intraocular pressure (IOP). This is most commonly accomplished through medical therapy. However, when medical management fails, or is not practical, glaucoma surgery is indicated. Medical and surgical therapies cannot restore established optic nerve damage due to glaucoma, but treatments, either medical or surgical, reduce the absolute risk of progression by slowing and/or delaying visual field loss.

Surgical treatments are often safe and are effective in:

(a) Eliminating or reducing the necessity for anti-glaucomatous medications and their side effects
(b) Alleviating compliance problems and the ongoing cost of disease treatment

Surgical indications for glaucoma are progressive visual field loss on maximal medical therapy, intolerance of glaucoma medications, and poor adherence to treatment plans.

Glaucoma surgery is divided into laser therapies and incisional therapies.

Laser Therapies

Laser therapy may be a good option for treating many types of glaucoma. Laser treatment is generally less invasive, carries fewer risks, and results in fewer complications than incisional therapies. These therapies can target the trabecular meshwork, iris, and/or ciliary body to achieve reduced intraocular pressure.

Trabecular Meshwork

Laser Trabeculoplasty
Laser trabeculoplasty (trabecular meshwork laser treatment, LTP), a relatively uncomplicated office procedure, enhances aqueous humor outflow in most forms of open-angle glaucoma by treating the trabecular meshwork with laser energy. Laser applications cause either a burn in the trabecular meshwork to pull on the adjacent meshwork, thus opening intervening drainage spaces, or cause a renewal of trabecular meshwork cells and accelerate the turnover of extracellular matrix, depending on the type of laser used (Fig. 20.1).

E. Göktas, MD
Department of Ophthalmology, Columbia University Irving Medical Center, Edward S. Harkness Eye Institute, New York, NY, USA

L. A. Al-Aswad, MD, MPH (✉)
Columbia University Irving Medical Center, New York, NY, USA

Department of Ophthalmology, Edward S. Harkness Eye Institute, Columbia University Vagelos College of Physicians and Surgeons, New York, NY, USA
e-mail: laa2003@cumc.columbia.edu

© Springer Nature Switzerland AG 2019
D. S. Casper, G. A. Cioffi (eds.), *The Columbia Guide to Basic Elements of Eye Care*,
https://doi.org/10.1007/978-3-030-10886-1_20

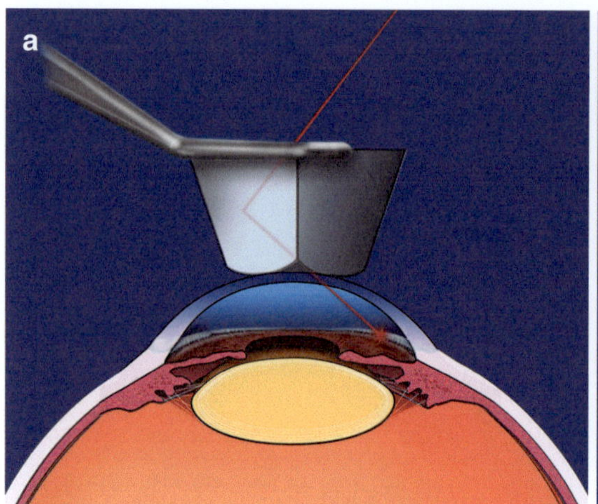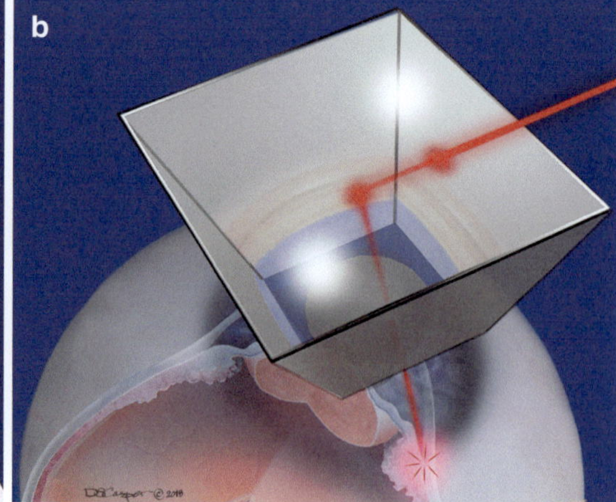

Fig. 20.1 LTP laser application technique using a four-mirror gonioscopy contact lens. (**a, b**) Schematically show the beam directed to the mirror directly opposite the area to be treated, thereby focusing the energy on the trabecular meshwork

These tissue changes restore trabecular function and improve aqueous drainage. LTP is indicated in patients with mild-to-moderate glaucoma poorly controlled with medical therapy, poor compliance with medical regimens, or difficulty using eye drops due to intolerance, allergic reaction, lifestyle considerations, or financial issues. LTP is also employed by some physicians as a first-line treatment for open-angle glaucoma, rather than using daily topical drop therapy. The maximum IOP-lowering effect of LTP typically does not appear until 6–12 weeks posttreatment.

Effective LTP can provide IOP lowering up to 20–30% from baseline. If the patient needs a greater reduction in IOP because of severe, pre-existing glaucomatous damage, filtering surgery should be considered first (see below). The long-term outcomes of LTP have been extensively reported in the literature. In approximately 77% of eyes treated with laser trabeculoplasty, IOP was significantly lower 1 year postoperatively. However, efficacy of LTP treatment decreases significantly over time; the success rate drops to 49% after 5 years. Repeat treatments can be performed after the first LTP if necessary.

In rare cases, IOP can be transiently, but significantly, elevated immediately after the procedure is performed. For this reason, an alpha agonist drop is usually given at the time of surgery to prevent any such brief spikes in IOP.

Generally, ophthalmologists use three types of laser systems for trabeculoplasty: argon laser (ALT), selective laser (SLT), and micropulse diode laser (MLT). Currently, SLT and ALT are the most common types of LTP preferred. Studies have demonstrated that both laser treatments are good options, with similar potential to reduce IOP, and relatively few side effects. Nevertheless, SLT is the preferred choice due ease of use and the lack of subsequent scarring.

An alternative treatment to SLT and ALT is MLT. Several studies have shown that MLT is effective in reducing IOP with less post-laser inflammation and side effects, compared with ALT. Early results report the success rate of MLT is 75%, with >20% reduction in IOP and medication requirement during 6–12 months of follow-up. Additional studies are currently ongoing to determine the long-term efficacy of MLT.

LTP may prove to be more cost-effective than lifelong topical glaucoma medication use.

Iris

Laser Peripheral Iridotomy

Laser iridotomy is the preferred method for managing all forms of angle-closure glaucoma involving pupillary block and as a prophylactic measure for patients with high-risk anatomic narrow angle. If a patient with narrow-angle anatomy presents with red, painful eye and extremely high pressures, this usually indicates acute angle-closure glaucoma, an ophthalmic emergency which can be confirmed with slit-lamp examination. The immediate, critical action in an episode of narrow-angle glaucoma is to "break" the attack as rapidly as possible. This can usually be accomplished with topical and/or system medications; once the attack is broken, ophthalmologists usually perform laser iridotomy in both eyes to prevent further attacks.

Laser iridotomy is the creation of a small hole through the peripheral iris to improve aqueous flow from the area posterior to the iris into the anterior chamber, thereby bypassing the pupil, thus deepening the anterior chamber and permitting the angle to reopen (Fig. 20.2). Argon and neodymium:YAG (yttrium aluminum garnet) laser is used for the creation of iridotomies. This procedure can be performed in the office under topical anesthesia, is safer than incisional surgical iridotomies (the only option prior to the introduction of laser iridotomy), and achieves similar results. Complications of laser iridotomy are rare but may include pressure elevation, hyphema, corneal epithelial injury, endothelial damage, cataract, retinal burn, and complaints of glare and double vision.

Laser Iridoplasty (Gonioplasty)

The main indications for laser iridoplasty are the conditions plateau iris syndrome and pseudoplateau iris caused by iridociliary cysts (Fig. 20.3). After a successful peripheral iridotomy, if angle closure without peripheral adherent scars within the angle (anterior synechiae) persists, the most probable diagnosis is plateau iris, a condition most typically found in younger patients, where the ciliary body inserts into the posterior iris more anteriorly than normal, resulting in a forward arching of the peripheral iris in relation to adjacent trabecular meshwork. This anatomic

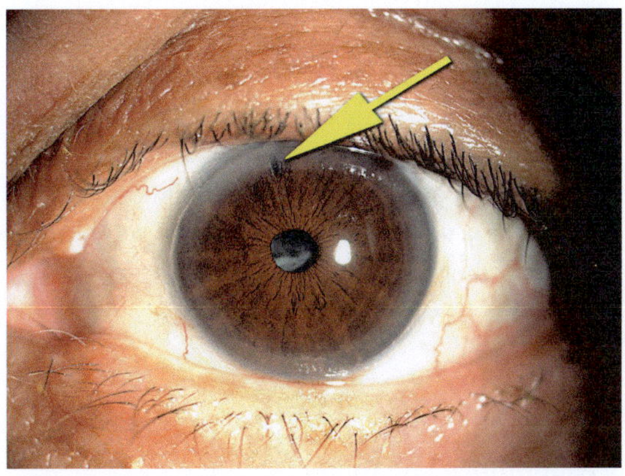

Fig. 20.2 Peripheral iridotomy seen in the iris at approximately 12:00 (yellow arrow)

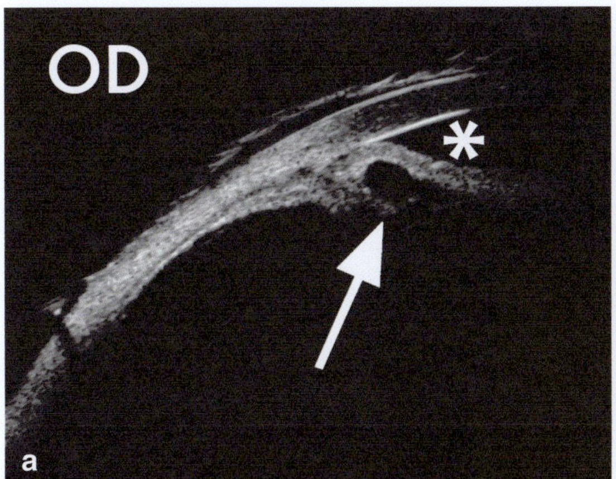

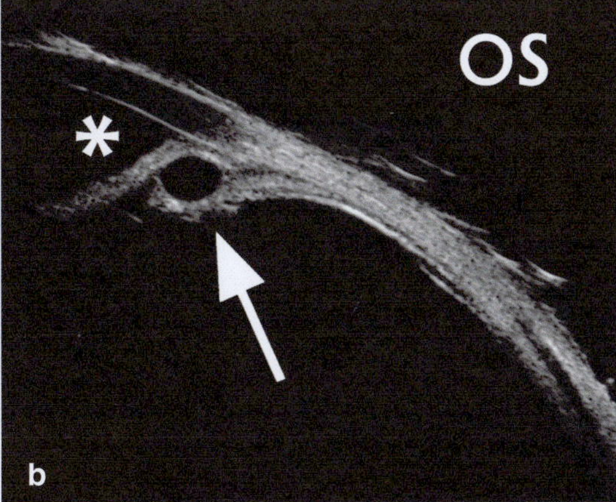

Fig. 20.3 Ultrasound biomicroscopy (UBM) image showing closed angles in a 27-year-old female with normal intraocular pressure (10 mmHg) and normal anterior chamber depth. Routine exam noted narrowed angles in both eyes. UBM exam demonstrated retroiridial cysts in all quadrants of both eyes, most prominent temporally and inferiorly. The images show the temporal aspect of the anterior segment of both eyes where large cysts result in angle closure. Arrows, retroiridial cysts; asterisks, closed angles. (Images courtesy of Dr Ronald Silverman)

anomaly can be confirmed with ultrasound. Medical treatment can decrease IOP but will not address the actual problem, which is the bowed iris configuration and resultant angle blockage. Laser iridoplasty is an effective and safe treatment for plateau iris syndrome. Typically, 20 or more laser burns distributed over 360° of the peripheral iris are sufficient to reposition the iris diaphragm to a more normal contour, with correction of the angle blockage, and subsequent improved aqueous outflow.

Other Iris Laser Procedures

Pupilloplasty and pupillary sphincterotomy employ lasers to enlarge, reshape, or reposition a small or adherent pupil, either of which can contribute to reduced aqueous fluid outflow. Goniosynechiolysis is a technique that uses laser energy to sever adhesions present in the angle between the peripheral iris and peripheral cornea (synechiae), which restrict access of aqueous to the angle, thereby reducing outflow.

Ciliary Body

Cyclophotocoagulation

Whereas most laser and incisional therapies are employed to increase aqueous outflow, the goal of cyclodestructive procedures is to reduce aqueous production by destroying elements of the ciliary body, with resultant lower IOP. These procedures are performed as either trans-scleral laser or endoscopic laser cyclophotocoagulation (TSCP or ECP). In TSCP, laser energy is applied externally through the anterior sclera. ECP, however, requires an invasive, intraocular approach which directly treats ciliary processes. TSCP is indicated in cases of refractory glaucoma after failure of previous trabeculectomies or tube shunt procedures, patients with limited vision and highly elevated IOP despite maximum medical therapy, and painful eyes due to uncontrolled high IOP with no visual potential. ECP can also be considered in patients with medically controlled glaucoma undergoing cataract surgery, because of the potential for reduction in dependence on medical glaucoma treatment.

Cyclophotocoagulation complications, which can be severe, may include surface burns, pain, inflammation, anterior chamber bleeding, changes in visual acuity, sympathetic ophthalmia (a rare, bilateral uveitis which occurs after unilateral eye trauma and is presumed to be auto-immune in nature), and malignant glaucoma (also referred to as aqueous misdirection syndrome).

Incisional Surgery (Filtration Surgery)

If a glaucoma patient has progressive visual field loss and optic nerve damage or uncontrolled IOP despite maximum tolerated medical and laser surgical therapies, the next course of treatment is incisional surgery (Table 20.1).

The most common forms of incisional glaucoma surgeries are trabeculectomy and tube shunt device implantation. These so-called filtration operations provide an alternate, low-resistance pathway from the anterior chamber to the subconjunctival space for augmented aqueous fluid egress. Normal aqueous outflow occurs via the angle, through Schlemm's canal to collector channels that drain into the venous circulation. The greatest resistance to aqueous humor outflow is presumed to be at the trabecular meshwork; therefore, the primary goal of filtration surgery is to eliminate the meshwork obstruction to aqueous fluid outflow. The success rate of incisional glaucoma surgery in reducing IOP and preserving vision is 70–80%; it carries risks of significant but mostly treatable complications.

Table 20.1 Indications for glaucoma surgery

Failure of medical therapy due to ineffectiveness, intolerance, poor compliance, or side effects
Progression of glaucoma on maximal tolerated glaucoma medications
Uncontrolled intraocular pressure
The coexistence of glaucoma and visually significant cataract

Trabeculectomy

Trabeculectomy with mitomycin C is widely considered the "gold standard" surgical procedure for glaucoma. This surgery is performed in the operating room, usually under local anesthesia (either topical anesthesia with eye drops, total akinesia with retrobulbar injections, or partial akinesia with peribulbar or subtenon injections). The basic trabeculectomy was supplemented by addition of the antimetabolite mitomycin C approximately 25 years ago, which decreases scarring, thereby significantly increasing chances of operative success. Preoperative evaluation of patients is very important for these procedures. For example, a common, minor condition such as blepharitis may increase the risk of post-trabeculectomy endophthalmitis, and poor compliance with postoperative instructions greatly increases the risk for surgical failure.

A variety of different techniques are used to perform trabeculectomy with mitomycin C, but the basic procedure is same. A conjunctival flap is performed superiorly, followed by creation of a partial-thickness scleral flap. A small piece of combined sclera and trabecular meshwork is removed, and the scleral flap and overlying conjunctiva are closed with sutures (Fig. 20.4). Mitomycin C is either injected in the superior subconjunctival space before surgery or applied directly to the sclera before or after flap creation.

Aqueous flows through the new pathway to the subconjunctival space, creating a blister-like elevation, referred to as a bleb (Fig. 20.5). From there, aqueous enters subconjunctival vessels and then empties into the venous circulation.

Modifications to trabeculectomy surgery include the use of different types of antimetabolites and various surgical modifications. The adjunctive use of antimetabolite drugs (5-fluorouracil or mitomycin C) with trabeculectomy surgery can delay the healing process and provide lower long-term IOP control. However, antimetabolites must be used with care, as they may cause a variety of complications, including scleral melting, wound leak, endophthalmitis, and prolonged low IOP (hypotony) (Fig. 20.6). While frequently successful, complications can occur, both in the early and late postoperative periods, such as endophthalmitis, blebitis, persistent hypotony, and cataract (Figs. 20.7 and 20.8).

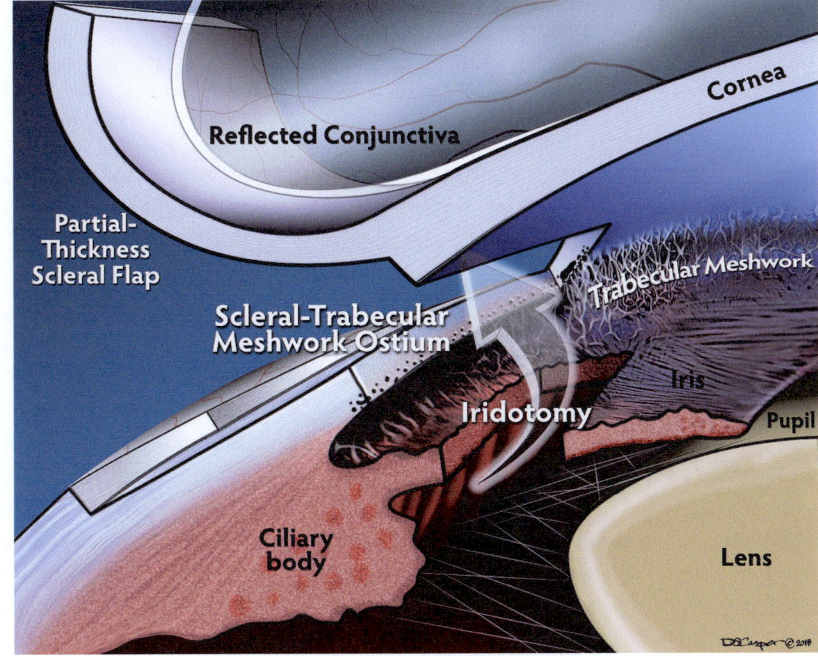

Fig. 20.4 Schematic of trabeculectomy architecture. The arrow shows how after trabeculectomy has created a new outflow pathway, aqueous fluid bypasses the trabecular meshwork and instead exits the anterior chamber through the surgical opening, to drain into the subconjunctival space

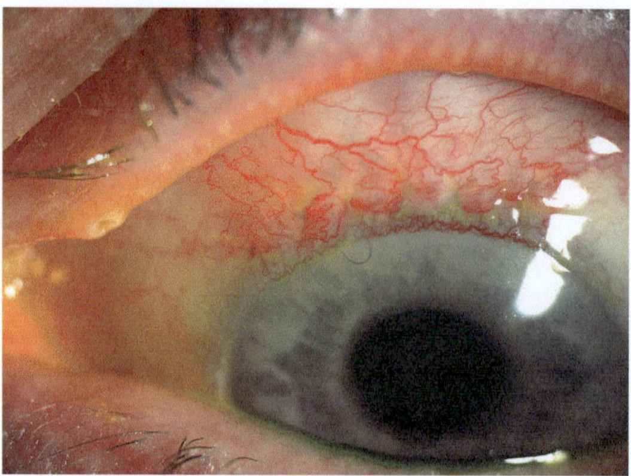

Fig. 20.5 A recent postoperative trabeculectomy bleb

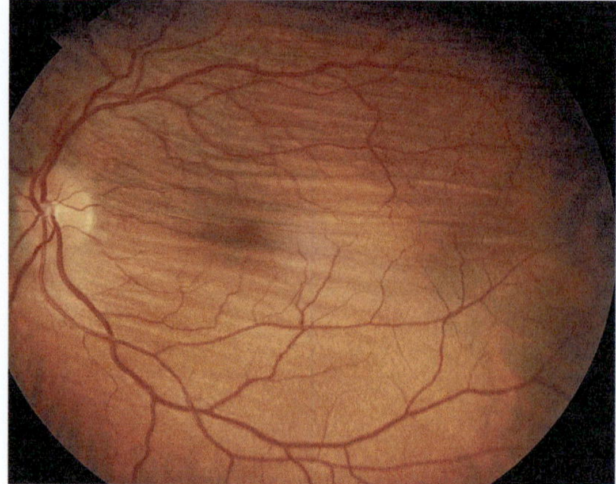

Fig. 20.6 Prominent choroidal folds in a hypotonous eye subsequent to trabeculectomy. (Courtesy of Dr Hermann Schubert)

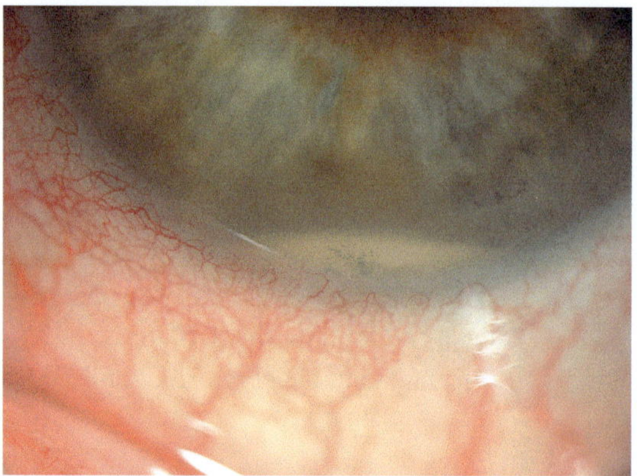

Fig. 20.7 A recent trabeculectomy with "blebitis" showing a small, layered hypopyon inferiorly

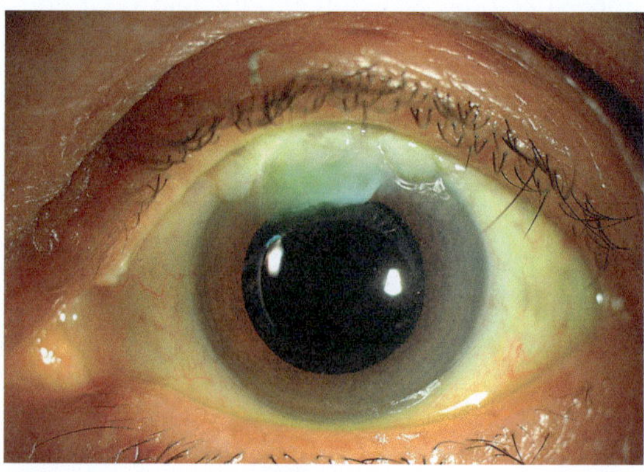

Fig. 20.8 A cystic bleb that is no longer functional due to scar formation. Note also that the patient has undergone cataract surgery as well

Sometimes the surgery is not successful, resulting in pressure that remains high, requiring reinstitution of glaucoma medications, or additional glaucoma surgery. Conversely, IOP may become too low (hypotony) causing a shallow anterior chamber or hypotony maculopathy. In these situations, additional surgery may be necessary.

Glaucoma Drainage Devices

Tube shunt (or aqueous shunt) surgeries are another commonly performed incisional procedure for the management of glaucoma. These procedures can be applied to patients who previously had failed trabeculectomy, or in cases with poor prognosis with filtering surgery (such as neovascular or uveitic glaucomas), or in patients with preexisting, extensive perilimbal conjunctival scarring. Recent studies demonstrated that the proportion of practitioners using tube shunts is increasing due to the lower complication rate compared with trabeculectomy surgery. Various aqueous drainage devices have been developed for management of refractory glaucoma; the most commonly used tube shunt implants can be classified into two categories: flow-restrictive (valved) or non-flow-restrictive (nonvalved).

Ahmed Glaucoma Implant (Flow-Restrictive)

The Ahmed glaucoma implant (AGI) is the most frequently employed glaucoma drainage device worldwide (Fig. 20.9). AGI is designed with a venturi-based flow restrictor mechanism which activates below 7 mmHg to forestall postoperative hypotony and shallow anterior chambers. AGI allows aqueous outflow through a small tube, toward a plate placed on the posterior sclera in the subtenon space. Topical anesthesia is sufficient in most cases. Different types of glaucoma drainage devices can be performed with a similar surgical technique. After an incision of the conjunctiva and Tenon's capsule is made, the plate of the AGI is sutured to the sclera approximately 8–9 mm posterior to the limbus. The tube, which is trimmed to an appropriate length, is inserted into the anterior chamber, covered with patch graft, and then the overlying conjunctiva and Tenon's capsule are closed with absorbable sutures.

Many studies have been designed to evaluate the short- and long-term results of the AGI, and typically they have reported that the success rates of AGI in the IOP control are approximately 80% at 1 year, 75% at 2 years, and 65% at 5 years.

Table 20.2 Complications of glaucoma drainage devices

Hypotony
Choroidal detachments
Obstruction of tube by fibrin, blood, iris, vitreous
Corneal decompensation (corneal edema)
Cataract acceleration
Endophthalmitis
Retinal detachment
Motility problems
Epithelial down-growth

Baerveldt Glaucoma Implant (Non-flow Restrictive)

The Baerveldt glaucoma implant (BGI) consists of a silicone tube attached to a silicone plate which is larger than that in the AGI. The implantation technique is similar to the AGI, but BGI requires special maneuvers to create a temporary tube ligature to obstruct flow in the early postoperative period because of its non-valved mechanism. The BGI achieves successful IOP control because of its wide end-plate surface area. However, when the ligature is dissolved or removed, there is a risk of hypotony due to inadequate wound healing around the implant. The success rates of BGI reported in studies range from about 70% to 90% at 12 months and from 60% to 80% at 48 months. Recently, many studies have compared Ahmed and Baerveldt implants. In these studies, similar rates of success were demonstrated with both implants at 5 years. The BGI implantation had greater IOP reduction requiring fewer medications than the AGI implantation, but BGI implantation also had a slightly higher complication rate.

Significant potential complications may occur after tube shunt surgeries, although many cases can be treated effectively (Table 20.2).

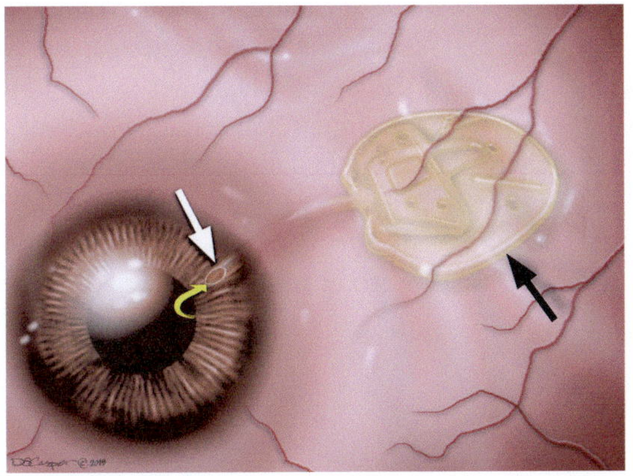

Fig. 20.9 An illustration of an Ahmed valve glaucoma drainage implant (black arrow). The valve itself is seen located subconjunctivally, and the drainage tube can be seen entering the anterior chamber (white arrow). Aqueous exits via the tube (yellow arrow), bypassing the normal drainage system

Cataract and Glaucoma Surgery

Glaucoma and cataract often develop together, especially in the aging population. In fact, each condition has a strong correlation with age. Both diseases can also affect management of the other. For example, cataract can contribute to narrowing of the anterior chamber angle, which can lead to angle-closure glaucoma. On the other hand, glaucoma medications and surgery can significantly increase the risk of cataract development. For this reason, both diseases must be considered during treatment planning. Faced with this situation, there are surgical alternatives, such as a variety of minimally invasive procedures, or combined phacoemulsification and trabeculectomy.

Minimally Invasive Glaucoma Surgeries (MIGS)

Minimally invasive procedures for glaucoma have recently been introduced and can be performed with or without cataract surgery. These have quicker recovery times and are much safer than standard glaucoma surgeries. MIGS are generally indicated for mild-to-moderate glaucoma stages, but not for advanced disease.

Microstent

Microstent (iStent) implantation is a surgical modification of the trabecular portion of the outflow system. This device creates a new channel from the anterior chamber to the trabecular meshwork and is performed in combination with cataract surgery. Studies show the rates of mean IOP reduction were approximately 25% with 1.6 fewer drops at 1 year, 24% with 1.1 drop reduction at 2 years, 19% with 0.8 fewer drops at 3 years, and 16% with 0.5 drop reduction at 5 years. Inserting more than one iStent is associated with enhanced IOP lowering; however, insertion of only one iStent is currently FDA approved. The most common adverse events in iStent application are transient lumen occlusion and device malpositioning. Hydrus is a trabecular microstent made of nickel-titanium recently approved by the FDA. Early studies demonstrated more than 20% reduction in IOP at 24 months with fewer glaucoma medications.

Trabectome and Kahook Dual Blade

The trabectome is another surgical treatment considered in glaucoma patients with or without coexisting cataract. In this procedure, a piece of trabecular meshwork and inner wall of Schlemm's canal are removed via electro-ablation with simultaneous infusion of fluid and aspiration of tissue debris. This technique increases aqueous access to Schlemm's canal and the collector channels. Trabectome is considered a safer procedure compared to other incisional surgeries. After trabectome surgery, the mean IOP reduction has been reported to be 30–40% at 1 year and 40–50% at 4 years. The most common complication after trabectome surgery is hyphema (blood in the anterior chamber). The kahook dual blade removes the trabecular meshwork (TM) without the need for additional hardware. Early studies demonstrated 40% reduction of IOP at 6 months with fewer glaucoma medications.

XEN Gel-Stent

The XEN implant, recently introduced in the United States, is a valve-free collagen tube that is implanted from the anterior chamber to the subconjunctival space without requiring a conjunctival incision. XEN implantation can be combined with cataract surgery. In preliminary studies, IOP-lowering effect of XEN was found to be 35%, with 90% fewer drops required 1 year postoperatively.

CyPass Microstent

The supraciliary CyPass, also recently made available in the United States, is a microstent implanted from the anterior chamber to the supraciliary space for enhanced suprachoroidal outflow of aqueous. This procedure is minimally invasive and less traumatic than standard, full-thickness incisional surgeries. According to the recent COMPASS trial results, supraciliary microstenting with cataract surgery significantly decreased IOP (77%) and hypotensive ocular medication use, compared with cataract surgery alone (60%) at 24 months postoperatively. The CyPass has low complication rates, the most common being transient hypotony, outflow obstruction, and postoperative IOP elevation. The CyPass was withdrawn from the market in 2018 due to increased endothelial cell loss.

Combined Phacoemulsification and Trabeculectomy

Trabeculectomy and cataract surgeries can be carried out together as a combined procedure (phacotrabeculectomy). This surgical method is especially useful for elderly patients who have glaucoma and coexisting cataract. Isolated trabeculectomy increases the risk of consequent cataract development by up to 78%. Additionally, subsequent cataract surgery may increase failure of a prior trabeculectomy. For this reason, the combined procedure is the most popular among current surgical techniques. Another advantage of phacotrabeculectomy is that it is more cost-effective than two separate procedures. Combined phacoemulsification and trabeculectomy can generally be performed utilizing standard techniques. IOP outcomes of phacotrabeculectomy are similar to trabeculectomy alone but with more rapid visual recovery.

Suggested Reading

Budenz DL, Barton K, Gedde SJ, Feuer WJ, Schiffman J, Costa VP, Godfrey DG, Buys YM, Ahmed Baerveldt Comparison Study Group. Five-year treatment outcomes in the Ahmed Baerveldt comparison study. Ophthalmology. 2015;122(2):308–16.

Damji KF, Bovell AM, Hodge WG, Rock W, Shah K, Buhrmann R, Pan YI. Selective laser trabeculoplasty versus argon laser trabeculoplasty: results from a 1-year randomised clinical trial. Br J Ophthalmol. 2006;90(12):1490–4.

Jea SY, Francis BA, Vakili G, Filippopoulos T, Rhee DJ. Ab interno trabeculectomy versus trabeculectomy for open-angle glaucoma. Ophthalmology. 2012;119(1):36–42.

Samuelson TW, Katz LJ, Wells JM, Duh YJ, Giamporcaro JE, US iStent Study Group. Randomized evaluation of the trabecular micro-bypass stent with phacoemulsification in patients with glaucoma and cataract. Ophthalmology. 2011;118(3):459–67.

Samuelson TW, Chang DF, Marquis R, Flowers B, Lim KS, Ahmed IIK, Jampel HD, Aung T, Crandall AS, Singh K, HORIZON Investigators. A schlemm canal microstent for intraocular pressure reduction in primary open-angle glaucoma and cataract: the HORIZON Study. Ophthalmology. 2019;126(1):29–37.

Sheybani A, Dick HB, Ahmed II. Early clinical results of a novel Ab interno gel stent for the surgical treatment of open-angle glaucoma. J Glaucoma. 2016;25(7):e691–6.

Vold S, Ahmed II, Craven ER, Mattox C, Stamper R, Packer M, Brown RH, Ianchulev T, CyPass Study Group. Two-year COMPASS trial results: supraciliary microstenting with phacoemulsification in patients with open-angle glaucoma and cataracts. Ophthalmology. 2016;123(10):2103–12.

Part IV

Posterior Segment and Retina

Age-Related Macular Degeneration

21

Victoria North and Srilaxmi Bearelly

Age-related macular degeneration (AMD), or the progressive degeneration of the central portion of the retina, is one of the leading causes of blindness in the United States (USA) and the developed world. Among white individuals in the USA, it is the leading cause of blindness, accounting for 54.5% of cases. In 2004 it was estimated that over 7 million individuals in the USA had large subretinal deposits (drusen) consistent with moderate AMD and that approximately 1.75 million had advanced disease. By 2020, it is expected that nearly three million Americans will have advanced AMD.

AMD is characterized by a spectrum of degenerative changes in the macula that affect multiple structures including the outer retina, retinal pigment epithelium (RPE), Bruch's membrane, and choriocapillaris. Though the etiology of AMD is not fully understood, risk factors include age greater than 50, smoking, Caucasian race, family history, hypercholesterolemia, and cardiovascular disease. Additionally, several genetic poly-

morphisms have been implicated, most notably those of complement factor H (CFH) and other components of the complement pathway including complement factor B and C3.

AMD is typically classified as either non-neovascular or neovascular, commonly referred to as "dry" and "wet" AMD, respectively. All patients with AMD start with non-neovascular features; they may or may not be symptomatic, which is why individuals over age 50 are encouraged to have a baseline dilated exam. In its late forms, AMD may be either neovascular and/or develop into geographic atrophy. It is in the late forms, also known as advanced disease, that vision loss typically becomes symptomatic. Clinical features and management of each type are detailed in this chapter.

Early Non-neovascular AMD

Clinical Features

The defining clinical feature of non-neovascular AMD is the presence of subretinal deposits called drusen. These lipid-rich deposits of extracellular material lie beneath the RPE and appear as round, yellow lesions on funduscopic exam (Figs. 21.1, 21.2, and 21.3a). Drusen are differentiated by their size and appearance: they may be small, intermediate, or large and hard, soft, or confluent. Hard drusen have sharp, well-demarcated

V. North, MD (✉)
Department of Ophthalmology, Harvard Medical School, Boston, MA, USA
e-mail: vsn2104@caa.columbia.edu

S. Bearelly, MD, MHS
Columbia University Irving Medical Center, New York, NY, USA

Department of Ophthalmology, Edward S. Harkness Eye Institute, Columbia University Vagelos College of Physicians and Surgeons, New York, NY, USA

© Springer Nature Switzerland AG 2019
D. S. Casper, G. A. Cioffi (eds.), *The Columbia Guide to Basic Elements of Eye Care*,
https://doi.org/10.1007/978-3-030-10886-1_21

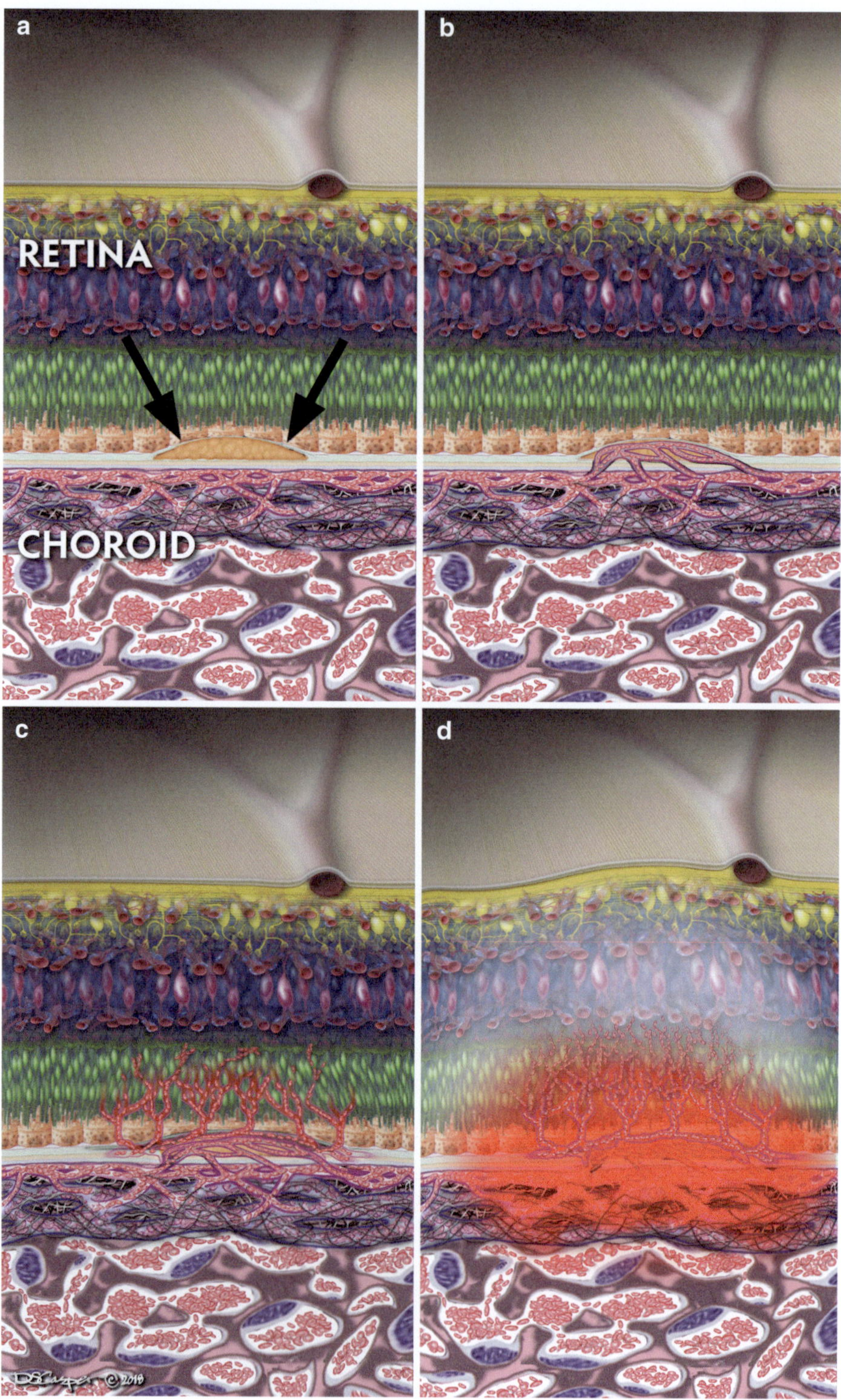

Fig. 21.1 Schematic illustration showing location of drusen and subretinal neovascularization (see Fig. 1.30a). (**a**) Drusen deposited beneath the retinal pigmented epithelium (arrows). (**b**) Early neovascularization originating from the choriocapillaris. (**c**) Further neovascularization, extending through the pigment epithelium and into the outer retinal layers. (**d**) Hemorrhage originating from the neovascular vessels, with adjacent retinal edema

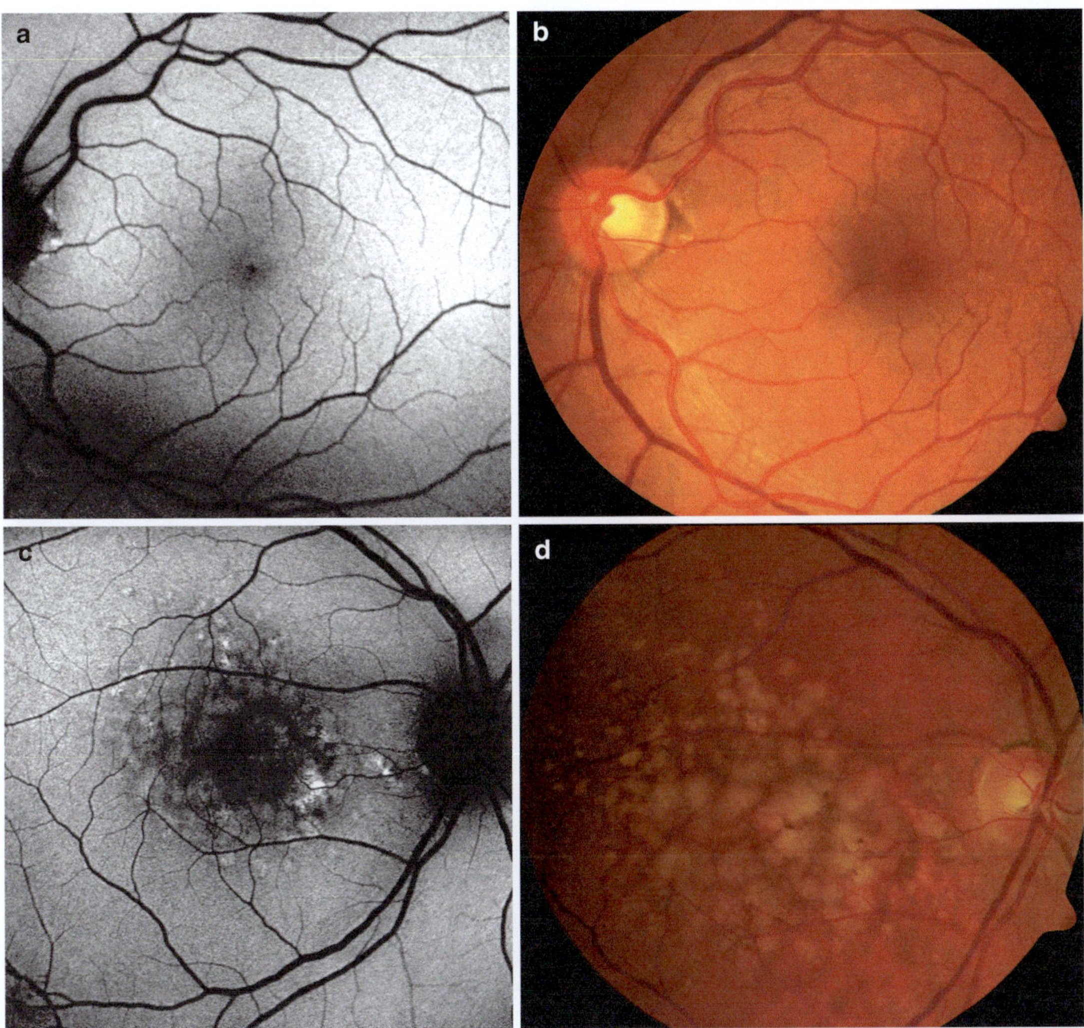

Fig. 21.2 Early AMD. Autofluorescence (left column) and color fundus photographs (right column): (**a, b**) normal; (**c, d**) early AMD with diffuse drusen

borders, whereas soft drusen are amorphous with poorly defined borders. Multiple soft drusen may coalesce and become confluent.

In addition to drusen deposits, there may also be abnormalities of the RPE, which may appear as focal areas of *hyper*pigmentation or else as larger, noncontiguous areas of *de*pigmentation known as *non*geographic atrophy. On funduscopic exam, nongeographic atrophy has a mottled or speckled appearance. More extensive damage to the RPE that results in contiguous atrophy, often involving the fovea, is termed geographic atrophy (GA) and is consistent with late-stage AMD (discussed separately). Fluorescein angiography (FA) can be a useful tool to assess features of AMD: drusen typically stain in late views, whereas areas of focal hyperpigmentation appear as blockages.

Drusen can be clinically silent depending on their size and location, but when they are large or involve the fovea, they may affect vision. Even smaller drusen may cause damage to overlying photoreceptors, which results in some vision loss or disruption of dark adaptation. Due to the variability of clinical presentation, it is helpful to classify patients with drusen based on risk of

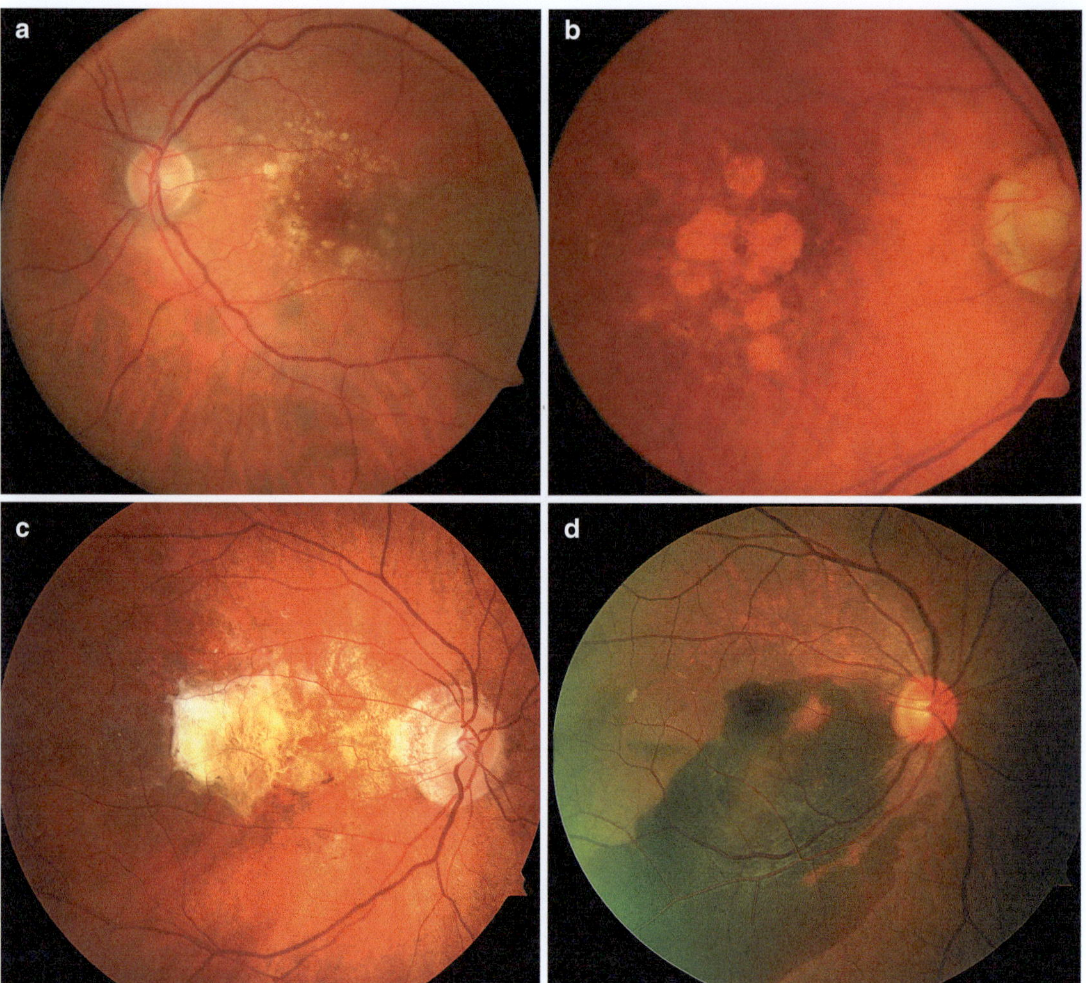

Fig. 21.3 AMD. (**a**) Early AMD with drusen, (**b**) Classic AMD with areas of hyperpigmentation, (**c**) AMD with macular scar, (**d**) AMD with large subretinal hemorrhage inferiorly

progression to late AMD. The Age-Related Eye Disease Study (AREDS) followed participants with mild-to-moderate AMD to assess progression to advanced disease, which they defined as the presence of GA involving the center of the macula or any choroidal neovascularization (CNV). Patients with fewer than five small drusen were considered disease-free, those with multiple small or single intermediate drusen had mild disease, and those with at least one large druse, multiple intermediate drusen, or GA not involving the center of the macula had moderate disease. The risk of progression to advanced AMD in 10 years was very low in participants with no disease or mild disease (0% and 1.5%, respectively) and higher in those with bilateral intermediate drusen at enrollment (13.8%). Participants with bilateral large drusen had the highest risk (36.1%) of developing advanced AMD in at least one eye within 10 years.

Another high-risk feature is the presence of reticular pseudodrusen (RPD). These drusenoid deposits are located above the RPE, unlike true drusen. Like drusen, they are composed of membranous deposits, cholesterol, and complement. On funduscopic exam, RPD appear as a reticular pattern of yellow-white lesions (Fig. 21.4). They are often best seen with infrared or autofluorescence imaging. Though not specific to AMD, the

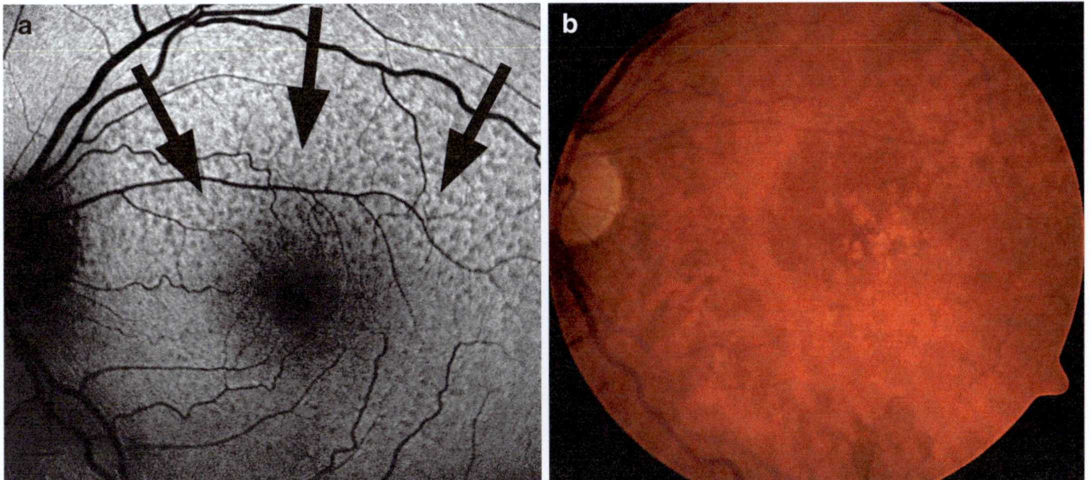

Fig. 21.4 Reticular pseudodrusen (RPD). Autofluorescence (**a**) and color fundus photograph (**b**) of early AMD with RPD (arrows)

presence of RPD is a strong risk factor for progression to advanced AMD, particularly GA, in a similar fashion as the presence of focal pigmentary abnormalities and large drusen.

Management

As there is no direct treatment for non-neovascular AMD, focus is on early detection and prevention of progression to advanced disease. This is especially true in the primary care setting. Various strategies for detection and prevention are outlined below.

Amsler Grid and Follow-Up

Patients with drusen or those at high risk for developing AMD should be followed with regular dilated eye exams to assess for progression of disease. In addition, it is important to educate patients about symptoms of advanced disease such as scotoma, loss of central vision, or metamorphopsia. One simple and effective method patients can use to evaluate these symptoms is the Amsler grid, a test card with a central dot and a black grid on a white background. Testing each eye individually, patients fixate on the central dot and assess whether the surrounding grid has any new distortions, blind spots, or breaks (Fig. 21.5).

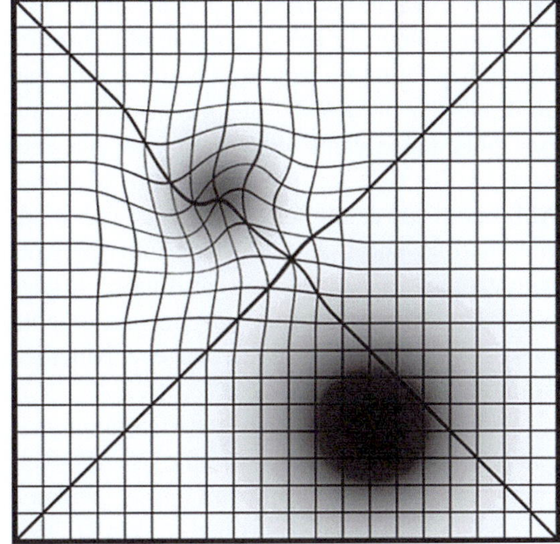

Fig. 21.5 Amsler grid, showing an area of metamorphopsia superiorly, and a scotoma inferiorly

Lifestyle Modifications

While many risk factors for AMD such as race, age, light iris color, and genetic polymorphisms are not modifiable, certain lifestyle modifications such as weight loss and smoking cessation may be beneficial. Smoking carries a particularly strong association with advanced AMD: the Blue Mountains Eye Study found that current smokers had a fourfold higher risk of having advanced

AMD than never smokers even after controlling for factors such as age and sex. In addition, they found that former smokers had a threefold higher risk of GA. Therefore, counseling patients on smoking cessation is an important aspect of management of early AMD. UV light may be retinotoxic and is thought to be one potential mechanism of AMD progression. Therefore, many ophthalmologists also recommend UV-protective eyewear to their patients.

Micronutrients

Several studies have investigated the association between micronutrients and risk of AMD. In a multicenter, randomized controlled trial, the AREDS group evaluated the effect of high-dose antioxidants (vitamin C, vitamin E, beta-carotene) and zinc on AMD progression. Subjects aged 55–80 were randomly assigned to receive antioxidants, zinc, antioxidants plus zinc, or placebo and were followed over an average of 6.3 years. While they found no benefit in patients who had no disease or mild AMD at time of enrollment, zinc plus antioxidants, compared with placebo, lowered the risk for progression to advanced AMD or visual acuity loss in patients with moderate and advanced AMD. Specifically, patients with extensive intermediate size drusen, at least one large druse, noncentral GA in one or both eyes, or advanced AMD in one eye benefited from treatment.

An important caveat to the AREDS findings is that beta-carotene may increase the risk of developing lung cancer in current and former smokers. A second randomized controlled trial, AREDS2, assessed the value of eliminating beta-carotene. They also assessed the addition of carotenoids (lutein and zeaxanthin) and omega-3 fatty acids (DHA and EPA). They saw no further reduction in progression to advanced AMD with addition of carotenoids or omega-3 fatty acids or both. Importantly, they also saw no negative effect in eliminating beta-carotene from the formulation, while they did note more lung cancers in the beta-carotene group, particularly in former smokers. Overall, they concluded that lutein and zeaxanthin could be an appropriate substitution for beta-carotene in the original AREDS formulation.

Late AMD

Clinical Features

Late or advanced AMD is typically defined as vision-threatening geographic atrophy (GA) involving the center of the macula or the presence of choroidal neovascularization (CNV). Each form of advanced AMD is discussed below, with emphasis on CNV and its treatments.

Geographic Atrophy

Approximately one million Americans have GA, which is characterized by cell-death in adjacent regions of RPE and photoreceptors that appear as sharply demarcated areas of hypopigmentation on funduscopic exam. Atrophy of overlying RPE and photoreceptors unmasks choroidal vessels, and the choriocapillaris may be attenuated or atrophied as well. Advanced imaging techniques can help identify these lesions, which are characterized by choroidal signal enhancement on optical coherence tomography (OCT). This is seen due to loss of absorbing pigment and thinning of outer retinal layers. Additionally, atrophy of the RPE reduces fluorophores and leads to markedly reduced signal, or "window defect," on FA. Autofluorescence imaging is another imaging modality commonly used to assess extent of RPE loss in the setting of GA (Fig. 21.6a, b).

Clinically, GA may not affect central vision until late in the course, and thus visual acuity is not a good marker of disease progression. Atrophic areas typically coalesce into a horseshoe and later a ring surrounding the fovea, but peripheral spread often occurs more quickly than that toward the center. When the parafoveal region and fovea become involved, the patient may experience a dense visual scotoma and, ultimately, irreversible central vision loss.

Neovascular AMD

Dry AMD progresses to wet AMD when neovascularization occurs within the choroidal or subretinal space. Drusen and other changes such as thickening of the inner aspect of Bruch's membrane render the membrane susceptible to breaks.

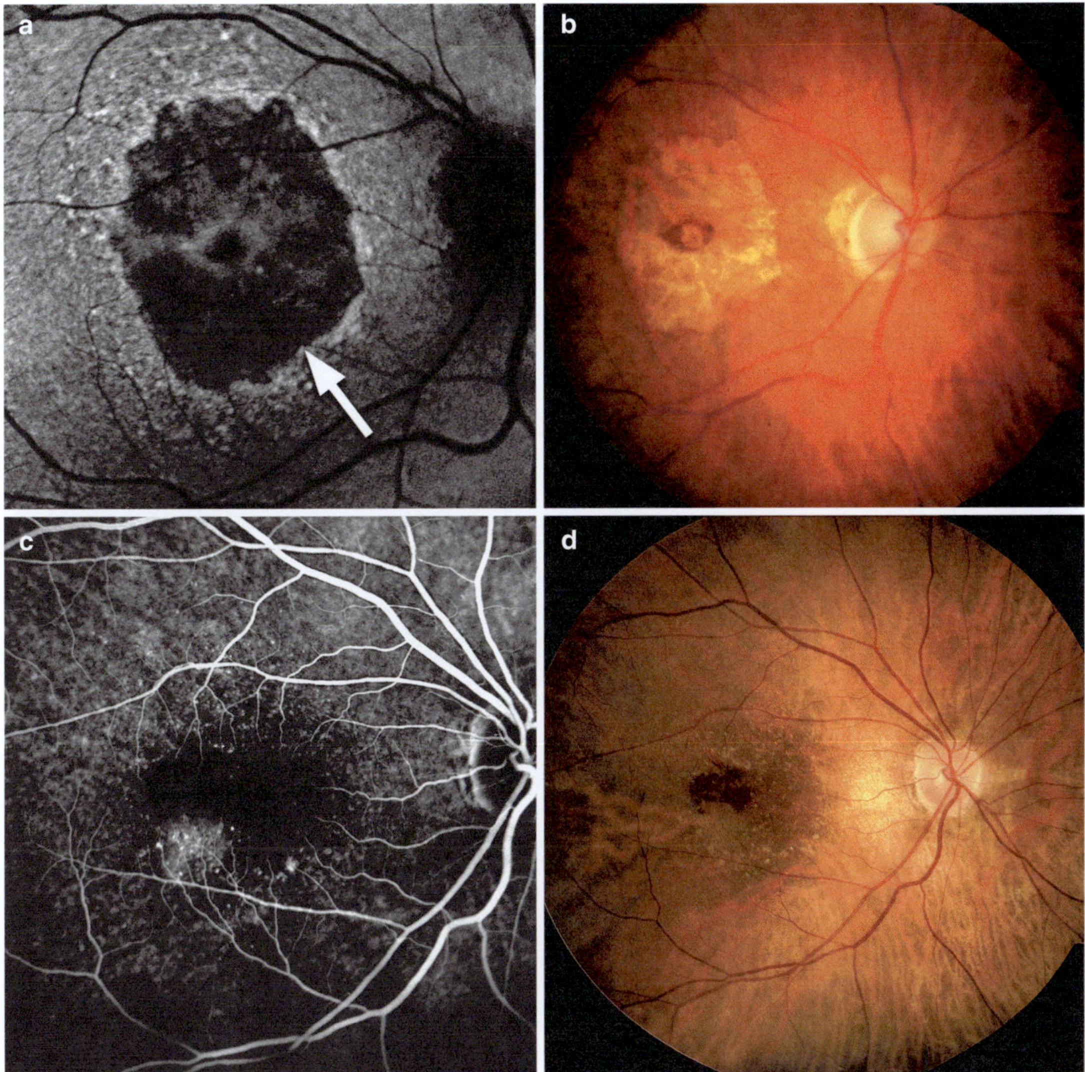

Fig. 21.6 Late AMD. Autofluorescence (left column) and color fundus photographs (right column): (**a**, **b**) late AMD with geographic atrophy (white arrow) and RPD; (**c**, **d**) neovascular AMD with subretinal hemorrhage

In this setting, capillary buds and fibroblasts from the underlying choriocapillaris extrude through breaks in the membrane, causing choroidal neovascularization (CNV). The presence of fibrovascular complexes in the subretinal space leads to multiple complications such as leakage of fluid or blood, detachment of the RPE, and in more serious cases, the formation of scars (Fig. 21.3c, d). Clinically, patients typically experience loss of vision that is much more rapid in onset than with GA. With neovascular AMD, there may be a sudden decrease in visual acuity, a new metamorphopsia or a central scotoma.

A variety of changes may be present on funduscopic exam, including subretinal fluid or blood, elevation or tear of the RPE, cystoid macular edema (CME), or a gray-white subretinal lesion corresponding to a disciform scar (Figs. 21.6c–d and 21.7). Advanced imaging techniques, particularly fluorescein angiography (FA), are helpful in visualizing the neovascular changes associated with AMD. CNV can be categorized by

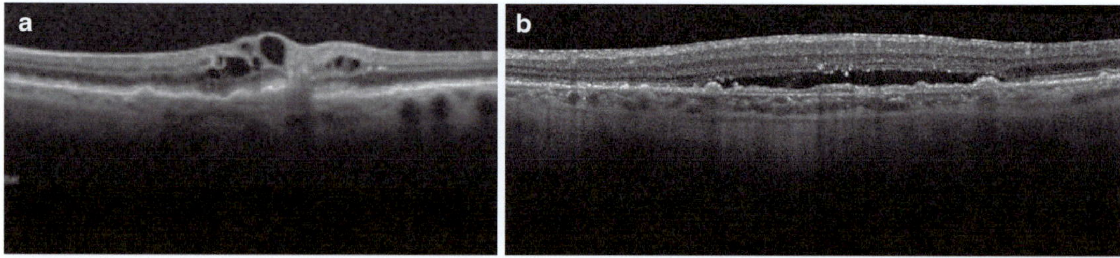

Fig. 21.7 Late AMD. Optical coherence tomography (OCT) images of (**a**) CME, (**b**) subretinal fluid

appearance on FA: classic lesions are well defined in early frames and display late leakage, whereas occult lesions are ill defined early and display late leakage. OCT is another useful imaging modality that demonstrates the presence of subretinal fluid, RPE elevation, or CME (Fig. 21.7).

Management

Pharmacotherapy

The discovery of vascular endothelial growth factor (VEGF) and its role in angiogenesis has greatly impacted the treatment of neovascular AMD. Formation of new blood vessels in the choroid, as elsewhere in the body, depends on multiple pro- and anti-angiogenic factors. VEGF expression is increased in RPE cells early in AMD and is therefore implicated in the initiation of new vessel growth. The majority of pharmacotherapy for neovascular AMD has focused on intravitreal injections of anti-VEGF molecules.

The first of these therapies to be approved by the FDA was pegaptanib, an aptamer that binds the 165 isoform of VEGF. Though the VISION clinical trial showed that visual acuity in subjects treated with pegaptanib was better than in those treated with sham injections, newer anti-VEGF therapies are more effective, and thus pegaptanib is rarely used.

More success has been seen with ranibizumab, a recombinant monoclonal antibody fragment that binds to and inhibits all active forms of VEGF. Two separate randomized controlled trials, MARINA and ANCHOR, demonstrated a statistically significant benefit with monthly injections of ranibizumab versus sham injections.

Importantly, these trials showed both that subjects lost fewer than 15 letters from baseline visual acuity (94–96% in treatment group vs. 62–64% in placebo group) and that they were more likely to gain more than 15 letters from baseline as well (25–40% vs. 5–6%).

Bevacizumab is a full-length monoclonal antibody against VEGF that is similar to ranibizumab but differs in that it has an additional antigen-binding domain and a longer half-life. Importantly, there is a substantial cost difference between the two. Bevacizumab, which is FDA approved for the treatment of metastatic colorectal cancer and currently used "off-label" for intravitreal injections, costs significantly less than ranibizumab.

Most recently approved by the FDA for treatment of neovascular AMD is aflibercept, a recombinant fusion protein that competes for binding of VEGF. This drug therefore acts as a VEGF trap.

Thermal Laser

Historically, the treatment of choice for classic CNV lesions was photocoagulation with thermal laser, which can be performed perifoveally, or of the entire CNV lesion. Though laser photocoagulation of CNV slows the progression of visual loss in patients with neovascular AMD, it is associated with an increased risk of visual loss immediately after treatment, particularly in patients with subfoveal AMD. Thus with the advent of anti-angiogenic therapies, thermal laser photocoagulation of subfoveal CNV is no longer recommended. This technique may still be useful in small lesions outside the central macula.

Photodynamic Therapy

Another treatment approach used less commonly with the advent of pharmacotherapy is photodynamic therapy (PDT). This technique involves systemic administration of a photosensitizing drug, verteporfin, just prior to targeted light therapy. This two-step process leads to a localized photochemical reaction that damages neovascular tissue and is safer for use in the fovea than thermal laser photocoagulation. Trials investigating the benefit of PDT saw lower rates of visual loss compared to placebo at 1 and 2 years after treatment, though the size of this effect was modest. PDT is mainly used in patients who fail to respond to anti-VEGF therapies.

Conclusion

Age-related macular degeneration (AMD) is one of the leading causes of blindness in the developed world. AMD can be non-neovascular or neovascular, and either type can progress to irreversible central vision loss. In the primary care setting, emphasis is on early detection of disease and prevention of progression to advanced disease when possible. This requires close follow-up, education, and lifestyle modification. Supplementation with antioxidants and zinc may be useful for patients with moderate disease. For patients with neovascular AMD, treatment with intravitreal injection of anti-VEGF molecules such as ranibizumab can slow disease progression and may even improve vision from baseline presentation. Finally, there are many promising areas of ongoing research with the potential to influence treatment and prognosis. These include intraocular implants that may provide sustained delivery of biologics, complement factor inhibitors, retinoid inhibitors, RPE or stem cell transplantation, and many more.

Suggested Reading

Age-Related Eye Disease Study Research Group. A randomized, placebo-controlled, clinical trial of high-dose supplementation with vitamins C and E, beta carotene, and zinc for age-related macular degeneration and vision loss: AREDS report no. 8. Arch Ophthalmol. 2001;119(10):1417–36.

Age-Related Eye Disease Study Research Group. Lutein + zeaxanthin and omega-3 fatty acids for age-related macular degeneration: the Age-Related Eye Disease Study 2 (AREDS2) randomized clinical trial. JAMA. 2013;309(19):2005–15.

Chakravarthy U, Adamis AP, Cunningham ET, et al. Year 2 efficacy results of 2 randomized controlled clinical trials of pegaptanib for neovascular age-related macular degeneration. Ophthalmology. 2006;113(9):1508. e1–25.

Chew EY, Clemons TE, Agrón E, et al. Ten-year follow-up of age-related macular degeneration in the age-related eye disease study: AREDS report no. 36. JAMA Ophthalmol. 2014a;132(3):272–7.

Chew EY, Clemons TE, Sangiovanni JP, et al. Secondary analyses of the effects of lutein/zeaxanthin on age-related macular degeneration progression: AREDS2 report No. 3. JAMA Ophthalmol. 2014b;132(2):142–9.

Congdon N, O'Colmain B, Klaver CC, et al. Causes and prevalence of visual impairment among adults in the United States. Arch Ophthalmol. 2004;122(4):477–85.

Finger RP, Chong E, McGuinness MB, et al. Reticular pseudodrusen and their association with age-related macular degeneration: the Melbourne collaborative cohort study. Ophthalmology. 2016;123(3):599–608.

Friedman DS, O'Colmain BJ, Muñoz B, et al. Prevalence of age-related macular degeneration in the United States. Arch Ophthalmol. 2004;122(4):564–72.

Holz FG, Strauss EC, Schmitz-Valckenberg S, van Lookeren Campagne M. Geographic atrophy: clinical features and potential therapeutic approaches. Ophthalmology. 2014;121(5):1079–91.

Kaiser PK, Brown DM, Zhang K, et al. Ranibizumab for predominantly classic neovascular age-related macular degeneration: subgroup analysis of first-year ANCHOR results. Am J Ophthalmol. 2007;144(6):850–7.

Rosenfeld PJ, Brown DM, Heier JS, et al. Ranibizumab for neovascular age-related macular degeneration. N Engl J Med. 2006;355(14):1419–31.

Tan JS, Mitchell P, Kifley A, Flood V, Smith W, Wang JJ. Smoking and the long-term incidence of age-related macular degeneration: the Blue Mountains Eye Study. Arch Ophthalmol. 2007;125(8):1089–95.

Virgili G, Bini A. Laser photocoagulation for neovascular age-related macular degeneration. Cochrane Database Syst Rev. 2007;3:CD004763.

Wormald R, Evans J, Smeeth L, Henshaw K. Photodynamic therapy for neovascular age-related macular degeneration. Cochrane Database Syst Rev. 2007;3:CD002030.

Diabetic Eye Disease

Daniel S. Casper and Jonathan S. Chang

Epidemiology

In the year 2000, the number of patients in the United States known to have diabetic retinopathy was believed to be about 4 million. Recent National Eye Institute studies estimated that among people older than 40 years of age, there were approximately 8 million known cases in 2010 and project that the number of cases of diabetic retinopathy in the United States will most likely double over the next 40 years, to an estimated 15 million in 2050. In 2007, the estimated number of diabetics in the United States was approximately 24 million (NIDDK), yet the prevalence of undiagnosed diabetes cases was estimated to be close to 6 million people; one can assume that the numbers for undiagnosed diabetic eye disease are similarly underestimated.

D. S. Casper, MD, PhD (✉)
Columbia University Irving Medical Center,
New York, NY, USA

Department of Ophthalmology, Edward S. Harkness
Eye Institute, New York, NY, USA

Naomi Berrie Diabetes Center, Columbia University
Vagelos College of Physicians and Surgeons,
New York, NY, USA
e-mail: dsc5@cumc.columbia.edu

J. S. Chang, MD
Department of Ophthalmology and Visual Sciences,
University of Wisconsin School of Medicine and
Public Health, Madison, WI, USA

Diabetic retinopathy is cited as the leading cause of new cases of blindness in persons aged 20–74, and about 12% of new cases of blindness yearly are attributed to diabetes. It is believed that in 60–90% of those cases, visual loss could have been prevented with early detection and management. Despite this, it has been estimated that about one-third of US diabetic patients have never had an eye exam, and only two-thirds of those with high-risk proliferative retinopathy or clinically significant macular edema have had an ophthalmic evaluation within 2 years.

Pathophysiology

With continually improving treatments for diabetes, expanded patient lifespan has resulted in increased frequency of macro and microvascular complications. Prior to the 1980s, there was very little that ophthalmologists could offer patients with diabetic retinopathy, and blindness due to retinal detachments or macular edema was a common complication. With the development of laser phototherapy at the end of the last century and anti-neovascular compounds at the beginning of this century, there is more reason than ever for patients with diabetic eye disease to be identified, as there are now effective treatments for early and late manifestations of diabetic eye disease.

Although current teaching presumes an initial hyperglycemia-induced lesion at the retinal

© Springer Nature Switzerland AG 2019
D. S. Casper, G. A. Cioffi (eds.), *The Columbia Guide to Basic Elements of Eye Care*,
https://doi.org/10.1007/978-3-030-10886-1_22

capillary pericytes, there is evidence that an earlier effect may occur in retinal neurons. If true, this lesion is not easily identified with current ophthalmic examination techniques, while evidence of early capillary damage is relatively easily seen, without the need for special research instrumentation. The hypothesis of capillary damage invokes early pericyte death and loss of blood-retinal barrier integrity, followed by endothelial cell injury and death, with resultant non-functional capillary beds. These "acellular capillaries" are incapable of nourishing surrounding retinal tissues, and eventually, ischemia leads to death of inner retinal neurons, with identifiable and potentially devastating effects on visual acuity.

This cascade of damage may be partially visualized with ophthalmoscopy: capillary closure is seen as microaneurysms ("dots"), cotton wool spots (localized areas of retinal ischemia, rendering the normally transparent retina opaque), dilated capillaries, vascular loops, and venous beading. Blood-retinal barrier dysfunction results in capillary leakage ("blot" hemorrhages), hard exudates (extravascular lipoprotein deposits), and retinal edema, manifested as macular thickening, cyst formation, and surface distortion (Fig. 22.1).

Capillary dropout and retinal edema are difficult to visualize directly, and classically, intravenous fluorescein angiography (FA) administered by antecubital venipuncture and recorded by high-speed photography has been used extensively to characterize the extent of these findings. More recently, the introduction of optical coherence tomographic (OCT) imaging has simplified obtaining and quantifying resulting information, employing a rapid, noninvasive technology (Fig. 22.2 and see Appendix 1).

The visible sequellae of early diabetic retinopathy, listed above, were previously referred to as "background" retinopathy. Newer terminology refers to this level of retinal pathology as *non-proliferative*, to distinguish it from the subsequent stage, *proliferative* retinopathy, which is much more worrisome and usually necessitates urgent intervention.

Non-proliferative diabetic retinopathy (NPDR) does not usually require ophthalmic treatment and is typically asymptomatic. If the patient's diabetes is in poor control, with hemoglobin A_1c levels above 7%, the patient is educated as to the importance of blood glucose control and the likelihood of worsening diabetic eye disease if chronic hyperglycemia persists. Most ophthalmologists also stress good blood pressure and lipid control, with smoking cessation as well, to reduce the risk of developing NPDR, or to limit worsening of disease already present.

After NPDR has been present for a number of years, and usually in the face of persistent poor control, the next phase of diabetic retinopathy, proliferative diabetic retinopathy (PDR), may develop. Proliferation refers to the growth of new, abnormal, neovascular (NV) fronds that pierce the internal limiting membrane and proceed into the vitreous compartment. NV is described by location, occurring either at the *disc* (NVD) or *elsewhere* (NVE) (Fig. 22.3).

These neovascular tufts are quite delicate and friable, and frequently bleed, either directly into the vitreous body (a vitreous hemorrhage) or in the potential space between the vitreous and the retinal surface (a preretinal hemorrhage) (Fig. 22.4). The patient will often notice a sudden diminution or total loss of vision in the affected eye. These hemorrhages may resolve spontaneously, over a period of months, or may require surgical removal (vitrectomy, see below).

With repeated hemorrhagic episodes, a fibrous component develops along the arcades affected by neovascular changes, and on the retinal surface, and these fibrovascular proliferations tend to contract over time (Fig. 22.5). As that occurs, the retina pulls away from the layer posterior to it, the pigmented epithelium, resulting in a *tractional* retinal detachment (TRD) (Fig. 22.6). If the detached portion of the retina is not

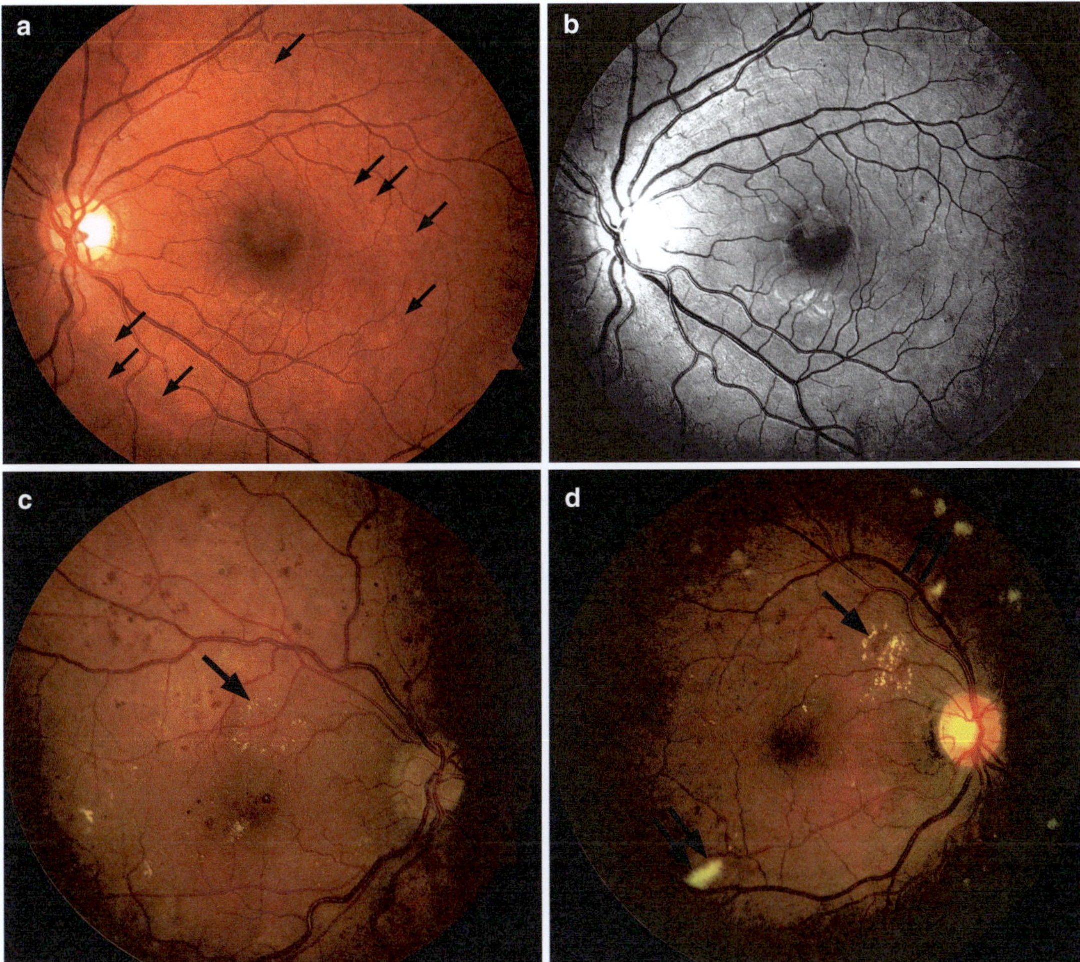

Fig. 22.1 (**a–g**) Very mild non-proliferative diabetic retinopathy (NPDR), showing scattered microaneurysms (MAs). (**a**) A color fundus photograph, with arrows indicating some of the MAs. (**b**) Is a "red-free" image, produced using a green filter (such as that found on most direct ophthalmoscopes) which increases contrast and makes small diabetic lesions easier to identify. (**c, d**) Show more severe NPDR, with lipid deposits ("hard exudates," single arrows) and areas of retinal ischemia ("cotton wool spots," double arrows). In addition to the small microaneurysms noted in (**a, b**), larger, blot hemorrhages are also scattered throughout. (**e**) Moderate NPDR, with lipid adjacent to the fovea, and macular thickening with surface distortion visible as radiating folds. Figure (**f**) is an OCT of a patient with foveal cystic macular edema in the right fundus, and a few lipid deposits in the left perifoveal region, without cysts or foveal distortion. (**g**) The inferior temporal arcade in a left eye, with severe NPDR with microaneurysms, blot hemorrhages, vascular loops (single black arrows), and venous beading (double arrows). The single white arrows demonstrate arteriovenous crossing abnormalities in this patient, who also had uncontrolled hypertension. Superiorly, in the macula, hard exudates and a cotton wool spot are also present

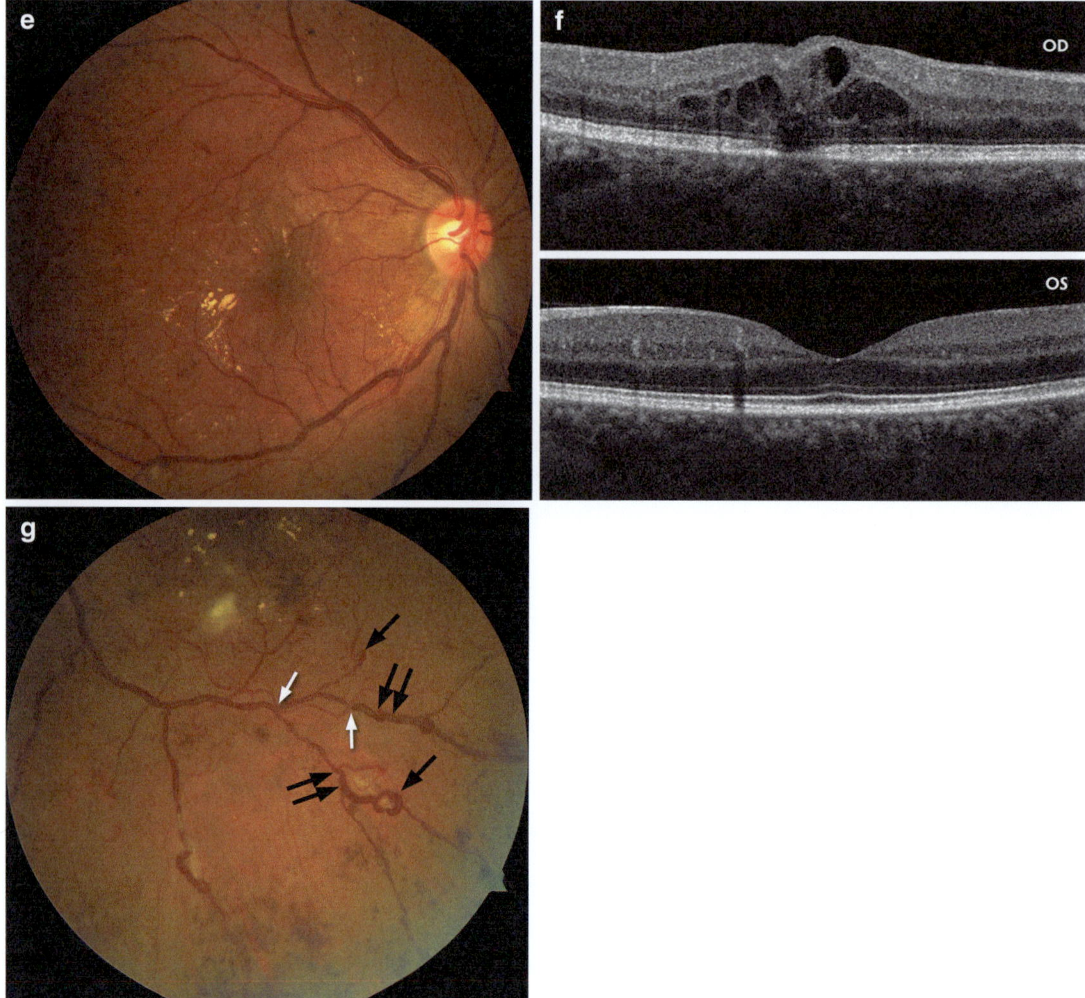

Fig. 22.1 (continued)

repositioned in contact with the posterior layers (specifically the pigmented epithelium and underlying choriocapillaris), eventually permanent vision loss occurs. A tractional detachment can be partial or total. A total retinal detachment often assumes a funnel-like configuration, with the retina attached at the optic nerve head posteriorly, and anteriorly at its termination, the ora serrata, but otherwise completely separated from the previously underlying pigmented epithelium, and therefore incapable of sustaining vision (Fig. 22.7a–d).

The other mechanism by which vision is lost with diabetic retinopathy is the development of diabetic macular edema (DME), with fluid extravasating into the macula, often accompanied by lipoprotein precipitates ("hard exudates") and overall thickening of the central retina as the blood-retinal barrier loses its integrity (Figs. 22.2 and 22.8). Central vision occurs at the macula, so irregularity of the macular surface and cystic edema of the retinal layers leads to distortion of central vision, a condition known as metamorphopsia (see Fig. 21.5), and resultant decreased visual acuity. As this can impair central vision, DME, particularly if it is bilateral, can severely limit the ability to drive, read or even continue normal daily activities.

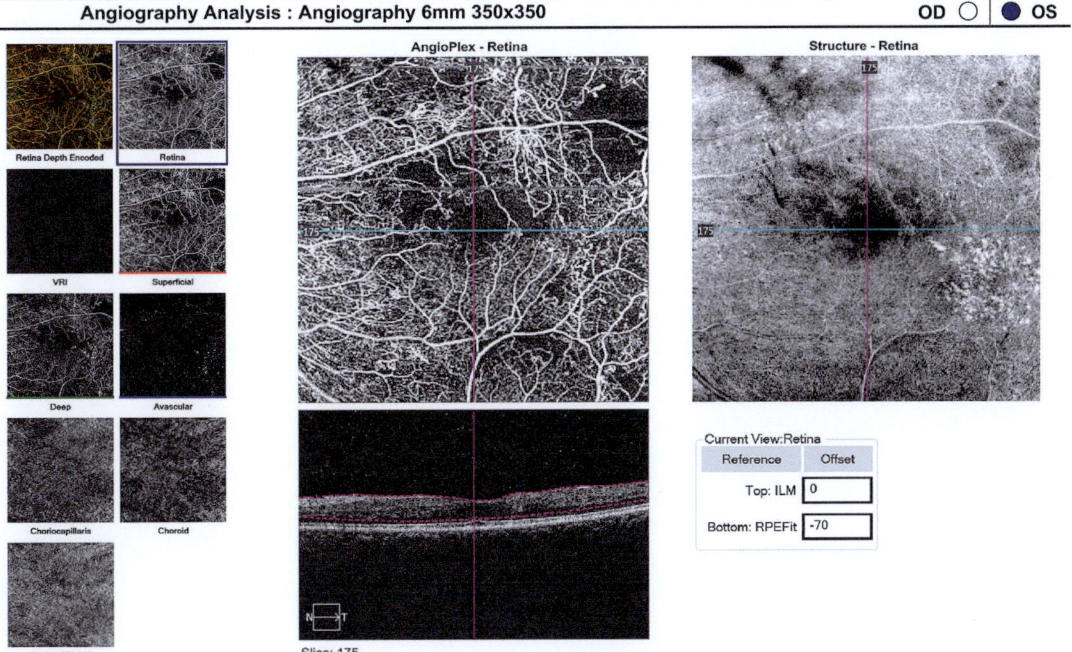

Fig. 22.2 An optical coherence tomography angiogram (OCTA), a new, noninvasive technique which shows the capillary bed without requiring injection of intravenous dye, as is done with fluorescein angiography. The central upper image shows significant capillary dropout in the perifoveal area, resulting in an enlargement of the normal foveal avascular zone (FAZ) with resultant loss of central acuity (A normal FAZ, demonstrated using traditional fluorescein angiography, is shown in Fig. 1.29b)

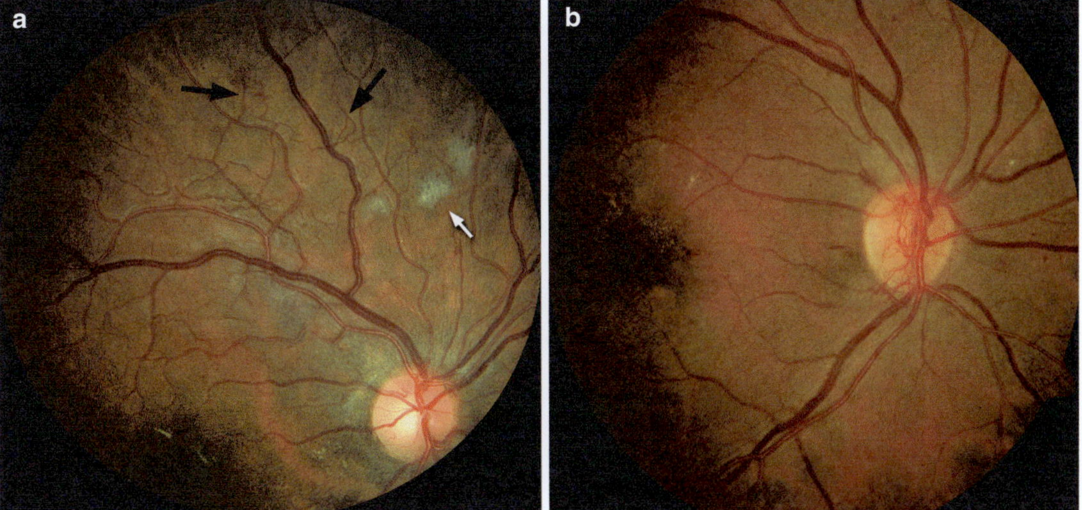

Fig. 22.3 (**a–d**) Proliferative diabetic retinopathy (PDR). (**a**) Early neovascularization elsewhere (NVE, black arrows) is seen in the superior temporal quadrant, adjacent to a cluster of three cotton wool spots (white arrow). (**b**) Early neovascularization at the disc (NVD) is seen as a network of fine vessels just anterior to, and emanating from, normal disc vessels. (**c**) Increasing NVE (white arrows), with NVD OU. A cotton wool spot is seen just external to the superior temporal arcade OD; small, old macular laser burns, previously applied to treat focal macular leakage, are noted in the perifoveal regions OU (black arrows). Figure (**d, e**) shows a patient with severe bilateral NVD extending upwards into the vitreous; the upper images are standard color photographs, the lower ones are red-free images to better demonstrate the neovascular fronds (white arrow, NVE not well-visualized in color photograph)

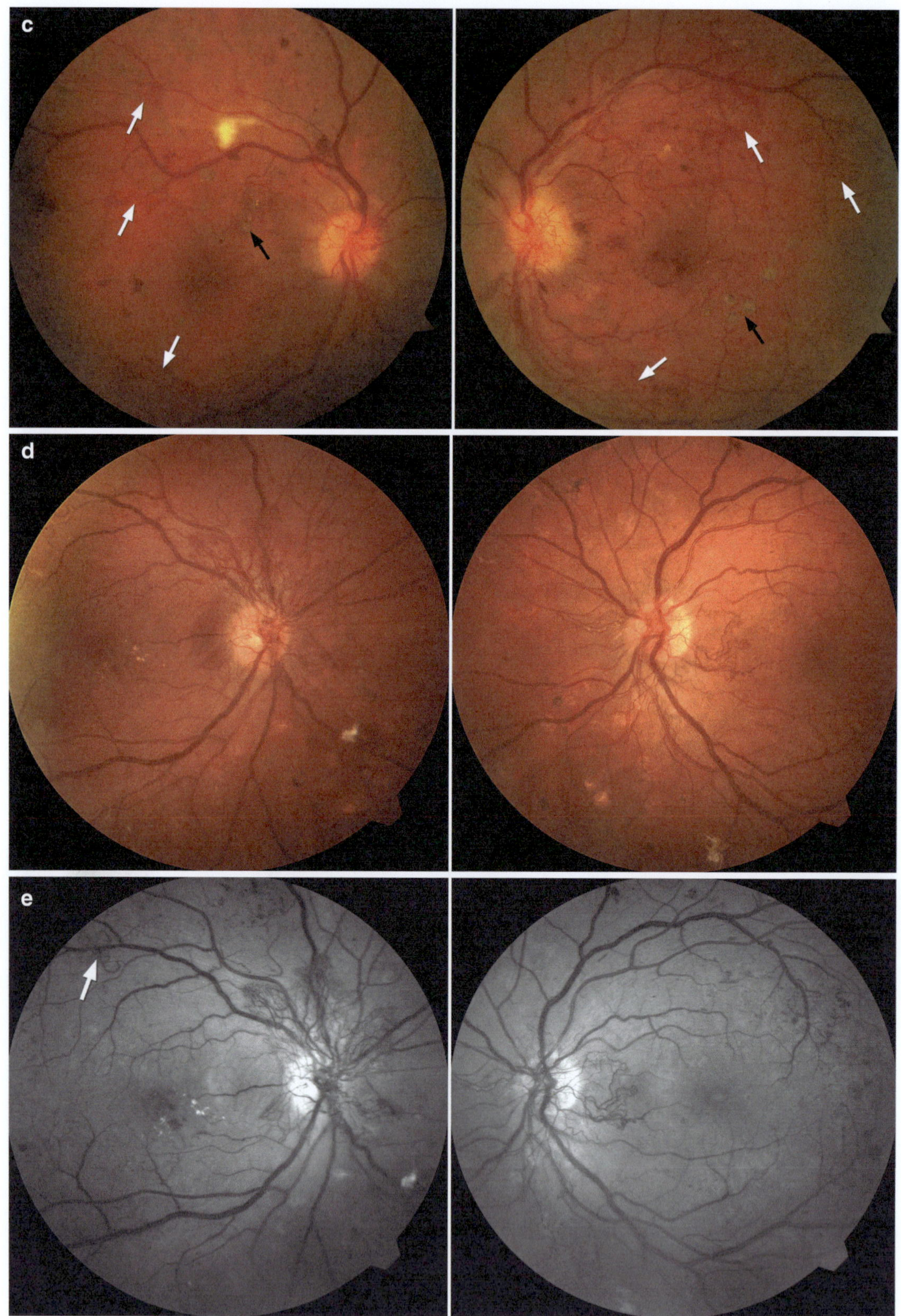

Fig. 22.3 (continued)

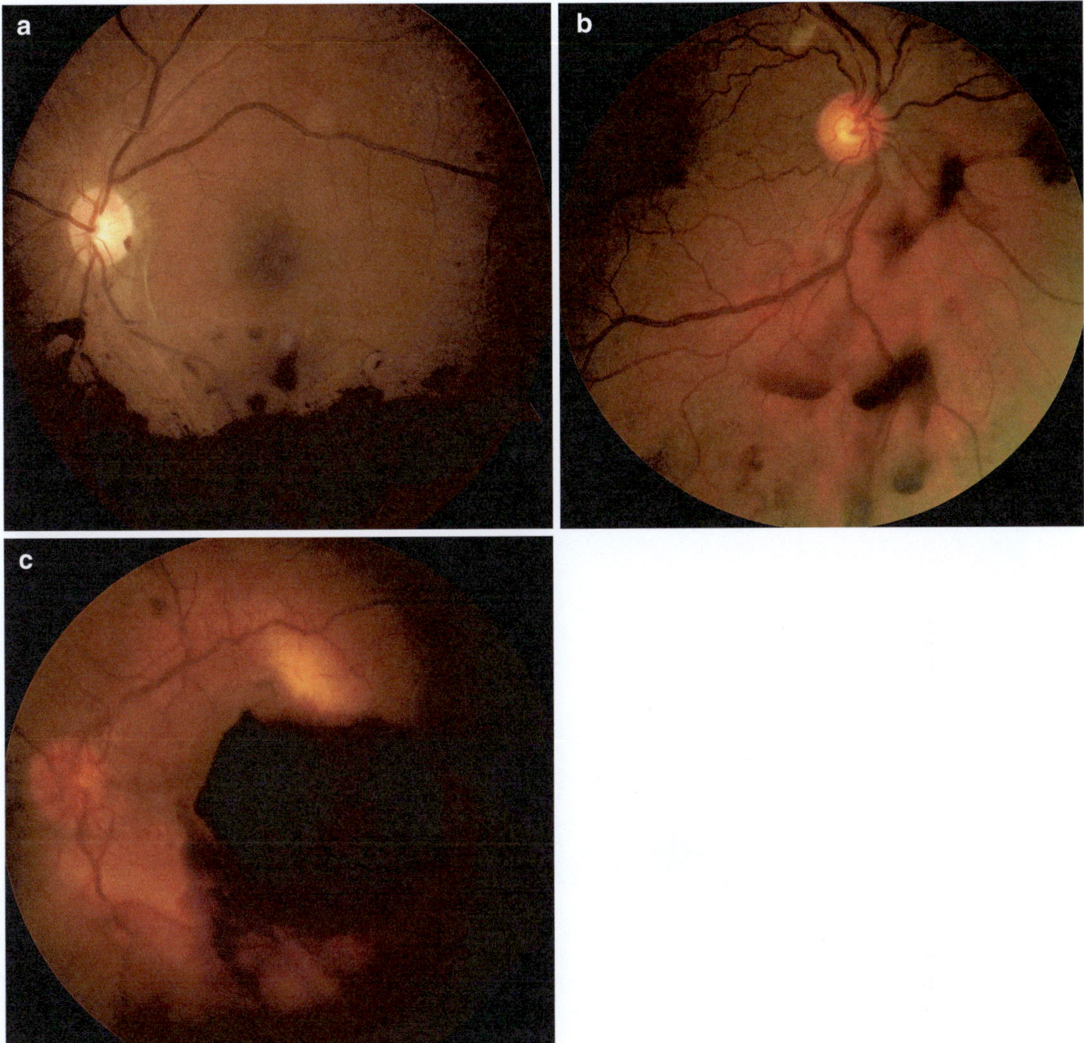

Fig. 22.4 (**a–c**) Typical diabetic hemorrhages. (**a**) A pre-retinal ("scaphoid" or boat-shaped) hemorrhage seen in the lower half of the image, where it has settled due to gravity, and is confined by the potential space it fills between the retina and the posterior vitreous face. (**b**) A mild vitreous hemorrhage is noted, with blood scattered through the vitreous compartment. When mild, the patient may not even be aware of these hemorrhages or may complain of "floaters" in their visual field. An extensive, dense vitreous hemorrhage is shown in (**c**). As this overlies the macula, this patient experienced sudden, severe loss of central vision. If slow to resolve, or in monocular patients, such hemorrhages may require surgical intervention (a vitrectomy) to restore central acuity

A complication of diabetes which may also occur in nondiabetic eyes spontaneously or after trauma or inflammation is an alteration of the interface between the posterior vitreous face and the anterior retinal surface, which often occurs in the macular area. Thickening and distortion causes traction on the normally smooth inner retinal face, with resultant metamorphopsia as occurs with macular edema (Fig. 22.9). This surface distortion can be due to development of a fibrous sheet, known as an epiretinal membrane (ERM), macular pucker or cellophane maculopathy, or to abnormal adhesion between the vitreous and the retina, a condition known as

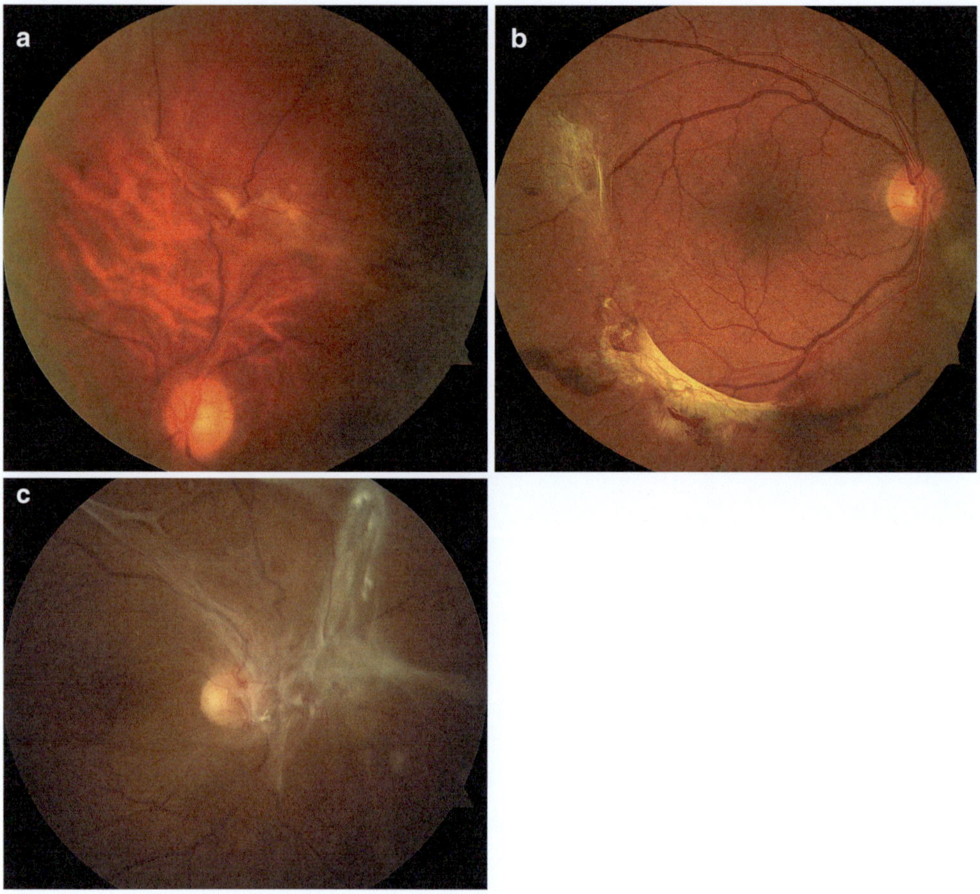

Fig. 22.5 (**a–c**) Development of a fibrous component seen along the neovascular fronds of PDR, which act as a scaffolding on which this abnormal tissue proliferates. (**a**) Early fibrous growth at NVE superonasally; (**b**) fibrous component with associated hemorrhage predominantly along the inferior temporal quadrant. (**c**) A fibrous proliferative component sheathes a large intravitreal segment of NVD

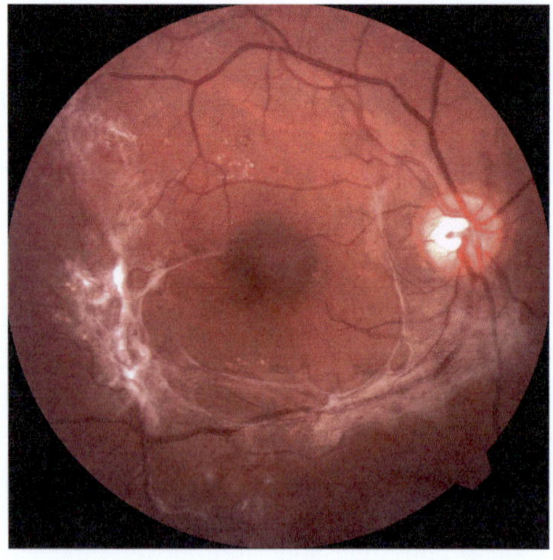

Fig. 22.6 Extensive fibrous proliferation partially encircles the macula, producing a partial tractional retinal detachment inferiorly

vitreomacular traction (VMT). The two conditions may also co-exist. Identification and treatment of these conditions has been greatly enhanced by the introduction and rapid improvement in optical coherence tomography imaging (see below).

It is believed that the underlying mechanism for both forms of retinopathy, NPDR/PDR and DME (which can occur together or independently) is essentially the same, and related to the intraocular production of vasoactive compounds such as vascular endothelial growth factors (VEGF). These compounds, normal constituents in the bloodstream which are overexpressed in diabetes, disrupt the blood-retinal barrier, leading to retinal edema, and promote proliferative neovascular growth as well. An inflammatory

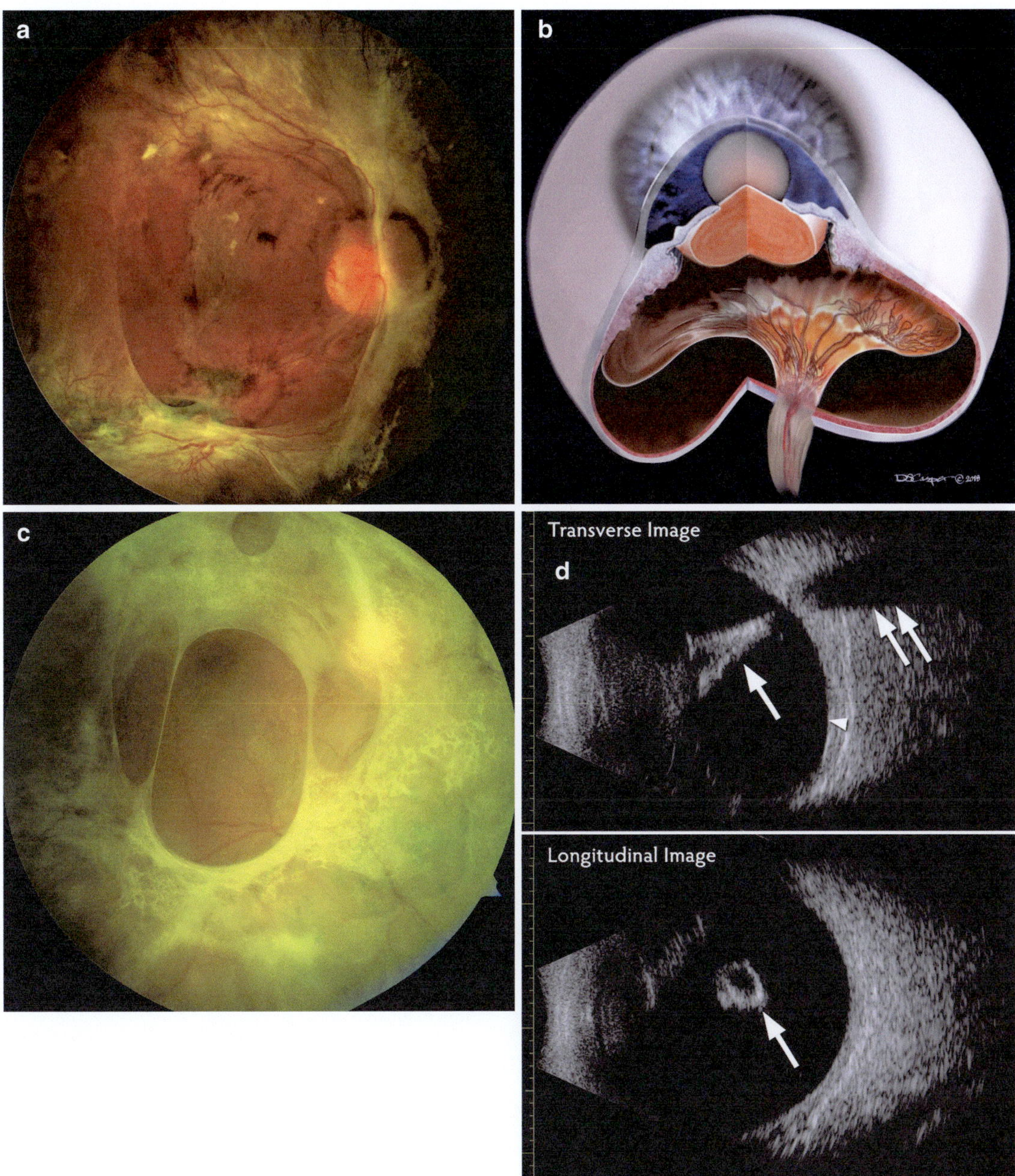

Fig. 22.7 (**a**, **b**) A purse-string-like encirclement and contraction of the proliferative fibrous tissue, which creates a funnel-shaped distortion of the retina, leaving the posterior portion attached at the optic nerve head, but otherwise displacing the remainder of the retina into the mid-vitreous space, resulting in a complete tractional detachment. Active proliferation and bleeding are visible. (**c**) An old total tractional detachment is seen, with dense and thickened fibrous tissue within the vitreous compartment, and the pale, nonfunctional retina visible through the central aperture; active proliferation and bleeding are absent. (**d**) Ultrasound images in the transverse and longitudinal planes show the funnel-like configuration of a chronically detached retina within the central globe, and the circular profile the funnel produces when viewed in cross section. Single arrow, funnel detachment; double arrows, optic nerve; arrowhead, posterior globe. ((**d**) Courtesy of Dr. Ronald Silverman)

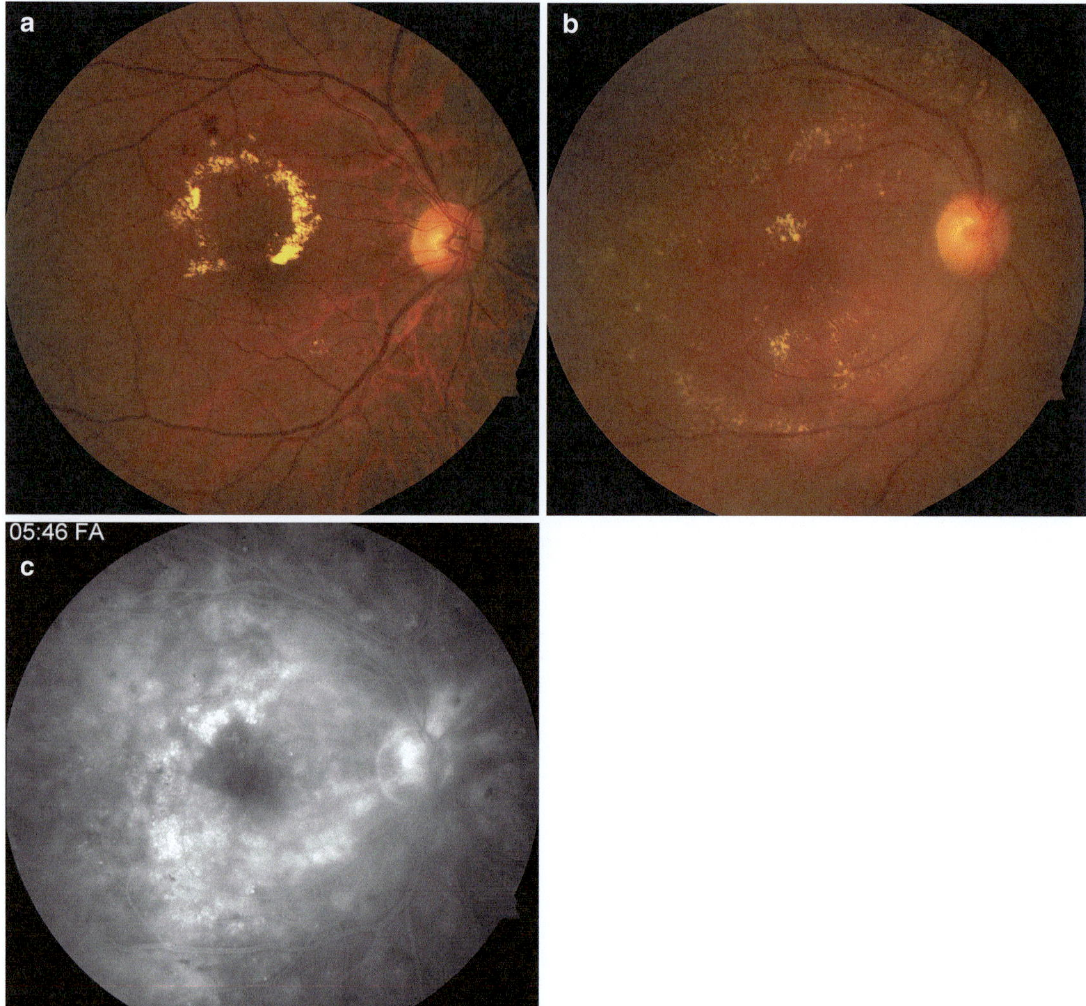

Fig. 22.8 Loss of blood-retinal barrier integrity can produce macular edema. (**a**) Focal leakage of lipoprotein which precipitates out in a "circinate ring" around the leaking vessel(s). (**b**, **c**) The entire macula is diffusely edematous, with scattered areas of lipid deposition, and a grayish, yellow appearance to the fundus visible in the color image. The accompanying fluorescein angiogram (FA), taken 5 minutes and 46 seconds after the injection of dye shows extensive leakage throughout the region, indicating extensive loss of vascular integrity. More commonly now, an optical coherence tomogram (OCT) is obtained to indicate the location and extent of fluid leakage and allow for quantification of edema or thinning, which greatly aids in assessing progression or response to treatment. Although the fundus photograph (**d**) shows only minimal perifoveal lipid and some retinal pallor, the OCT (**e**) shows clinically significant central thickening and cyst formation

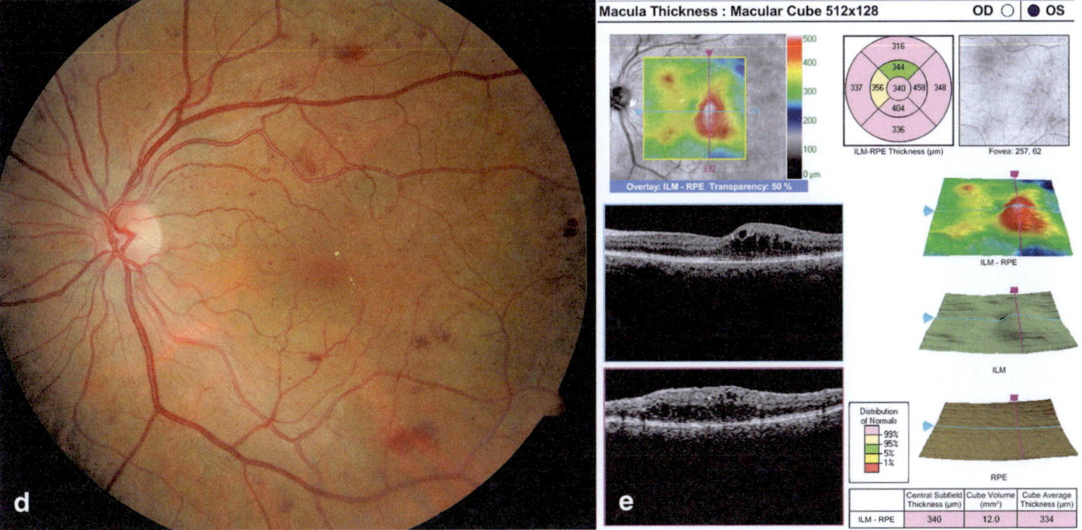

Fig. 22.8 (continued)

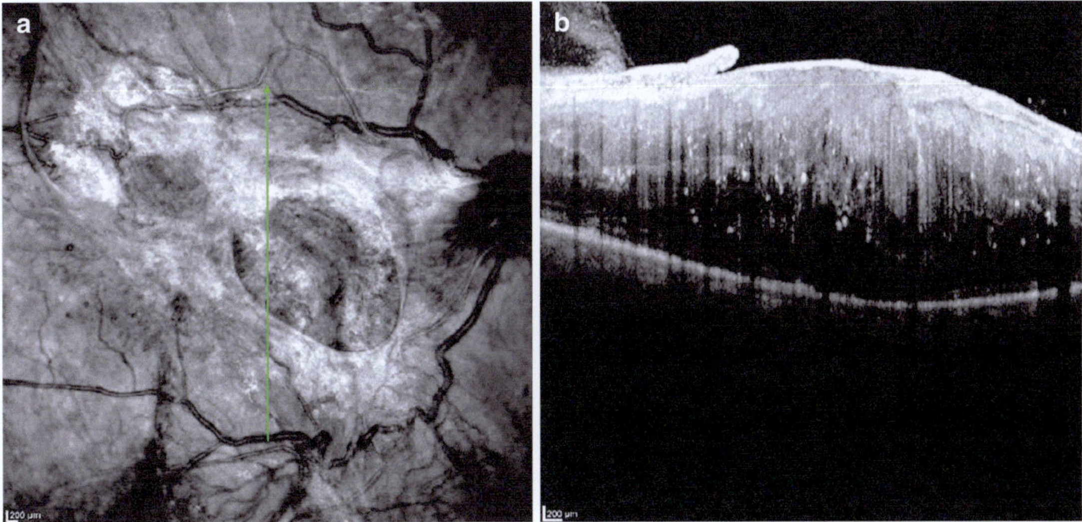

Fig. 22.9 (**a**, **b**) OCT image of the right eye in a 49-year-old diabetic man. (**a**) *en face* image of macular surface, with disc to the right; (**b**) OCT sectional image in the plane of the green arrow seen in (**a**). Fibrosis associated with proliferative diabetic retinopathy has created a thick epiretinal membrane that is causing macular distortion with obliteration of the normal foveal contour with vision loss. Contraction of the fibrotic membrane can lead to traction retinal detachment. Surgical intervention may be indicated in this patient to prevent detachment, although there is a significant risk of bleeding and iatrogenic retinal hole formation when removing this tissue

component may also contribute to the advancement of diabetic retinopathy.

Emphasis on regular eye examinations and education for diabetic patients is paramount in preventing the development of diabetic complications that may threaten vision and require treatment. When complications requiring intervention do develop, the options and potential benefits are vastly improved at earlier disease stages. In the last few years, however, available treatments have greatly increased and improved, compared to what was available only 10 or 20 years ago.

Management of Diabetic Retinopathy

The gold-standard treatment for PDR was, until recently, extensive laser photocoagulation of the retina. Of note, this photodestructive therapy was not directed at the neovascular fronds, as such treatment leads to increased bleeding and fibrous contraction. Rather, treatment is directed to ischemic peripheral retina, outside of the large temporal arcades, sparing the macular area (Fig. 22.10). The mechanism by which this worked was obscure for many years, but is now felt to be explained by the VEGF-induced nature of DR development. It is believed that the obliteration of peripheral retinal tissue reduces metabolic demand produced by ischemic retinal areas; reducing the volume of tissue demanding perfusion results in the cessation of VEGF production, and thereby involution of early NVD and NVE. Fluorescein angiography can be used to confirm neovascular proliferations and leakage and to locate areas of capillary non-perfusion (see Fig. 22.11) and thereby guide laser therapy. In the last decade, direct anti-VEGF compounds have been introduced directly into the vitreous, with encouraging results; their effect may also be synergistic when combined with photocoagulation. A recent study suggested that over 2 years, direct intravitreal injection of anti-VEGF compounds may provide similar benefit to laser photocoagulation in preventing the complications of PDR. Because these medications have a shorter

duration, how this affects long-term management of PDR is still unknown.

In severe PDR, the patient may develop a vitreous hemorrhage with resultant symptoms ranging from mild, such as floaters, to severe, with significant drop in acuity to hand motions or finger counting. Because a hemorrhage can opacify the normally transparent virtreous media, which limits the ability for examination, diagnostic ultrasonography is often used to determine the presence of a concurrent TRD (Fig. 22.7d). If the ultrasound is suggestive of TRD, then prompt vitrectomy surgery is recommended. If a TRD is not present, then the hemorrhage may be observed, as most will naturally clear over time. As the hemorrhage subsides, laser photocoagulation can be applied to visible peripheral retina in order to decrease the drive for neovascularization. If the hemorrhage persists for a period of 1–3 months, then vitrectomy may be performed to remove it and laser photocoagulation can then be applied.

Blood thinners can be safely continued for patients with vitreous hemorrhage secondary to PDR, regardless of the need for surgery. Intravitreal anti-VEGF agents may be used as an adjunct to either surgery or observation, to allow for more rapid clearing of hemorrhage and application of laser, although in a recent study the final percentage of patients requiring vitrectomy was not reduced by administration of intravitreal medications.

When a tractional retinal detachment is present, surgery is required in order to reattach the retina. In these cases, vitrectomy is performed with peeling of the fibrous membranes to relieve traction and allow for retinal reattachment. Because the fibrotic membranes are quite adherent, iatrogenic holes may occur and can add to surgical complexity. Laser photocoagulation is concurrently performed and a tamponade agent may be used to facilitate reattachment in the immediate post-operative period. Detachments affecting the macula cause the most significant vision loss and usually require prompt management. Some patients with fibrovascular proliferation and neovascularization may have surgery as prophylaxis for TRD.

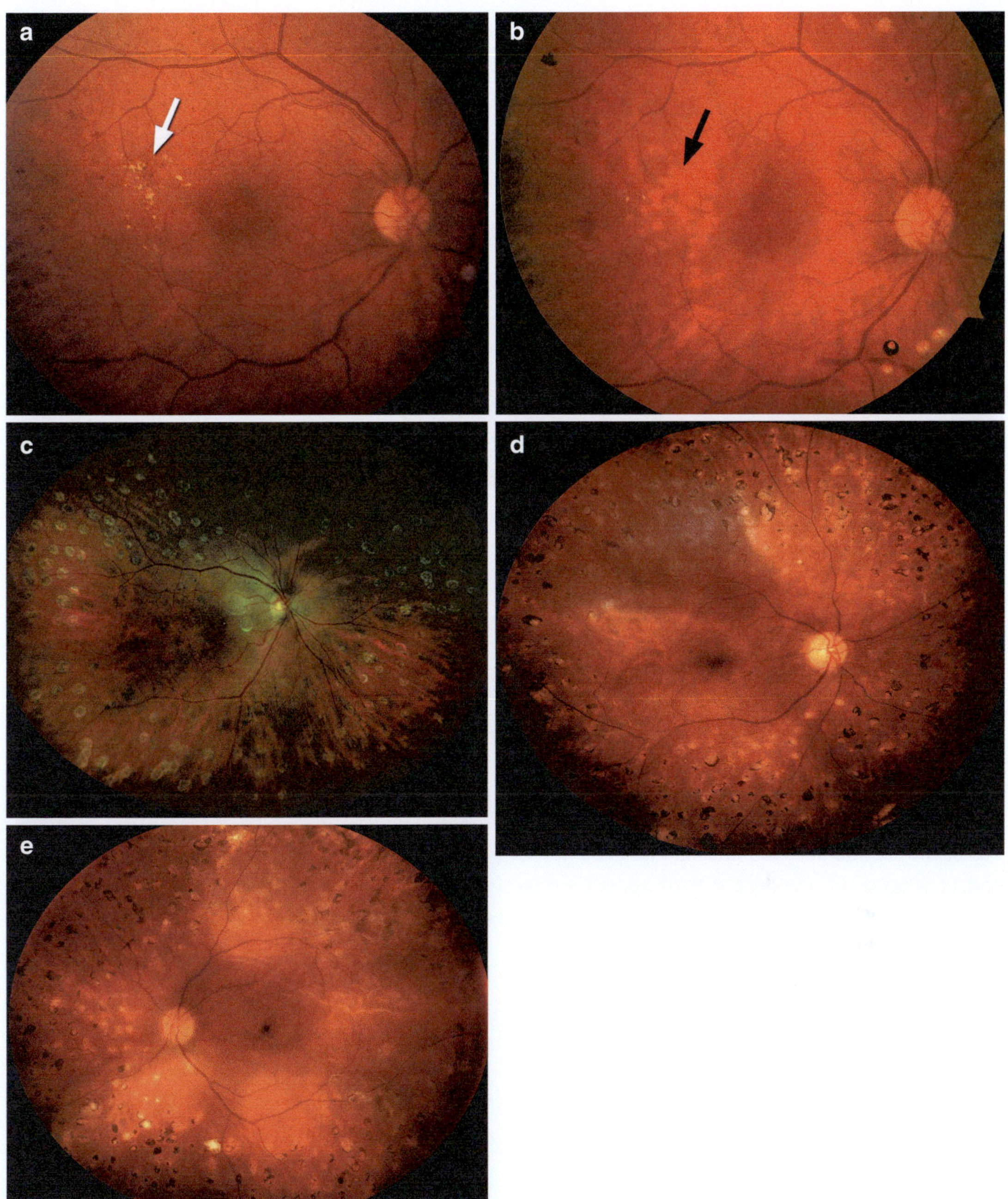

Fig. 22.10 (**a–d**) Laser photocoagulation treatment has been the mainstay of diabetic eye disease treatment for many years, although newer techniques are rapidly growing in popularity. (**a, b**) An area of leakage is seen with localized lipid deposition just temporal to the fovea (white arrow). The second image, post laser treatment, shows a cluster of focal laser burns which have been directed to the vessels shown to be leaking on FA (black arrow). Incidentally noted are some peripheral laser burn scars external to the arcades. (**c**) A full panretinal photocoagulation (PRP) treatment is shown in a wide-field image. Note that the macular area is spared, but the majority of the retina external to the temporal arcades has been treated. (**d, e**) shows wide-field right and left images of the patient shown in Fig. 22.3d, e; note that the extensive PDR visible in that figure has resolved here, subsequent to full PRP treatment

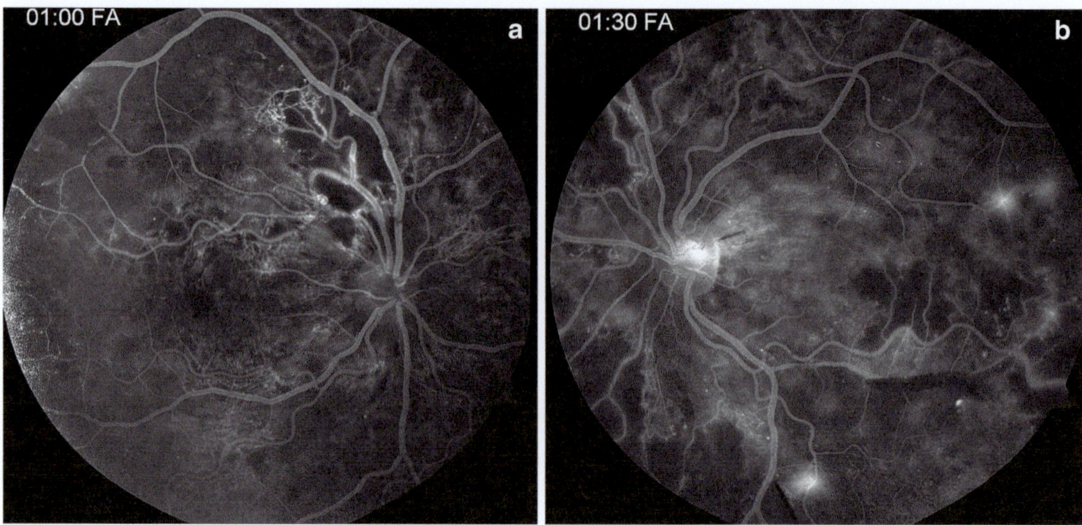

Fig. 22.11 (**a**, **b**) Right and left fluorescein angiograms from a patient with PDR, macular edema, and areas of capillary non-perfusion. The non-perfused, ischemic areas can be identified by the absence of fluorescein staining, while areas of PDR show dye leaking into the surrounding vitreous

Vitrectomy surgery is a safe outpatient procedure currently used for many retinal conditions. The surgical technique uses three microsurgical incisions as small as 27-gauge through the avascular pars plana, to access the retina and posterior segment. Tamponade agents, either intraocular gas or intraocular silicone oil, may be used at the end of surgery to maintain retinal apposition to the pigment epithelium. If silicone oil is required, then a second procedure may be required several months later for maximal visual recovery. The major risks of surgery include re-detachment of the retina, recurrent bleeding, cataract formation and endophthalmitis (intraocular infection or inflammation).

The processes associated with DME are more chronic in nature, and often patients may have small areas of DME without significant symptoms. Once symptomatic, patients should be evaluated, although treatment can usually be initiated on an elective basis. Therapeutic options for DME have undergone significant evolution over the last decade. Focal (or grid) laser was the previous gold standard, where light photocoagulation was used to reduce vascular permeability. While laser is still used in DME management, it has been relegated to a secondary role as the use of intravitreal anti-VEGF agents, guided by OCT results, has become the most common initial treatment (Fig. 22.12). Additionally, steroids can be administered to the vitreous for DME management. Treatment results in resolution of macular fluid and cysts, presumably resulting in renewed blood-retinal barrier competency, and consequent restoration of normal macular and foveal anatomy, although vision may not return to pre-edematous levels. Anti-VEGF therapy requires repeated intraocular injections, often as frequently as every month. Steroid injections are given less frequently but carry a slightly higher risk of glaucoma development and cataract formation. Newer steroid injections use implantable, depot drug delivery devices that degrade and release medication for months or years. Neither steroid nor anti-VEGF medications have been found to have any significant systemic impact or complications, although these medications are likely absorbed into the systemic circulation in low concentrations. In some recalcitrant cases, DME is thought to be exacerbated by abnormal adhesions and interactions at the vitreoretinal interface, and vitrectomy surgery, with removal

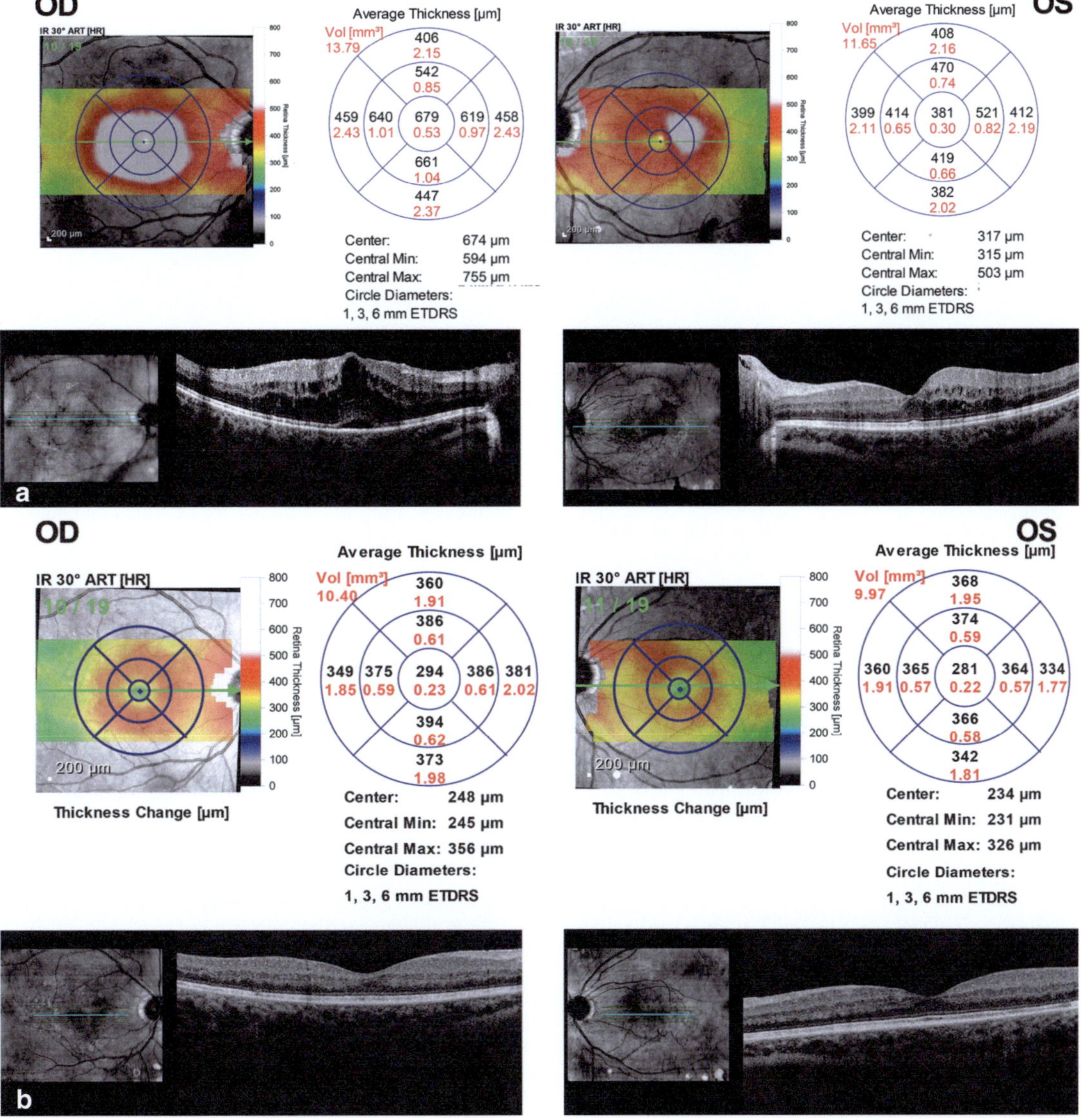

Fig. 22.12 (a, b) OCT images from the same patient as seen in Fig. 22.10, obtained before and after intravitreal injections of anti-VEGF medication. (a) From 2015, there is bilateral macular edema, right significantly worse than left, with central foveal thickness readings of 679 and 381 μ, respectively. (b) Taken in 2017, approximately 1.5 years after therapy was instituted, the edema appears to be completely resolved OU, with central foveal thicknesses of 294 μ OD and 281 μ OS

("peeling") of the internal limiting membrane, may provide some relief and restoration of retinal anatomy.

Although retinopathy is the most well-known consequence of diabetes, there are other ocular effects, some of which should be mentioned. Corneal desensitization, a phenomenon probably similar to peripheral neuropathy, can result in severe corneal abrasions which produce relatively little pain, particularly with contact lens overwear (see Fig. 12.6). Diabetic papillopathy, edema of the optic nerve, is discussed in Chap. 36 (see Fig. 36.3a). A dreaded complication is mucormycosis, which is a potentially fatal condition and usually requires extensive surgical excision, often including full exenteration of the orbit

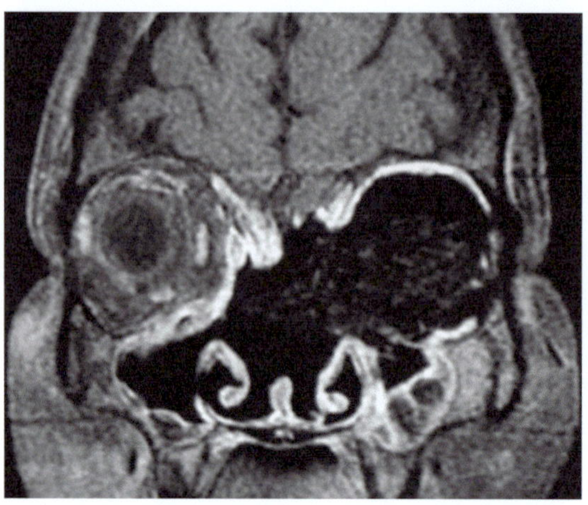

Fig. 22.13 A case of mucormycosis associated with poorly controlled diabetes, which required complete unilateral orbital exenteration, as well as removal of periorbital sinuses. (Courtesy of Dr. Michael Kazim)

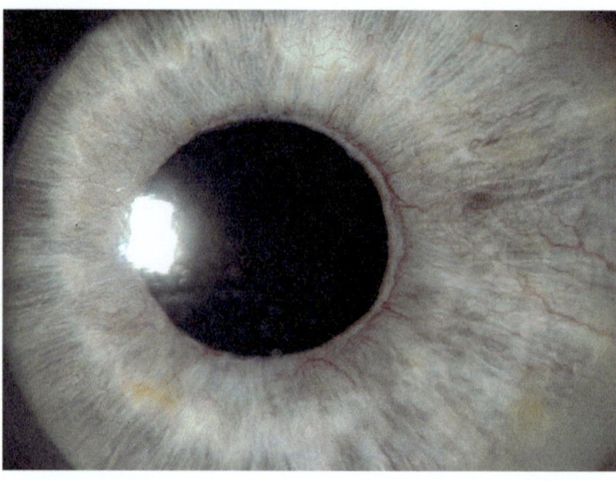

Fig. 22.14 A case of rubeosis iridis. Fine neovascular vessels can be seen proliferating along the pupillary margin and the iris surface; these vessels will usually invade the angle as well, reducing aqueous outflow and cause a secondary glaucoma

and surrounding contiguous sinuses (Fig. 22.13; see Chap. 32).

Various types of cataract occur with increased frequency with diabetes, particularly snowflake, coronary, posterior subcapsular, and cortical cataracts (see Fig. 11.3). In general, diabetic patients tend to develop cataracts at a younger age than nondiabetic patients, and progression of these cataracts tends to be relatively faster.

Finally, iris neovascularization, also known as rubeosis iridis, is a process similar to that seen with retinal neovascularization, where new, abnormal blood vessels grow in the anterior chamber, on the iris surface, and typically invade the angle (Fig. 22.14; see Chap. 16). There, aqueous outflow is restricted by the neovascular growth, and intraocular pressure rises, in a rare complication known as neovascular glaucoma. The association of diabetes and progressive open-angle glaucoma is controversial; there are those who feel there is increased risk and others who disagree.

While the potential for severe vision loss persists in diabetic retinal disease, there are more treatment options than ever available to clinicians. With proper monitoring and therapy, along with tight glucose and blood pressure control, even severe cases can undergo a reversal of disease, with subsequent maintenance of good, useful vision.

Suggested Reading

Cheung N, Mitchell P, Wong TY. Diabetic retinopathy. Lancet. 2010;376(9735):124–36. https://doi.org/10.1016/S0140-6736(09)62124-3. Epub 2010 Jun 26.

Chew EY, Klein ML, Murphy RP, Remaley NA, Ferris FL 3rd. Effects of aspirin on vitreous/preretinal hemorrhage in patients with diabetes mellitus. Early treatment diabetic retinopathy study report no. 20. Arch Ophthalmol. 1995;113(1):52–5.

Diabetic retinopathy study. Report number 6. Design, methods, and baseline results. Invest Ophthalmol Vis Sci. 1981;21:147–226.

Early Treatment Diabetic Retinopathy Study R. Photocoagulation for diabetic macular edema. Early Treatment Diabetic Retinopathy Study report number 1. Early Treatment Diabetic Retinopathy Study research group. Arch Ophthalmol. 1985;103:1796–806.

Elman MJ, Bressler NM, Haijing Qin MS, et al. Expanded 2-year follow-up of ranibizumab plus prompt or deferred laser or triamcinolone plus prompt laser for diabetic macular edema. Ophthalmology. 2011;118(4):609–14.

Frank R. Diabetic retinopathy. NEJM. 2004;350:48–58.

Moss SE, Klein R, Klein BE. Factors associated with having eye examinations in persons with diabetes. Arch Fam Med. 1995;4:529–34.

Writing Committee for the Diabetic Retinopathy Clinical Research Network. Panretinal photocoagulation vs intravitreous ranibizumab for proliferative diabetic retinopathy: a randomized clinical trial. JAMA. 2015;314(20):2137–46.

Other Retinal Vascular Diseases

Ahmet M. Hondur and Tongalp H. Tezel

Retina has the highest metabolic activity in the human body and consumes a much higher amount of oxygen and nutrients per weight than any other organ. Its oxygen consumption is several folds greater than that of the central nervous system. The main reason for high oxygen demand is to fuel ionic pumps that continuously move positively charged electrolytes out of photoreceptors in the dark. This high oxygen demand gives rise to two separate vascular networks: retinal and choroidal. The presumed reason for such a privileged oxygen supply is the evolutionary need of vision for survival. Retina is highly sensitive to systemic vascular events that block the supply of oxygen and other nutrients, despite the fact that it has approximately 100 times more photoreceptors than are required for seeing. Thus, systemic vasculopathies that may alter retinal blood flow, such as hypertension, atherosclerosis, and diabetes, almost always constitute a risk for retinal dysfunction.

The perfusion border between retinal and choroidal vasculature is the outer plexiform layer

(Figs. 23.1 and 1.1). Photoreceptors, which lie in the outer third of the retina, receive oxygen from the choroidal vascular system. Oxygen extraction from this high flow vascular bed is quite low, resulting in venous oxygen saturation higher than in any other vascular bed in the body. On the other hand, the inner two-thirds of the retina is supplied by the retinal arterial system. In contrast to choroidal vessels, blood flow within the retinal vasculature is low, resulting in high extraction of oxygen. In about 25% of the population, a cilioretinal artery supplied by the choroidal vasculature can cross into retina around the temporal aspect of the optic nerve and contribute to retinal blood supply.

The 5.5 mm circular portion of the retina between the inferior and superior temporal arcades is called the macula (Fig. 23.2). In this portion of the retina, ganglion cells make up multiple layers and the retina is the thickest. A central depression of about 1.5 mm in the macula is called the fovea. The fovea contains cone photoreceptors specialized for high visual acuity and color vision. This area evolved to be free of blood vessels, preventing any interference between photoreceptors and incipient light. This anatomical arrangement makes the fovea solely dependent on choroidal blood circulation. Surrounding the fovea, inner retinal neurons are arranged in multiple layers to preprocess the central visual information generated by densely packed foveal photoreceptors. This thickened

A. M. Hondur, MD
Department of Ophthalmology, Gazi University
Medical School, Ankara, Turkey

T. H. Tezel, MD (⊠)
Department of Ophthalmology, Edward S. Harkness
Eye Institute, Columbia University Vagelos College
of Physicians and Surgeons, New York, NY, USA
e-mail: tht2115@cumc.columbia.edu

© Springer Nature Switzerland AG 2019
D. S. Casper, G. A. Cioffi (eds.), *The Columbia Guide to Basic Elements of Eye Care*,
https://doi.org/10.1007/978-3-030-10886-1_23

Fig. 23.1 Schematic anatomy of retina showing retinal and choroidal vasculature perfusion border

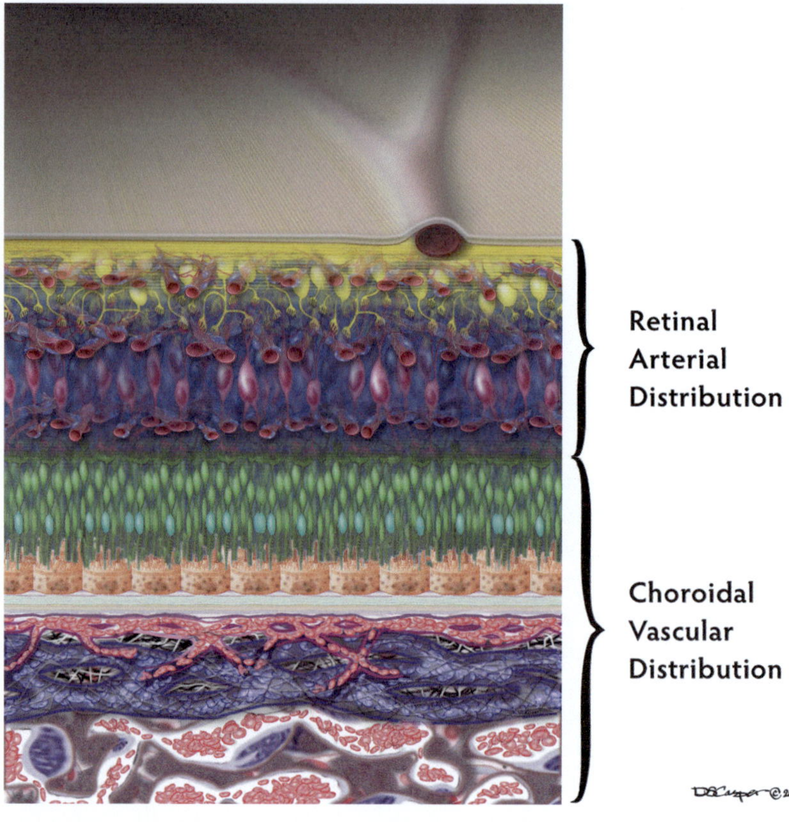

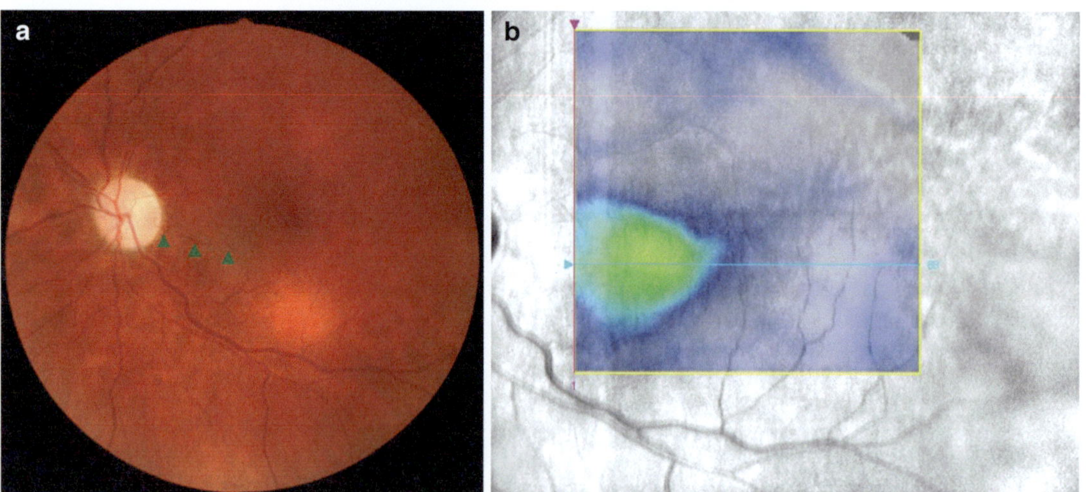

Fig. 23.2 A 76-year-old patient with recanalized cilioretinal artery occlusion (green arrowheads) of the left eye. (**a**) Fundus exam reveals slight graying of the area perfused by the occluded cilioretinal artery. Note the slightly pale color of the temporal half of the optic disc, indicating partial atrophy of the papillomacular nerve bundle. (**b**) Retinal thickness map in optical coherence tomography reveals retinal thickening (colored area) along the occluded vessel

parafoveal region demands the most oxygen in accordance with the greater density of the retinal neurons and the highly complex task they perform. For this reason, the earliest effects of impaired blood flow appear at this vulnerable part of the retina.

The only human artery and vein visible to the human eye by direct visualization is the central retinal artery and vein. The central retinal artery maintains its arterial structure for just a short distance and then loses its internal elastic lamina and becomes an arteriole. As all other blood vessels in the body, retinal vessels are affected by systemic vasculopathies like atherosclerosis, diabetes, and hypertension. This allows physicians to gauge the extent of pathologies in different vascular beds by simply inspecting the retinal vessels.

Retinal blood circulation can be better viewed with angiography. Instead of using radio-opaque materials as in other vascular beds of the body, fluorescent dyes are used for this purpose. These dyes emit a longer wavelength light upon stimulation with an excitation light. Fluorescein and indocyanine green are two dyes used for angiography. Recently, Doppler technology has been applied to visualize the retinal vasculature without the need of any fluorescent dyes. This motion contrast technology is called optical coherence tomography (OCT) angiography (see Appendix 2). With retinal angiography fine details and structural abnormalities of the retinal and choroidal vascular beds can be visualized. Thus, it permits identification of areas of capillary loss, plasma leakage, aneurysmal dilation, telangiectasis, and new vessel formation, which cannot be delineated easily with direct ophthalmoscopy.

The most common retinal vascular disease is diabetic retinopathy (see Chap. 22), followed by retinal vein occlusions. Retinal arterial occlusion, although much less common, leads to very severe visual loss and requires immediate medical attention. Other major vascular diseases of retina include retinal artery macroaneurysms and sickle cell retinopathy.

Retinal Arterial Occlusions

Central Retinal Artery Occlusion

Central retinal artery occlusion leads to a sudden interruption of blood supply to inner retina. It results in acute and severe vision loss, which may remain permanent if not treated immediately. At presentation visual acuity is usually at the level of finger counting or worse. If there is a patent cilioretinal artery feeding the fovea, central vision may not be affected. Due to the cessation of axoplasmic flow through the papillomacular bundle, an afferent pupillary defect is usually present. The visual field is also compromised, most commonly presenting as a central scotoma, since the thin peripheral retina may receive oxygen from the underlying choroid, resulting in some preservation of the outermost field.

Initial ophthalmoscopic changes may be subtle; however, attenuation of arteries and veins, with slow flow ("sludging") and segmentation of the blood column ("cattle trucking" or "boxcarring") may be seen, and retinal edema usually will develop later. Inner retinal edema develops mainly due to stagnated axoplasmic flow in the nerve fiber layer. It manifests itself as macular whitening. The foveal center, lacking ganglion cells and other inner retinal cellular elements, remains edema-free; therefore, its preserved transparency allows visualization of the underlying pigment epithelium and perfused choroid, producing the typical "cherry-red spot" appearance (Fig. 23.3a–d) characteristic of this condition. Intraluminal emboli may be seen in only 20–40% of non-arteritic cases.

The occluded retinal artery may eventually recanalize due to breakdown or peripheral dislodging of the embolus. Ischemic retina can also be reperfused by development of collateral anastomoses. However, late restoration of blood flow often does not help restore central vision due to irreversible ischemic damage to inner retinal neurons. Fifteen percent of the cases are further complicated with the development of iris neovascularization and subsequent neovascular glaucoma.

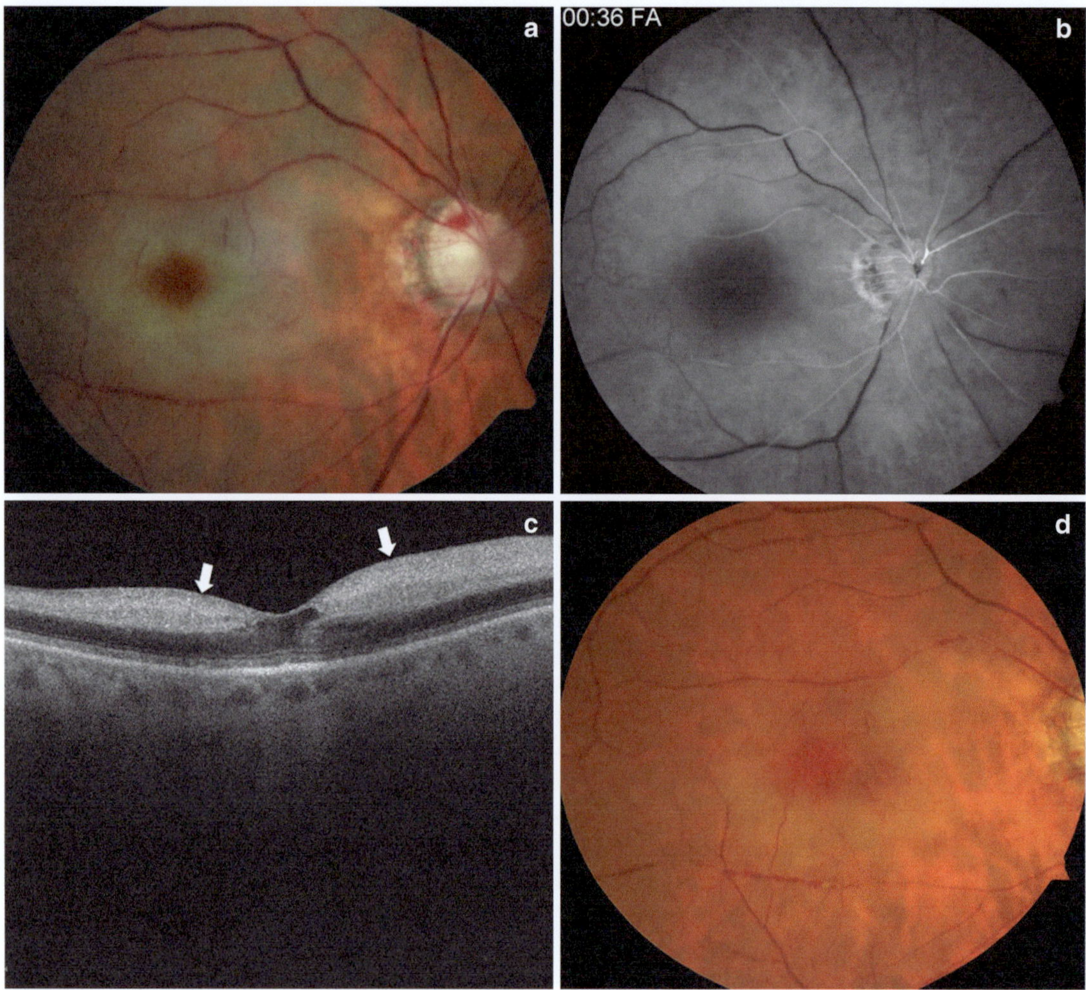

Fig. 23.3 A 70-year-old patient with central retinal artery occlusion of the right eye. Patient's presentation visual acuity was at "light perception" level. (**a**) Fundus exam reveals typical whitening of the retina and cherry-red spot. (**b**) The occluded retinal artery reveals delayed filling (seen here at 36 s) in fluorescein angiography. Fluorescein (white) could reach only to few proximal branches of the central retinal artery after being injected into the antecubital vein. The upper limit of arterial filling should not exceed 28 s. (**c**) An optical coherence tomography scan reveals hyperreflectivity (white arrows) of the inner retina due to the edema and opacification in the inner retinal layers. Cessation of the axoplasmic transport and building of the axoplasmic material is responsible for inner retinal edema. (**d**) Fundus exam of the same eye 2 weeks after 27-gauge pars plana vitrectomy and intravitreal triamcinolone injection. Visual acuity improved from light perception to finger counting at 1 ft. Note alleviation of the edema

Etiology and Management

One to two percent of central retinal artery occlusions can be due to giant cell arteritis, which is a systemic autoimmune disease characterized by inflammation and occlusion of medium- and large-sized arteries (See Chap. 36). Early recognition of giant cell arteritis is important to prevent permanent visual loss and severe systemic complications, which can usually be prevented by early initiation of immunosuppressive treatment. Typical symptoms of giant cell arteritis include temporal headache, scalp tenderness, jaw claudication, anemia, and an elevated erythrocyte sedimentation rate. However, 1/5 of giant cell arteritis cases can be without any of these symptoms, and a high index of suspicion is required to diagnose.

The source of emboli in non-arteritic central retinal artery occlusion can be an atherosclerotic plaque in the carotid artery or cardiac valvular disease. Retinal emboli can be detected in only 20–40% of cases, despite the embolic nature of the occlusion. This is due to the entrapment of the embolus at the narrowest part of the central artery, located where it pierces the optic nerve behind the lamina cribrosa. Thus, only fragmented pieces can be seen before they further break into smaller emboli that are pushed distally in the retinal vascular tree. Careful examination of the retinal periphery may reveal these small fragments of the cholesterol emboli, which indicate a previous embolic event.

Embolic occlusion of central retinal artery is analogous to ischemic cerebral stroke. However, 74% of the emboli (clots) in central retinal artery occlusions are composed of cholesterol, and only 15% are made up of fibrin. Thus, the majority of central retinal artery occlusion cases do not respond to conventional thrombolytic (clot lysing) treatment, which is efficacious in treatment of cerebral stroke. The pathophysiologic events that occur after central retinal artery occlusion are similar to what happens in the brain after an ischemic stroke. Upon cessation of the blood supply, inner retinal neurons hold non-vital metabolic activities to adapt to the new hypoxic environment, and conserved energy is used to carry out only basic cellular functions required for cell survival. Among many processes, the visual cycle is also shut off and contributes to the loss of vision at presentation. Diffusion of oxygen from the underlying choroid may provide the minimal amount of oxygen required to maintain cell viability, especially in the thin peripheral retina. This temporary vegetative state due to occlusion can be reversed by any therapeutic method that increases inner retinal oxygenation. Eventually, prolonged ischemia depletes cellular energy sources and stops ionic pumps that are required to maintain electrolyte gradients across cell membranes. Consequently, fluid influx into the cell results in cytotoxic edema and cell death. Experimental models of central artery clamping indicate a critical period of 97 min after clamping of central retinal artery during which restoration of blood flow can provide recovery of central vision. Beyond this period irreversible retinal damage commences, and after 240 min vision loss becomes permanent.

Despite this experimental data, there are anecdotal reports of visual recovery beyond the critical period in patients with central retinal artery occlusion. Some of these reports may reflect the natural history of central retinal artery occlusion history, since approximately 1/5 of patients that present within the first week of symptoms may experience visual improvement.

There is no medical treatment for central retinal artery occlusion. Ocular massage to dislodge the thrombus with cyclic pressure changes; aspirin, intravenous acetazolamide, heparin, isovolemic hemodilution, sublingual isosorbide dinitrate, intravenous mannitol or oral glycerol, anterior chamber paracentesis, intravenous methylprednisolone followed by streptokinase, and retrobulbar injection of alpha-adrenergic receptor antagonist tolazoline have all proved to have limited efficacy. Various surgical approaches have been tried to restore blood flow in central retinal artery occlusion. The surgical goal has traditionally been to destroy, remove, or dislodge the visible embolus. Local infusion of a fibrinolytic agent, embolysis with neodymium-yttrium-aluminum-garnet (Nd:YAG) laser, surgical embolectomy, and surgical cannulation of the central retinal artery have been tried without any measureable benefits.

A new hope for retinal arterial occlusions may be immediate vitrectomy with or without manual dislodging of the embolus. In a recent case series, immediate vitrectomy within 36±25 h was reported to restore retinal blood flow in all cases, accompanied by >3 lines of visual improvement. Vitrectomy may work by restoring retinal blood flow and by exposing ischemic retina to ionic oxygen carried through convectional currents within the eye. Presumably, increased oxygenation restores metabolic activity, resolves intracellular edema, and helps remaining retinal neurons to regain their function. Vitrectomy may also remove inflammatory and pro-apoptotic mediators.

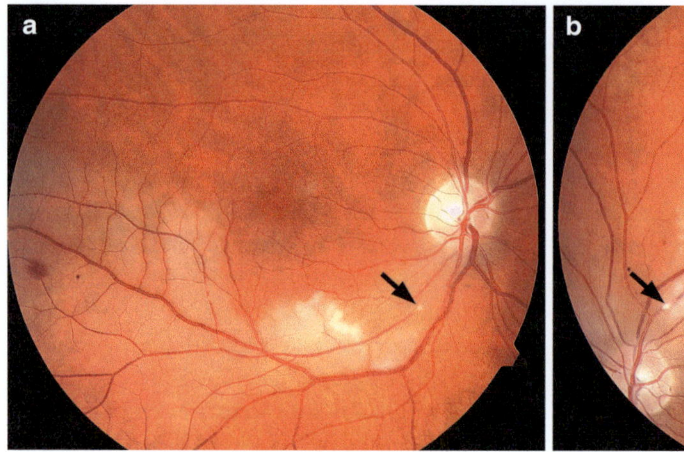

Fig. 23.4 A 39-year-old man with history of polysubstance abuse and multiple episodes of endocarditis who presented after a suicide attempt with bacteremia and a vegetation on his tricuspid valve. Chest CT revealed multiple septic emboli, s/p PICC placement for antibiotic treatment. He subsequently complained of blurry vision and was found to have bilateral emboli (arrows) causing branch retinal artery occlusions, inferotemporally in the right, and superotemporally in the left. Retinal whitening, indicative of ischemia, is noted bilaterally. The emboli were assumed to have originated from cardiac valve vegetations. (**a**) Right fundus; (**b**) left

Branch Retinal Artery Occlusion

Branch retinal artery occlusion affects the function of the retinal segment supplied by the occluded arteriole and thus results in less severe visual loss compared to central retinal artery occlusion. Visual blurring and field loss are limited by clearly circumscribed borders. Visible emboli in branch retinal arteries can be observed much more often in branch retinal artery occlusion than with central retinal artery occlusion (Fig. 23.4).

The visual prognosis in branch retinal artery occlusion is generally favorable, with final visual acuity of 20/40 or better in 80–90% of eyes. Some degree of macular perfusion through neighboring arterioles can prolong the "critical period" for retinal survival and increase the chance for spontaneous visual recovery.

Management

An embolic event with underlying atherosclerosis is almost always the cause for a branch retinal artery occlusion. Rarely, giant cell arteritis can be the cause of a branch retinal artery occlusion. Aggressive therapy is required only for branch retinal artery occlusion cases involving the fovea.

Surgical embolectomy and Nd:YAG embolysis have been attempted to restore the blood flow. However, serious intraoperative complications and the lack of any demonstrable functional benefits limit the use of these treatment modalities. Based on results of immediate vitrectomy following central retinal artery occlusion, eyes with branch retinal artery occlusion affecting the fovea may also benefit from early vitrectomy with or without manual dislodging of the embolus.

Retinal Venous Occlusions

Retinal vein occlusions are the second most common retinal vascular disease after diabetic retinopathy. The combined prevalence of central and branch vein occlusions is 1–2% in people older than 40 years of age, with branch retinal vein occlusion being four times as common as central retinal vein occlusion.

In contrast to the embolic nature of retinal arterial occlusions, retinal vein occlusions are thrombotic in nature. The pathophysiology follows the principles of thrombogenesis, which involves changes in blood flow dynamics (stasis, turbulence) and resultant endothelial injury.

Arteriovenous crossing points are more vulnerable for such changes to occur. At these points, the artery and vein share the same outer sheath. Thus, in case of an atherosclerotic artery, the underlying vein wall is compressed, and the blood flow will become turbulent. This leads to endothelial cell damage and subsequently clot formation due to the exposure of the subendothelial matrix to coagulation factors. The site of occlusion is readily visible in branch vein occlusion. However, in central retinal vein occlusion, it is within the nerve and cannot be visualized with routine ophthalmoscopy.

Although both branch and central retinal vein occlusions are thrombotic diseases, the importance of local and systemic factors in predisposing to these conditions are quite different. Increased blood pressure, hyperopia, and atherosclerosis are more common in branch retinal vein occlusion, whereas high intraocular pressure seems to play a more important role in development of central retinal vein occlusion. Hematologic risk factors for general venous thrombosis seem to occur sporadically in retinal vein occlusions and are not very prevalent. However, in young patients (<45 years old) without systemic hypertension, presence of a coagulopathy must be kept in mind. This may be due to several factors, including resistance to activated protein C, antiphospholipid antibodies, and deficiency of the anticoagulant proteins such as Factor V Leiden mutation or hyperhomocysteinemia. Other hypercoagulable states, such as polycythemia, lymphoma, leukemia, sickle cell disease, multiple myeloma, macroglobulinemia, and use of oral contraceptives, can result in central retinal vein occlusion.

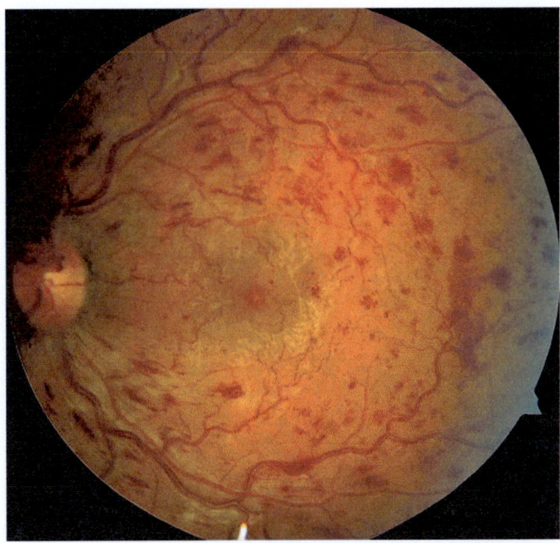

Fig. 23.5 A 73-year-old patient with central retinal vein occlusion of the left eye. Tortuosity of the central vein and scattered retinal hemorrhages dominate the clinical picture

blurring of vision. Ischemic cases can lead to subsequent new vessel development in the iris and at the iridocorneal juncture. Such neovascular proliferation in the aqueous outflow path can cause blockage of the aqueous drainage path, which may result in a type of increased intraocular pressure known as neovascular glaucoma. Ophthalmoscopically, all tributaries of central retinal vein demonstrate tortuosity and dilation along with edema of the macula and optic nerve head, retinal hemorrhages, and cotton wool spots throughout the fundus (Fig. 23.5). In nonischemic cases, vascular anastomoses, or so-called collateral vessels, may open around the optic disc between retinal and choroidal venous circulations, thereby shunting away stagnant venous blood.

Central Retinal Vein Occlusion

Patients with central retinal vein occlusion describe blurring of vision in the affected eye. The onset of symptoms can be insidious, and mild occlusions may even go unnoticed. Visual acuity less than 20/400 and an afferent pupil defect, if present, typically imply the ischemic occlusive form and are associated with severe

Branch Retinal Vein Occlusion

Branch retinal vein occlusions present with sectoral visual field defects. Visual loss is mild compared to that seen with central retinal vein occlusion. Macular edema and ischemia are the two major etiologies of visual loss. Retinal hemorrhages, cotton wool spots, and dilated and

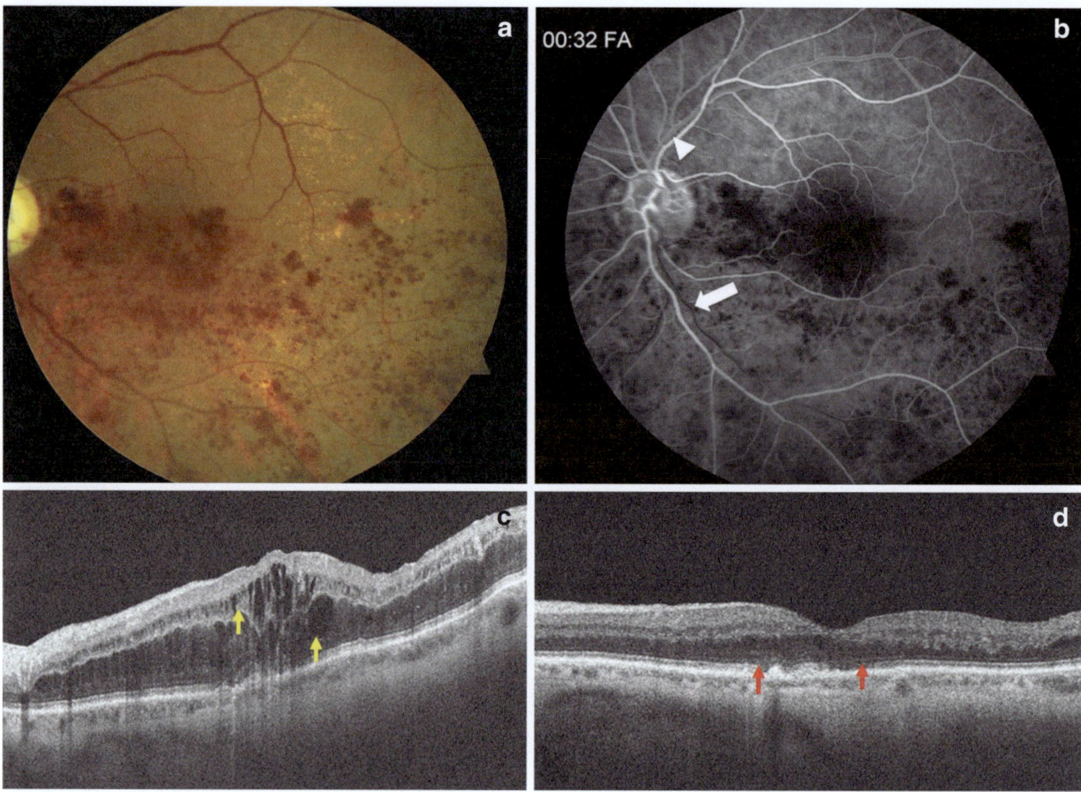

Fig. 23.6 A 73-year-old patient with branch retinal vein occlusion of the left eye. (**a**) Posterior segment exam reveals inferior temporal branch retinal vein occlusion. There are scattered retinal hemorrhages along the area that is supposed to be drained by the occluded retinal vein. (**b**) Fluorescein angiography of the same eye. Note the absence of fluorescein (white arrow) in the occluded inferotemporal vein, whereas its presence in the supero-temporal branch (white arrowhead) is clearly visible. This delay in the filling of the occluded vein results from the high intraluminal resistance due to occlusion. (**c**) Horizontal optical coherence tomography scan crossing the fovea shows areas of cystoid edema (yellow arrows) as optically empty dark areas. (**d**) Two months after treatment with intravitreal dexamethasone implant, the edema resolved. Areas of photoreceptor damage are apparent as interruption of the ellipsoid band between red arrows

tortuous veins are main features of branch retinal vein occlusions and are restricted to the segment of the retina drained by the occluded vein (Fig. 23.6). Retinal neovascularization may develop in ischemic cases, but it is rare to see neovascularization in the iris. Vascular anasto-moses can develop across the horizontal raphe between neighboring venous branches in order to drain pooled blood away from the occluded vein.

Management of Retinal Vein Occlusions

Pooling of blood distal to the occluded vein inevitably increases the hydrostatic pressure within the capillary bed leading to endothelial cell death and ischemia, as well as leakage through capillaries and retinal edema. These two events also trigger other pathogenic pathways, including upregulation of vascular endothelial growth factor (VEGF) production, new vessel formation, and an inflammatory response. Moderate to severe macular edema is a part of the clinical picture in 87% of central retina vein occlusions and 51% of the branch retinal vein occlusions. It resolves spontaneously in 51% of the cases in 2 years. Favorable visual outcome is associated with shorter duration of macular edema. Prevention and/or treatment of macular edema and retinal ischemia are the mainstays of retinal vein occlusion management. Although macular ischemia cannot be cured, complications secondary to ischemia-induced neovascularization can be treated. Scatter laser photocoagulation for eyes that develop neovascularization of the optic disc, retina, or iris can decrease the risk of vision loss.

Although grid laser treatment is an accepted treatment for macular edema secondary to branch retinal vein occlusions, it has largely been replaced with intravitreal injection of pharmacologic agents within the last 10 years, due to more favorable anatomic and functional outcomes with these agents. Various studies have shown that macular edema can be controlled with intraocular injections of anti-VEGF agents and/or steroid implants. Despite good initial response, multiple intravitreal injections may be needed to prevent the recurrence of macular edema.

For intractable macular edema due to both central and branch retinal vein occlusion, pars plana vitrectomy appears to be the most widely embraced surgical treatment, relieving traction on the macula by severing vitreomacular adhesions. Additional benefits of vitrectomy may include increased oxygenation and removal of cytokines that increase vascular permeability, such as VEGF and related compounds.

Retinal Arterial Macroaneurysm

A retinal artery macroaneurysm is a localized and acquired dilation in a retinal arteriole within the initial three orders of arterial bifurcation (Fig. 23.7). It usually occurs in elderly patients with systemic hypertension and atherosclerosis, and in 10% of cases, it is bilateral.

Retinal arterial macroaneurysms may present in one of the two patterns: exudative and hemorrhagic. In the exudative form, visual loss is gradual, due to leakage through the aneurysmal vessel wall or surrounding remodeled capillary bed. Leakage of plasma results in exudative retinal detachment and/or intraretinal exudation. In contrast, the hemorrhagic form manifests itself with sudden visual loss due to rupture of the aneurysm and massive bleeding in, under, and above the retina.

Most retinal arterial aneurysms thrombose and close spontaneously, leading to visual recovery. However, visual prognosis may be poor in eyes that present with long-standing exudation or

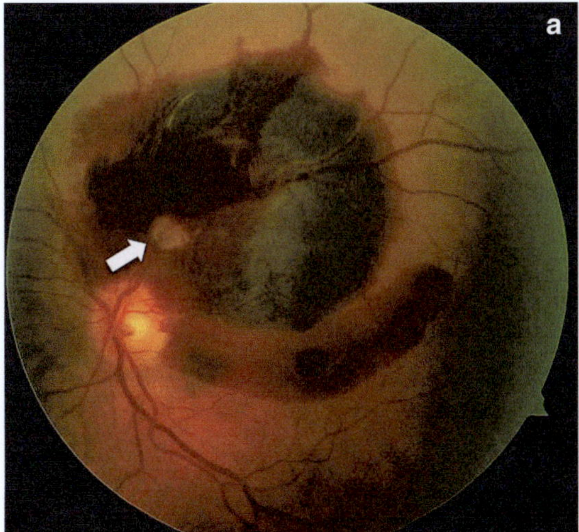
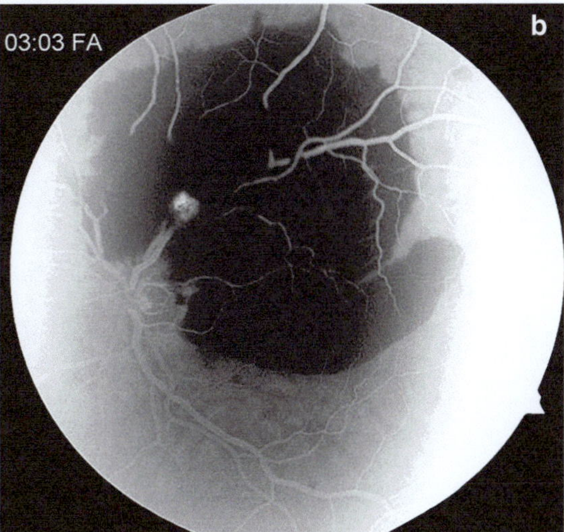

Fig. 23.7 A 75-year-old patient with a hemorrhagic retinal arterial macroaneurysm in left superotemporal retinal artery. (**a**) The image reveals a macroaneurysm (arrow) with preretinal, intraretinal, and subretinal hemorrhage. (**b**). Retinal arterial macroaneurysm fills with fluorescein during angiography and appears hyperfluorescent. Note that preretinal hemorrhage blocks the view of superotemporal retinal vessels

massive subretinal bleeding. In cases with massive subretinal bleeding, vitrectomy with pneumatic displacement and use of tissue plasminogen activator may help to clear blood underneath the fovea and preserve central vision. Intraretinal and vitreous hemorrhages usually clear spontaneously. If lipid exudation involves the foveal center, direct laser photocoagulation can be performed with care to avoid occlusion of the artery.

Management of a retinal artery macroaneurysm should also involve treatment of underlying systemic medical problems, such as systemic hypertension.

Sickle Cell Retinopathy

Sickle cell disease is the most common inherited blood disorder, with an incidence of 1/500 among African Americans and 1/36,000 among Hispanic Americans. Paradoxically, homozygous sickle cell disease (SS), which has the highest rate of systemic vascular complications, carries the lowest risk for retinopathy. This is because of the relatively lower hematocrit level in SS patients due to higher incidence of sickling in peripheral macrovessels, which in turn decreases the micro-vascular complications of the sickle cell disease. Consequently, retinopathy most commonly manifests in patients with sickle cell hemoglobin C (SC) and sickle cell thalassemia (SThal) where peripheral macrovascular complications are relatively less.

Mutation of the globin gene in sickle cell disease results in a tendency of the mutant hemoglobin molecule to polymerize in the deoxygenated state. This results in loss of erythrocyte flexibility under hypoxia, acidosis, or dehydration and, hence, causes arteriolar and capillary occlusions. Intraretinal hemorrhages are typically seen in the non-proliferative stage of the disease. These hemorrhages can be fresh ("salmon patch hemorrhages") or partially resorbed ("refractile spots"). Localized areas of secondary retinal pigment epithelial hyperplasia and intraretinal pigment migration ("black sunburst lesions") can also be seen. In the proliferative stage, extensive peripheral non-perfusion can lead to dilation of pre-existing capillaries ("arteriovenular anastomoses"). After prolonged ischemia, highly branching new vessels emerge on the inner retinal surface. These vessels are named "sea-fan" neovascularization due to their characteristic appearance (Fig. 23.8). Traction on these vessels may cause vitreous hemorrhage and resultant

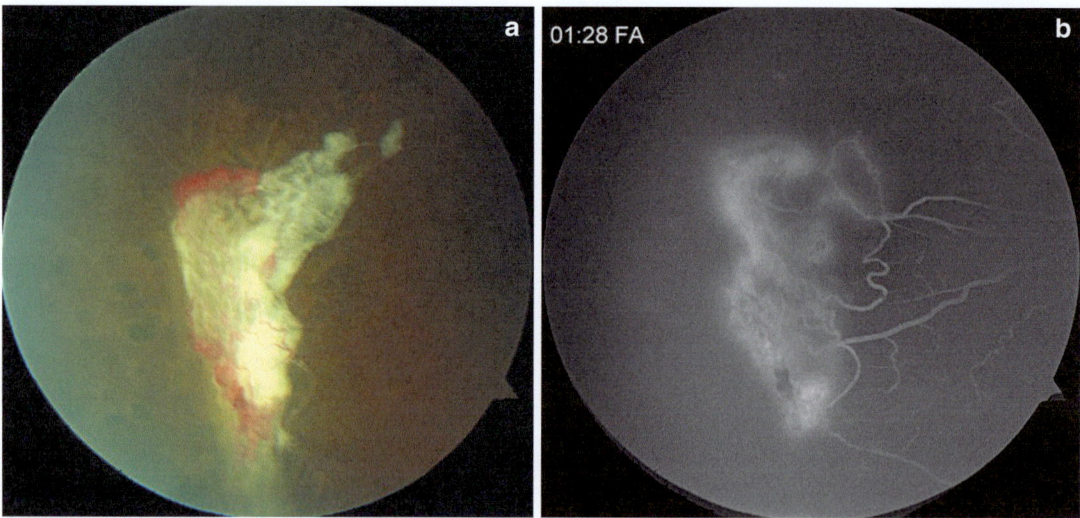

Fig. 23.8 A 39-year-old patient with sickle cell retinopathy in the right eye. Posterior segment exam (**a**) and fluorescein angiography (**b**) reveal sea-fan neovascularization

tractional retinal detachment. Another posterior segment manifestation is dilated, dark-colored capillaries on the optic disc surface, which appear as small red dots ("the disc sign of sickling").

In most cases, careful biomicroscopy reveals saccular dilatations of small conjunctival vessels. These occur due to occlusion and redirection of blood within the capillary bed as a result of microthrombi. They may also lead to segmentation of blood in conjunctival capillaries ("comma sign"). Segmental iris ischemia and necrosis can result in iris atrophy and pupil abnormalities. Iris neovascularization is a natural consequence of anterior segment ischemia.

Management of retinopathy involves ablation of the ischemic retinal areas with scatter laser photocoagulation and clearing of vitreous hemorrhage with vitrectomy. Any fibrovascular tissue pulling and detaching the retina can be removed with vitrectomy. Blood in the anterior chamber (hyphema) requires aggressive treatment of ensuing intraocular pressure elevation to avoid optic nerve damage. Carbonic anhydrase inhibitors should be avoided, since drug-induced acidosis may worsen sickling.

Retinopathy of Prematurity

Retinopathy of prematurity (previously referred to as "retrolental fibroplasia") is characterized by the development of new retinal vessels in premature infants exposed to high oxygen concentration. Risk factors for this vasoproliferative retinopathy include gestational age less than 30 weeks and a birth weight of less than 1500 g. It is the leading cause of blindness in childhood and accounts 14% of childhood blindness in the USA.

In developing retina, blood vessels begin to sprout radially from the optic nerve at the fourth month of the gestational age, and full maturation of the vasculature occurs just before full term birth. Premature birth results in exposure of developing retinal vessels to relatively higher ambient oxygen concentrations compared to in utero oxygen levels (50 vs 160 mmHg), which results in downregulation of physiologic vasculogenesis signaling via VEGF and IGF-1, halting progression of normal retinal vessel sprouting. As a result, peripheral retina remains avascular and releases vast amounts of angiogenic cytokines after birth, due to the inadequate oxygen available to supply increasing retinal metabolism. Stimulation of angiogenesis from retinal vessels toward the ischemic peripheral retina results in bleeding, fibrosis, tractional retinal detachment, and eventually blindness.

Clinical staging and management planning for retinopathy of prematurity is based on the *location*, *severity*, and *extent* of retinal neovascularization.

Location is expressed in "zones" (Fig. 23.9). Zone I is defined as a circular area centered at the optic disc and has a diameter of twice the distance between the fovea and the optic disc. Zone II covers a circular area outside Zone I centered at the optic disc and extends to cover the nasal ora serrata, and Zone III is the temporal area outside Zone II.

Severity indicates the stage of retinal neovascularization. Stage 1 is a white-gray demarcation line between vascularized and avascular retina. In Stage 2 a ridge develops at the vascular–avascular border. In Stage 3 newly developed retinal vessels extend into the vitreous or avascular retina, and in Stage 4 the retina is pulled away from the eye wall due to the contraction of fibrovascular tissue. With contraction, a partial tractional retinal detachment occurs. If this detachment remains in the periphery of the retina, it is referred to as Stage 4A, whereas if it involves the fovea, it is called Stage 4B. Stage 5 refers to a total retinal detachment.

The *Extent* of retinal pathology is expressed by clock hours which are affected by the pathologic process. Special emphasis is given to the dilation and tortuosity of the retinal vasculature, since these factors carry a risk for progression of the retinopathy of prematurity, which is referred to as *plus disease*.

Dilated fundus examination should be done in all infants born earlier than 30 weeks of gestational age or less than 1500 g of weight to determine retinal vascular development and the presence of retinopathy of prematurity. Follow-up

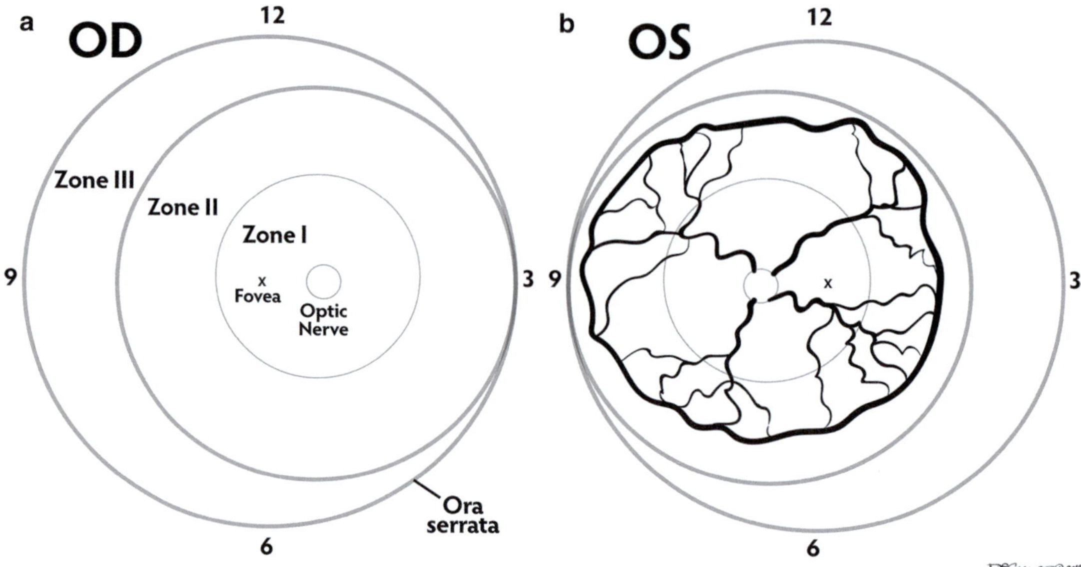

Fig. 23.9 (**a**) The International Classification of Retinopathy of Prematurity (ICROP) according to the *location*, *severity*, and *extent* of the disease. The *location*, *extent*, and *severity* of the disease are determined by evaluating the development of retinal vasculature in three concentric retinal zones. Zone I and II are centered on the optic nerve where retinal vasculature originates. Zone I has a radius twice the distance between the fovea and the center of the optic disc. Zone II is the area outside the Zone I with a radius extending from the center of the disc to the nasal ora serrata (3 o'clock in the right and 9 o'clock in the left eye). Remaining crescentic area outside of Zone II that extends to the temporal ora serrata is called Zone III. The *extent* of the disease is expressed as the number of clock hours involved, whereas *staging* of the disease is recorded as the status of the abnormal vascular development at the junction of the vascular and avascular retina. Additionally, venous dilatation and arteriolar tortuosity of the posterior retinal vessels is marked *plus disease* (+) since it has prognostic and therapeutic significance. (**b**) An example of a drawing of Zone II (+) disease in the left eye

exams are required to ensure full maturation of the retinal vasculature, ensuring that treatment is not required. Employment of telemedicine for remote areas has been demonstrated to yield similar accuracy for detection of those infants that require treatment.

Treatment of ROP is aimed at destruction of areas of ischemic retina in order to stop production of angiogenic chemokines such as vascular endothelial growth factor (VEGF). To accomplish this treatment in these very young babies, cryotherapy or laser photocoagulation has been employed. A newer approach is to neutralize the effects of VEGF with intravitreal injection of anti-VEGF drugs. Studies with cryotherapy found a 50% risk of subsequent retinal detachment in certain ROP patients, and these patients are described as having *threshold disease.* Threshold disease is defined as five contiguous clock hours of stage 3 ROP or eight noncontiguous clock hours of stage 3 ROP in zone I or II in the presence of plus disease. Because of the detachment risk in threshold disease, application of cryotherapy over ischemic areas is intentionally decreased, which reduces the probability (45% vs 64%) of unfavorable visual outcomes (<20/200) as well as unfavorable structural outcomes such as retinal folds or retinal detachment (30% vs 52%). The question whether earlier treatment with thermal laser may result in better preservation of vision and decrease unfavorable structural outcomes was tested in the Early Treatment for Retinopathy of Prematurity (ETROP) study. An analysis of the CRYO-ROP cohort identified high-risk groups with an unfavorable outcome which are referred to as *prethreshold disease.* Prethreshold disease is defined as Zone I disease less than threshold, Zone II

Stage 2 with plus disease; Zone II, stage 3 disease without plus disease; and Zone II, stage 3 with plus disease (Fig. 23.10). Laser ablation of the ischemic retina in prethreshold disease resulted in a similar reduction in unfavorable visual (19.8% vs 14.3%) and structural outcomes (15.6% vs 9.0%). Further analysis of the results revealed a clear benefit of laser photocoagulation in eyes with *Type I prethreshold disease*, which is defined as Zone I, any stage with plus disease; Zone I, Stage 3 without plus disease; and/or Zone II, Stage 2 or 3, with plus disease.

Failure of ablative treatments to completely prevent visual loss and the occurrence of significant complications such as peripheral visual loss or myopia induction resulted in rapid adaptation of anti-VEGF pharmacotherapy for retinopathy of prematurity. The BEAT-ROP study revealed that intravitreal injection of bevacizumab in Stage 3 retinopathy of prematurity in Zones I or II along with Plus disease can yield lower recurrence rates of Zone I disease (6% vs 42%) compared to laser photocoagulation. Intravitreal injection of bevacizumab did not cause any deficit in the normal neurodevelopment of the infants. Further studies have shown that similar benefits can be obtained with very low intravitreal doses of bevacizumab.

Progression of ROP to the fibrosis stage results in tractional retinal detachments that require surgery to preserve vision. The preferred surgical method is a lens-sparing vitrectomy, which is generally accepted to be superior to scleral buckling alone. Preoperative bevacizumab can be helpful to suppress angiogenesis and minimize or prevent intraoperative bleeding. Several adjuncts such as intravitreal triamcinolone and plasmin can aid surgical repair of ROP tractional detachments.

Suggested Reading

Anderson B Jr, Saltzman HA. Retinal oxygen utilization measured by hyperbaric blackout. Arch Ophthalmol. 1964;72:792–5.

Arruga J, Sanders MD. Ophthalmologic findings in 70 patients with evidence of retinal embolism. Ophthalmology. 1982;89:1336–47.

Fraser SG, Adams W. Interventions for acute non-arteritic central retinal artery occlusion. Cochrane Database Syst Rev. 2009;1:CD001989.

Hayreh SS. Ocular vascular occlusive disorders: natural history of visual outcome. Prog Retin Eye Res. 2014;41:1–25.

Hayreh SS, Zimmerman MB. Central retinal artery occlusion: visual outcome. Am J Ophthalmol. 2005;140:376–91.

Hayreh SS, Zimmerman MB. Fundus changes in central retinal artery occlusion. Retina. 2007;27:276–89.

Hayreh SS, Zimmerman MB. Fundus changes in central retinal vein occlusion. Retina. 2015;35:29–42.

Hayreh SS, Podhajsky PA, Zimmerman B. Occult giant cell arteritis: ocular manifestations. Am J Ophthalmol. 1998;125:521–6.

Hayreh SS, Zimmerman MB, Kimura A, Sanon A. Central retinal artery occlusion. Retinal survival time. Exp Eye Res. 2004;78:723–36.

Heiss WD. The ischemic penumbra: how does tissue injury evolve? Ann N Y Acad Sci. 2012;1268:26–34.

Jia Y, Bailey ST, Hwang TS, McClintic SM, Gao SS, Pennesi ME, Flaxel CJ, Lauer AK, Wilson DJ, Hornegger J, Fujimoto JG, Huang D. Quantitative optical coherence tomography angiography of vascular abnormalities in the living human eye. Proc Natl Acad Sci U S A. 2015;112:E2395–402.

Kuhli-Hattenbach C, Scharrer I, Lüchtenberg M, Hattenbach LO. Coagulation disorders and the risk of retinal vein occlusion. Thromb Haemost. 2010;103:299–305.

Liew G, Wang JJ, Mitchell P, Wong TY. Retinal vascular imaging: a new tool in microvascular disease research. Circ Cardiovasc Imaging. 2008;1:156–61.

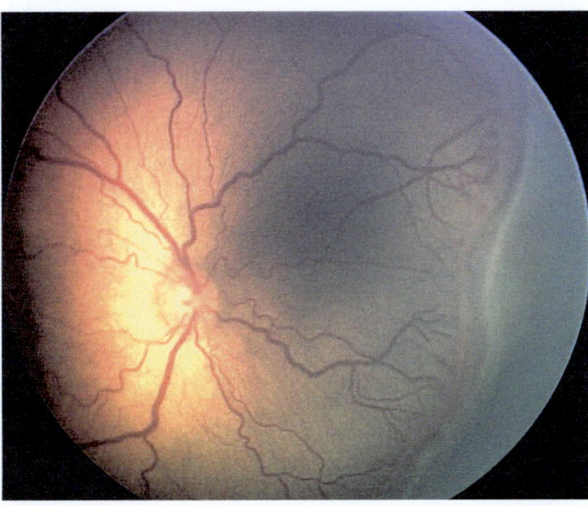

Fig. 23.10 *Stage 3 Retinopathy of Prematurity with Plus Disease.* Fundus photograph of the left eye of a premature baby reveals dilated and tortuous retinal vessels indicating the presence of "plus disease." Note new vessel formation at the ridge between avascular and vascularized retina

Mason JO 3rd, Nixon PA, Albert MA Jr. Trans-luminal nd:YAG laser embolysis for branch retinal artery occlusion. Retina. 2007;27:573–7.

Prager F, Michels S, Kriechbaum K, Georgopoulos M, Funk M, Geitzenauer W, Polak K, Schmidt-Erfurth U. Intravitreal bevacizumab (Avastin) for macular oedema secondary to retinal vein occlusion: 12-month results of a prospective clinical trial. Br J Ophthalmol. 2009;93:452–6.

Rogers S, McIntosh RL, Cheung N, Lim L, Wang JJ, Mitchell P, Kowalski JW, Nguyen H, Wong TY, International Eye Disease Consortium. The prevalence of retinal vein occlusion: pooled data from population studies from the United States, Europe, Asia, and Australia. Ophthalmology. 2010;117:313–9.

Schmidt D, Hetzel A, Geibel-Zehender A, Schulte-Mönting J. Systemic diseases in non-inflammatory branch and central retinal artery occlusion-an overview of 416 patients. Eur J Med Res. 2007;12:595–603.

Scholl S, Kirchhof J, Augustin AJ. Pathophysiology of macular edema. Ophthalmologica. 2010;224(Suppl 1):8–15.

Tezel T, Gunalp I, Tezel G. Morphometrical analysis of retinal arterial macroaneurysms. Doc Ophthalmol. 1994;88:113–25.

Tezel TH, Geng L, Lato EB, Schaal S, Liu Y, Dean D, Klein JB, Kaplan HJ. Synthesis and secretion of hemoglobin by retinal pigment epithelium. Invest Ophthalmol Vis Sci. 2009;50:1911–9.

Wong TY, Scott IU. Clinical practice. Retinal-vein occlusion. N Engl J Med. 2010;363:2135–44.

Wong TY, Larsen EK, Klein R, Mitchell P, Couper DJ, Klein BE, Hubbard LD, Siscovick DS, Sharrett AR. Cardiovascular risk factors for retinal vein occlusion and arteriolar emboli: the Atherosclerosis Risk in Communities & Cardiovascular Health studies. Ophthalmology. 2005;112:540–7.

Yuzurihara D, Iijima H. Visual outcome in central retinal and branch retinal artery occlusion. Jpn J Ophthalmol. 2004;48:490–2.

Retinal Detachment

Hermann Schubert

Retinal detachment is a sight-threatening condition which, prior to 1930, was rarely cured. Effective treatments are now available, and therefore, early (<4 days) diagnosis is important to reduce the risk of permanent visual loss. Failure to diagnose, refer, or treat a retinal detachment risks both visual and potential legal difficulties.

Anatomy

Anatomically, retinal detachment is a separation of neurosensory retina from the retinal pigment epithelium (RPE), which recreates a potential epithelio-retinal interspace. It "recreates," because this space previously existed, during formation of the optic cup in embryogenesis, and is only obliterated after cup invagination in the first month of organogenesis. This interspace eradication results in an apex-to-apex sensory-RPE epithelial arrangement at birth, but this normal arrangement may be reversed in pathologic states (Fig. 24.1).

It is "potential," because negative pumping action of the RPE preserves the apex-to-apex arrangement, unless there are major opposing forces to the natural epithelial apposition. Opposing forces include direct traction on the sensory retina and/or flow of vitreous or choroid fluid into the epithelio-retinal interspace, both of which can potentially overpower the ability of the RPE to pump fluid and maintain normal epithelial apposition. If the opposing forces do overwhelm the RPE pumping system, then fluid will accumulate in the potential interspace, and neurosensory retina will separate from underlying RPE, resulting in a detachment.

Presentation

Clinically, a detached retina appears to the patient as a shadow or visual field defect which is often noted a few days after the appearance of large vitreous floaters (motile spots, lines, or "cobwebs" which move along with eye movements). Biomicroscopically, the separation appears as a retinal "elevation," i.e., an out-of-focus area of the retina adjacent to attached retina which appears in sharp focus. The retinal elevation may occur in one or both eyes simultaneously and may appear first centrally or peripherally. If the detachment is of long duration, signs of inflammation (posterior uveitis) may appear, often combined with

H. Schubert, MD (✉)
Department of Ophthalmology, Edward S. Harkness Eye Institute, Columbia University Vagelos College of Physicians and Surgeons, New York, NY, USA
e-mail: hds1@cumc.columbia.edu

© Springer Nature Switzerland AG 2019
D. S. Casper, G. A. Cioffi (eds.), *The Columbia Guide to Basic Elements of Eye Care*,
https://doi.org/10.1007/978-3-030-10886-1_24

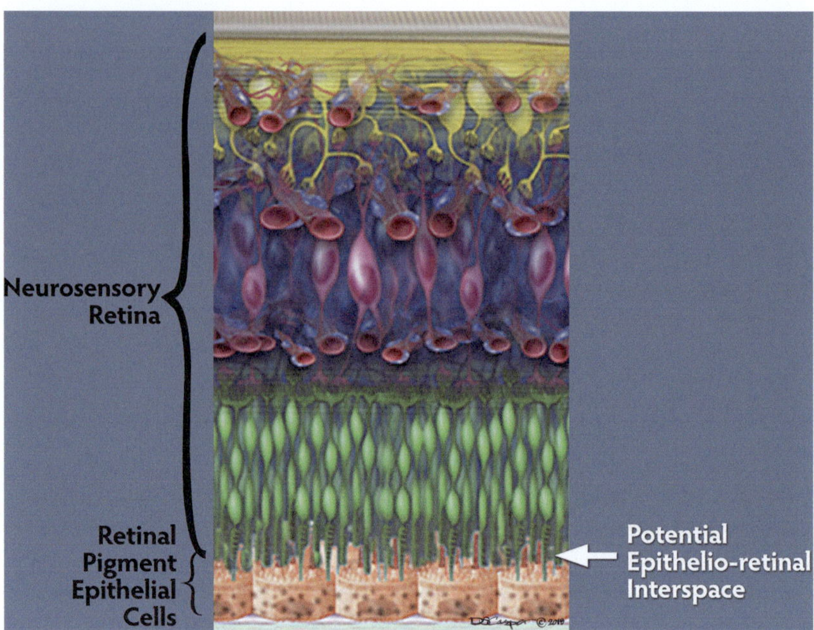

Fig. 24.1 A schematic illustration of the potential epithelio-retinal interspace. This space previously existed during formation of the optic cup in embryogenesis and is only obliterated after cup invagination in the first month of organogenesis, and its eradication results in an apex-to-apex sensory-RPE epithelial arrangement at birth

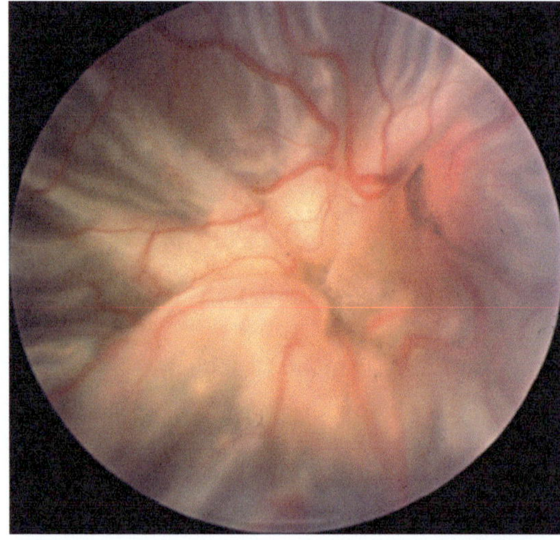

Fig. 24.2 Color photo of a chronically detached retina complicated by proliferative vitreoretinopathy. Note the folded and contracted retina assuming a closed funnel configuration. Disc and macula are obscured by epiretinal folds and membranes contracting circumferentially at the equator

significantly reduced intraocular pressure (hypotony) and ultimately, scarring of the retina and vitreous (proliferative vitreoretinopathy, PVR). (Fig. 24.2).

Retinal Elevation: Rhegmatogenous Detachment

The majority of detachments are caused by retinal tears or holes and are referred to as rhegmatogenous (derived from the Greek *rhegma*, referring to breakage) detachments.

In addition to causing peripheral visual field defects and central blind spots (scotomas), rhegmatogenous detachments are symptomatic in a manner related to the particular break formation which caused it to occur (see Lincoff's Rules (Fig. 24.3). Vitreous degeneration (syneresis) causes the appearance of floaters, and vitreous collapse and subsequent traction on the adjacent retina causes flashes (bursts of light visible to the patient). If vitreous traction exceeds the structural cohesiveness of the retina, tractional tears occur, and a rhegmatogenous separation may result. As the retina tears and detaches, blood vessels may be torn; therefore, retinal breaks may be associated with vitreous hemorrhage, which appears as large black floaters and peripheral shadows, usually associated with some decreased visual acuity. Biomicroscopically, the elevated, out-of-focus retina appears tan, rather than the

TYPICAL LOCATION OF RETINAL BREAKS
("Lincoff's Rules")

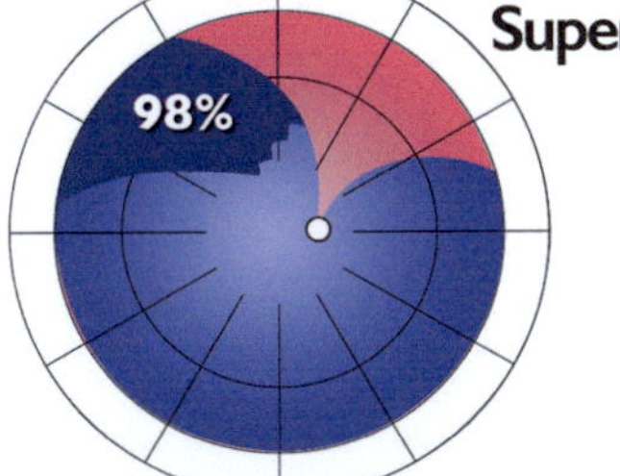

Superior temporal or nasal detachments:

In 98% of cases, the primary break lies within 1 1/2 clock hours of the highest border.

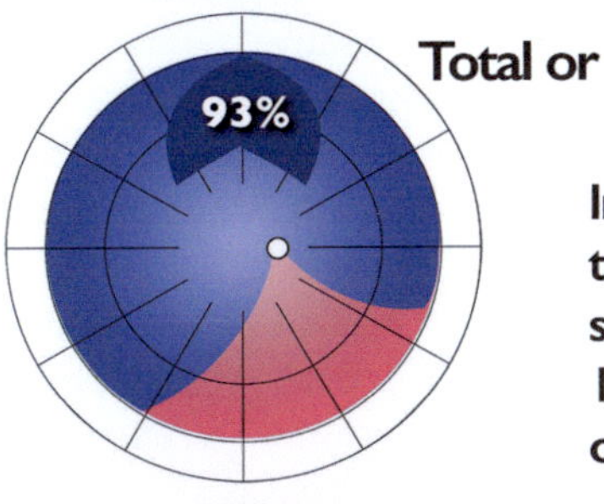

Total or superior detachments that cross the 12 o'clock meridian:

In 93%, the primary break lies within a triangle, the apex of which is at the ora serrata, and the side of which extends 1 1/2 clock hours to either side of 12 o'clock

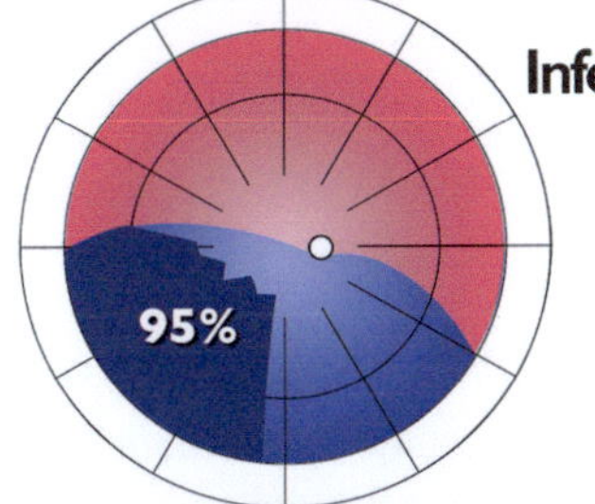

Inferior Detachments:

In 95% the higher side of the detachment indicates on which side of the disc an inferior break lies

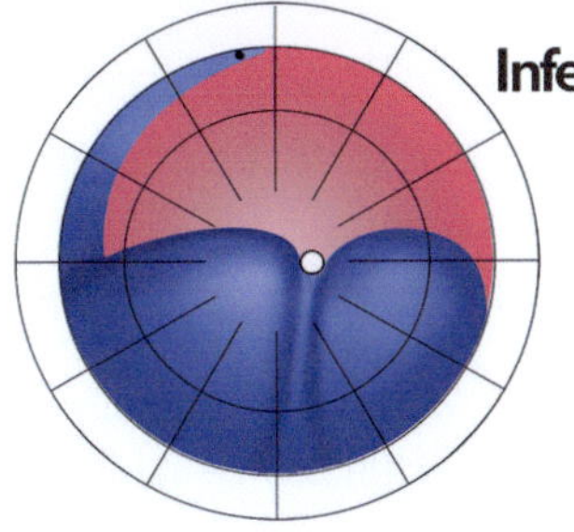

Inferior bullous detachments:

Inferior bullae in a rhegmatogenous detachment originate from a superior break

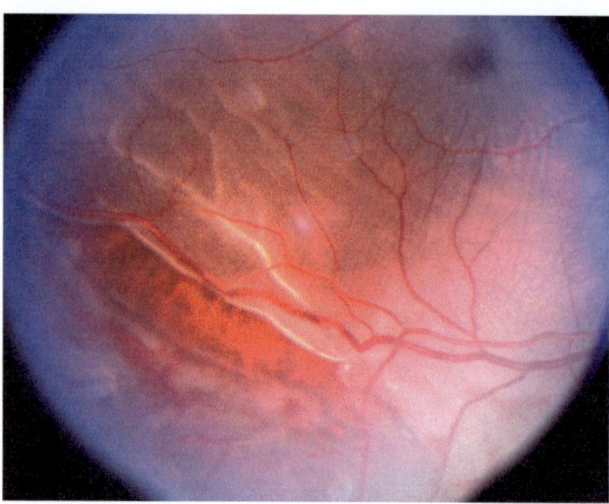

Fig. 24.4 Full-thickness neurosensory break associated with lattice degeneration. The surrounding retina is elevated by subretinal fluid. Note the two bridging retinal blood vessels

normal orange-pink color, but the detachment may initially be obscured by vitreous hemorrhage.

Full-thickness neurosensory retinal breaks which result in rhegmatogenous detachments most commonly occur at the posterior vitreous base, i.e., usually in the periphery (Fig. 24.4). At first, a symptomatic break will be surrounded by fluid, which may offer an opportunity to treat the break with direct application of laser coagulation (See Fig. 5.4). If not too large, the elevated area can be surrounded with laser burns, or, in some cases, the patient's eyes are both patched and immobilized for a day, which will often reduce the volume of subretinal fluid, which results in the need for less extensive laser demarcation. The laser burns act as a "welding" procedure, causing the retina to adhere firmly to underlying RPE, preventing the influx of more fluid, and returning the layers to their appositional arrangement.

Left untreated, subretinal fluid will progress in the area involved, and it will follow gravity.

- Large superior breaks will result in downward tracking of fluid, which causes overhanging, "bullous" retinal detachments.
- Small superior breaks may create a shallow peripheral sinus and inferior bullous detachment.

- Inferior breaks may cause a more shallow detachment, located inferior to the horizontal meridian but usually asymmetric, with the detachment extending higher on the side of the break.

These gravitational influences are the basis of the Lincoff Rules, developed by Dr. Harvey Lincoff at Cornell University in the 1970s (Fig. 24.3). These rules utilize the contours, borders, and characteristics of a particular detachment to guide the retinologist in locating the causative retinal break(s), which is critical for successful treatment.

In general, rhegmatogenous detachments are symptomatic, have convex borders, extend from the peripheral ora serrata to the optic disc, and often follow gravity. Treatment which focuses on closing the retinal breaks(s) within the first week is beneficial and frequently curative.

Retinal Elevation: Nonrhegmatogenous

Nonrhegmatogenous detachments fall into three groups: exudative, tractional, and schisis detachments.

Exudative Detachment

Exudative detachments lack the underlying pathologic basis of vitreous traction and therefore are often asymptomatic, except for central or peripheral visual loss and shadows seen in some cases.

As with rhegmatogenous detachment, the retinal elevation typically extends from the optic nerve head to the periphery and has convex borders. The borders will shift following gravity however, i.e., fluid will follow the gravitational center. The detachments are usually inferior and sometimes bilateral (Fig. 24.5).

If a retinal break cannot be found, history and ancillary testing are important to help determine

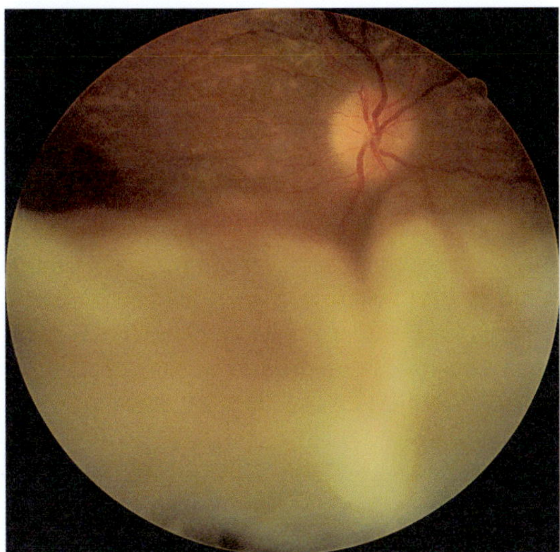

Fig. 24.5 Inferior bilobed exudative retinal detachment in uveal effusion syndrome, related to thickened sclera. The macula to the left of the optic disc shows chronic pigment epithelial changes

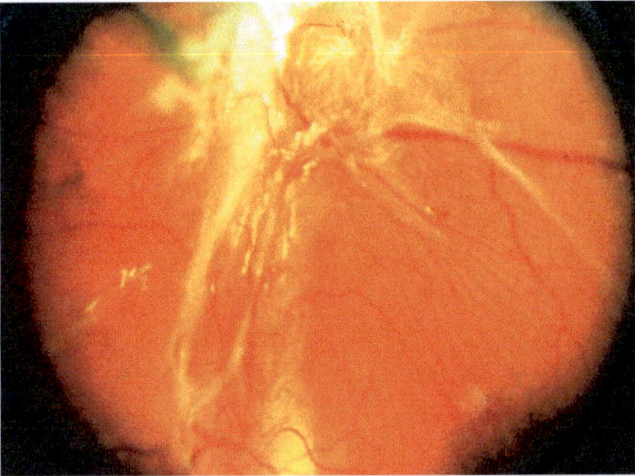

Fig. 24.6 Tractional retinal detachment along the superotemporal vascular arcade related to proliferative diabetic retinopathy. The disc is shown at 6 o'clock. Note the pigment demarcation line which differentiates the traction detachment from tractional retinal schisis in diabetes

the nature and cause of the detachment. Exudative detachments are often related to underlying systemic pathology and so are best approached with a blood pressure cuff to rule out systemic hypertension and retinal angiography to rule out central serous chorioretinopathy (CSR) and Harada's disease (granulomatous uveitis and exudative retinal detachments that may be accompanied by both neurologic and cutaneous manifestations). Ocular coherence tomography and ultrasound may help document choroidal thickening in Harada's disease and in scleritis. An added benefit of ultrasound examination in retinal elevations is to exclude choroidal metastatic or primary tumors, retinoblastoma in the young, and melanoma in the adult, all of which may present initially with exudative detachments. Uveal effusion syndrome is a rare condition related to thickened sclera and hyperopia, which can produce bilateral exudative detachments. The typical patient presenting with an exudative detachment therefore could be hypertensive, pregnant (eclampsia), 35 years old and male (CSR), and Asian or Hispanic (Harada's), have a painful eye (scleritis), or have a history of malignancy (metastatic retino-choroidopathy).

Tractional Detachment

Tractional detachments, which are often asymptomatic, result from vitreous strands pulling on the retina, without the presence of an associated hole or break. Vitreous traction elevates the retina, centrally or peripherally with a concave configuration, i.e., it usually does not extend from the ora serrata to the disc, as do fully developed rhegmatogenous or exudative detachments (Figs. 24.6 and 24.7). Central elevation is usually related to proliferative diabetic retinopathy, while peripheral elevation is typically seen with peripheral vascular occlusions and sickle cell disease. Tractional elevations can be complicated by retinal tears and may become rhegmatogenous and symptomatic.

Peripheral shadows and visual loss may also be caused by glaucoma, vascular occlusion, and intra- or preretinal hemorrhages. Retinal pallor with blood and an in-focus retina will facilitate the diagnosis. Difficult biomicroscopy in a non-diabetic patient is suspicious for retinal elevation and therefore needs ancillary testing, including angiography, optical coherence tomography, ultrasound, and even MRI scanning, if that is all that is available.

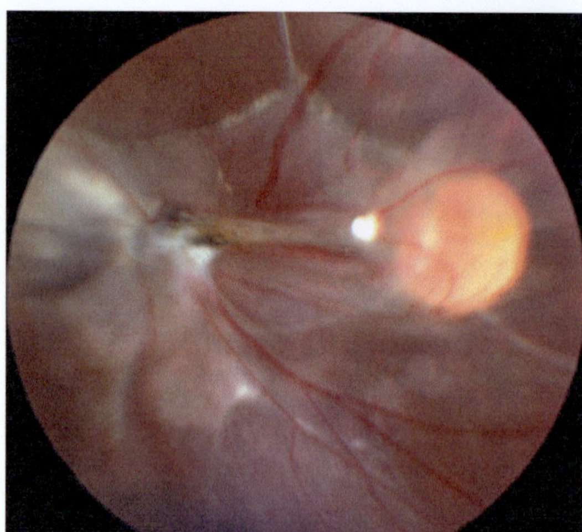

Fig. 24.7 Color photo of a macular scar and fold, resulting from repair of a traumatic retinal detachment. Note the distorted vasculature, pigment epithelial hyperplasia, and luteal pigment in the fold. The nerve head is to the right. Vision was counting fingers

Schisis Detachment

Schisis detachments involve a splitting of the retinal layers; this may be tractional, associated with diabetic retinopathy, vein occlusions, or sickle retinopathy, or it may be non-tractional, as occurs with degenerative peripheral schisis. As with tractional detachments, schisis elevations may become rhegmatogenous by hole formation in the internal or external layer. Such detachments will typically be symptomatic and reach from the ora serrata to the disc, their contour modified by associated vitreous traction.

Conclusion

Retinal detachment, of whatever etiology, is an important diagnosis to make. The primary diagnostic tool utilized by the retinologist is the indirect ophthalmoscope, although the examination is often enhanced by slit lamp biomicroscopy as well. Particularly with nonrhegmatogenous clues and history, all available ancillary tests should also be employed.

The treatment of retinal detachment is the subject of an entire ophthalmic subspecialty.

No retinal detachment is the same. Treatment involves precise identification of all retinal breaks, followed by chorioretinal adhesion.

Apposition is achieved by draining fluid (puncture), external indentation of the eyewall against the breaks (using either circumferential or localized scleral buckling), internal corking of the retinal break(s) (pneumopexy), and/or removal of the vitreous with internal drainage (vitrectomy). Often, these procedures are combined or applied sequentially.

Adhesion has classically been achieved using cautery, cryopexy, or laser surrounding the break. Most of these procedures focusing on the retinal breaks are successful; however vitrectomy and internal drainage of the detachment combined with generous endolaser have become the preferred initial treatment. Vitrectomy promotes cataract formation and glaucoma. It is preservation of the lens, of comfortable binocularity, accommodation, and avoidance of glaucoma that keeps pneumopexy and scleral buckling in the armamentarium of retinal surgeons. If the patient is young and phakic, scleral buckling may be an attractive option.

From the perspective of a patient who suddenly sees flashes and floaters or flashes and shadows, he or she should not panic, avoiding the "acute retinal panic syndrome" (Dr Norman Byer, personal communication).

Rather, immobilization and double patching should be employed until it is possible to schedule an examination with a skilled retinologist. Any movement of the head may further detach the retina and is therefore to be avoided. Subsequent timely treatment (be it buckling, vitrectomy, gas, or laser) as indicated will usually produce excellent results.

Suggested Reading

Kreissig I. A practical guide to minimal surgery for retinal detachment, vol. 1. Stuttgart: Thieme; 2000.

Kreissig I, editor. Primary retinal detachment. Options for repair. Berlin: Springer-Verlag; 2005.

Schubert HD, Buckling S. In: Saxena S, Meyer CH, Ohji M, Akduman L, editors. Vitreoretinal surgery. New Delhi: Jaypee Brothers Medical Publishers Ltd; 2012.

Posterior Segment Trauma

25

Jonathan S. Chang

Ocular trauma is a significant cause of vision loss, with over two million people affected each year. Trauma is one of the largest sources of vision loss in the developed world. The types of trauma are diverse, including sports-related, physical abuse, work-related or automobile accidents. In general, males tend to be affected by trauma to a greater degree than females. Injuries may be penetrating (causing a disruption in the sclera) or non-penetrating, and both can lead to significant ocular damage. Direct or indirect ocular trauma can cause vision loss.

In cases where ocular trauma is suspected, a thorough history and ophthalmic exam must be performed. In some incidents, the patient may not recall how the trauma occurred, and witnesses may be needed to provide necessary information. Some manifestations of ocular trauma may initially be quite subtle or accompany severe intracranial injury, so any suspicion of ocular injury warrants urgent ophthalmic evaluation, which may help prevent severe vision loss.

Since the extent of trauma can vary, it can be difficult to predict recovery and visual function. Typically, better initial visual acuity and injuries limited to the anterior segment have a better overall prognosis. Because the optic nerve and macula are critical for good vision, seemingly small or limited injuries that affect these essential areas may still have significant visual consequences.

Blunt Eye Injuries

Non-penetrating (the so-called closed globe) injuries can result from direct injury at the point of trauma, as well as indirect, contrecoup injury opposite to the impact site. The vitreous is adherent to the retina, and blunt trauma can transmit vitreous tractional forces onto the retina, resulting in retinal tears, macular holes, or shearing of retinal vessels, leading to intraocular hemorrhage (Fig. 25.1).

Although vitreous hemorrhage may resolve on its own, the presence of hemorrhage may suggest a concurrent occult retinal tear or detachment. Patients may notice increased floaters or flashing lights, and visual acuity can range from fairly good with a limited, mild hemorrhage to severely reduced with extensive bleeding. If vitreous hemorrhage does not resolve on its own, vitrectomy surgery may be indicated, depending on the clinical scenario and if additional retinal pathology is noted. B-scan ultrasonography may be useful in evaluation of the retina if the view through the vitreous is sufficiently opacified.

J. S. Chang, MD (✉)
Department of Ophthalmology and Visual Sciences,
University of Wisconsin School of Medicine
and Public Health, Madison, WI, USA
e-mail: jschang4@wisc.edu

© Springer Nature Switzerland AG 2019
D. S. Casper, G. A. Cioffi (eds.), *The Columbia Guide to Basic Elements of Eye Care*,
https://doi.org/10.1007/978-3-030-10886-1_25

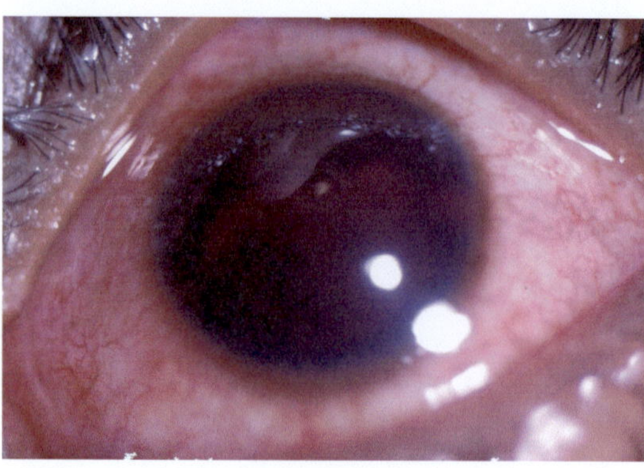

Fig. 25.1 Blunt trauma with hyphema. Slit lamp photograph of a total or "8-ball" hyphema after a snowball hit the eye. Patients can develop problems leading to long-term vision loss including elevated intraocular pressure and corneal blood staining. Individuals with sickle cell disease are at highest risk for these problems. A total hyphema such as this prevents direct fundus viewing; it is imperative to rule out posterior injuries, such as retinal detachment, or injuries to the optic nerve or sclera

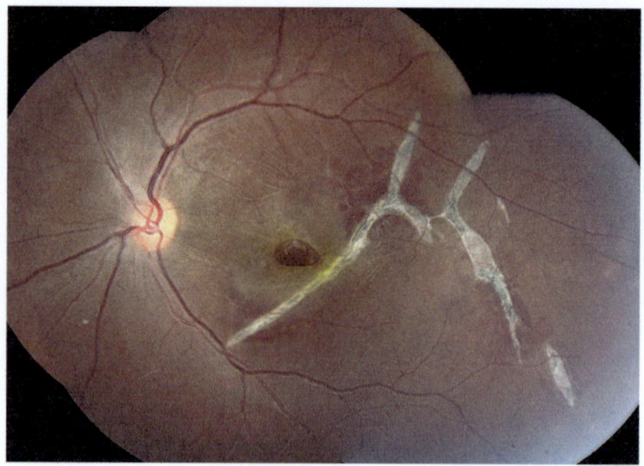

Fig. 25.2 Left fundus image of a woman who had a heavy box hit her in the eye. A macular hole is present, along with a choroidal rupture and subretinal hemorrhage. Despite attempt at surgical repair, the hole could not be closed, and the vision remained at counting fingers

Retinal tears are peripheral lesions that can lead to retinal detachment and are usually treated with laser prophylaxis. A giant retinal tear encompasses an area greater than three retinal clock hours and carries a higher morbidity than do smaller tears. Symptoms of retinal tear include a sudden increase in floaters or flashing lights. These full-thickness defects in the retina can allow liquid vitreous fluid to enter the subretinal space, leading to retinal detachment. A retinal dialysis, or disinsertion of the retina at its most anterior location (the vitreous base), is also a peripheral lesion associated with trauma and potential for retinal detachment. Retinal dialysis is more common in younger patients and sometimes has a very slow progression, with retinal detachment occurring months after the initial injury. Scleral buckle or vitrectomy surgery may be used alone or in combination for retinal detachment repair.

A macular hole is a full-thickness defect in the center of the retina (Fig. 25.2). In blunt trauma, it is believed that the retina is stretched tangentially, leading to the central defect. The strong attachment of the vitreous to the fovea may contribute to this pathophysiology. In some patients these may resolve with observation; however, others require vitrectomy. Surgery is usually performed promptly but in some cases can be deferred for several weeks or even months after the initial injury.

Deformation of the globe in blunt trauma can lead to disruption of Bruch's membrane and the inner choroid, causing a choroidal rupture (Fig. 25.2). The site of rupture is usually central and often forms a concentric arc around the optic disc. The highly vascular choroid may hemorrhage into the subretinal space following rupture, and both the blood and tissue disruption can lead to a permanent scotoma. There is no surgical or medical treatment for choroidal rupture. Because there is a defect in Bruch's membrane, these patients are at risk for developing future choroidal neovascularization, which may require treatment with anti-vascular endothelial growth factor injections, similar to the treatment for neovascular age-related macular degeneration.

Some of the most severe vision loss in blunt trauma is due to optic nerve damage. Traumatic optic neuropathy may be present due to sudden stunning of optic nerve axons. Visual acuity can vary in these cases but is often severely decreased. Traumatic optic neuropathy can be associated with compression of the nerve or orbit fracture. Intravenous or oral steroids have been utilized in these cases with limited and unproven effectiveness. In an optic nerve avulsion, the optic nerve is partially or completely severed due to a rapid torsional injury (Fig. 25.3). Visual acuity will be no light perception, and unfortunately no treatment

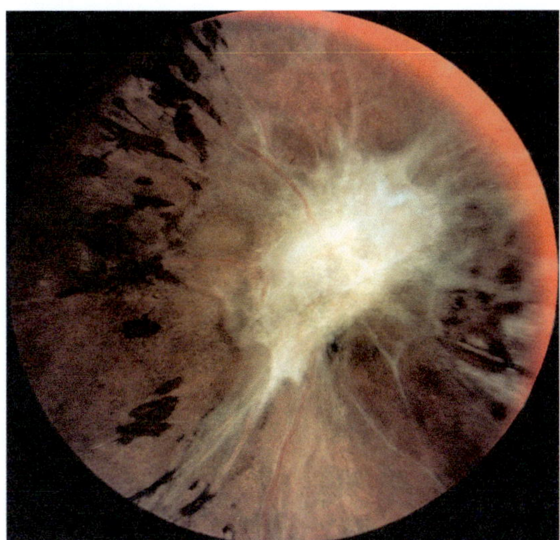

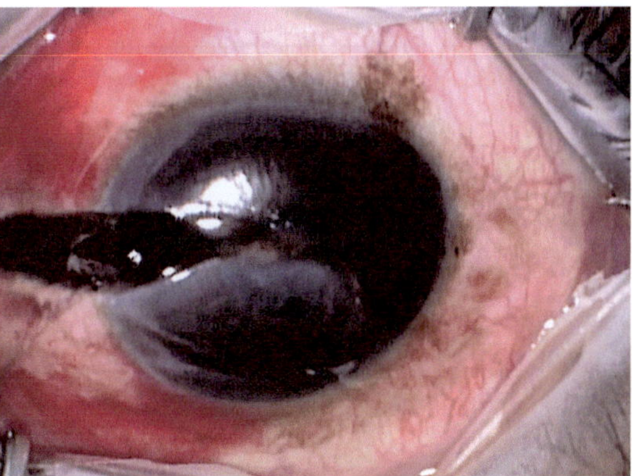

Fig. 25.4 Intraoperative photograph of a patient who had a trauma causing scleral and corneal laceration. Uveal tissue can be seen prolapsed through the wound

Fig. 25.3 Fundus photograph of a patient with chronic changes following optic nerve avulsion, with scarring of the optic disc, peripapillary chorioretinal scarring, and sclerotic vessels. (Courtesy of Dr. Jeffrey Odel)

exists to reattach the severed optic nerve to the globe and restore vision.

Commotio retinae is usually a mild injury to the retina associated with blunt trauma. It is very common, often asymptomatic, and often resolves within 2 weeks. Retinal examination reveals a retinal whitening that correlates with outer retinal damage on pathology. It is believed to occur due to contrecoup injury mechanisms. If this occurs in the macula, it may be symptomatic and is also known as Berlin's edema. A similar but uncommon condition, sclopetaria retinae, occurs when a high-velocity projectile (often a bullet) causes a shearing effect that leads to a retinal and choroidal rupture without penetrating injury. The effect on visual acuity will depend on the location of the actual pathology.

Penetrating and Perforating Eye Injuries

In a penetrating eye injury, a sharp or high-velocity object lacerates the cornea or sclera (Fig. 25.4). A perforating eye injury is a penetrating injury with both an entry and exit wound. The further posterior the location of the wound, the worse the visual prognosis because these wounds can be more difficult to access and repair. Posterior injuries also increase the chance for retinal detachment or optic neuropathy.

Prompt (within 24 hours) surgical closure of penetrating injuries is usually performed. Orbital CT can help rule out the presence of intraocular foreign bodies, concurrent orbit fractures, and other head traumas. Patients should also receive tetanus booster and systemic antibiotics. In these cases, concurrent ocular injuries can include corneal opacification, hyphema (blood collecting in the anterior chamber), iridodialysis (dislocation of the iris from its root), lens dislocation, vitreous hemorrhage, retinal detachment, choroidal detachment, and optic nerve avulsion. Typically, additional injuries are managed after closure of the primary laceration.

If a foreign body is present, removal may accompany primary wound closure. Some materials, such as glass or stone, may be inert, but wood and organic material have high rates of infection, and metals such as iron and lead may cause toxicity (Fig. 25.5). Vitrectomy surgery is typically performed in order to remove posterior segment foreign bodies.

Other Forms of Trauma

The ophthalmologist often plays an important role in evaluating children and babies with non-accidental trauma. In these cases, a dilated retinal

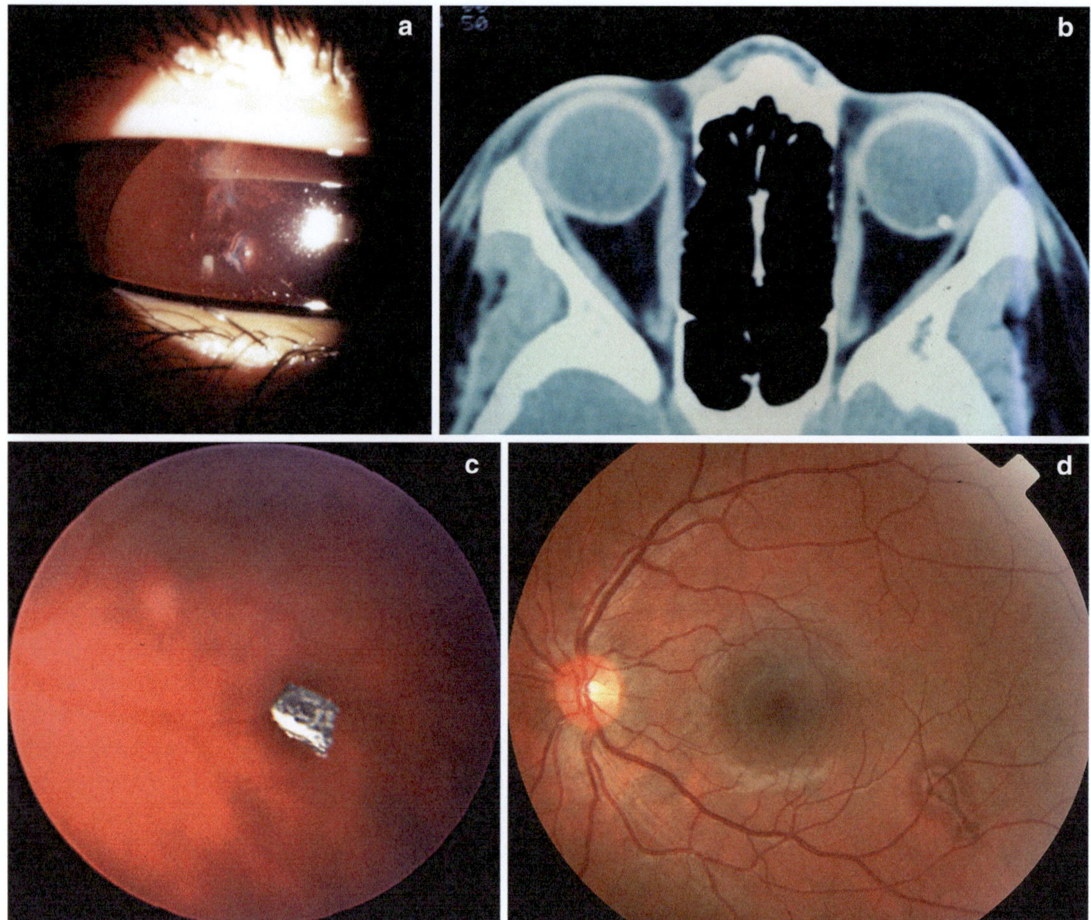

Fig. 25.5 Series of images associated with a metallic intraocular foreign body. (**a**) The anterior segment entry wound is seen, and a deep red reflex is suggestive of a vitreous hemorrhage. (**b**) CT scan shows a highly reflective foreign body in the posterior segment of the left globe. (**c**) Fundus image of a foreign body along a retinal blood vessel. (**d**) Fundus image of the left eye following vitrectomy and foreign body removal. A small scar and area of hemorrhage are noted along the retinal arcade, but the visual acuity was preserved because the impact was away from the fovea. (Courtesy of Dr. Hermann Schubert)

examination may demonstrate preretinal, intraretinal, and subretinal hemorrhages in multiple anatomical locations, which is suggestive of non-accidental etiology (Fig. 25.6). This may correlate with other non-ophthalmic clinical findings consistent with abuse, such as fractures and intracranial hemorrhage.

A severe Valsalva maneuver may lead to vitreous, subhyaloid, and intraretinal hemorrhage and vision loss. This is believed to occur because of sudden increase in intrathoracic pressure, leading to increased venous pressure and overload of the capillary system. Often, this may resolve spontaneously with observation, but vitrectomy surgery and Nd:YAG laser treatments to the internal limiting membrane have also been reported to be beneficial.

Because the crystalline lens is held in place by fragile fibers known as zonules, blunt trauma can result in dislocation of the natural lens or of a previously placed intraocular lens implant. Such an injury requires surgical repair. Patients with a history of Marfan syndrome or homocystinuria who have a risk for spontaneous lens dislocation

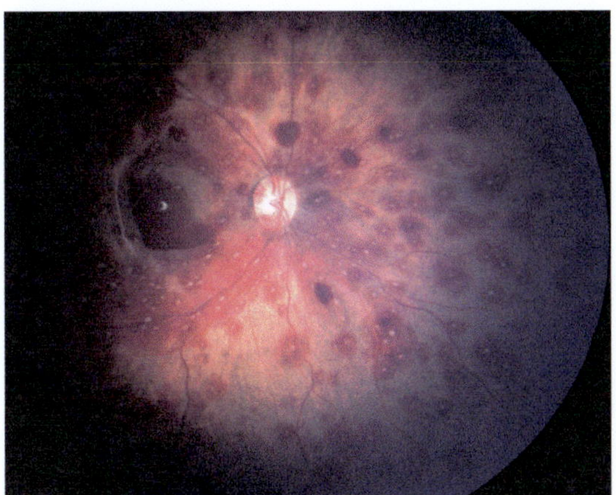

Fig. 25.6 Non-accidental trauma demonstrating multiple preretinal, intraretinal, and subretinal hemorrhages in a child, suggestive of non-accidental etiology. (Courtesy of Dr. Steven Brooks)

may exhibit such lens luxation after relatively minor trauma (Fig. 25.7a, b).

Two other forms of trauma can produce ocular consequences. In Terson's syndrome, a subdural or subarachnoid hemorrhage can lead to subretinal, intraretinal, and vitreous hemorrhage (Fig. 25.8). The specific mechanism of this is unknown. Purtscher retinopathy is a rare cause of sudden vision loss associated with trauma to either the head or thoracic cavity. Examination findings include multiple cotton wool spots, dot hemorrhages, and areas of retinal whitening called Purtscher flecken (Fig. 25.9). A Purtscher-like retinopathy has also been associated with acute pancreatitis, fat emboli, childbirth, and other systemic illnesses.

Conclusion

There are many potential causes of vision loss in trauma patients. To reduce morbidity, clinicians can advocate for the use of safety glasses and head protection, promote education concerning the risks involved when engaging in high-risk activities, and minimize the likelihood that such potentially devastating accidents occur. Unfortunately, not all trauma is preventable, but with prompt evaluation and treatment, many patients can retain vision. Because these injuries

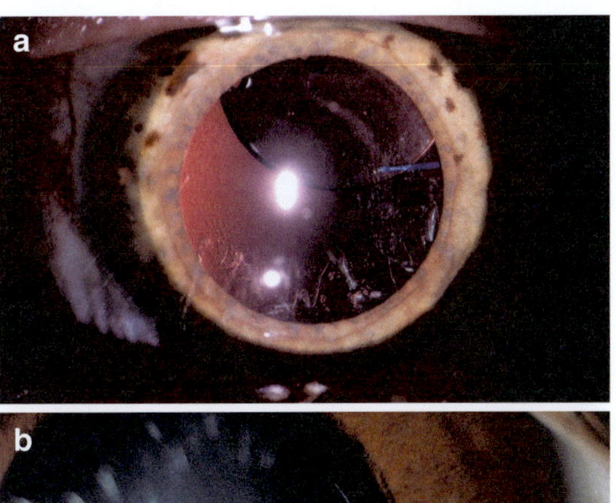

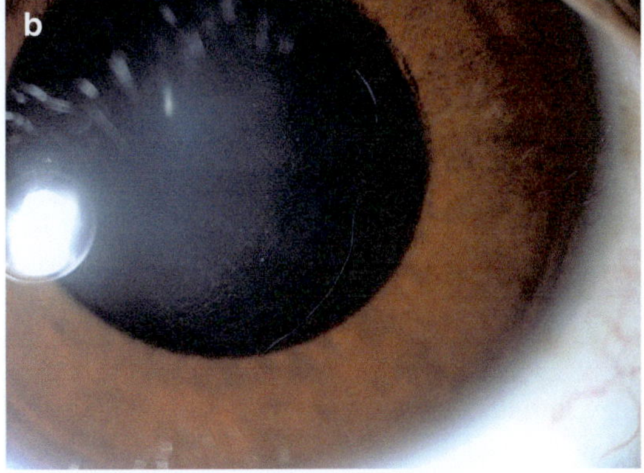

Fig. 25.7 (**a**) Post-traumatic superotemporally dislocated posterior chamber implanted intraocular lens. (**b**) Slit lamp photograph of a patient with Marfan syndrome and dislocated crystalline lens after minor trauma. The fine zonular fibers can be seen at the lens edge temporally

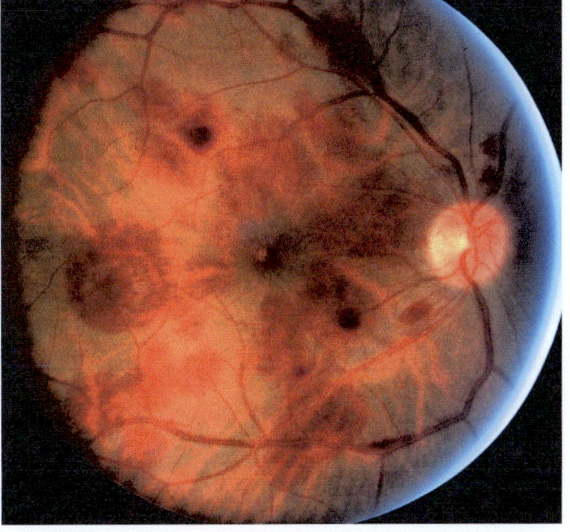

Fig. 25.8 Fundus image of a left eye in a patient with Terson's syndrome. Multiple subretinal, intraretinal, and preretinal hemorrhages are found with concurrent intracranial hemorrhage. (Courtesy of Dr. Hermann Schubert)

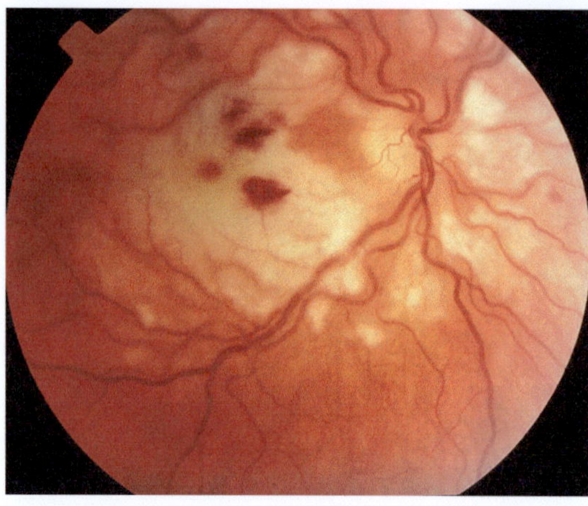

Fig. 25.9 Right eye fundus image of a patient with Purtscher retinopathy. The retina becomes whitened along with cotton wool spots and hemorrhages. Purtscher retinopathy usually accompanies head or thoracic trauma. A Purtscher-like retinopathy can also be seen in some systemic conditions. (Courtesy of Dr. Hermann Schubert)

may initially be asymptomatic, a high degree of suspicion and low threshold for referral should be considered with any patients who have a history of head injury, periorbital ecchymosis, or altered visual acuity.

Suggested Reading

Chaon BC, Lee MS. Is there treatment for traumatic optic neuropathy? Curr Opin Ophthalmol. 2015;26(6):445–9.

Gopal L, Sharma T, Bhende PS. Chapter 109: giant retinal tear. In: Wilkinson CP, Wiedemann P, editors. Retina, vol. 3. 5th ed. New York: Elsevier; 2013. p. 1844–51.

Kuhn F, Pieramici DJ. Ocular trauma principles and practice. New York: Thieme; 2002.

Kuhn F, Morris R, Witherspoon CD, Mann L. Epidemiology of blinding trauma in the United States Eye Injury Registry. Ophthalmic Epidemiol. 2006;13(3):209–16.

Recchia FM, Sternberg P Jr. Chapter 110: Surgery for ocular trauma, principles and techniques of treatment. In: Wilkinson CP, Wiedemann P, editors. Retina, vol. 3. 5th ed. New York: Elsevier; 2013. p. 1852–75.

Sabella P, Bottoni F, Staurenghi G. Spectral-domain OCT evaluation of Nd:YAG laser treatment for Valsalva retinopathy. Graefes Arch Clin Exp Ophthalmol. 2010;248(4):599–601.

Williams DF, Mieler WF, Gilliams GA. Posterior segment manifestations of ocular trauma. Retina. 1990;10:S35–44.

Inherited Retinal Dystrophies

26

Gregory Stein, Tarun Sharma, Thiago Cabral, Stephen Tsang, and Wendy Chung

Background

Inherited retinal dystrophies (IRDs) include a diverse group of retinal disorders, and our knowledge of these diseases has grown tremendously with advances in imaging and genetics. In some cases, the cause is an abnormality that affects the retina in isolation, whereas in others the retinal dystrophy may be part of a syndrome that affects multiple organ systems. This section will describe the evaluation of patients with suspected retinal dystrophies and will characterize some of the more common dystrophies encountered.

G. Stein, MD (✉)
Uptown Retina and Vitreous of New York, New York, NY, USA
e-mail: gstein@uptownretinany.com

T. Sharma, MD
Department of Ophthalmology, Edward S. Harkness Eye Institute, Columbia University Vagelos College of Physicians and Surgeons, New York, NY, USA

T. Cabral, PhD
Department of Ophthalmology, University Federal of Sao Paulo, Sao Paulo, Brazil

S. Tsang, MD, PhD
Departments of Ophthalmology and Pathology and Cell Biology, Harkness Eye Institute, Columbia University Vagelos College of Physicians and Surgeons, New York, NY, USA

W. Chung, MD, PhD
Department of Pediatrics, Columbia University Irving Medical Center, New York, NY, USA

History and Examination

Evaluation begins with a careful history of systemic and visual symptoms. Important parts of the history include age of onset, laterality, nyctalopia (night blindness), hemeralopia (day blindness), and visual distortion. A family history is critical and can help narrow the differential diagnosis and later guide genetic testing. Examination includes visual acuity and field testing, as well as a detailed fundus examination. The evaluation is often supplemented by imaging that includes color fundus photography, spectral domain ocular coherence tomography (OCT), blue autofluorescence (BAF), and near-infrared autofluorescence (NrAF). Electroretinography (ERG) and other electrodiagnostic modalities play an important role in the diagnosis and monitoring of retinal diseases. Electrodiagnostic testing can specifically pinpoint the location of a retinal abnormality by distinguishing dysfunctional rod photoreceptors, cone photoreceptors, and retinal pigment epithelium (RPE) cells. Lastly, confirmation with gene testing plays an increasingly critical role in diagnosis and management of IRDs.

© Springer Nature Switzerland AG 2019
D. S. Casper, G. A. Cioffi (eds.), *The Columbia Guide to Basic Elements of Eye Care*,
https://doi.org/10.1007/978-3-030-10886-1_26

Selected Common Inherited Retinal Dystrophies

Retinitis Pigmentosa

Retinitis pigmentosa (RP) is a degenerative retinal disease that primarily affects rod photoreceptors or light-sensing (primarily peripheral black and white light) cells. The estimated prevalence of RP in the USA and Europe is 1 in 3000–4000. As our understanding and ability to analyze retinal disease has increased, it has become apparent that RP is remarkably heterogenous, affecting different parts of photoreceptor cells differently and having different underlying causes. However, clinicians currently unify many of these different diseases under the umbrella diagnosis of RP.

More than 70 genes and over 3000 mutations are known to cause non-syndromic RP, leading to disease heterogeneity. Ultimately, these mutations cause rod photoreceptor death, which secondarily leads to death of cone photoreceptors (responsible for central color vision) and migration of retinal pigment epithelium. Mutations in the gene that encodes rhodopsin, the visual pigment in rods that mediates night vision, were among the first to be associated with RP. RP is inherited as autosomal dominant in approximately 10–20% of cases (26 gene mutations), autosomal recessive in 20% (over 50 genes), and X-linked recessive in 10% (2 genes). Around 40% of RP is sporadic, with no family history, and this presentation is known as RP simplex.

As RP has many different underlying causes, clinical features vary. The age of symptom onset varies from early childhood to adulthood, but it is common for people to notice vision impairment in the teenage years. Individuals with X-linked recessive RP usually have more severe disease and present with earlier onset; the converse is true for autosomal dominant RP, that is, they have less severe disease with later onset. Nyctalopia is a hallmark feature of the disease and is due to the rod photoreceptor defect. Patients may, for example, report trouble orienting themselves in a dark environment, such as finding seats in a crowded movie theater or driving at night. Peripheral visual field constriction is another important feature of this disease. Visual field constriction becomes very debilitating, and though acuity may be retained, the "tunnel vision" of advanced RP is often enough to qualify for legal blindness and preclude driving.

Clinical findings may vary significantly in terms of onset and severity; there are, however, some common findings. Visual field testing typically shows a constricted field early in the disease course, with gradual progression over time. Most patients retain good acuity until late in the disease, but vision is commonly affected to some degree. Some RP cases eventually result in no light perception (NLP, i.e., total blindness) vision.

The classic retinal findings in RP exhibit three components: retinal vessel attenuation, waxy pallor of the optic nerve, and intraretinal pigment migration producing a "bone-spicule" appearance (Fig. 26.1). These changes result from photoreceptor cell death. Cataracts, often the posterior subcapsular type, frequently form at an earlier age in patients with RP as compared with normal patients. Cystoid macular edema (CME) and a Coats-like response (an exudative vasculopathy which resembles Coats disease, showing telangiectasia, aneurysmal dilation and peripheral capillary dropout, and extravascular lipid deposits) may also occur simultaneously and contribute to reduced visual acuity in these patients at an earlier age.

Full-field ERG testing usually shows severely decreased rod function and diminished cone response that subsequently worsens over time.

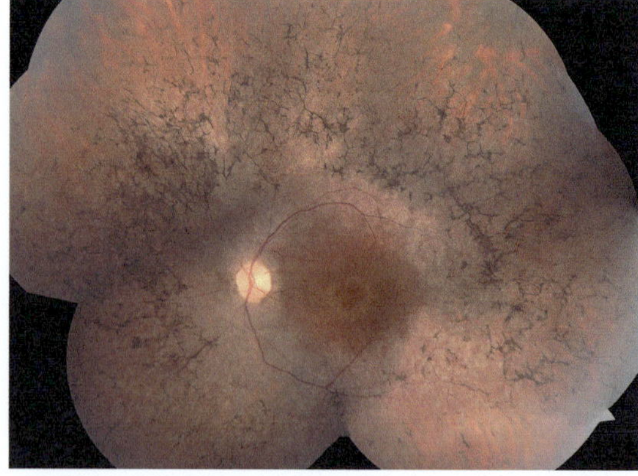

Fig. 26.1 Color photograph of the left eye of a patient with retinitis pigmentosa demonstrating pallor of the optic nerve, attenuation of the vasculature, and pigment abnormalities in the peripheral retina, which are also referred to as bone spicules

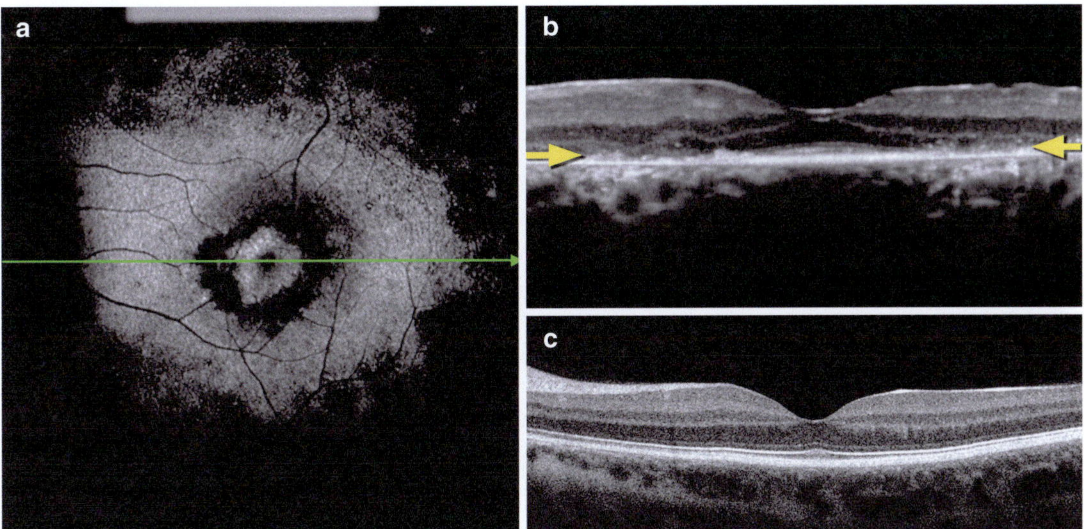

Fig. 26.2 (**a**) Autofluorescence of the left eye in the same patient demonstrating extensive loss of photoreceptors sparing the fovea. (**b**) An OCT-B scan which shows a retinal cross section corresponding to the green line seen in the left AF image. There is disorganization of outer retinal layers, including the outer nuclear layer and ellipsoid zone, in the region between the yellow arrows. (**c**) An OCT-B scan of a normal retina for comparison, to show normal outer retinal architecture

OCT imaging shows the extent of photoreceptor loss, with disorganization of outer retinal layers, including the outer nuclear and ellipsoid zone in regions of photoreceptor loss (Fig. 26.2). Autofluorescence (AF) imaging generally shows decreased autofluorescence in the regions of photoreceptor and retinal pigment epithelium (RPE) atrophy. A hyperautofluorescent ring delineates the abnormal retina from normal retina (Fig. 26.3). Serial longitudinal AF and OCT imaging show a progressively shrinking area of a healthy retina.

RP may be associated with disorders involving other organ systems. In Usher syndrome, RP is associated with varying degrees of congenital sensorineural hearing loss. In Bardet-Biedl syndrome, severe RP is associated with obesity, diabetes, polydactyly, and decreased cognitive function.

Annual follow-up is recommended after the diagnosis has been made. Serial electrodiagnostic testing and imaging can show the disease progression and help predict visual prognosis. There is evidence that supplementation with high-dose vitamin A may preserve some cone function. Dark sunglasses with UV filtering may also be protective. Patients with CME are monitored more frequently and treated with topical or systemic

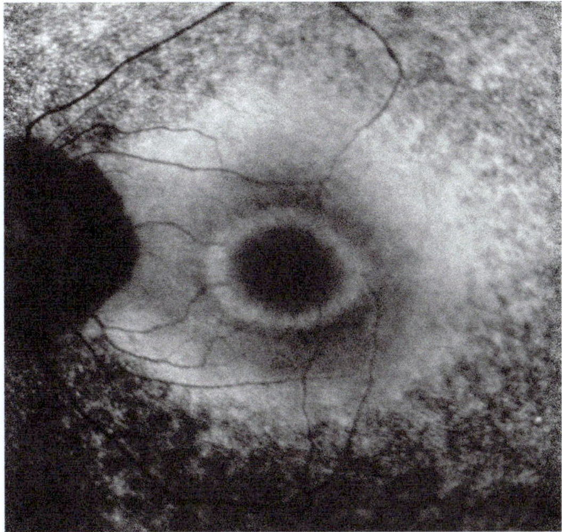

Fig. 26.3 Autofluorescence (AF) image of the left eye of a patient showing decreased AF in the periphery and a hyperautofluorescent ring in the macula, delineating normal retina from atrophic retina

carbonic-anhydrase inhibitors. These medications are effective, if indicated. Cataract surgery should be considered with caution. While every effort to optimize vision should be undertaken, cataract surgery will not result in improved acuity if the retina is severely compromised. Genetic testing and gene therapy are becoming more important in RP and will be covered later in the chapter.

Depending on the mutation, prognosis varies considerably. Visual field constriction often becomes severe enough to warrant a cane or guide dog, although a very narrow window of central acuity may be preserved. Central vision may, however, be affected directly by photoreceptor degeneration, or by CME, and in rare cases may progress to NLP vision.

Choroideremia

Choroideremia (CHM), an X-linked recessive disorder, is another common inherited retinal dystrophy. Symptoms are similar to those of retinitis pigmentosa. Patients have poor peripheral vision bilaterally (manifest as a ring scotoma), which deteriorates over time. The most notable clinical findings include severe chorioretinal atrophy, leaving behind visible bare sclera on ophthalmoscopy, and photoreceptor cell death; the choroid is involved primarily, with retinal degeneration occurring secondarily. Chorioretinal atrophy begins peripherally and encroaches centripetally on the macula, but most patients preserve central visual acuity (Fig. 26.4). End-stage

CHM can be indistinguishable from end-stage RP. ERG testing shows reduced rod and cone function. The diagnosis can be confirmed with a genetic test, as CHM is caused by a defect in Rab escort protein 1 (REP1) on the CHM gene on the X chromosome. Because of the X chromosome location, only males are affected in choroideremia. Gene therapy trials are ongoing.

Gyrate Atrophy

Gyrate atrophy is another retinal dystrophy that produces severe chorioretinal degeneration. A sharply defined, scalloped appearance of the peripheral atrophic border distinguishes it from choroideremia (Fig. 26.5); unlike in CHM, subjects with gyrate show areas of hyperpigmentation of the remaining RPE. Over time, these edges become less scalloped, and the retina takes on a more diffusely atrophic appearance. Similar to choroideremia and RP, patients will present with nyctalopia and peripheral vision loss. Gyrate atrophy is inherited in an autosomal recessive manner and is due to a defect in the enzyme ornithine-ketoacid aminotransferase, which leads to high levels of plasma ornithine. Limiting arginine intake and supplementation with vitamin B6 (pyridoxin) are recommended to reduce disease

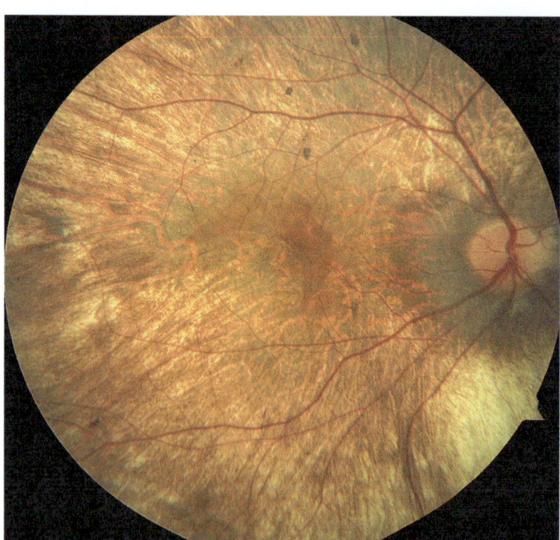

Fig. 26.4 Color fundus photo of the right eye of a patient with choroideremia showing a white-appearing fundus due to the loss of the retinal pigment epithelium and choroid, which permits visibility of the outer sclera

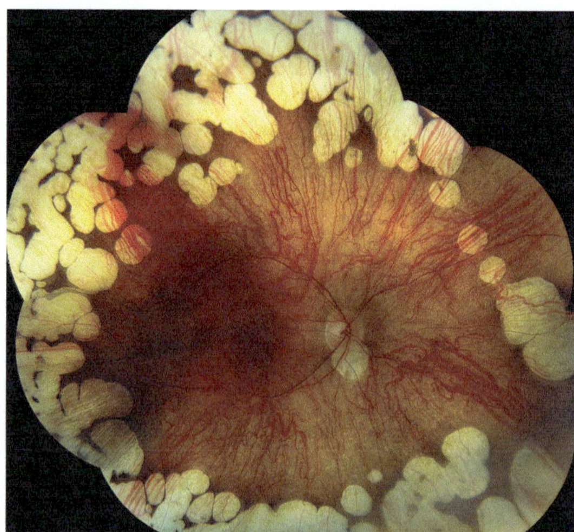

Fig. 26.5 Color fundus photograph of the right eye of a patient with gyrate atrophy showing confluent patches of atrophic retina and choroid in the peripheral fundus

progression. Gyrate atrophy is one of the better-known retinal dystrophies secondary to a metabolic derangement.

Leber Congenital Amaurosis

Leber congenital amaurosis (LCA) is a severe, progressive retinal dystrophy that appears at birth. Its prevalence ranges from 1/50,000 to 1/100,000. Classic features include an absence of fixation, which is usually noticed at around 6 weeks, sensory nystagmus, amaurotic or nonreactive pupils, high hyperopia, and marked dysfunction of both rod and cone photoreceptors on ERG. Vision is poor, ranging from 20/200 to no light perception. The oculodigital sign, in which infants repeatedly press on their eye with their fingers or knuckles, may be present. The fundus examination may be normal-appearing or have a range of abnormal findings such as attenuated vessels, macular atrophy, bone-spicule pigmentary changes, or clumping. LCA is inherited in an autosomal recessive fashion, and mutations in over 20 different genes have been identified. In December 2017, the FDA approved Luxturna (voretigene neparvovec-rzyl) for the treatment of patients with confirmed biallelic RPE 65 mutation-associated retinal dystrophy. Luxturna works by delivering a normal copy of the RPE 65 gene directly to retinal cells.

Achromatopsia

Achromatopsia, or rod monochromatism, is a hereditary, stationary retinal disorder that is characterized by abnormal function of cone photoreceptors; these subjects have normal rod function. Cone photoreceptors are responsible for color perception and fine detail discrimination under lighted conditions. Due to an apparent absence of all cone function, these patients see everything in shades of gray (total color blindness). The prevalence is approximately 1 in 30,000 people. It presents in infancy with pendular nystagmus, photosensitivity, and poor fixation and typically remains stable over time (hence, "stationary"). Examination shows poor visual acuity, and the fundus may be unremarkable or have macular atrophy or pigmentary mottling. Visual acuity is typically 20/200 or less, but it may be better if there is partial cone function. Electrophysiological testing shows abnormal cone function and normal rod function. Of note, the severity and prevalence of achromatopsia are different to red-green color blindness which impairs red- and green-sensing cones to varying degrees and is present in up to 8% of the male population. Patients with achromatopsia require special assistance from an early age, as with LCA, and benefit from red-tinted glasses or contact lenses. Gene therapy trials to treat achromatopsia caused by CNGA3 and CNGB3 are ongoing.

Cone Dystrophy

Cone dystrophy includes a group of progressive disorders that primarily affect cone photoreceptors, thus compromising central vision more than peripheral. While conditions which cause destruction of rod photoreceptors often secondarily affect cone photoreceptors, the reverse is not true, and rod functioning is maintained. Symptoms include hemeralopia (more difficulty seeing in bright light, the opposite of nyctalopia) and photosensitivity (photoaversion). In contrast to patients with rod dystrophies, who see poorly in the dark, these patients report that their night vision is actually much better and that using sunglasses enhances their quality of vision when in bright light. Patients may benefit from wearing tinted glasses in indoor environments as well. Visual acuity is impaired initially and deteriorates over time to 20/200 or even counting fingers. Color perception, which is determined by cone photoreceptors, will be diminished as well. The fundus examination typically presents with a mottled macula, giving it a bull's-eye appearance (bull's-eye maculopathy, BEM) (Fig. 26.6). ERG establishes the diagnosis by demonstrating abnormal cone function and preserved rod function. The fundus autofluorescence (FAF) shows alternating areas of hypo- and hyperautofluorescence in the early stage and more areas of hypofluorescence as RPE atrophy sets in. In some, rod photoreceptors also get involved, leading to cone-rod dystrophy (CORD).

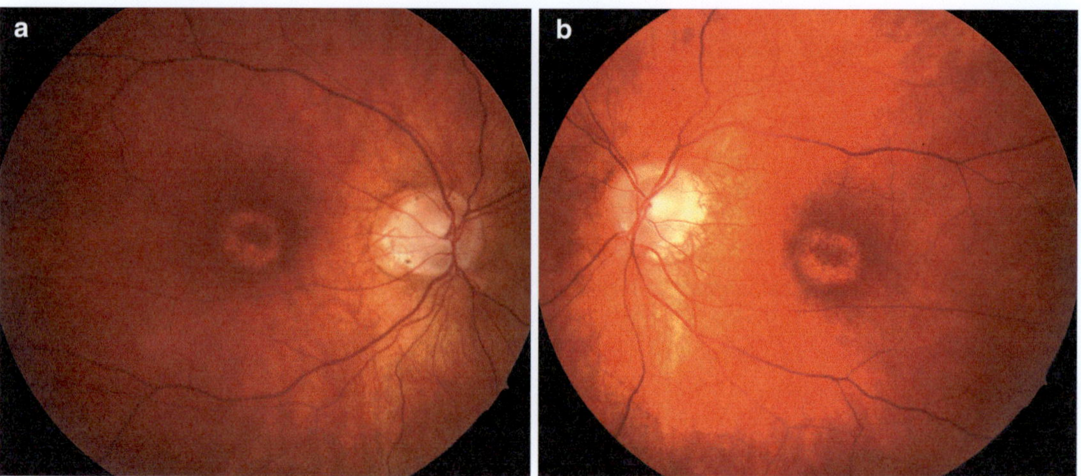

Fig. 26.6 Color fundus photos in cone dystrophy (**a** right eye and **b** left eye) showing a bull's-eye pattern of depigmentation in the macula, where cone photoreceptor concentration is the highest

Stargardt Disease

Stargardt disease (STGD) is the most common juvenile-onset macular dystrophy, with a prevalence of around 1 in 8000–10,000. It is an autosomal recessive disease caused by a mutation in the ABCA4 gene, which encodes a transport protein located in photoreceptor outer segments. The ABCA4 gene is long, and there are many known mutations, producing a spectrum of severity. Patients typically report blurred vision in early adolescence, and visual acuity deteriorates over time. End-stage acuity approaches 20/200 or worse in most people. While it is a disabling disease, patients usually maintain ambulatory vision. Clinical findings include yellow flecks at the level of the retinal pigment epithelium located in the macula; when flecks are seen all over the posterior pole, it is called fundus flavimaculatus. Those who develop STGD at a later age retain better vision for a longer period, and only 30% of them show flecks.

Flecks represent deposition of lipofuscin in the retinal pigment epithelium, a histological landmark of STGD. These pisciform, round or dotlike yellowish lesions change their distribution over time. Peripapillary sparing is one of the characteristics of STGD. The macula often has a bull's-eye pattern or beaten-bronze appearance, and in later disease stages, there may be large areas of macular atrophy (Fig. 26.7a). Classically, fluorescein angiography was used to diagnose the disease by demonstrating a "silent choroid," reflecting decreased identifiable fluorescence due to blockage by an accumulation of lipofuscin pigment. More recently, autofluorescence (AF), a noninvasive imaging technique, has been used. On fundus autofluorescence, newer flecks appear hyperautofluorescent, while older ones become hypoautofluorescent with time. This finding may also be highlighted by the presence of adjacent large areas of decreased, normal autofluorescence due to atrophy of the RPE and overlying photoreceptors (Fig. 26.7b). ERG testing may be helpful in categorizing the severity of Stargardt disease and determining prognosis. There is no known treatment. Genetic testing helps to confirm the diagnosis in many cases as clinical features can overlap with other retinal diseases. Some suggest that vitamin A supplementation, which is recommended in many types of retinitis pigmentosa, may be deleterious in Stargardt disease. As with any of the retinal dystrophies with pediatric onset, children with this disease may benefit from community and educational programs that are designed for the visually impaired. Since children with this disease have normal vision at birth and disease onset is gradual, diagnosis may be delayed, with subsequent poor school performance if it is not recognized

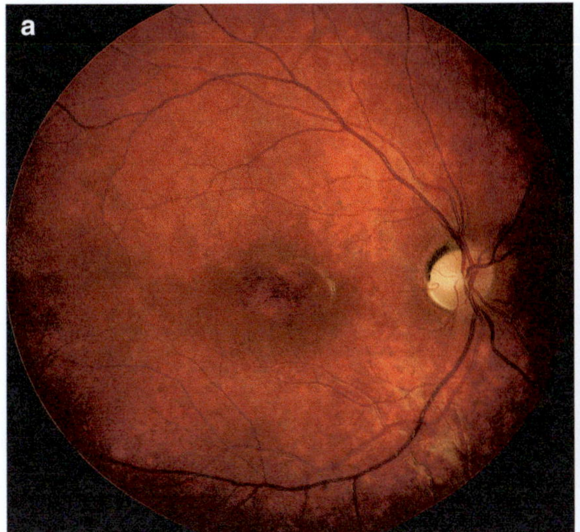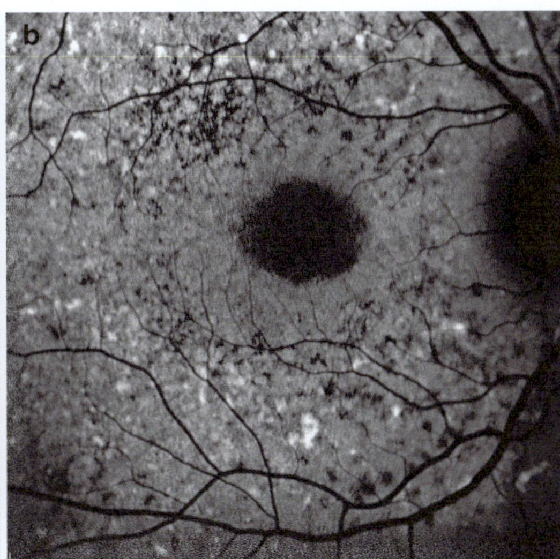

Fig. 26.7 (**a**) Color photograph showing a well-circumscribed, oval loss of pigment in the macula, and pale, pisciform flakes that extend from the paramacular area to the midperiphery in a patient with Stargardt dis-ease. (**b**) Autofluorescence (AF) image of the same patient which shows decreased AF in the macula in a bull's-eye pattern and peripheral flecks of increased and decreased AF

promptly and managed appropriately. Deuterium enrichment of vitamin A at the C20 position for the treatment of Stargardt disease is in clinical trials. Another drug, emixustat hydrochloride, is being evaluated to treat subjects with macular atrophy secondary to STGD.

Best Disease

Best disease is another common retinal dystrophy that primarily affects the macula. It is an autosomal dominant disease with a prevalence of 1/70,000. Caused by a mutation in the bestrophin gene, it typically manifests in the teenage years. Visual acuity may be better than the fundus examination would suggest and may range from minimal impairment to 20/200, but most patients have around 20/80 vision. The disease has a well-known and characteristic natural history. Initially, there are bilateral vitelliform lesions (round, yellowish spots resembling an egg yolk) present in the macula. Over time, this lesion fragments and loses its bright-yellow appearance. As the material breaks down, there is a clear fluid in the upper part and yellowish material in the lower part, giving a picture of "pseudohypopyon" (Fig. 26.8a).

Later in the disease, the vitelliform material disintegrates, leaving behind a mottled macula with damaged photoreceptors, described as vitelliruptive stage and later, eventually, an atrophic scar (Fig. 26.8b). In some patients the disease may be complicated by the formation of a choroidal neovascular membrane, which may subsequently hemorrhage. OCT shows hyperreflective material in the subretinal space. Fundus autofluorescence appearance varies with the clinical appearance: intense hyperAF is seen in the beginning, and usually the pattern changes as the lesion passes through various stages. The electrooculogram (EOG) in Best disease is pathognomonic, showing a "light-rise" pattern.

X-Linked Juvenile Retinoschisis

X-linked juvenile retinoschisis (XLRS) is another common macular dystrophy, with a prevalence of 1/5000–1/25,000. It occurs only in males and may present from birth to adolescence. The retinoschisis (splitting of the retinal layers) may extend outside of the macula, but peripheral vision is usually preserved. Examination is characterized by bilateral superficial cysts arranged in a stellate pattern

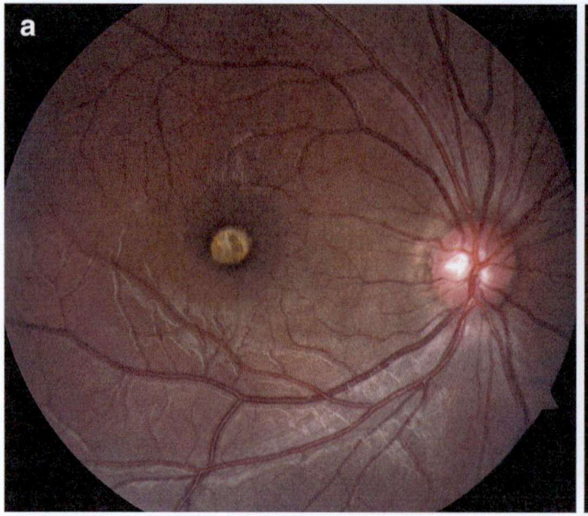

Fig. 26.8 (**a**) Color fundus photo in Best disease shows a vitelliform lesion in the central macula in the early phase of the disease. (**b**) Color fundus photo in long-standing Best disease shows central macular atrophy following breakdown of the vitelliform lesion

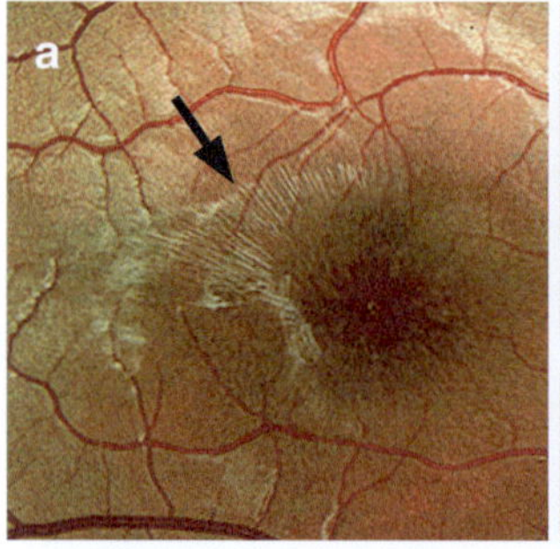
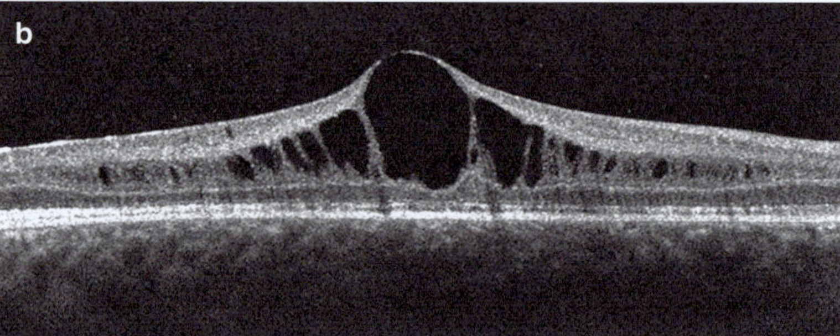

Fig. 26.9 (**a**) Color fundus photo of the right eye in X-linked retinoschisis demonstrating striae (arrows) consistent with foveal schisis and (**b**) SD-OCT-B scan showing retinoschisis in the fovea predominantly in the inner nuclear layers, extending from the optic nerve across the length of the macula

with fine retinal striae, extending outward from the fovea, known as foveal schisis (Fig. 26.9a). OCT demonstrates separation of the retinal layers (schisis) predominantly within the inner nuclear layer (Fig. 26.9b). Full-field ERG shows decreased b-wave amplitude with preserved a-wave, so the alteration of b/a ratio (a-wave amplitude exceeding the b-wave amplitude (negative waveform)) is an important diagnostic feature. XLRS is caused by a defect in the gene RS1, which encodes the protein retinoschisin, and is believed to lead to degeneration of retinal Müller cells. Visual acuity is typically around 20/80 but may be more severely affected over time. Possible complications include vitreous hemorrhage, retinal detachment, and macular hole development. Topical dorzolamide has been shown to decrease retinal edema in these patients. Vitreoretinal surgery is needed in those who develop vitreous hemorrhage or rhegmatogenous retinal detachment. Gene therapy trials are ongoing.

Gene Testing

As in other areas of medicine, genetic testing of retinal dystrophies has been transformative in our evaluation, diagnosis, and management of these diseases. Some of the named retinal dystrophies exhibit a range of phenotypes and severity and are associated with a number of different mutations. In these cases, only genetic testing can verify a diagnosis. In the years ahead, retinal dystrophy nomenclature will likely evolve, as the identification of gene mutations correctly distinguishes diseases that present similarly but can be attributed to different mutations.

In the past, genetic testing for retinal dystrophies may have been a purely academic exercise, but today, diagnosis is essential: not only may it establish a definitive diagnosis, but it may impact treatment. Gene therapy trials for many retinal dystrophies, including Leber congenital amaurosis, autosomal recessive RP, achromatopsia, X-linked recessive RP, Usher syndrome, choroideremia, Stargardt disease, and X-linked retinoschisis, are currently underway. Voretigene neparvovec, administered in the subretinal space, approved by the FDA in 2017, is the first gene therapy to treat Leber congenital amaurosis caused by mutation in RPE 65.

Unfortunately, genetic testing is still quite expensive and frequently not covered by insurance. Hopefully, this will change in the near future. To test most efficiently, it is best if a group of genes can be tested collectively; if these tests are negative, or if a disease is rare, one may then test for a broad range of retinal dystrophies or perform whole-exome or whole-genome sequencing, which usually requires samples from family members.

Only after a genetic mutation has been established can genetic therapy be considered. Gene therapy involves the delivery of an agent that can correct for a specific mutation. Current genetic medicine therapy trials for retinal dystrophies use a virus vector to introduce genetic material with the correct gene into host cells. In the future, gene therapy may use a new strategy that involves clustered, regularly interspaced, short palindromic repeats (CRISPR). While genetic medicine techniques introduce a new copy of the defective gene, the goal of CRISPR, also known as "genome surgery," is to repair a mutation, with resultant production of a functional protein.

Retinal dystrophies are unique among inherited diseases because of their great potential to benefit from gene therapy. The ability to easily visualize the retina and directly treat it with gene therapy is a feature not found elsewhere in the body. Extensive monitoring of the retina after intervention can be accomplished with physical examination and imaging, which are harmless, noninvasive procedures. Methods currently in clinical trials for the delivery of gene therapies include intravitreal and subretinal injections. These procedures are quick and relatively inexpensive and have a low risk of systemic side effects (See Appendix 1).

Stem cell therapy for retinal dystrophies is also being investigated. Currently, there are stem cell clinical trials for the treatment of Stargardt disease and retinitis pigmentosa, as well as other retinal diseases including age-related macular degeneration.

Whereas the goal of gene therapy is to halt progression of disease, the goal of stem cell therapy is to restore retinal function with new retinal tissue. For this to take place, several difficult steps must occur: Implanted stem cells must differentiate into operative neurosensory tissue and, posteriorly, must establish appropriate connections with the RPE and choroidal blood supply. On the inner retinal side, implanted cells must develop functioning connections with neural retina to transmit information to the visual pathway via ganglion cell axons that constitute the optic nerve. Only when construction of this complex chain is achievable will such therapies offer hope for reversing the visual impairments of these devastating diseases.

Suggested Reading

Chapter 3: Retinal physiology and psychophysics, in the basic and clinical science course: section 12. Am Acad Ophthalmol. 2012–2013.

Lin MK, Tsai YT, Tsang SH. Emerging treatments for retinitis pigmentosa: genes and stem cells, as well as new electronic and medical therapies, are gaining ground. Retin Physician. 2015;12:52–70.

Tsui I, Song B, Lin CS, Tsang SH. A practical approach to retinal dystrophies. Retin Physician. 2007;4:18–26.

Michael Jay Weiss and Albert J. Hofeldt

Uveitis, strictly defined, represents inflammation of the uveal tract, which includes the iris, ciliary body, and choroid. However, the term uveitis, as used by clinicians, is more commonly an all-encompassing term for inflammation anywhere within the eye. To illustrate this point, ocular toxoplasmosis, the most common cause of posterior "uveitis" in North America, is actually a primary "retinitis" and therefore would not be considered a true uveitis. Scleritis, a disease commonly managed by uveitis specialists, is also technically not a uveitis, as the sclera is not a uveal tract component.

The impact of uveitis varies globally and is region-dependent. In the United States, uveitis is only the fifth or sixth leading cause of blindness, but because it can occur in all age groups, uveitis may lead to more years of vision loss than other age-related ocular diseases. In a population-based study known as the Northern California Epidemiology of Uveitis Study, the prevalence and incidence of uveitis were 115.3/100,000 and 52.4/100,000, respectively.

Presumed Pathogenesis of Uveitis

When attempting to establish an etiology for uveitis, there are three broad differential diagnostic categories: infectious, noninfectious (also referred to as autoimmune or auto-inflammatory) with or without associated systemic disease, and masquerade syndromes (such as carcinoma or other entities which mimic uveitis). In stud antibodies which ies looking at uveitis prevalence, 80–90% of cases were noninfectious. Clinical and experimental evidence suggests that immunological mechanisms (either autoimmune or immune-mediated) are involved in the pathogenesis of most cases of noninfectious uveitis.

Due to the developmental origin and physiologic factors that modulate immune responses, the eye is considered immunologically privileged. In the mid-twentieth century, Peter B. Medawar discovered that tumor tissue from one animal grafted subcutaneously into another was quickly destroyed, whereas similar tissue placed within the anterior chamber of the eye survived for an indefinite period. Investigators concluded that the combination of absence of lymphatic drainage and physiologic ocular barriers prevented the immune system from becoming aware of, and responding to antigens in such "privileged" sites. However, in 1987, Streilein observed that foreign tissue placed into the anterior chamber of rabbit and rat eyes did induce serum antibodies, which would not be possible if antigens in privileged sites were truly sequestered. Thus, it was concluded that immune

M. J. Weiss, MD, PhD (✉)
Department of Ophthalmology, Edward S. Harkness
Eye Institute, Columbia University Vagelos College
of Physicians and Surgeons, New York, NY, USA
e-mail: mjw2@cumc.columbia.edu

A. J. Hofeldt, MD
AMA Optics, Miami Beach, FL, USA

© Springer Nature Switzerland AG 2019
D. S. Casper, G. A. Cioffi (eds.), *The Columbia Guide to Basic Elements of Eye Care*,
https://doi.org/10.1007/978-3-030-10886-1_27

privilege does not lead to immunologic ignorance of the antigen but rather an altered immunologic response in the eye; this has been termed Anterior Chamber-Associated Immune Deviation (ACAID). Ocular features felt to confer this unique regional immunology include:

- Deficient efferent-draining *lymphatics*, aqueous fluid that has crossed the trabecular meshwork directly enters the blood vasculature via aqueous veins.
- *Blood-ocular barriers*, which include the blood-aqueous barrier provided by the nonpigmented ciliary body epithelium and the endothelium of iris capillaries and the blood-retinal barrier, consisting of the retinal pigment epithelium and retinal vascular endothelium.
- *Minimal MHC class II molecule* expression on intraocular cells.
- A microenvironment of *immunosuppressive soluble factors* secreted by macrophages and dendritic cells that lead to unique processing of antigens by the eye.

The major consequences of ACAID include activation of T-regulatory cells that suppress induction of delayed-type hypersensitivity (DTH), unimpaired cytotoxic T-cell responses, and altered humoral immunity with upregulation of non-complement binding antibodies and impaired production of complement-fixing antibodies. Streilein called ACAID a "dangerous compromise," as DTH generally provides an overall better immune defense but is also capable of causing severe intraocular inflammation. Teleologically, ACAID can be thought of as an evolutionary trait that evolved to preserve the visual system from potentially damaging effects of inflammation while still permitting selective immunity. Immune privilege is not absolute. When confronted with a serious challenge, patients with uveitis experience breakdown of the blood-ocular barrier and loss of immune privilege.

Evaluation of a Uveitis Patient

Evaluation of a patient with uveitis begins with a thorough history, followed by a complete ocular examination. Based on the history and physical exam, a differential diagnosis is generated, leading to a targeted laboratory work-up to help establish a specific diagnosis. Depending on the final diagnosis, the safest and most effective treatment strategy is devised and implemented.

History

A complete and detailed medical history is essential in the evaluation of uveitis. This begins with the age, gender, geographic location of residence and travel, and ethnic origins of the patient – information that may prove extremely helpful in diagnosis. For example, sarcoid uveitis is more prevalent in black females with a regional predilection in the southeastern part of the United States, Behçet's disease has a male preponderance and is more commonly seen in the Middle East and Eastern Asia, and Vogt-Koyanagi-Harada disease (VKH, or uveomeningitis syndrome) has a predilection for dark-skinned patients of Hispanic, Asian, and Native American ancestry.

The chief ocular complaint is identified. Uveitis may present with or without symptoms, and this is important to establish, to help determine appropriate follow-up care intervals. If present, symptoms in anterior uveitis include ocular pain, tenderness, erythema, and photophobia. Posterior segment uveitis patients tend to complain more of floaters and blurred vision. A list of symptoms and potentially associated uveitic/systemic conditions are listed in Table 27.1.

Chronology and course of the present problem and any prior treatment are explored in detail, along with other relevant past ocular history. It is especially important to determine the presence of preexisting glaucoma or cataract, since corticosteroids, the mainstay of uveitis treatment, may raise intraocular pressures in some patients and accelerate cataract formation.

A careful review of the patient's past medical history is made. Although uveitis may be a local disorder restricted to the eye (such as Fuchs' heterochromic iridocyclitis (FHI), birdshot chorioretinopathy (BSCR), or pars planitis), it is often a manifestation of underlying systemic disease. Examples of systemic diseases associated with

Table 27.1 Symptoms and potentially associated uveitic/systemic conditions

Physical signs/symptoms	Potential associated uveitic/systemic conditions
Arthritis/joint pain	Ankylosing spondylitis, inflammatory bowel disease, Behçet's, sarcoidosis, reactive arthritis, psoriasis, Lyme, JIA
Diarrhea/bloody stools	Inflammatory bowel disease, reactive arthritis, Whipple's
Cutaneous	
Mouth or genital sores	Behçet's, reactive arthritis, syphilis
Skin rash	Syphilis, sarcoidosis, Lyme, SLE
Vitiligo, alopecia poliosis	VKH, sympathetic ophthalmia
Skin nodules	Sarcoidosis, leprosy, onchocerciasis
Weakness, numbness	Demyelinating disease, steroid-induced myopathy
Shortness of breath, cough	Sarcoidosis, tuberculosis, malignancy, vasculitis
Headaches, meningismus, hearing loss	VKH, sarcoidosis, vasculitis, Behçet's
Hematuria, UTI	Reactive arthritis, vasculitis

uveitis include rheumatoid arthritis, sarcoidosis, Behçet's disease, demyelinating disease, HLA B27-related spondyloarthropathies, Sjögren's syndrome, inflammatory bowel disease (IBD), and vasculitides. Careful attention to a patient's medical status is also important in determining the potential safety profile of any intended treatment decisions.

Factors which may predispose to the development of uveitis and should be identified include:

Past Medical History
- Joint pain or arthritis (consider juvenile idiopathic arthritis (JIA), sarcoidosis, ankylosing spondylitis, or reactive arthritis (Reiter's syndrome))
- Gastrointestinal symptoms such as abdominal pain, bloody stools, or chronic diarrhea (consider inflammatory bowel disease (IBD), reactive arthritis, Whipple's Disease, or *giardia*)
- Skin disease, including rashes, ulcers, or vitiligo (consider VKH, psoriasis, sarcoidosis, syphilis, Behçet's, Kawasaki's, or Lyme)
- Pulmonary symptoms such as coughing, hemoptysis, fevers, or shortness of breath (consider sarcoidosis, *Mycobacterium tuberculosis* or granulomatous polyangiitis (GPA or Wegener's syndrome))
- Tick bite or hiking in wooded areas (consider Lyme, Babesiosis, anaplasma, or ehrlichiosis)
- Neurological symptoms (consider VKH, sarcoidosis, Behçet's disease, syphilis, Lyme, or multiple sclerosis)
- Urethral discharge (consider reactive arthritis)

Travel History
- Lyme is most common in the mid-Atlantic and New England area but has also become common in north-central states (Wisconsin and Minnesota) and northern California.
- Histoplasmosis is endemic in the Ohio-Mississippi-Missouri valley region.
- Coccidiomycosis is endemic in the San Joaquin Valley in California.
- Cysticercosis, amebiasis, and onchocerciasis are primarily found in Central and South America and Africa.

History of Exposure to Pets
- Exposure to cats/cat feces, contaminated sandbox, and pica (consider toxoplasmosis and *Bartonella*)
- Exposure to dogs/dog feces, contaminated sandbox, and pica (consider toxocariasis)

Dietary History
- Ingestion of undercooked meat or unwashed vegetables (consider toxoplasmosis and cysticercosis)

Sexual History
- If the patient is sexually active, the examiner must determine the number of sexual contacts, sexual orientation, and history of venereal disease(s) (consider human immunodeficiency virus (HIV), syphilis, human T-cell lymphotropic virus (HTLV), and hepatitis C).

Drug History
- History of IV drug use (consider HIV and endogenous infections)
- History of medications associated with uveitis, i.e., topical prostaglandin analogues, bisphosphonates, rifabutin, cidofovir, and sulfonamides

Family History of Uveitis

- Although uveitis is generally not inherited, a family history should be sought because certain autoimmune diseases and uveitides have strong HLA associations.

Ophthalmic Examination

After obtaining a thorough medical and ophthalmic history, a complete eye exam is performed.

External Exam

The exam begins with an external examination of the ocular adnexa, with emphasis on the lids and periorbital area, looking for cutaneous findings such as nodules, poliosis (whitening of eyelashes), vitiligo, vesicular lesions, or parotid or lacrimal gland swelling. The integument and mucosal surfaces are examined when appropriate. Evidence of joint swelling or tenderness should be noted. Some of the more common cutaneous associations include erythema nodosum in Behçet's disease and sarcoidosis; vitiligo, alopecia, and poliosis in VKH; skin nodules in lepromatous uveitis; chronic, indurated skin lesions (lupus pernio) seen in sarcoidosis; mucosal ulcers in herpes, Behçet's, and reactive arthritis; parotid or lacrimal swelling in sarcoidosis, Sjögren's syndrome, or lymphoma; and joint swelling in JIA, IBD, reactive arthritis, RA, acute sarcoidosis, or ankylosing spondylitis.

The cranial nerves are evaluated by examining the pupils, extraocular muscle actions, and corneal sensitivity. Sarcoidosis and Lyme disease are common causes of seventh nerve palsies. VKH neurosyphilis and Behçet's can present with cranial nerve palsies. Ocular involvement with herpetic viruses commonly leads to decreased corneal sensitivity, which may result in a neurotrophic corneal ulcer (see Fig. 12.4).

Slit-Lamp Examination

A slit-lamp exam is performed with emphasis on the pertinent findings seen in ocular inflammatory disease, which include:

Conjunctiva and Sclera

- Hyperemia of the conjunctiva, a nonspecific finding, is a common sign of anterior uveitis. In contradistinction to "conjunctivitis," which can also present with conjunctival hyperemia, there is typically no associated discharge when uveitis is the underlying cause. Conjunctival hyperemia uniformly surrounding the limbus (so-called ciliary flush) is highly suggestive of uveitis with ciliary body involvement (cyclitis) (Fig. 27.1). The conjunctival fornices are evaluated for evidence of a follicular reaction, which can be a manifestation of sarcoidosis. Subconjunctival tissues are examined for evidence of superficial and/or deep capillary plexus erythema. Whereas *episcleritis* is only associated with superficial episcleral plexus involvement, the more serious *scleritis* usually involves both the superficial and deep episcleral plexuses. (Fig. 27.2). In patients

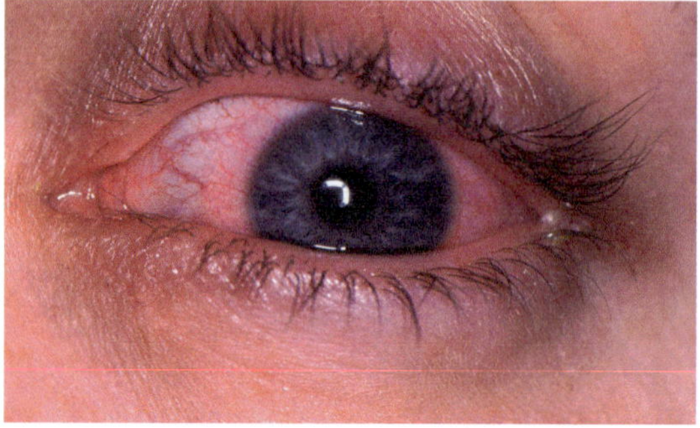

Fig. 27.1 Limbal flush associated with intraocular inflammation

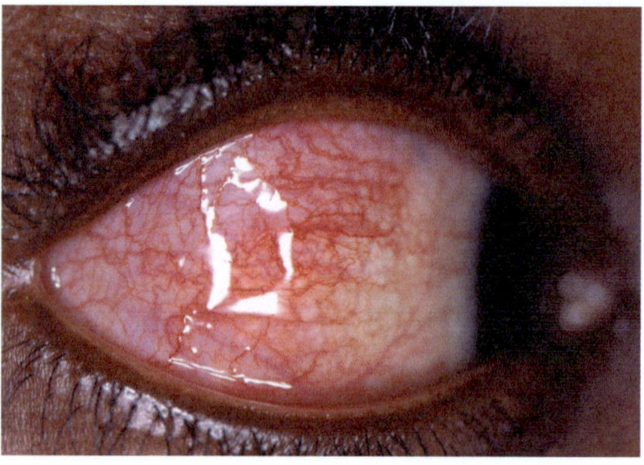

Fig. 27.2 Deep episcleral plexus erythema in anterior diffuse scleritis

suspected of having scleritis, careful inspection for areas of scleral necrosis is mandatory, as necrotizing scleritis may be a harbinger of potentially life-threatening illnesses such as granulomatous polyangiitis or polyarteritis nodosa. Left untreated, necrotizing scleritis can result in globe perforation.

Cornea

- Band keratopathy is the deposition of calcium in Bowman's layer of the cornea, seen frequently in patients with chronic uveitides such as JIA, sarcoidosis, and pars planitis (Fig. 27.3).
- Keratic precipitates (KPs) are aggregates of inflammatory cells which, due to convection currents in the anterior chamber, typically deposit on the lower half of the corneal endothelium in a base-down triangular configuration (Arlt's triangle) (Fig. 27.4). Keratic precipitates are classified as granulomatous or non-granulomatous. The more commonly seen non-granulomatous KPs are generally well circumscribed, small, and relatively fine and represent collections of lymphocytes and polymorphonuclear lymphocytes (PMNs). In contrast, granulomatous or so-called mutton fat KPs are generally larger and greasy appearing and consist of lymphocytes, PMNs, and macrophages, the latter cellular component responsible for the greasy appearance.

- Epithelial dendrites can be seen in cases of viral uveitis such as infection with HSV and VZV.
- Stromal corneal infiltrates (interstitial keratitis) can be seen in syphilis (congenital and acquired), Lyme, Cogan's syndrome (a rare, probably autoimmune condition in which the cornea and ears are subject to recurrent inflammatory episodes with vertigo and other

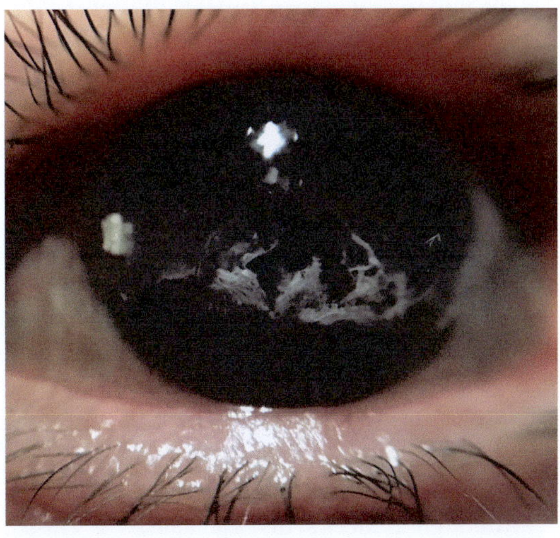

Fig. 27.3 Band keratopathy involving visual axis. (Courtesy of Harvey Schneier, MD)

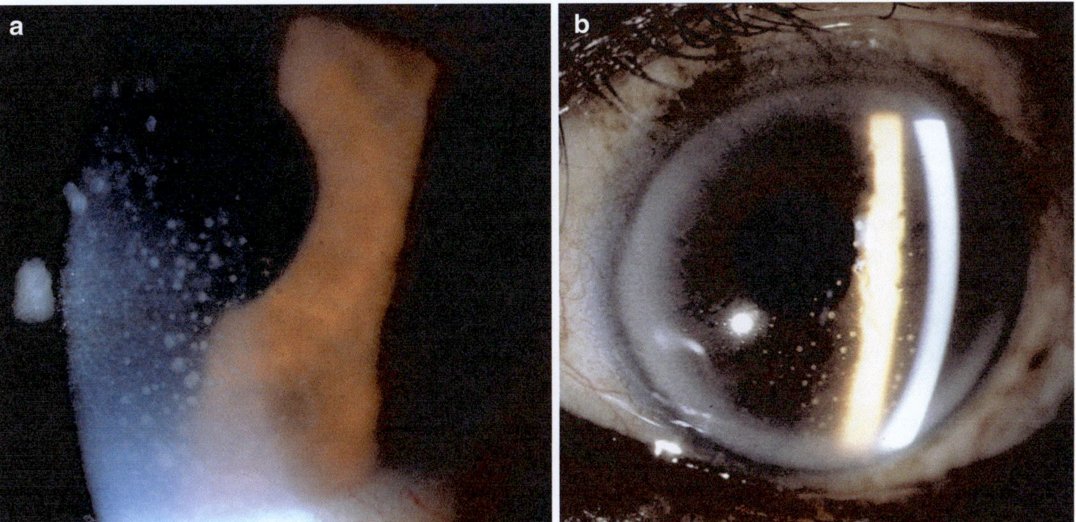

Fig. 27.4 (**a**) Diffuse granulomatous keratic precipitates. (**b**) Non-granulomatous keratic precipitates in a base-down triangular, inferior distribution (Arlt's triangle)

systemic signs, including vasculitis), tuberculosis, and leprosy.

- Stromal keratitis in association with peripheral ulcerative keratitis typically occurs in patients with RA but is also seen in granulomatous polyangiitis (GPA, or Wegener's syndrome), polyarteritis nodosa, systemic lupus, and relapsing polychondritis (Fig. 27.5).

Anterior Chamber (AC)

- The anterior chamber, which is normally optically empty (i.e., appears clear when viewed in the slit lamp), is examined for evidence of protein (a hazy appearance referred to as flare) and white blood cells (seen as small white opacities floating in the AC). Flare and cells occur due to breakdown of the blood-aqueous barrier and is an indication of inflammation involving the iris and/or ciliary body (Fig. 27.6).
- When inflammation is severe, the cells may settle in the inferior angle leading to formation of a hypopyon (Fig. 27.7). In North America, the most common cause of uveitis with hypopyon is HLA-B27–related anterior uveitis. Although Behçet's disease causes a classic "hypopyon uveitis," hypopyon secondary to Behçet's disease only occurs in approximately 1/3 of patients and appears only transiently. To determine the extent of inflammatory disease activity and response to treatment, various grading systems have been proposed over the years to quantify anterior chamber cellular activity. Each grading system has its own merits and deficits, but whichever scoring system is decided upon, it is critical that the examiner consistently use the same scoring system to be able to determine a patient's clinical status and response to treatment. With effective treatment, there is gradual reconstitution of the blood-aqueous barrier, and the number of cells and their size will decline until the aqueous regains optically clarity.
- Flare is caused by protein leaking from the iris and ciliary vasculature into the aqueous fluid and may remain despite effective treatment. Persistence of flare represents incomplete reconstitution of the blood-aqueous barrier,

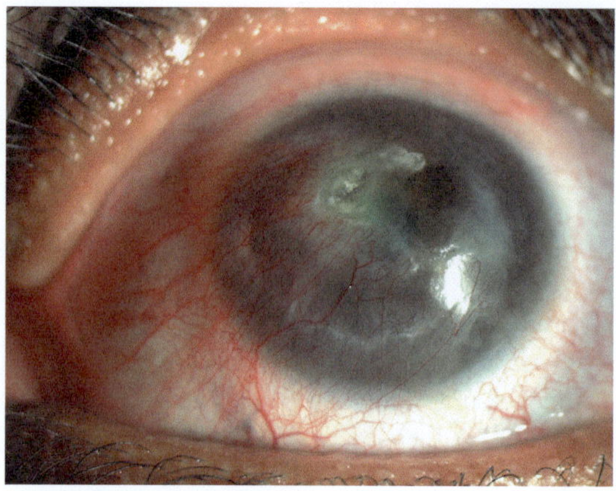

Fig. 27.5 Active necrotizing sclerokeratitis in a patient with rheumatoid arthritis

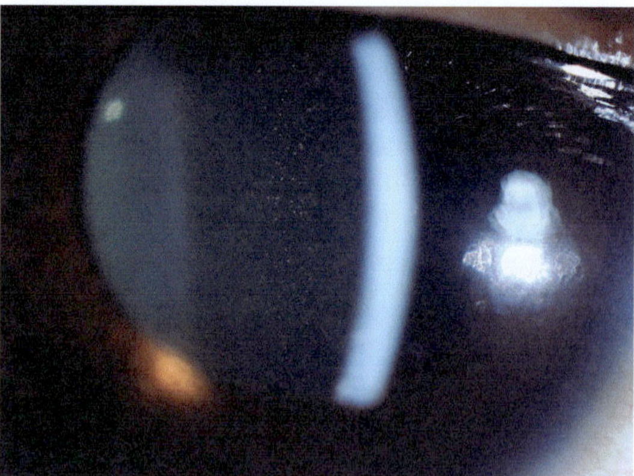

Fig. 27.6 Cell (seen as small white dots) and flare (protein leakage, seen as diffuse haze) present in the anterior chamber

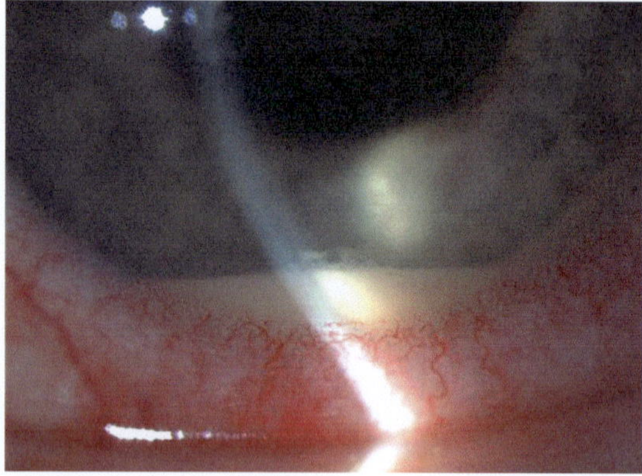

Fig. 27.7 Hypopyon (layered cells appearing in the inferior angle)

which continues to permit leakage of low molecular weight proteins while blocking extravasation of cellular blood components. Flare can also be clinically graded, but flare alone without cells is not regarded as a sign of active intraocular inflammation and therefore does not require treatment.

- The iris is examined for evidence of potential inflammatory sequela. Posterior synechiae (PS) represent inflammation-related adhesions that develop between the iris and the underlying anterior lens capsule at the pupillary margin and present a potentially significant complication of anterior uveitis (Figs. 27.8 and 27.17). The presence of PS is usually an indication of poorly controlled or undiagnosed chronic anterior segment inflammation and/or inadequate pupil management with topical cycloplegics

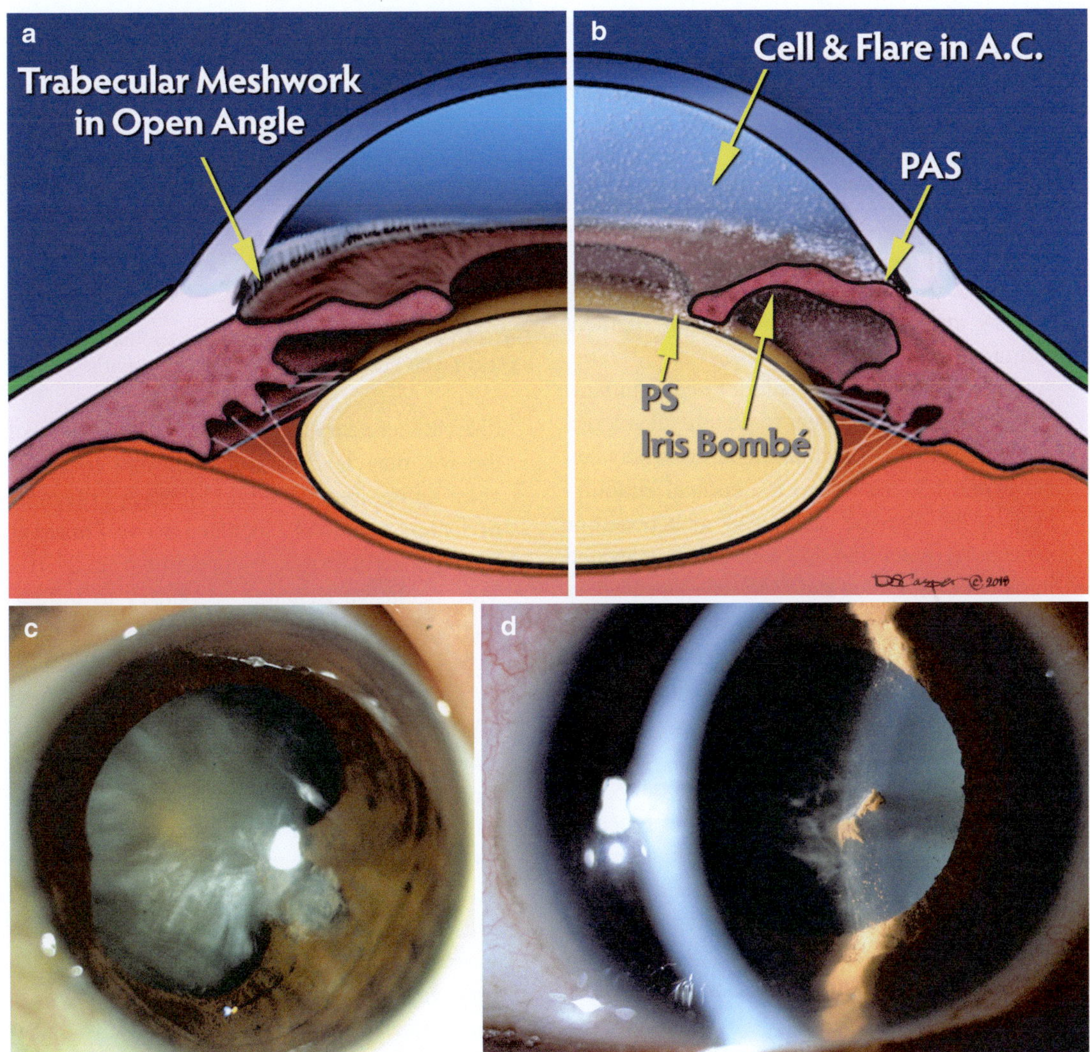

Fig. 27.8 (**a**) Normal anterior segment anatomy. (**b**) Artist's depiction of anterior segment uveitis findings. *A.C.* anterior chamber; *PS* posterior synechiae; *PAS* peripheral anterior synechiae. (**c**) Iris adhesions to underlying lens surface (posterior synechiae). (**d**) Lysis of posterior synechiae after intensive dilating therapy

(see "Treatment of NonInfectious Anterior Iritis"). Topical, short-acting cycloplegic agents are routinely used in patients with anterior uveitis to keep the pupil moving and somewhat distant from the anterior lens surface to prevent PS formation. Extensive PS prevent normal aqueous fluid egress from the posterior to anterior chambers via the pupil due to iridopupillary adhesions (a "secluded pupil"). This leads to the development of iris bombé and pupillary block angle-closure glaucoma. Occasionally, repeated use of strong dilating drops will lyse PS and allow normal aqueous flow to resume. For patients who have developed extensive, irreversible PS, a prophylactic laser iridotomy, which relieves pupillary block by reestablishing aqueous communication between the posterior and anterior chambers, is performed to prevent angle closure. Extensive posterior synechiae also prevent normal pupil dilation, thereby impeding adequate posterior segment examination.

- Another complication of anterior ocular inflammation is the development of peripheral anterior synechiae (PAS), which are adhesions between peripheral iris tissue and the corneal endothelium at the chamber angle. As with posterior synechiae, extensive PAS result in elevated intraocular pressures and eventual glaucoma; in this case, elevated pressure is due to blocked aqueous egress at the trabecular meshwork and Schlemm's canal, the normal physiologic drainage pathway of aqueous from the eye.

- The iris surface is examined for the presence of inflammatory nodules. Koeppe's nodules are small elevations found at the pupillary margin which can be present in both granulomatous and non-granulomatous inflammation (Fig. 27.9); Busacca nodules are pathognomonic for granulomatous inflammation, generally larger than Koeppe's, and found in the iris stroma. Berlin's nodules, typically seen with ocular sarcoid, are found on the peripheral iris or angle.

- Stromal atrophy of the iris may occur due to inflammatory-induced vaso-occlusive ischemia leading to diffuse or zonal sector atrophy (see Fig. 2.4) and is highly suggestive of a viral cause for uveitis, such as that seen with herpetic

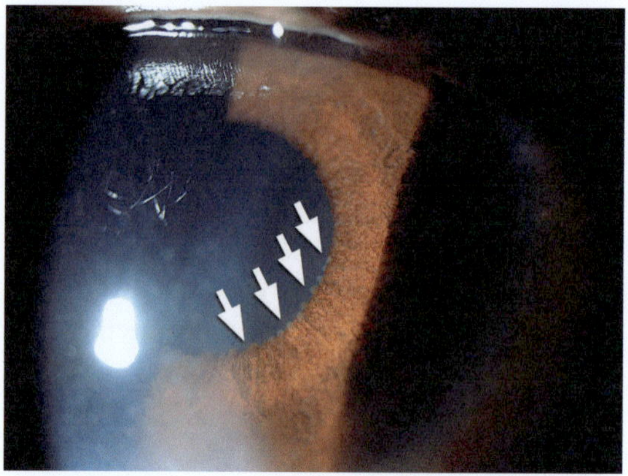

Fig. 27.9 Koeppe nodules seen at pupillary sphincter margin (arrows)

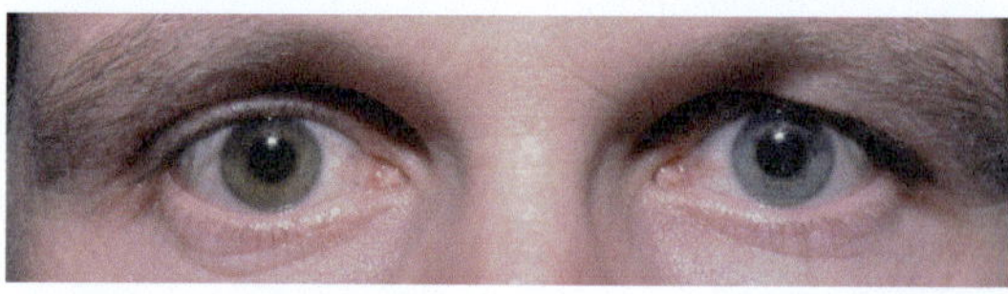

Fig. 27.10 Heterochromia due to iris stromal atrophy in a patient with Fuchs' heterochromic iridocyclitis

disease secondary to HSV and VZV. Atrophy of the iris may lead to heterochromia (one eye color lighter than the other) which is a diagnostic feature commonly seen in a uveitis known as Fuchs' heterochromic iridocyclitis (Fig. 27.10). Vaso-occlusive ischemia secondary to inflammation can also lead to the development of neovascular vessels on the iris surface (NVI) and/or in the angle (NVA). If left untreated, NVI and NVA can lead to dangerously elevated intraocular pressure (neovascular glaucoma), which may result in a blind, painful eye. The pathophysiologic basis of neovascular vessel formation is ischemia, the same underlying mechanism that leads to development of proliferative diabetic retinopathy. Peripheral anterior synechiae, angle nodules, and NVA are identified on slit-lamp examination by a technique known as gonioscopy, which utilizes a mirrored contact lens that provides for 360° visualization of angle structures (Fig. 27.11) (See Chap. 15).

Lens

- The crystalline lens is examined for evidence of cataract formation, i.e., areas of lens

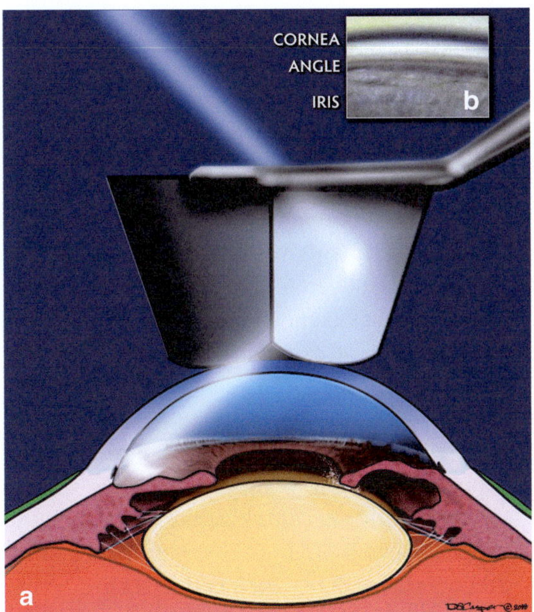

Fig. 27.11 (**a**) Gonioscopy demonstrating normal angle anatomy. (**b**) Gonioscopic view of angle anatomy

opacity. Ocular inflammation is potentially cataractogenic via several mechanisms. The avascular lens is nourished by the aqueous, and with ocular inflammation, ciliary body aqueous production is decreased. Inflammatory cells deplete the aqueous nutrient content, and cytokines secreted by inflammatory cells may be toxic to the lens epithelium. It is significant that uveitis treatment, which almost always involves the use of steroids, also promotes cataract formation. Therefore, both inflammation and its major treatment modality (corticosteroids) predispose to cataract formation, posterior subcapsular cataracts being the most common subtype. Some patients fearful of cataract formation may consider low-grade, smoldering inflammation to be preferable to long-term treatment with steroids, but on balance, uncontrolled inflammation is felt to be significantly more cataractogenic than the use of topical steroids. However, every effort is made to limit the amount of steroid use with chronic uveitis. Pigment deposition on the lens surface may also be noted, a common finding following successful medical lysis of posterior synechiae.

Intraocular Pressure (IOP)

- Intraocular pressure measurements are crucial, as uveitic glaucoma is a frequent complication of inflammatory eye disease. In addition, as previously mentioned, the use of steroids will often lead to IOP elevation. For most uveitides, acute inflammation leads to a transient lowering of pressure, although over time, chronic IOP elevation and glaucoma typically ensues.

Vitreous

- Normal vitreous is composed of collagen fibrils and hyaluronic acid and is devoid of inflammatory cells. Inflammation in the vitreous, "vitritis," is characterized by the presence of cells and flare (protein) that may arise from the retina, choroid, or ciliary body. So-called vitreous "snowballs" represent collections or clumps of inflammatory cells; a vitreous strand connecting several snowballs is termed a "string of pearls." Clumps of inflammatory cells may settle inferiorly on the peripheral retina or pars plana leading to the formation of pars plana exudates or a fibroglial mass known as a "snowbank."

- The quantification of vitreous cells and flare is more difficult compared to anterior chamber cells and flare, and a number of grading systems have been proposed. Whereas cells noted in the anterior chamber always indicate active inflammation, the presence of cells in the vitreous may not, since vitreous cells may signify old inflammatory cells trapped within the vitreous matrix. Findings on slit-lamp examination can help the clinician distinguish active from inactive vitritis.

Retina

Examination of the retina is performed using a combination of techniques, including direct ophthalmoscopy, slit lamp with a 90-diopter lens for posterior pole evaluation and a three-mirror contact lens, and indirect ophthalmoscopy with scleral depression to visualize peripheral retinal pathology. Critical observations must include:

- Is there evidence of retinitis? Retinitis usually appears as superficial, granular, yellow-white inner retinal infiltrates, which are frequently associated with hemorrhage and exudation.

- Is there evidence of an associated serous retinal detachment (i.e., not due to retinal tears, exudation, or tractional causes)? Inflammatory serous retinal detachments can be the result of a compromised retinal pigment epithelium (RPE, the outer retinal barrier) leading to accumulation of fluid beneath the retina. Uveitic entities that can manifest as a serous retinal detachment include VKH, sympathetic ophthalmia (a rare, bilateral, diffuse uveitis following uniocular trauma or surgery), posterior scleritis, toxoplasmosis, and syphilis.

Optic Nerve

- Is there evidence of optic nerve swelling with blurred margins (papillitis)?
- Is there evidence of optic disc or choroidal neovascularization (NVD and CNV, respectively, both complications of inflammation-induced ocular ischemia)?
- Is there optic nerve cupping (a sign of glaucoma)?

Macula

- Cystoid macula edema is one of the most common sight-threatening complications of uveitis and is caused by inflammatory cytokines that cause breakdown of perifoveal capillary tight junctions with resultant accumulation of macular fluid (See Fig 11.11).

Retinal Vasculature (see Chap. 28)

- True retinal vasculitis (as seen on histopathologic analysis of biopsies in systemic vasculitides) is usually not seen. Rather, the term *retinal vasculitis* refers to the ophthalmoscopic visualization of retinal inflammatory cells which create a perivascular cuff (Fig. 27.12) or vascular occlusion. Vascular occlusion may lead to retinal edema, hemorrhages, exudates, and retinal neovascularization. In the majority of cases, retinal veins are more commonly involved than arterioles. In active retinal vasculitis, retinal vessels appear engorged and, on imaging studies, demonstrate vascular leakage and/or occlusion. It is important to determine if the vasculitis involves central or peripheral retinal vasculature, as more central disease carries a much

higher potential for subsequent visual impairment.

Choroid

- The choroid is examined with the same techniques as used for the retinal exam. Focal or multifocal choroidal lesions are a common finding in patients with posterior uveitis. The appearance of certain choroidal lesions allows for a specific diagnosis, but for most choroidal lesions, a broad differential diagnosis needs to be considered. Lesions can vary in size from 50 to 500 μm in diameter. Active lesions generally have a yellowish-gray, creamy appearance with poorly defined or diffuse margins, whereas old, inactive lesions tend to appear as well-circumscribed atrophic chorioretinal scars (Figs. 27.13 and 27.14).

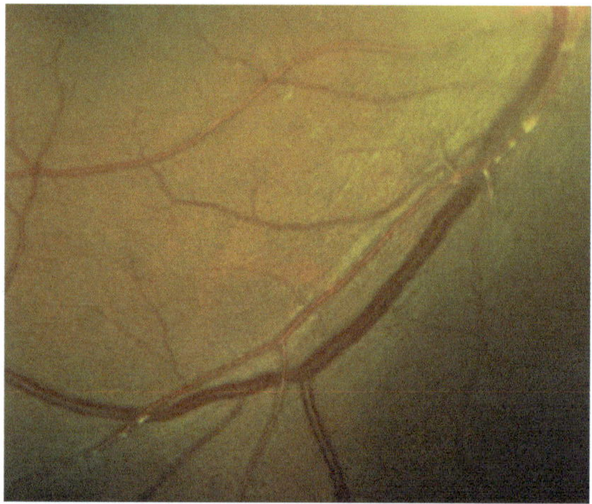

Fig. 27.12 Perivascular cuffing in sarcoid periphlebitis

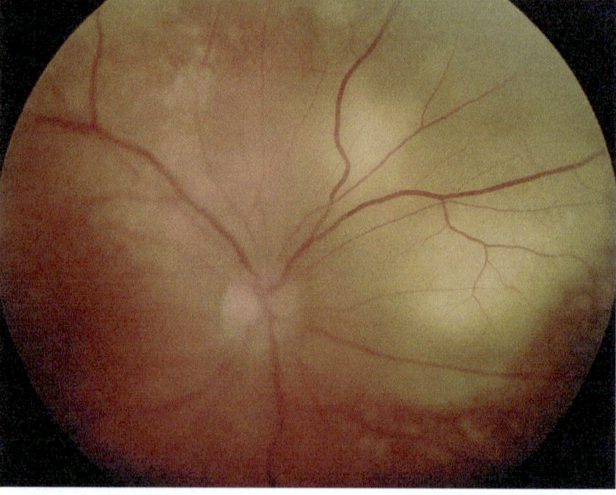

Fig. 27.13 Subretinal lesions seen with intraocular B-cell lymphoma

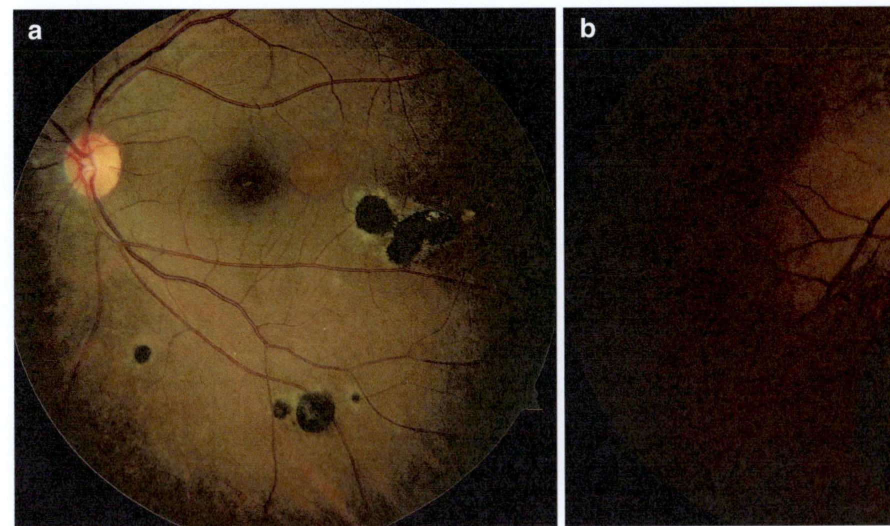

Fig. 27.14 (**a**, **b**) Old chorioretinal scars in a patient with congenital ocular toxoplasmosis

Uveitis Classification

Following the physical exam, the classification of the uveitis helps establish potential etiologies. The most clinically helpful classification system is anatomic classification, which is based on the eye compartment where inflammation is predominantly located.

- *Anterior* uveitis, the most common form, primarily involves the anterior chamber and can be further subclassified as an iritis or iridocyclitis. Iritis indicates inflammation confined to the anterior chamber, while iridocyclitis includes white blood cells in the deeper retrolental space, indicative of ciliary body involvement.
- *Intermediate* uveitis primarily affects the vitreous and peripheral retina. As described above, a subset of intermediate uveitis includes a fibroglial mass usually located in the retinal periphery and pars plana and referred to as a "snowbank;" idiopathic intermediate uveitis with or without a snowbank is termed pars planitis.
- *Posterior* uveitis is confined to the retina or choroid and can be further subclassified as focal or multifocal.
- When all components of the uveal tract are involved, the term *panuveitis* is used.

Some clinicians classify uveitis as "granulomatous" or "non-granulomatous." This system has less utility, however, as granulomatous inflammation can be present in non-granulomatous cases and vice versa, and on occasion one can observe a mix of both features in the same patient. It should be noted that keratic precipitates (see "Slit-Lamp Examination") are usually described as being either granulomatous or non-granulomatous, which is not necessarily related to the uveitic type, making the classification systems somewhat confusing.

Testing

Once the patient's uveitis has been anatomically classified, a differential diagnosis can be more easily generated, which provides the basis for a focused laboratory evaluation (Table 27.2). In addition to testing for the purpose of establishing a diagnosis, ancillary testing may also be necessary to determine to what extent the ocular inflammation is potentially sight-threatening. Frequently, one sees nonspecific, "shot-gun work-ups" employed to assist in uveitis diagnosis; such approaches are wasteful and unnecessary and should be discouraged.

The first goal of the work-up is to exclude any infectious etiology and masquerade syndromes. There is a wide spectrum of bacterial, viral, fungal, and parasitic agents to consider; the likelihood of any one being the causative agent will

Table 27.2 Causes of anterior, intermediate, and posterior uveitis

Common causes of anterior uveitis
  Autoinflammatory/autoimmune
    Sarcoidosis
    HLA-B27 with or without associated systemic disease
    Ankylosing spondylitis
    Psoriatic arthritis
    SLE with scleritis
    RA with scleritis
    GPA (Wegener's) with scleritis
    Polyarteritis nodosa with scleritis
    Sjögren's
    Autoimmune hepatitis
    Fuchs' heterochromic iridocyclitis
    Behçet's
    TINU (tubulointerstitial nephritis and uveitis)
    JIA
    Inflammatory bowel disease
    Posner-Schlossman syndrome (glaucomatocyclitic crisis)
    Kawasaki's
  Drug/medication induced
  Infectious
    Herpetic viruses (HSV, VZV, CMV)
    Syphilis
    Tuberculosis
    Toxoplasmosis
    Lyme
  Masquerades
    Leukemia
    Juvenile xanthogranuloma
    Pigment dispersion syndrome
    Ocular ischemia
    Intraocular foreign body
    Chronic retinal detachment
Common causes of intermediate uveitis
  Autoinflammatory
    Idiopathic pars planitis
    Sarcoidosis
    Demyelinating disease
    Inflammatory bowel disease
    TINU
  Infectious
    Lyme
    Tuberculosis
    Syphilis
    HTLV
    Hepatitis C
    Toxocara
    Bartonella henselae (cat scratch)
    Tropheryma whipplei (Whipple's)

Table 27.2 (continued)

  Masquerade:
    Intraocular lymphoma
    Intraocular foreign body
    Amyloidosis
Common causes of posterior uveitis
  Autoinflammatory
    Sarcoid
    VKH
    Birdshot chorioretinopathy
    Behçet's
    Acute posterior multifocal placoid pigment epitheliopathy (APMPPE)
    Serpiginous chorioretinopathy
    Multifocal choroiditis and panuveitis
    Sympathetic ophthalmia
    Immune recovery uveitis
    Multiple evanescent white dot syndrome (MEWDS)
  Infectious
    Toxoplasmosis
    Toxocariasis
    Acute retinal necrosis
    Syphilis
    Tuberculosis
    CMV retinitis
    Progressive outer retinal necrosis
    Bartonella henselae
    Endogenous infectious endophthalmitis
    Presumed ocular histoplasmosis syndrome (POHS)
  Masquerade
    Intraocular lymphoma
    Posterior scleritis
    Metastatic malignancy
    Intraocular foreign body
    Chronic retinal detachment

vary geographically and will be affected by the patient's past medical history and overall immune status. Laboratory tests that are commonly obtained to exclude potential infectious causes of uveitis include:

- Complete blood count with differential
- Quantiferon gold (or purified protein derivative test (PPD, or Mantoux test) with anergy panel if no history of prior Bacillus Calmette-Guérin (BCG) injection) for tuberculosis evaluation

- Chest X-ray (CXR) for tuberculosis and sarcoidosis evaluation
- Venereal disease research laboratory (VDRL) test and fluorescent treponemal antibody absorption (FTA-ABS) test for syphilis evaluation
- Serum antibody titers to identify exposure to Lyme, leptospirosis, toxoplasmosis, toxocara, HIV, HTLV, *Bartonella henselae* (the most commonly recognized cause of neuroretinitis), and *Herpesviridae* (including herpes simplex virus (HSV), varicella-zoster virus (VZV), cytomegalovirus (CMV), and Epstein-Barr virus (EBV))

If an endogenous infectious process is considered, appropriate fluids including blood, urine, and sputum should be cultured. It is important to note that immunoglobulin G (IgG) serum titers to an infectious agent only support a history of past exposure but do not necessarily indicate that this is the cause of uveitis. In certain circumstances, to secure the diagnosis of an infectious uveitis, sampling of aqueous and vitreous fluids to assay for pathogen-specific local antibody production (using the Goldmann-Witmer coefficient test) and/or DNA sequences (by polymerase chain reaction (PCR)) can be invaluable in establishing a definitive diagnosis attributable to pathogens such as herpes, toxoplasmosis, tuberculosis, and syphilis. Erythrocyte sedimentation rate (ESR) and C-reactive protein (CRP), although nonspecific indicators of systemic inflammation, may point in the direction of an occult, underlying systemic disease triggering a patient's uveitis.

If an infectious etiology can be excluded, uveitis is presumed to be of immune-mediated/autoinflammatory origin or, uncommonly, a masquerade syndrome. Most uveitis work-ups consider the possibility of sarcoid uveitis, and approximately 40% of patients with sarcoidosis have ocular involvement. Common laboratory testing employed to confirm sarcoidosis includes checking angiotensin-converting enzyme (ACE), lysozyme, serum calcium levels, and CXR. If there is a strong suspicion for sarcoid, testing can also include a chest CT scan and/or gallium scan to determine the extent of organ system involvement. Although an elevated ACE as an isolated finding is not a sensitive predictor of sarcoid, the combination of a positive chest CT and/or gallium scan and elevated ACE is 98% specific for sarcoidosis. A definitive diagnosis of sarcoid requires a histopathologic diagnosis from biopsy sites which may include the skin, conjunctiva (if nodules are present), lacrimal gland, lung, or liver.

If vasculitis is a major feature of the uveitis presentation, a search for an underlying systemic vasculitis is warranted. Common autoimmune investigations might include an antinuclear antibody (ANA); anti-extractable nuclear antigens (ENA); rheumatoid factor (RF); anti-cyclic citrullinated peptide (CCP); anti-double-stranded DNA (anti-dsDNA); perinuclear and cytoplasmic anti-neutrophil cytoplasmic antibodies (ANCAs); urinalysis with microscopic evaluation looking for protein, blood, and beta2-microglobulin (to exclude tubulointerstitial nephritis and uveitis syndrome (TINU)); and C3 and C4 complement levels. It has become almost reflexly routine when obtaining uveitis laboratory testing to include an ANA and RF. In fact, ANA testing is rarely helpful, except if a systemic vasculitis is suspected or when establishing frequency of JIA patient monitoring for possible iritis development. JIA patients that are most likely to develop complicating iritis are the pauciarticular (four or fewer joints involved) ANA-positive subgroup. This subgroup has an overall 25% likelihood of developing iritis, and patients need to be examined every 3 months, as JIA-related iritis may be asymptomatic. Rheumatoid factor testing is rarely helpful, except if scleritis is in the differential diagnosis, as the most common cause of scleritis is RA.

Some class I and II human leukocyte antigen (HLA) haplotypes have strong associations with certain ocular inflammatory disease. Confirming the presence of a specific HLA haplotype increases the likelihood of a particular uveitis entity and can therefore be helpful in supporting a tentative diagnosis. Common associations include HLA-

B27, with acute recurrent uveitis, HLA-A29 with birdshot chorioretinopathy, HLA-B*5 locus with Behçet's disease (HLA B51), and DR4 (subtype 0405) with VKH.

Diagnostic Imaging Tests

Fundus Photography

Color fundus photography is essential to document the appearance of the retina and choroid as well as to monitor the longitudinal evolution of any noted pathology. Fundus photography also serves as a clinical reference necessary for the accurate interpretation of angiographic findings (see below).

Fluorescein Angiography (FA)

Angiography is critical in defining the extent of structural damage caused by ocular inflammation as well as to help monitor response to treatment. When doubt exists, FA can objectively confirm the presence of sight-threatening disease. Fluorescein, the most commonly used dye to study retinal vasculature, does not flow through occluded vessels, and since it is a low molecular weight molecule, it leaks from inflamed retinal vessels; these abnormal patterns are readily seen with angiography. FA allows the clinician to determine the presence of perivascular staining, leakage due to retinal vasculitis, optic nerve leakage due to papillitis, cystoid macula edema, and areas of ischemia due to vascular occlusion. In addition, FA is vital in determining the presence of complicating retinal and choroidal neovascularization secondary to inflammation-induced ischemia.

Indocyanine Green Angiography (ICGA)

ICGA is used primarily to visualize choroidal, rather than retinal, vasculature. In contrast to fluorescein, ICGA dye is a larger compound and more plasma lipoprotein-bound and therefore does not normally leak from the fenestrated choroidal vasculature. In addition, ICGA dye fluoresces in the infrared spectrum, which allows for better imaging through hemorrhagic lesions, and

is more visible through the RPE, which helps determine the extent of choroidal involvement in posterior uveitides.

Optical Coherence Tomography

OCT imaging provides high-level, micron-resolution, cross-sectional imaging of the retina. OCT's main application in uveitis patients is demonstrating the presence of macular pathologies such as macular edema and CNV, as well as its ability to longitudinally monitor response to treatment.

B-Scan Ultrasonography (USG)

Ultrasound is used to image both anterior and posterior segment structures when opacified ocular media prevent direct visualization. Examples of conditions that might require ultrasound evaluation include an opacified cornea, hyphema, miotic pupil, posterior synechiae preventing adequate pupil dilation, dense cataract, vitreous hemorrhage, and extensive vitreous inflammatory debris. USG is helpful in assessing the degree of vitreous opacification and to determine if a choroidal or retinal detachment is present. USG is an essential imaging modality for diagnosing posterior scleritis, which manifests as thickening of the chorioscleral layer and adjacent edema (Fig. 27.15).

Fundus Autofluorescence (FAF)

As retinal photoreceptor outer segments undergo turnover and renewal, toxic byproducts can accumulate in RPE cell lysosomes, forming lipofuscin granules. FAF is a noninvasive imaging technique that assesses the health of the RPE layer based on the amount of accumulated lipofuscin. FAF patterns can help establish a definitive diagnosis as well as determine and monitor the amount of RPE damage in patients with posterior uveitis.

X-Ray (XR), Computed Tomography (CT), and MRI (Magnetic Resonance Imaging)

Plain XR studies of the chest may be ordered to screen for sarcoidosis and help rule out tuberculosis. X-rays of sacroiliac and other joints help establish the diagnosis of a spondyloarthropathy;

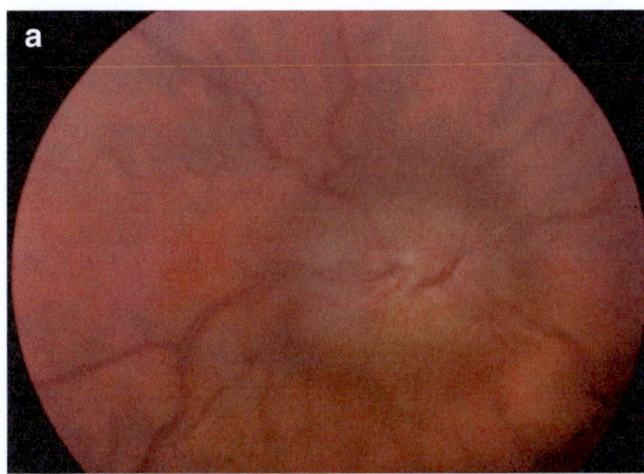

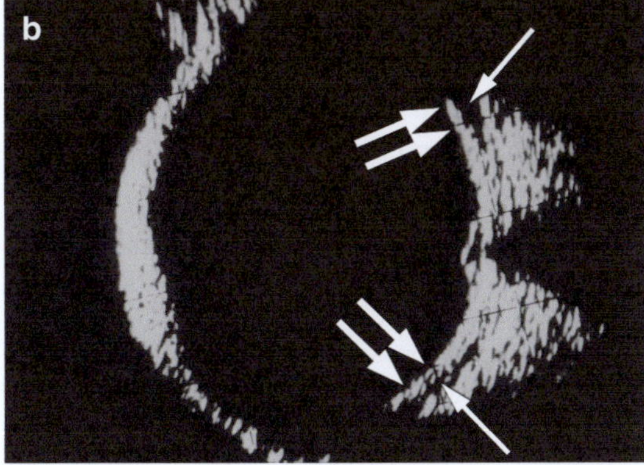

Fig. 27.15 (**a**) Marked disc swelling in a patient with posterior scleritis. (**b**) B-mode ultrasound demonstrating thickened chorioscleral layer (double arrows) and fluid in Tenon's space (single arrow)

in cases of necrotizing scleritis, sinus XR studies can help diagnose granulomatous polyangiitis. CT scanning is used primarily to look for pulmonary findings when there is a high index of suspicion for sarcoidosis. MRI scanning of the CNS is used in cases of intermediate uveitis when there is a suspicion for underlying demyelinating disease and to help exclude a diagnosis of CNS B-cell lymphoma, when ocular lymphoma is suspected.

Clinical Electroretinography (ERG)

Full-field ERG represents a mass electric response of the entire retina to light stimulation and is useful in uveitis conditions causing diffuse retinal damage. Focal or multifocal ERG (mERG) are employed to assess discrete areas of the posterior retina, in cases of uveitis that demonstrate localized, rather than diffuse, pathology; mERG is used to detect macular disease affecting outer retinal layers. ERG testing can be helpful both in determining the underlying retinal defect causing visual loss and in assessing clinical response to therapy.

Tissue Biopsy

When a definitive diagnosis cannot otherwise be made, tissue biopsy is warranted. Anterior chamber paracentesis involves the removal of a small amount of aqueous fluid to assist in the diagnoses of suspected infectious uveitis; this is a quick procedure, usually done at the slit lamp, using a small-gauge needle. Studies performed on the aqueous specimen may include gram stain, culture, and PCR, which is especially useful in the diagnosis of infectious uveitis secondary to HSV, VZV, CMV, and toxoplasmosis, even when inflammation is posteriorly located in the eye. Aqueous fluid can also be analyzed for the presence of antibody levels to presumed organisms; however, breakdown of the blood-aqueous barrier in uveitis patients can lead to passive diffusion of antibodies into the aqueous, resulting in a misleading diagnosis; therefore, it is essential to also measure serum immunoglobulin and specific serum antibody titers to confirm intraocular production of antibody (Goldmann-Witmer coefficient).

Retinal and chorioretinal biopsies can be considered in extreme sight-threatening pathology, usually bilateral cases that have been unresponsive to treatment and which presumably have eluded accurate diagnosis despite extensive routine evaluation.

Vitreous Tap

Diagnostic vitrectomy to obtain a vitreous specimen may be considered when other methods have failed to deliver a definitive diagnosis. Vitreous sampling is especially helpful in cases of exogenous and endogenous endophthalmitis, as well as when intraocular malignancy masquerading as uveitis is suspected (Fig. 27.16).

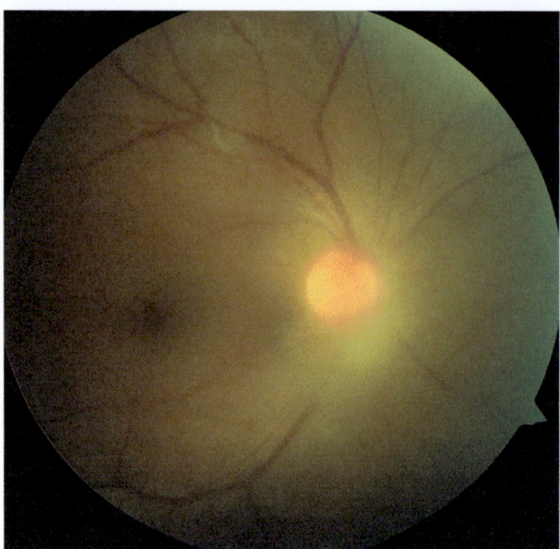

Fig. 27.16 Syphilitic chorioretinopathy with vitreous inflammation (vitritis)

Treatment

To decide on the most appropriate treatment plan and care, the ophthalmologist must answer five questions:

- What is the laterality of the uveitis?
- Is the uveitis associated with underlying systemic disease?
- What is the clinical course (acute, chronic, or recurrent)?
- Is the uveitis symptomatic or asymptomatic?
- Is the inflammation potentially sight-threatening?

Laterality

Uveitis may be exclusively unilateral, but more commonly, eventually involves both eyes. HLA-B27-related uveitis typically presents unilaterally, but recurrent attacks can present in either eye. It is important to establish laterality because patients with unilateral disease (especially those without an associated systemic disease) may be candidates for local therapy, i.e., topical medications and periorbital or intravitreal injections.

Symptomatic Versus Asymptomatic

Patients with uveitis may present with or without symptoms. When planning long-term management, it is helpful to determine whether the presentation is reliably symptomatic or asymptomatic. Symptoms typically associated with anterior segment uveitides include pain, redness, and photophobia, whereas posterior segment disease is more likely to present with blurred vision, flashing lights, and floaters. Paradoxically, asymptomatic presentations are more sinister because patients tend to present much later in the disease process, at which time smoldering chronic inflammation may have already led to permanent anatomic changes and corresponding visual deficits. Asymptomatic cases require more follow-up at regular intervals to insure the absence of occult, recurrent inflammation. In contrast, patients whose uveitis reliably presents with symptoms can be followed less closely but still need to be instructed to call immediately should they experience any symptoms suggestive of recurrent activity.

Acute Versus Chronic

The term *acute uveitis* generally refers to sudden onset uveitis that readily responds to treatment, which allows the patient to discontinue all medications within 3 months, absent recurrent inflammation for at least a 90-day interval following discontinuation. In *chronic uveitis*, persistent or recurrent inflammatory activity in the eye occurs during attempted tapering or upon discontinuation of therapy, which then requires an ongoing maintenance dose of medicine to keep the eye inflammation-free. Somewhat confusingly, both acute and chronic inflammation can be recurrent. Acute recurrent uveitis refers to recurrent inflammation occurring at least 90 days after the patient was deemed inflammation-free, off all medicine. Chronic recurrent inflammation refers to recurrent inflammation despite a maintenance dose of medicine that previously was adequate to control active inflammation. Patients with chronic and chronic recurrent uveitis are much more likely to require long-term therapy with steroid-sparing agents compared to acute and acute recurrent uveitis.

Sight-Threatening Disease

The treatment of uveitis is designed to prevent structural damage and vision loss. However, there are certain relatively benign ocular inflammatory conditions, e.g., pars planitis, which can be safely monitored if the inflammation is well tolerated by the eye, without evidence of sight-threatening complications. Prior to initiating therapy, it is important to establish that potential sight-threatening disease is present and that the benefits of treatment outweigh any risks.

Uveitis Treatment Strategies

The overwhelming majority of uveitis patients benefit from treatment. As a general rule, the earlier in the disease course that treatment is initiated, the better overall visual prognosis. Due to damaging effects of intraocular inflammation, the purpose of treatment is to eliminate all signs of inflammation and prevent recurrent inflammation. In the ophthalmic uveitis community, there is zero tolerance for any ocular inflammation, as even low-grade inflammation can cause extensive structural damage to the eye. The comorbidities resulting from ocular inflammation include, but are not limited to, glaucoma, cataracts, cystoid macula edema, and retinal detachment. These potential uveitic complications each have their own individual management requirements, separate from control of intraocular inflammation. The purpose of uveitis treatment is to prevent irreversible vision loss and, when possible, improve visual function. However, in cases with severe, end-stage, irreversible vision loss, the risks of immunosuppressive treatment must be weighed against potential visual benefits.

As previously mentioned, to establish an appropriate treatment strategy, it is essential to determine, to the extent possible, whether the uveitis falls in the infectious vs. immune-mediated vs. masquerade syndrome category. Uveitides of infectious origin will require specific anti-infectious therapy appropriate for the offending etiologic agent. However, even in the setting of an infectious uveitis, it is frequently necessary to use concomitant corticosteroids or immunomodulatory therapy (IMT) to protect the eye from structural damage caused by the accompanying inflammatory reaction. Furthermore, in uveitides of infectious origin, residual intraocular antigens may stimulate a secondary inflammation that requires concomitant, nonspecific immunosuppressive treatment.

"Masquerade syndromes" refer to malignant and nonmalignant disorders that present with intraocular inflammation simulating a chronic, idiopathic uveitis. Since half of all masquerade syndromes are neoplastic in origin, prompt diagnosis and treatment is essential. Patients classified as having chronic idiopathic uveitis should always be evaluated for the possibility of a masquerade syndrome. Common causes of masquerade syndromes can include primary central nervous system lymphoma and intraocular lymphoma (the overwhelming majority being non-Hodgkin's, diffuse B-cell lymphoma), metastatic malignancy with spread to the eye, leukemia, chronic retinal detachment, intraocular foreign body, paraneoplastic disorders such as carcinoma associated retinopathy (CAR), bilateral diffuse uveal melanocytic proliferation (BDUMP), and melanoma-associated retinopathy (MAR). In the pediatric age group, considerations include juvenile xanthogranuloma and retinoblastoma. Treatment of masquerade syndromes depends on the specific underlying etiology.

The treatment of uveitides caused by an autoinflammatory mechanism will involve some form of either local (topical drops or periocular or intravitreal injections) or systemic (PO, IM, IV) immunosuppression with steroids and/or immunomodulating agents. It is important to emphasize that topical treatment is only effective for uveitis affecting the anterior segment; topical steroids do not, to any significant degree, penetrate beyond the anterior chamber and, therefore, when used alone, are ineffective for intermediate or posterior uveitis treatment.

If disease is in the acute or acute recurrent category, treatment generally requires an induction phase followed by a slow taper with the expectation that patients will be off all anti-inflammatory medication within 3–4 months. For this category of uveitides, steroids are the best treatment option, as no other medicine works better or has a more rapid onset of action than corticosteroids. In the induction phase of treatment, dosage must be adequate to achieve rapid control of intraocular inflammation, thereby quickly eliminating the immediate danger to sight. For cases with severe and immediate sight-threatening disease, this could involve initial treatment for 3 days with IV Solu-Medrol to achieve rapid control of the inflammatory process, followed by conversion to oral steroids. We generally continue induction doses until all signs of active intraocular inflammation have resolved prior to initiating the tapering phase of treatment. A slow taper over several months is generally recommended to decrease the chances of "rebound" inflammation.

For uveitides that are in the chronic and chronic recurrent category, patients usually require long-term anti-inflammatory therapy. In these cases, treatment is divided into an induction phase followed by a long-term maintenance phase. As with acute disease, intraocular inflammation is brought under initial control with induction doses followed by a slow taper, establishing the lowest effective maintenance dose that keeps the eye quiet and prevents recurrent inflammatory episodes. Establishing the inflammatory threshold dose (i.e., the lowest possible maintenance dose needed to keep the eye inflammation-free) is determined empirically using a slow taper with frequent follow-up examinations. As one searches for the lowest maintenance dose that controls inflammatory activity, it is not uncommon to trigger recurrent disease as one dips below the threshold dose. When this occurs, induction doses are resumed until inflammatory activity is adequately controlled, followed by a slow taper to the previous maintenance dose documented to control smoldering or recurrent activity. Patients are generally kept on a consistent maintenance dose without further tapering for 1–3 years. After a prolonged period of mainte-

nance treatment, if a patient has had no intervening recurrent inflammatory episodes, attempts can then be made to attempt a taper and discontinue treatment, following carefully during the process for evidence of recurrent inflammation. Using this strategy, it is estimated that up to 1/3 of patients with chronic and chronic recurrent uveitis can achieve long-term, drug-free remission. As a general rule, the longer the patient has not had recurrent activity prior to tapering, the greater the chances of establishing prolonged drug-free remission.

Although steroids are very effective for the treatment of uveitis, long-term use, whether administered locally or systemically, is associated with a litany of well-known, unacceptable side effects, both ocular and systemic. Hence, for the expected long-term treatment of chronic and chronic recurrent uveitis, steroid-sparing agents are routinely employed to decrease and/or eliminate the need for steroid use. Ideally, we aim to totally eliminate the need for steroids, although in practice a dose below the "Cushing dose" (0.1 mg/kg body weight) is considered acceptable. The addition of steroid-sparing immunosuppressive agents for the treatment of uveitis has several indications including:

- Lowering or eliminating the need for steroid use for cases of noninfectious uveitis requiring long-term management.
- Unacceptable adverse effects from steroids.
- Uveitides such as Behçet's and serpiginous choroidopathy that have been shown to respond better when steroid-sparing agents are introduced early in the management strategy.

With the exception of adalimumab, the use of IMT for the treatment of uveitis remains off-label. Clinical studies evaluating and comparing the efficacy of different steroid-sparing agents for the treatment of uveitis are sparse, and most of the information available comes from anecdotal case report series.

When employing IMT there are generally two clinical approaches used by uveitis specialists: *bottom-up* or *top-down* treatment algorithms. In the traditional bottom-up approach, medicines with the lowest toxicity profile are used, gradually increasing doses as needed to eliminate inflammatory activity. If, however, clinical response is judged inadequate, either a more potent drug with a potentially less favorable toxicity profile is added to the regimen or the original medicine, if judged to be ineffective, is discontinued and replaced. The disadvantage of the bottom-up approach is that many steroid-sparing drugs can take 2–6 weeks to reach steady-state kinetics; during that induction period, irreversible damage can occur to the visual axis, especially when the starting dose is too low or if the drug will not end up being effective at any dose. With this in mind, especially when there is an immediate and significant threat to vision, many uveitis specialists prefer a top-down approach, which instead starts at high doses that are reduced over time. When using steroid-sparing agents, monotherapy that controls chronic inflammation is a desirable goal. However, in clinical practice, combination therapy is commonly used with double or even triple immunosuppression needed to adequately control inflammation. Potential advantages of combination therapy include being able to employ a lower dose of each medicine compared to the higher doses frequently needed with monotherapy and the potentially synergistic effect of using drugs with different mechanisms of action.

Prior to initiating treatment with steroids and/or steroid-sparing agents, it is essential to assess the patient's overall health to insure they are appropriate candidates for systemic IMT. The role of the uveitis specialist is not only to monitor response to treatment but to monitor for potential iatrogenic side effects induced by IMT, and comanagement with a patient's internist or rheumatologist is highly recommended. Prior to starting any IMT, patients should undergo the standard work-up necessary to institute this treatment. Baseline bone density measurements are considered for patients likely to be on a long course of steroids, and pregnancy must be excluded in all females of child-bearing age. Once started on IMT, routine monitoring of potential drug-induced toxicity should be performed every 1–3 months. Trough drug levels (cyclosporin and tacrolimus) can also be periodically checked to help insure target serum levels.

Treatment targets must be clearly delineated to establish if the patient's response is adequate to justify continued therapy. Proper monitoring of treatment efficacy includes periodic follow-up ocular examinations as previously described. Monitoring exams which may potentially be required include serial visual field testing, fundus photography, FA and ICGA imaging, OCT, and ERG testing. Medications that fail to meet pretreatment clinical criteria set for establishing efficacy should be discontinued in favor of other drug options.

Immunosuppressive drugs modulate the immune system by varied mechanisms of action and can be categorized into four main groups:

- Antimetabolites that interfere with purine nucleotide synthesis and include methotrexate, azathioprine, and mycophenolate mofetil.
- Calcineurin inhibitors interfere with T-cell activation and include cyclosporine and tacrolimus.
- Alkylating agents cause DNA damage by cross-linking of DNA bases and include cyclophosphamide and chlorambucil.
- Biologics are monoclonal antibodies or receptors directed against specific cytokines and cytokine receptors and include, but are not limited to, infliximab, adalimumab, tocilizumab, rituximab, and abatacept.

Treatment of Noninfectious Anterior Uveitis

Anterior uveitis accounts for the majority of cases seen by comprehensive ophthalmologists. A significant predisposing factor to the development of anterior uveitis is the presence of the HLA-B27 class I HLA haplotype, with or without associated systemic diseases such as ankylosing spondylitis, reactive arthritis, inflammatory bowel disease, and psoriatic arthritis. Other entities to consider include sarcoidosis, Fuchs' heterochromic iridocyclitis, JIA, Kawasaki's,

Behçet's, demyelinating diseases, TINU, and ocular trauma.

Most cases of noninfectious, acute anterior uveitis require only topical steroid treatment. In cases with severe inflammation not adequately responding to frequent steroid drops, it may become necessary to add a short course of systemic prednisone or a periocular steroid injection. As previously discussed, intraocular inflammation can lead to adhesions of the posterior iris to the underlying lens (posterior synechiae). To prevent this potential complication, in addition to controlling intraocular inflammation, "pupil management" with a topical cycloplegic-mydriatic agent such as cyclopentolate is essential. The consequences of posterior synechiae (PS) include inability of the pupil to properly dilate, a potential cosmetic issue, and, more importantly, limits (or completely blocks) visualization of the posterior segment. In addition, as discussed above, extensive PS may result in angle-closure glaucoma (Fig. 27.17).

In cases of chronic anterior uveitis which require long-term treatment, it is generally con-sidered acceptable to leave patients on steroid drops at a frequency of one to two times a day, if that controls intraocular inflammation. In cases requiring a higher maintenance topical steroid dose, uveitis specialists generally recommend adding a systemic immunomodulating drug to permit discontinuation of steroid drops in order to prevent steroid-induced cataracts and glaucoma. As previously mentioned, systemic immunomodulating therapy may offer the potential advantage of being able to induce prolonged, drug-free remission of uveitis.

Treatment of Noninfectious Intermediate Uveitis

In the absence of concomitant anterior segment involvement, there is no role for topical corticosteroids in the management of intermediate uveitis. Topically administered drops do not penetrate into the vitreous cavity in sufficient concentrations to be therapeutic. Not all cases of intermediate uveitis require treatment; some may have a relatively benign, non-sight-threatening course, in which case patients need only be carefully followed for evidence of potentially sight-threatening complications that would then mandate intervention. For unilateral cases of sight-threatening intermediate uveitis requiring treatment, the involved eye can be treated with periocular corticosteroid injections, which act as slow-release depot reservoirs. Injections can be repeated every 4–6 weeks depending on the clinical response. Alternatively, to circumvent the potential need for multiple injections, slow-release steroid implants can be placed directly into the vitreous cavity. A commonly used, commercially available biodegradable dexamethasone implant (Ozurdex) is injected into the eye in a routine office procedure and maintains adequate steroid levels in the vitreous cavity for 4–6 months. For cases of intermediate uveitis with a pars plana snowbank, additional treatment with peripheral cryotherapy or laser photocoagulation to the area of snowbanking with or without vitrectomy can be effective in achieving long-term control of intraocular inflammation.

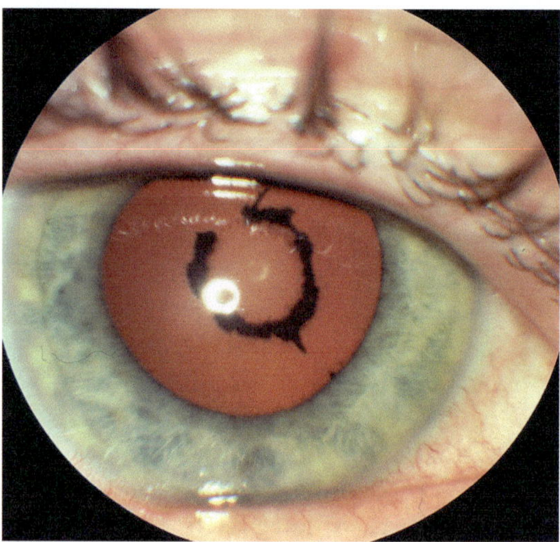

Fig. 27.17 Lysed 360° synechiae, leaving residual iris pigment ring adherent to anterior lens surface. Complete posterior synechia such as this can result in the condition known as a secluded pupil, where the iris-lens adhesion separates anterior and posterior chambers. This pupillary block will typically lead to buildup of aqueous posterior to the iris (iris bombé) and secondary angle-closure glaucoma

If local therapy is ineffective, or in bilateral cases with or without an associated systemic disease, systemic treatment can be employed in a manner similar to the treatment of posterior uveitis (see below).

Treatment of Noninfectious Posterior Uveitis and Panuveitis

Due to its effectiveness and rapidity of action, the first line of therapy for posterior uveitis or panuveitis is systemic prednisone. For patients with sight-threatening uveitis, when a more rapid onset of action is desirable, treatment can begin with IV methylprednisolone for 3 days prior to starting induction doses of oral prednisone. Induction doses need to be continued until an adequate response is obtained, followed by a slow taper as permitted by the patient's inflammatory status. If long-term, high-dose (usually greater than 7.5–10 mg/day) maintenance steroid therapy is required, steroid-sparing agents are added to reduce or eliminate the need for oral steroids. As previously discussed, there are few evidence-based recommendations from randomized clinical trials to help choose the IMT agent of choice. When the clinical situation permits, a bottom-up approach (as described above) can be used, with the goal being to ultimately use the lowest doses of the safest drugs that adequately control intraocular inflammation. When combination therapy is needed, "recipe building" combines agents that impact different arms of the inflammatory cycle to achieve synergistic effects. Despite the effectiveness of the newer biologics agents, they are generally added last, due to high cost and difficulty obtaining insurance approval for off-label use in uveitis patients. To avoid the systemic risks of IMT, local ocular therapy may be considered, especially in unilateral cases not associated with a systemic disease. Options include periocular injections of steroids or intravitreal placement of steroid implants. Currently, the two available steroid implants include Ozurdex (see above) and Retisert, a fluocinolone acetonide, non-biodegradable implant which is surgically placed in the posterior segment and provides intraocular steroid for approximately 30 months.

Suggested Reading

Dick AD, Okada AA, Forrester J. Practical manual of intraocular inflammation. New York: Informa Healthcare; 2008.

Durrani K, Zakka FR, Ahmed M, Memon M, Siddique SS, Foster CS. Systemic therapy with conventional and novel immunomodulatory agents for ocular inflammatory disease. Surv Ophthalmol. 2011;96(6):474–510.

Foster CS, Vitale AT. Diagnosis and treatment of uveitis. 2nd ed. New Delhi: Jaypee-Highlights Medical Publishers Inc.; 2013.

Jabs D, Rosenbaum JT, Foster CS, et al. Guidelines for the use of immunosuppressive drugs in patients with ocular inflammatory disorders: recommendations of an expert panel. Am J Ophthalmol. 2000;130:492–513.

Jaffe GJ, Dick AD, Brezin AP, et al. Adalimumab in patients with active noninfectious uveitis. N Engl J Med. 2016;375:932–43.

Nussenblatt RB, Whitcup SM. Uveitis fundamentals and clinical practice. 4th ed. St. Louis: Mosby; 2010.

Streilein JW. Anterior chamber associated immune deviation: the privilege of immunity in the eye. Surv Ophthalmol. 1990;35(1):67–73.

Weiss MJ, Hofeldt AJ. Uveitis. In: Gallin P, editor. Practical pediatric ophthalmology. New York: Thieme Medical Publishers, Inc.; 1999.

Infectious and Inflammatory Chorioretinopathies

Royce W. S. Chen

As discussed in the previous chapter, uveitis is a state of intraocular inflammation that may be either infectious or noninfectious (autoimmune) in nature. Broadly, uveitis can be classified into four categories depending on the primary site of inflammation:

- Anterior uveitis – affects the iris and ciliary body; inflammation primarily present in anterior chamber
- Intermediate uveitis – affects the vitreous and pars plana of the ciliary body
- Posterior uveitis – affects retina and choroid
- Panuveitis – affects all three sites

A heterogeneous group of disorders, both infectious and noninfectious, uveitides may result in inflammation that manifests as whitish-yellowish lesions of the retina and choroid, inflammation of the retinal vessels, and necrosis of retinal tissue that may lead to retinal detachment, macular edema, ischemia of the retina and choroid, and retinal and choroidal neovascularization. While several of the disorders discussed in this chapter may also manifest as an anterior uveitis or intermediate uveitis, herein we focus on the manifestations present in the setting of posterior or panuveitis.

R. W. S. Chen, MD (✉)
Columbia University Irving Medical Center, New York, NY, USA

Department of Ophthalmology, Edward S. Harkness Eye Institute, Columbia University Vagelos College of Physicians and Surgeons, New York, NY, USA
e-mail: rc2631@cumc.columbia.edu

Infectious Retinopathies

Infectious agents, including bacteria, fungi, viruses, and parasites, may spread to the eye either from direct inoculation (e.g., penetrating injury, perforated corneal ulcer) or from hematogenous spread, leading to one or more foci of infection in the retina and choroid.

Endophthalmitis

Bacteria and fungi may infect the retina and choroid by direct inoculation (e.g., cataract surgery or penetrating trauma) or hematogenous spread from another source in the body, such as an infected cardiac valve. When infections arise directly from contiguous structures, there is typically significant inflammation in the anterior segment, as well as vitritis, thus limiting the view of the retina and choroid. In cases of endogenous spread, septic emboli from other sites in the body may travel to the retinal or choroidal circulation, resulting in a subretinal or choroidal abscess. Vitreous and anterior inflammation may or may not be present. Endophthalmitis is treated with a combination of systemic and intravitreal antibiotics or antifungal agents with varying degrees of success, depending upon the causative organism and promptness of treatment. Surgical treatment with pars plana vitrectomy may also be required (Figs. 28.1 and 28.2).

© Springer Nature Switzerland AG 2019
D. S. Casper, G. A. Cioffi (eds.), *The Columbia Guide to Basic Elements of Eye Care*,
https://doi.org/10.1007/978-3-030-10886-1_28

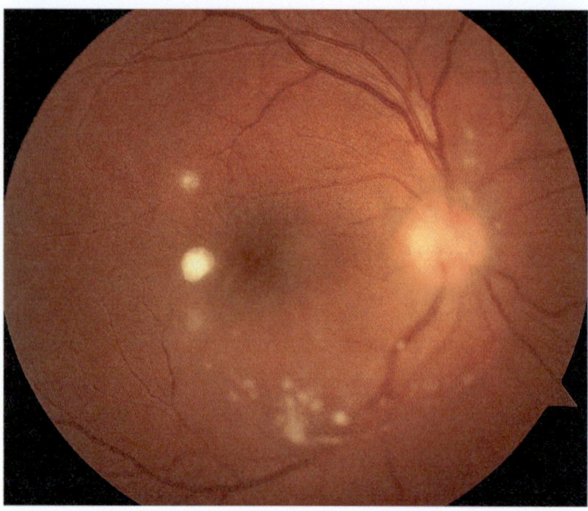

Fig. 28.1 Fungal endophthalmitis from hematogenous spread. Typical "fungus ball" infiltrates are seen within the vitreous, with mild associated vitritis

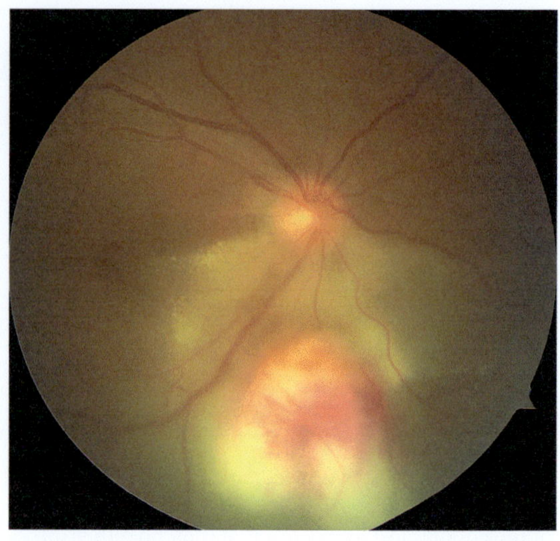

Fig. 28.2 Subretinal fungal abscess with associated sub-retinal fluid and hemorrhage in a patient with acute myelogenous leukemia

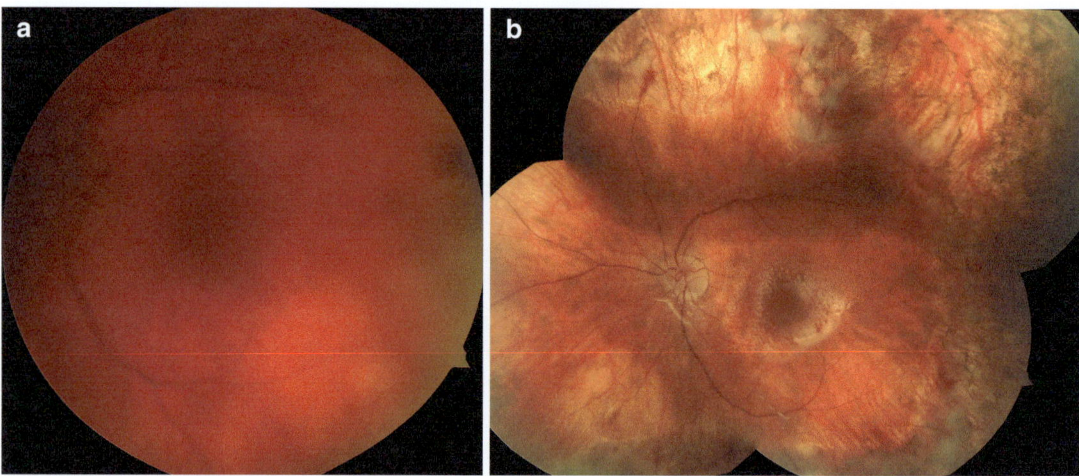

Fig. 28.3 (**a**) Acute retinal necrosis (ARN) OS in an otherwise healthy, 47-year-old man. There are severe vitritis, optic neuritis, and retinal necrosis present. Diagnosed as ARN and believed to be of herpetic etiol-ogy. (**b**) 2 months after treatment with acyclovir and prednisone. The patient underwent surgery with vitrectomy and silicone oil to repair a retinal detachment

Acute Retinal Necrosis

The herpesviruses, including varicella-zoster virus, herpes simplex virus 1 and 2, and cyto-megalovirus, may cause a destructive retinitis in immunocompetent individuals termed acute retinal necrosis (ARN). This condition is characterized by the development of anterior and intermediate uveitis, often accompanied by pain. An occlusive vasculitis occurs in the retina, with necrosis typically affecting the periph-ery, eventually coalescing and moving centripetally toward the macula as the disease progresses. Optic neuritis may accompany the retinal necrosis, leading to a worsened visual prognosis. Retinal detachment is common due to the formation of retinal breaks in necrotic tissue, affecting up to 70% of eyes with ARN. Treatment consists of intravitreal antiviral agents, systemic antivirals, systemic steroids, possible laser retinopexy, and vitrectomy as necessary (Fig. 28.3a, b).

Progressive Outer Retinal Necrosis

A related condition associated with the herpesviruses is progressive outer retinal necrosis (PORN), a syndrome in which rapid destruction of the retina occurs in immunocompromised individuals (e.g., those with acquired immune deficiency syndrome (AIDS) or transplant patients on chronic systemic immunosuppression). Unlike acute retinal necrosis (ARN), there is usually minimal vasculitis and vitritis, and the posterior pole is involved early in the course of disease. There are multifocal deep yellowish-whitish retinal lesions that become confluent with disease progression. Prognosis is poor in this condition, despite antiviral treatment.

Other Causes of Viral Retinitis

Globalization has resulted in the ability and desire of humans (and viruses) to intermix with unprecedented levels of freedom. In the past decade, this freedom of human migration has led to increasingly large outbreaks of Ebola (spread by direct bodily fluid contact), Zika (transmitted by *Aedes* mosquitos), West Nile (most commonly spread by various mosquito species), and chikungunya viruses (most often transmitted by *Aedes* mosquitos), among others. Although still relatively little is known about the pathophysiology of uveitis in these cases, all of these viruses may cause a multifocal retinitis and/or choroiditis in infected individuals.

Toxoplasmosis

Toxoplasma gondii is an obligate, intracellular protozoan that is responsible for one of the most common causes of posterior uveitis. Humans may be infected through ingestion of oocysts from infected cats or raw or undercooked meats. Individuals may also be infected via transmission through mucosal surfaces. Both acquired and congenital infections may result in toxoplasmic *retinochoroiditis* (retinochoroiditis because the retina is preferentially affected over the choroid). In cases of congenital infections with reactivation, there is typically a large atrophic scar in the macula, with an adjacent area of active focal retinitis. There may be minimal-to-significant vitritis overlying the area of retinitis. Occasionally, there will be vascular sheathing and associated retinal hemorrhages in the area of the active lesion. Newly acquired infections have similar presentations to reactivation of a congenital lesion, except that the foci of retinal inflammation are not adjacent to a chorioretinal scar. Vision loss in toxoplasmic retinochoroiditis may be secondary to vitreous inflammation, macular involvement, optic neuritis, retinal detachment, epiretinal membrane, and rarely, macular hole. If the macula is not involved in disease, vision may return to baseline levels after resolution of the infection. Controversy exists regarding the use of antibiotic agents and systemic steroids in the treatment of this condition, but many practitioners believe that the use of these agents will hasten visual recovery. In some cases of recurrent uveitis, long-term prophylactic antibiotic use may be indicated (Figs. 27.15a, b and 28.4a–c).

Cat Scratch Disease

Bartonella henselae, a gram-negative rod, is responsible for cat scratch disease, a condition characterized by regional lymphadenopathy, fever, and malaise, usually associated with a cat bite or scratch. When affecting the retina, cat scratch disease may lead to a characteristic set of findings including macular star formation (exudative), macular fluid, optic nerve head swelling, mild vitritis, and, often, small yellow-white retinal infiltrates (Fig. 28.5). Together, this constellation of findings has been termed Leber's idiopathic stellate neuroretinitis. Although vision may decrease to worse than 20/400 at presentation, the clinical prognosis is generally good, with or without antibiotics or steroid treatment.

Syphilis

Syphilis, often considered a masquerade-type syndrome due to its protean manifestations that mimic other infections, is a bacterial infection caused by the spirochete *Treponema pallidum*.

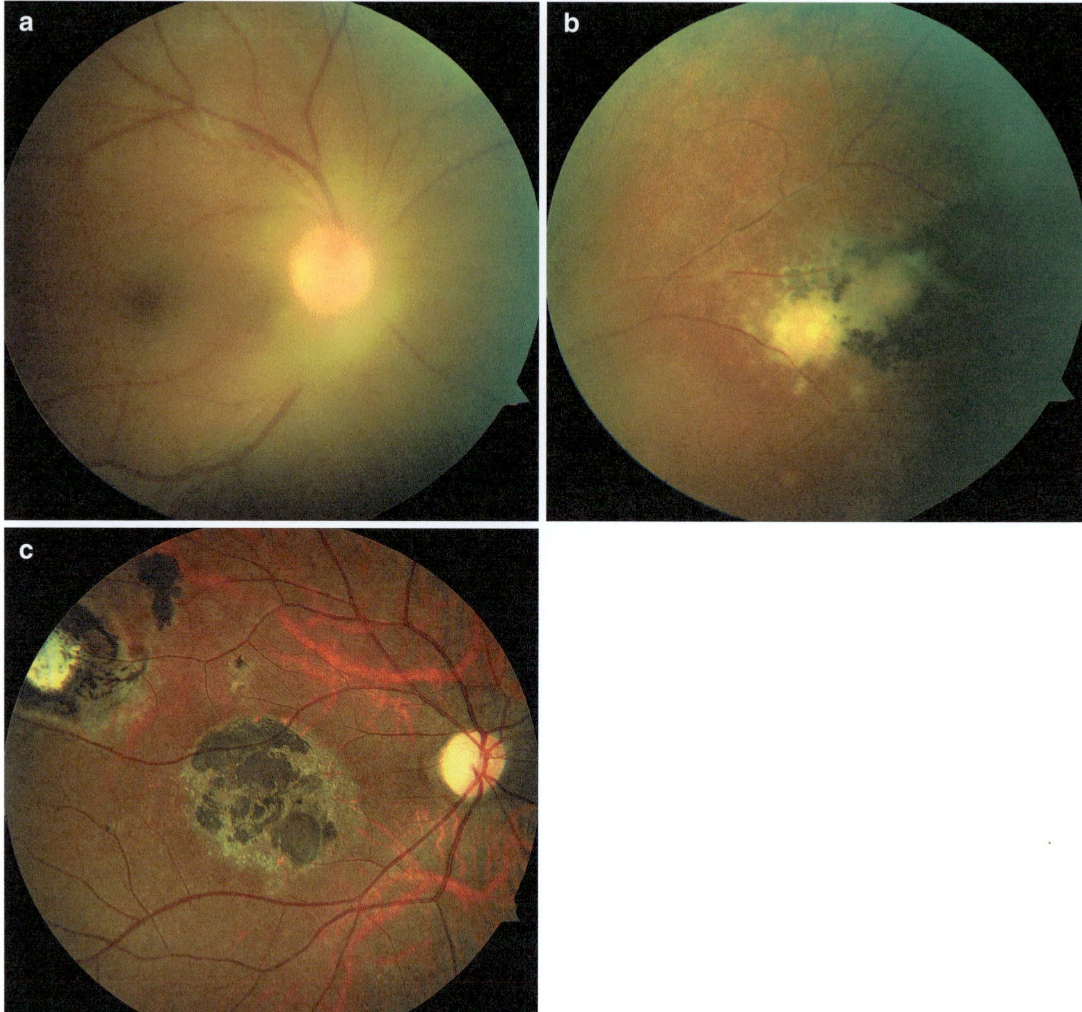

Fig. 28.4 (**a**) A 40-year-old woman with reactivated toxoplasmosis OD, showing uveitis with vitritis centrally. (**b**) A peripheral old, hyperpigmented lesion adjacent to an area of acute reactivation, with associated vascular sheathing also noted. (**c**) A 43-year-old woman found to have intra- and extramacular extensive old toxoplasmosis scars in her right eye

Just as its systemic manifestations are varied, the ocular manifestations of syphilitic uveitis are wide-ranging, and therefore this condition is one of the few diagnoses that must be considered in every case of uveitis. Although syphilitic uveitis may accompany any stage of systemic infection, it is more likely to occur with secondary or tertiary syphilis. Posterior ocular manifestations may include vitritis, vasculitis, exudative detachment, optic neuritis, neuroretinitis, and both non-necrotizing and necrotizing chorioretinitis. Syphilitic uveitis responds favorably to penicillin therapy. Periocular or systemic corticosteroids are useful adjuncts in the management of inflammation (Figs. 28.6 and 28.7). Syphilitic infection is often accompanied by other concurrent sexually transmitted infections such as HIV and gonorrhea, and concurrent infection must therefore be ruled out (Figs. 28.8 and 28.9).

Tuberculosis

Another masquerade-type syndrome, tuberculosis, is a condition that must be considered in all cases of uveitis. As *Mycobacterium tuberculosis* is an obligate aerobe, it has an affinity for highly oxygenated tissues, and the most highly oxygenated ocular structure is the choroid. Posterior uveitis may manifest as solitary or multifocal choroidal tubercles (granulomas), which appear as deep yellow-white lesions that originate in the choroid.

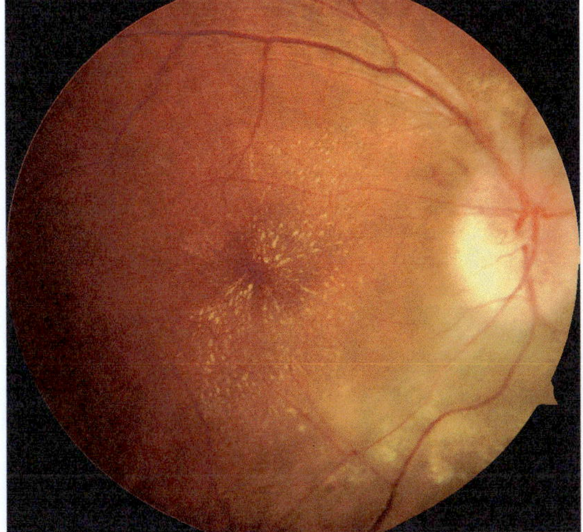

Fig. 28.5 Macular star with optic disc edema and subretinal fluid in a patient with neuroretinitis

Tuberculous chorioretinitis may be accompanied by serous retinal detachment, vasculitis, vitritis, and papillitis. Treatment follows the same regimens as indicated for pulmonary disease.

Noninfectious Retinopathies

White Dot Syndromes

The white dot syndromes comprise a group of noninfectious retinopathies that are usually transient in nature. Each condition has its own characteristic presentation, which manifests with small-to-large whitish lesions in the deep retina to choroid, accompanied by visual disturbances. The following conditions have been classified as white dot syndromes:

- Multiple evanescent white dot syndrome
- Acute posterior multifocal placoid pigment epitheliopathy
- Birdshot retinochoroidopathy
- Serpiginous choroidopathy
- Multifocal choroiditis and panuveitis
- Punctate inner choroidopathy
- Acute zonal occult outer retinopathy
- Acute retinal pigment epitheliitis
- Acute macular neuroretinopathy
- Acute idiopathic blind spot enlargement

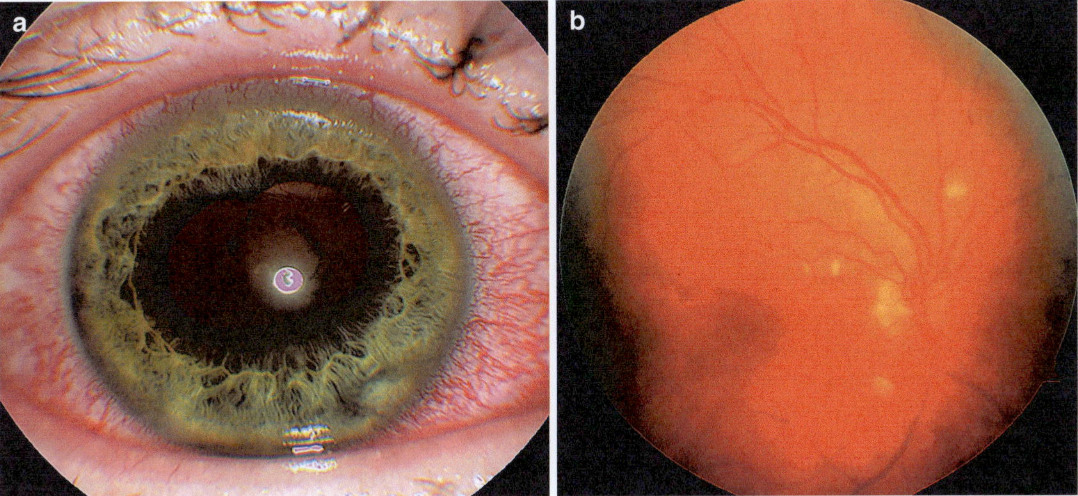

Fig. 28.6 A patient with syphilitic panuveitis. (**a**) Conjunctival injection with posterior synechiae formation. (**b**) Fundus photograph shows hazy media due to vitreous inflammation and multifocal yellow-white retinal lesions

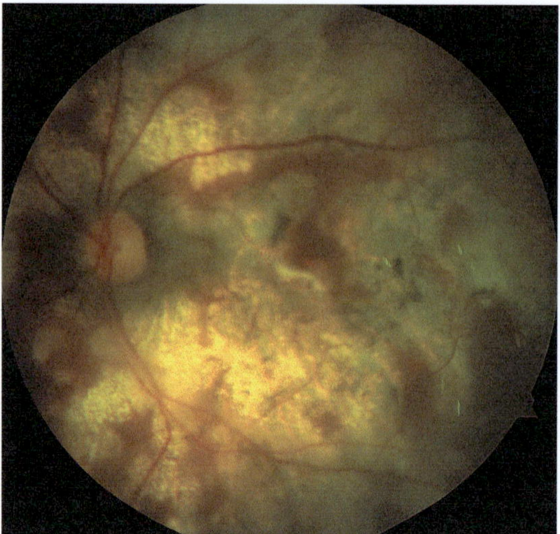

Fig. 28.7 A 62-year-old woman with placoid syphilitic chorioretinitis, originally thought to be serpiginous choroiditis, not responsive to prednisone treatment. This fundus image is status-post IV and IM Penicillin, showing resolution of acute chorioretinitis. Residual atrophic chorioretinal scars, yellow-white subretinal infiltrates centered around the disc, and peripheral salt and pepper pigmented lesions are now present

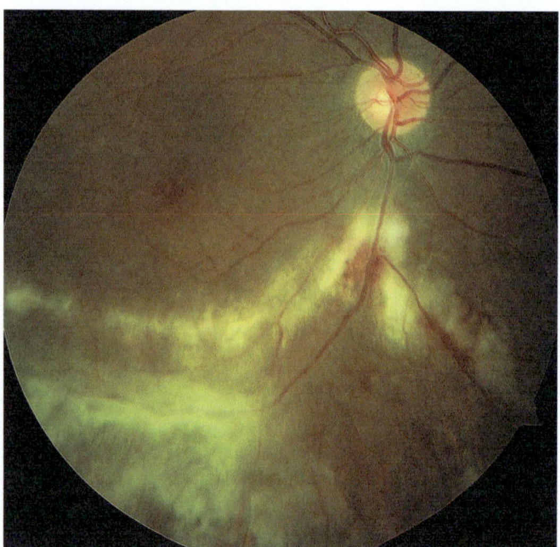

Fig. 28.9 Acute HIV-related CMV retinitis in a 35-year-old woman. Typical yellow-white lesions follow the vasculature, with associated hemorrhages, but minimal vitritis is present

Visual prognoses in this condition range from excellent to poor. Vision loss may occur secondary to macular inflammatory and ischemic changes, as well as the development of choroidal neovascularization (Figs. 28.10, 28.11, and 28.12).

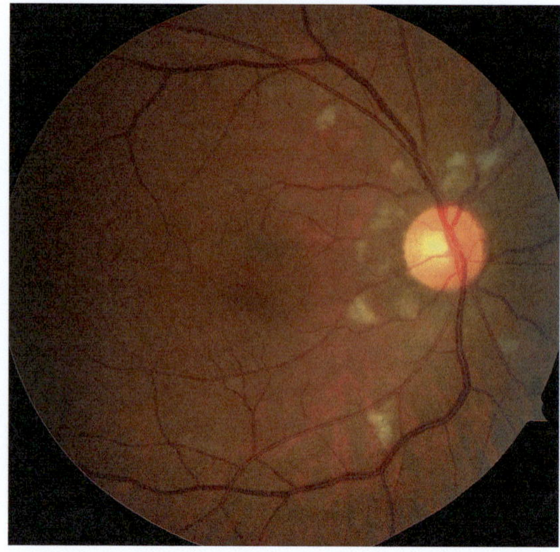

Fig. 28.8 A 62-year-old man with HIV/AIDS with HIV retinopathy. There are cotton wool spots along the arcades bilaterally, without hemorrhages, and no evidence of active CMV retinitis

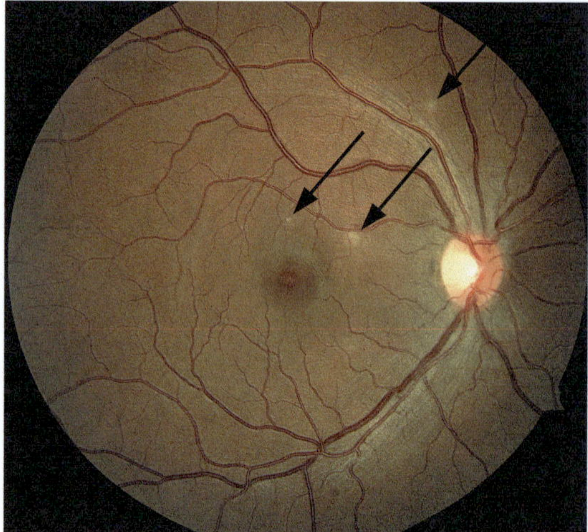

Fig. 28.10 Multiple evanescent white dot syndrome (MEWDS) in a 27-year-old woman. The black arrows show three macular and extramacular lesions in a mild case without associated macular edema, vitritis, or optic neuropathy

Behçet's Disease

Behçet's disease is a chronic, recurrent systemic inflammatory disorder characterized by the triad of oral ulcers, genital ulcers, and uveitis. Skin lesions are often present. Ocular disease typically follows the onset of systemic disease by a few years. In addition to significant anterior uveitis, frequently accompanied by hypopyon, posterior uveitis may present

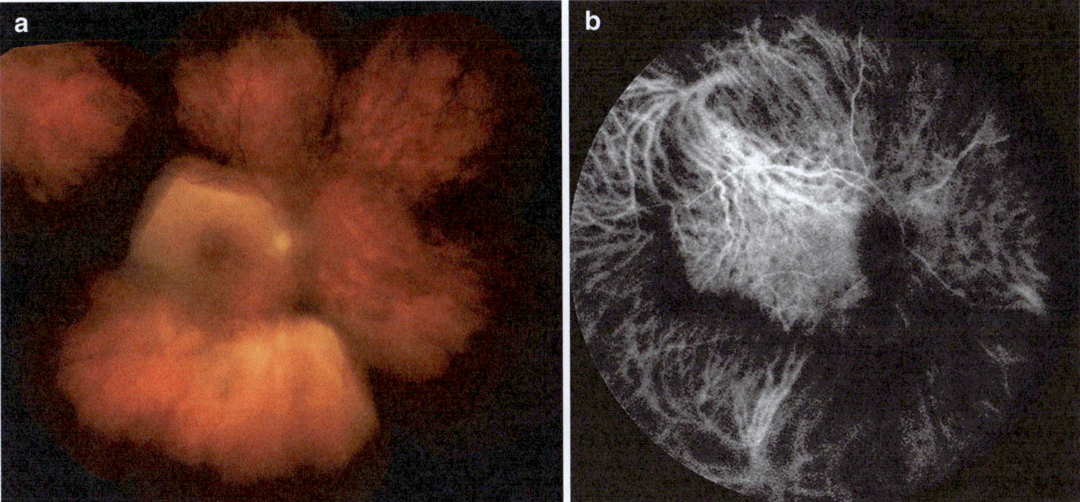

Fig. 28.11 An HLA-A29-positive patient with birdshot retinochoroidopathy. (**a**) Montage color fundus photo demonstrating small yellow lesions that extend radially from the optic nerve. (**b**) Corresponding indocyanine green angiography image showing blocked fluorescence in the areas of the yellow lesions

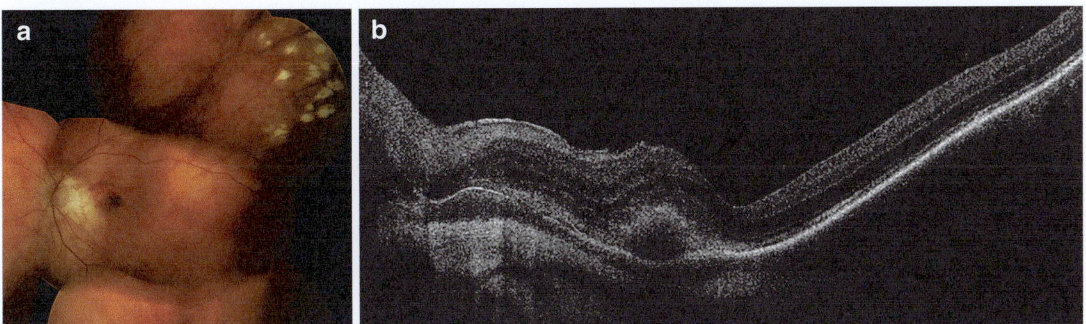

Fig. 28.12 A patient with multifocal choroiditis. (**a**) Montage color fundus photo demonstrating retinal hemorrhage and choroidal neovascular membrane in the macula and yellow punched-out lesions in the superotemporal periphery. (**b**) Corresponding macula spectral domain optical coherence tomography image showing subretinal elevation and hyperreflectivity from the choroidal neovascular membrane

with occlusive vasculitis, vitritis, retinal hemorrhages, macular edema, and ischemic optic neuropathy. The recurrent retinal vaso-occlusive episodes often lead to irreversible visual loss. If neovascularization occurs, recurrent vitreous hemorrhages and retinal detachment may develop. Because of the severity of recurrent occlusive attacks, long-term systemic immunosuppression is indicated.

Lupus Vasculitis

Systemic lupus erythematosus is a common autoimmune disorder characterized by immune complex deposition that may result in ocular disease. In milder forms, cotton wool spots may be the only visible retinal change, but the disease may present with severe vaso-occlusive injury to the retina and choroid. Neovascularization may result, as well as serous detachments of the retina and retinal pigment epithelium. In addition to systemic immunosuppressive therapy, plasmapheresis and systemic anticoagulation may be indicated. Panretinal photocoagulation may be employed for control of ischemic sequelae (Fig. 28.13).

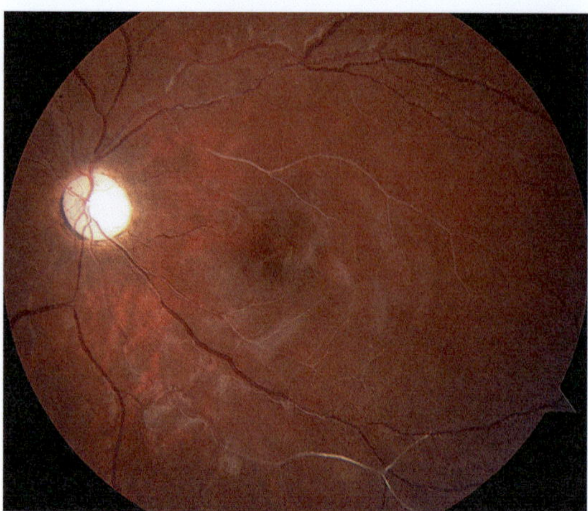

Fig. 28.13 A 16-year-old female with severe retinal lupus vasculitis who presented with loss of vision bilaterally. Fundus examination showed temporal disc pallor, arteriolar thinning, and sclerosis with venous dilation. Fluorescein angiography showed severe macular ischemia with absent capillary filling

Specific Ocular Effects of Anti-inflammatory Medications

Many medications have deleterious effects on the visual system, but perhaps the two most well-known toxicities are due to corticosteroid and plaquenil (hydroxychloroquine) use. The effects of steroids, primarily cataract formation and elevation of intraocular pressure in susceptible persons, have already been mentioned in the introductory uveitis chapter. Plaquenil is used for the treatment of many autoimmune conditions, including lupus, sarcoidosis, rheumatoid arthritis, and Sjögren's, all of which may also cause significant ocular pathologies, as has been discussed. Plaquenil-induced ocular effects are much rarer than those seen with corticosteroid use but may be significantly more vision-threatening. The ocular toxicity is poorly understood but is believed to be related to cumulative dosage and specifically causes a retinal lesion that occurs centrally and is known as "bull's-eye maculopathy" (Fig. 28.14a–f). Long-term use of the medication, at higher doses, is related to more likely occurrence of plaquenil maculopathy. Of great concern is the fact that once the lesion has been identified, and the medication stopped, further progression of retinal degeneration may still continue. Regular eye exams for patients taking plaquenil are strongly recommended, although the frequency of examination and the particular methods used to detect early toxicity are not uniformly agreed upon. Color vision and central visual field assessment and optical coherence are commonly used to assess plaquenil-induced maculopathy. A macular electroretinogram may sometimes be obtained depending on the findings of the more common tests.

Conclusion

Many conditions, both infectious and noninfectious, may lead to inflammation of the retina and choroid. The entities discussed in this chapter are presented to provide a broad survey of conditions encountered by the uveitis and retinal specialist, but this list is by no means comprehensive. A nuanced approach that considers medical and ocular history, constitutional symptoms, ocular manifestations, and targeted ancillary testing is required to provide patients with appropriate therapies and follow-up. Close collaboration with infectious disease specialists, rheumatologists, and other medical professionals is usually a critical aspect of care in these often complicated cases.

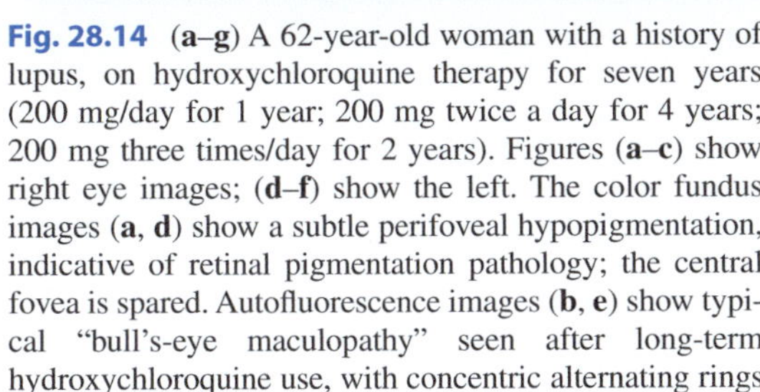

Fig. 28.14 (**a–g**) A 62-year-old woman with a history of lupus, on hydroxychloroquine therapy for seven years (200 mg/day for 1 year; 200 mg twice a day for 4 years; 200 mg three times/day for 2 years). Figures (**a–c**) show right eye images; (**d–f**) show the left. The color fundus images (**a, d**) show a subtle perifoveal hypopigmentation, indicative of retinal pigmentation pathology; the central fovea is spared. Autofluorescence images (**b, e**) show typical "bull's-eye maculopathy" seen after long-term hydroxychloroquine use, with concentric alternating rings of hyper- and hypopigmentation; the hyperpigmented perifoveal areas, which correspond to the fundus image perifoveal hypopigmentation, are believed to represent areas of photoreceptor damage. Central (10–2) Humphrey visual fields (**c, f**) show dense, bilateral perifoveal ring scotomas, with sparing of the most central fields. (**g**) Spectral-domain OCT images of hydroxychloroquine retinopathy show bilateral parafoveal thinning and disruption (yellow arrows) with relative sparing of the central foveal anatomy. (Images courtesy of Dr Srilaxmi Bearelly)

Suggested Reading

Freund KB, Sarraf D, Mieler WF, Yannuzzi LA, editors. The retinal atlas. Philadelphia: Elsevier; 2017.

Jabs DA, Busingye J. Approach to the diagnosis of the uveitides. Am J Ophthalmol. 2013;156:228–36.

Marmor MF, Kellner U, Lai TYY, Melles RB, Mieler W. Recommendations on screening for chloroquine and hydroxychloroquine retinopathy (2016 revision). Ophthalmology. 2016;123:1386–94. 2016 by the American Academy of Ophthalmology.

Nussenblatt R, Whitcup SM. Uveitis: fundamentals and clinical practice: expert consult. 4th ed. Philadelphia: Mosby; 2010.

Quillen DA, Blodi BA. Clinical Retina. Chicago: AMA Press; 2002. Chapter 9.

Part VI

Oculoplastics and Orbit

Thyroid Eye Disease

Ashley A. Campbell and Michael Kazim

Thyroid eye disease (TED) is an autoimmune disease most commonly associated with immune thyroid disorders, causing enlargement of orbital fat and muscle. Also known as Graves' orbitopathy or Graves' ophthalmopathy, TED is the most common cause of unilateral or bilateral proptosis in adults. The clinical phenotype of the disease is diverse, with symptoms and manifestations varying from mild to severe. In most patients, the disease presents with mild lid retraction, minimal proptosis, and dry eye symptoms. In a smaller subset of patients, however, the disease produces severe, often disfiguring proptosis, leading to corneal ulceration, limited extraocular motility, debilitating diplopia, and optic neuropathy.

Epidemiology

The annual age-adjusted incidence of TED in the United States is 16 in 100,000 women and 3 in 100,000 men. Females are affected six times more frequently than males, except in the older age group, where the female to male ratio decreases. Among patients diagnosed with TED, approximately 90% have Graves' disease (GD), 1% have primary hypothyroidism, 4% have Hashimoto's thyroiditis with hypothyroidism, and 5% are euthyroid. Depending on the report, between 20% and 50% of patients with Graves' hyperthyroidism will develop TED, and 85% of these will be diagnosed within 18 months of diagnosis of the dysthyroid state. The diagnosis of TED precedes the diagnosis of hyperthyroidism in 20% of patients, is made at the time of diagnosis of hyperthyroidism in 40% of patients, and occurs after the diagnosis of TED in another 40%. The most prominent modifiable risk factor for the development of TED is cigarette smoking, which increases the risk of developing TED in patients who are diagnosed with GD by sevenfold. Moreover, smokers have been shown to develop more severe forms of TED and suffer active-phase orbitopathy for 2–3 years, whereas the active phase spontaneously remits within 1 year in non-smokers. Treatment with radioactive iodine (RAI) for Graves' hyperthyroidism is an additional, albeit significantly smaller risk, to the development of TED or worsening of preexisting active-phase TED. There is a significant incidence of other coexisting autoimmune conditions, including ocular myasthenia gravis (approximately 5%), rheumatoid arthritis, colitis, vitiligo, and idiopathic thrombocytopenia.

A. A. Campbell, MD (✉)
Wilmer Eye Institute, Johns Hopkins School of Medicine, Baltimore, MD, USA
e-mail: Ashley.campbell@jhmi.edu;
acampb23@jhmi.edu

M. Kazim, MD
Edward S. Harkness Eye Institute, Columbia University Vagelos College of Physicians and Surgeons, New York, NY, USA

© Springer Nature Switzerland AG 2019
D. S. Casper, G. A. Cioffi (eds.), *The Columbia Guide to Basic Elements of Eye Care*,
https://doi.org/10.1007/978-3-030-10886-1_29

Pathogenesis

TED is related to the autoimmune process that drives the dysthyroid state of Graves' disease and Hashimoto's thyroiditis. It is believed that auto-antibodies against thyroid-stimulating hormone receptor (TSHR) expressed on orbital fibroblasts contribute to the expansion of orbital soft tissues. Enlargement and fibrosis of the extraocular muscles and orbital fat leads to the signs and symptoms of TED as exophthalmos develops and venous outflow is impeded. The disease evolves from the active to inactive phase, over a period of 1 year, on average, in a non-smoker and as much as 3 years in smokers. Concurrently, the inflammatory process within extraocular muscles and orbital fat leads to fibrosis and fat proliferation, resulting in stable strabismus, eyelid retraction, and fixed proptosis.

Typical Clinical Manifestations

One of the most common presenting symptoms of patients with TED is foreign body sensation and ocular irritation. Patients also complain of pulling or tightness in the orbit, especially when attempting to look upward. The patterns of TED presentation vary with age. Typically, those younger than 40 demonstrate expansion of the orbital fat compartment and proptosis. Conversely, patients older than 40 suffer primarily with significant enlargement of extraocular muscles. Those older than 65 years are at highest risk of the development of compressive optic neuropathy.

The most common ophthalmic sign of TED is unilateral or bilateral upper lid retraction, most often associated with temporal flare (Fig. 29.1). Patients may also present with unilateral or bilateral proptosis due to the expansion of orbital tissues within the confines of the non-expansible bony orbit (Fig. 29.2). Orbital congestion, from reduced venous outflow from the orbit, manifests as conjunctival chemosis, erythema over the insertions of the rectus muscles, and fluctuating eyelid/periorbital edema or erythema (Fig. 29.3a, b). Lid swelling usually has a diurnal pattern, with symptoms worse in the morning, after nighttime recumbency with resulting dependent edema.

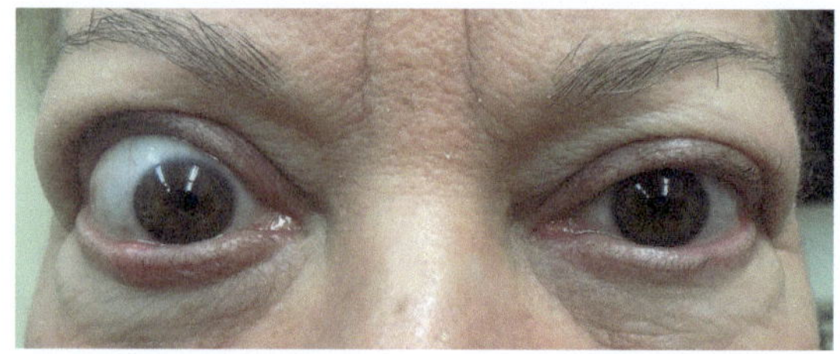

Fig. 29.1 Unilateral upper eyelid retraction of the right eye in a patient with TED in the inactive phase. The patient subsequently had surgery to correct the lid retraction so that the lid height is symmetric with the left eye

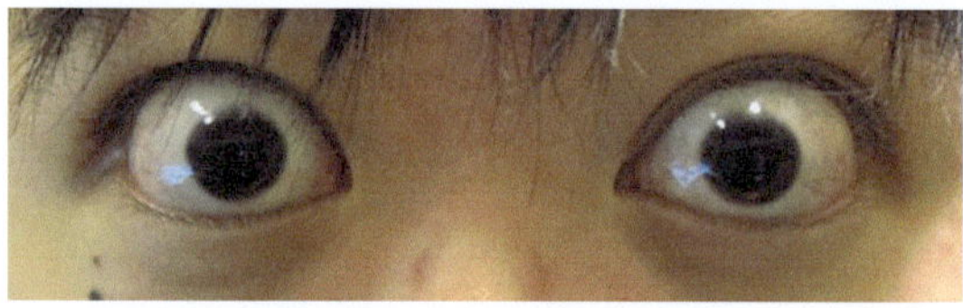

Fig. 29.2 Significant bilateral proptosis in a young patient with severe TED

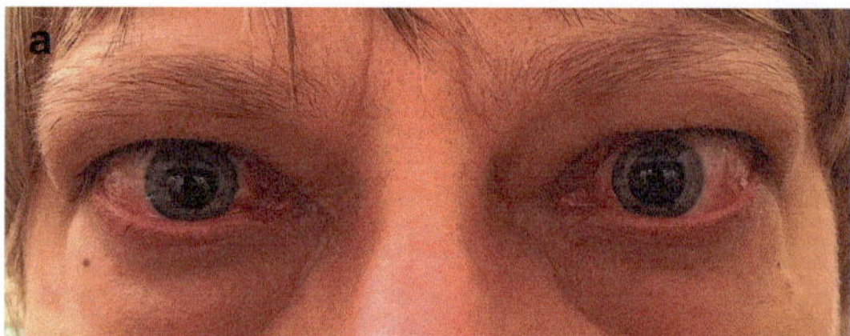

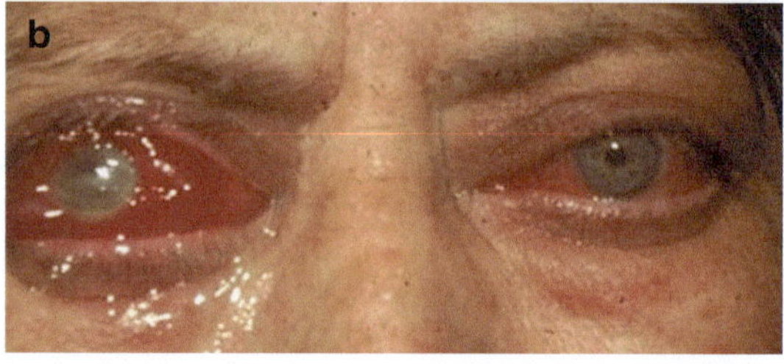

Fig. 29.3 (**a**, **b**) Conjunctival chemosis in patients with severe TED with enlargement of extraocular muscles on CT imaging, limitation of eye movements and compressive optic neuropathy. (**a**) Bilateral mild chemosis; (**b**) unilateral severe chemosis

Patients with asymmetric or significant enlargement of the extraocular muscles can develop double vision from misalignment of the eyes (Fig. 29.4). While most patients have a relatively mild course of the disease, about 10–15% develop a more severe form of TED with constant diplopia, significant exposure keratopathy due to incomplete lid closure, and a dramatic change in appearance. In about 5% of patients, optic neu-

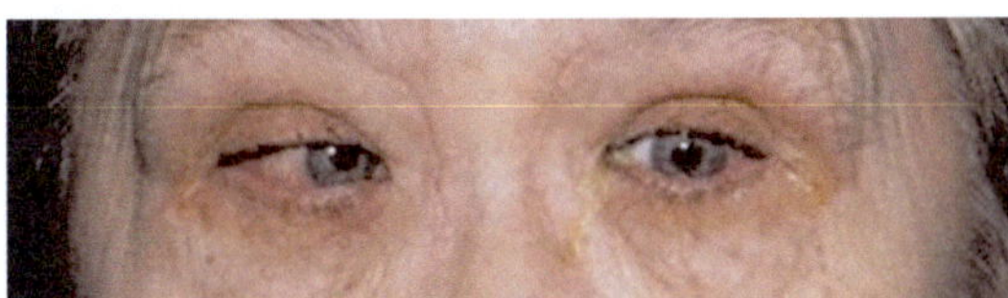

Fig. 29.4 A large angle esotropia in a patient with severe TED from enlargement of the extraocular muscles, leading to diplopia

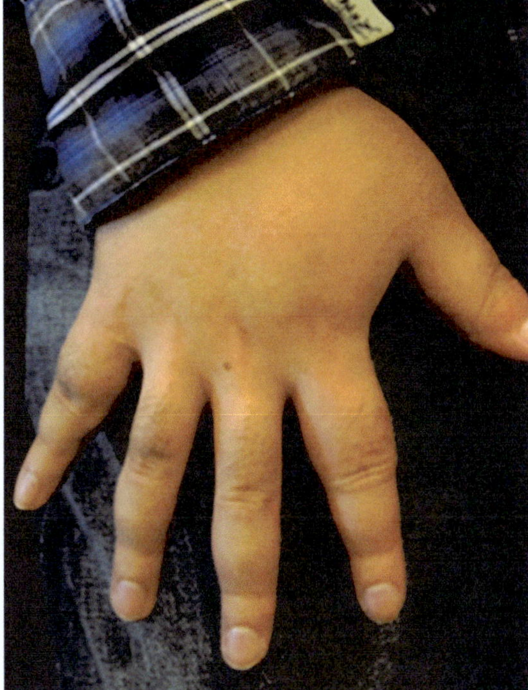

Fig. 29.5 Example of acropachy of the fingers in a patient with severe TED. The patient also had associated pretibial myxedema and elephantiasis of the feet

ropathy develops. In this form of the disease, decreased visual acuity, loss of the ability to differentiate certain colors, pupillary abnormalities, and visual field defects are typical findings.

Patients can also develop dermopathy. This includes pretibial myxedema (swelling of the soft tissue in the pretibial area) and acropachy (periosteal changes which produce swelling of the fingers and toes) (Fig. 29.5). The presence of coexistent dermopathy is associated with a worse prognosis of the TED.

Diagnostic Criteria and Assessment

The diagnosis of TED is established in the presence of two of the following criteria:

1. Radiographic (MRI or CT) evidence of fusiform enlargement of the rectus muscles without involvement of the muscle insertion, most commonly the superior rectus/levator muscle complex and/or inferior and medial recti (Fig. 29.6a, b)
2. Concurrent or prior history of autoimmune thyroid disease
3. Typical clinical features including upper eyelid retraction with temporal flare, bilateral proptosis, or restrictive strabismus

In a euthyroid patient, the presence of TSHR-binding antibodies, TSHR-stimulating antibodies, and thyroid-peroxidase antibodies can provide supportive but not conclusive evidence of TED.

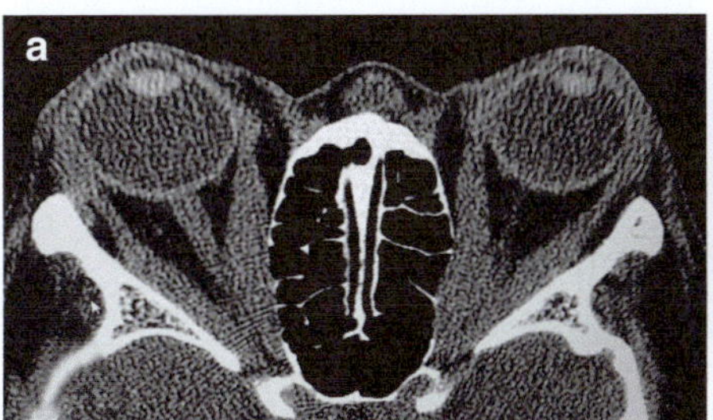
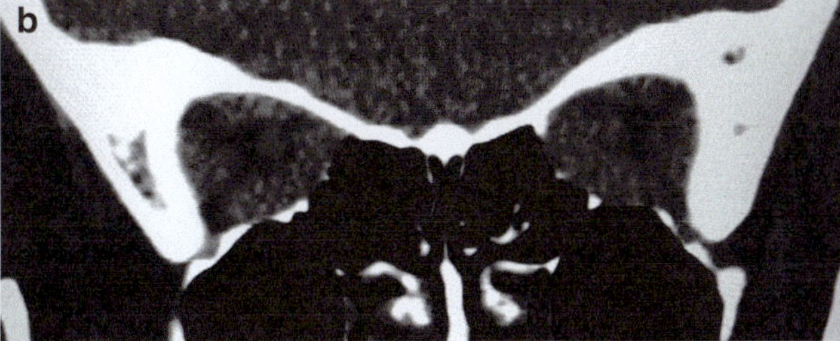

Fig. 29.6 (**a, b**) Enlargement of the extraocular muscles in a patient with severe TED and compressive optic neuropathy. (**a**) Axial computed tomography (CT) scan showing enlarged extraocular muscles. (**b**) Coronal CT scan demonstrating crowding of the optic nerve at the orbital apex, likely leading to compressive optic neuropathy

When evaluating a patient with TED, it is important to establish the duration, phase, and severity of disease. The disease course is best illustrated by Rundle's curve (Fig. 29.7), which schematically depicts the worsening of signs and symptoms of the disease before a peak is reached, followed by variable improvement, and then a long period of stability. Most patients can recall the time during which they first noted eye changes and can detail subsequent deterioration. Changes in eye symptoms over the prior 1–2 months and duration of disease less than 1 year in nonsmokers (2–3 years in smokers) are a strong indication of acute-phase disease. Conversely, clinical stability lasting 6 or more months is generally considered an indication of stable-phase disease. The goal of management varies depending upon which part of Rundle's curve the patient is on (namely, active versus inactive) and the height of the peak (i.e., whether the disease is mild or severe). The severity of TED can be established at each examination based on the presence of compressive optic neuropathy, restrictive diplopia, eyelid retraction, and exophthalmos. Predicting which patients will develop more severe manifestations of TED, especially early in the course of the active disease, can be more challenging. Doing so aids in the stratification of therapeutic options for acute-phase patients. Risk factors for development of more severe disease include smoking, rapidly progressive TED, and the presence of dermopathy. It is critical to identify optic neuropathy without delay, as this can lead to irreversible vision loss.

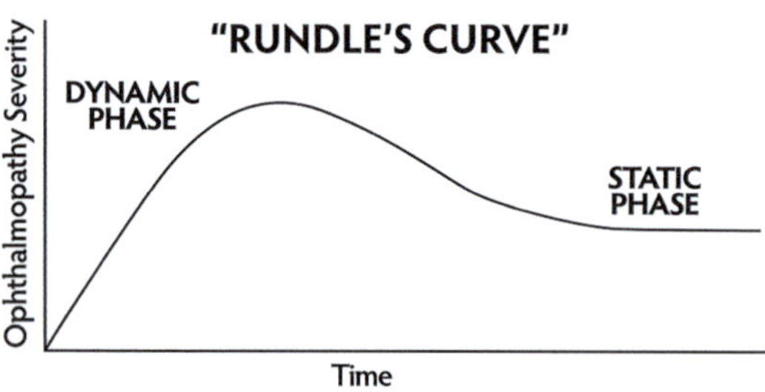

Fig. 29.7 Rundle curve plotting disease severity over time. There is an initial active phase with worsening of signs and symptoms before a peak is reached. This is followed by an inactive phase with variable improvement and then a long period of stability

Differential Diagnosis

When evaluating a patient with concern for TED, there are alternate diagnoses to consider. Orbital congestion can also be caused by an intracranial dural cavernous fistula, nonspecific orbital inflammatory disease, or even allergic or infectious conjunctivitis. Myositis or IgG4-related disease can also lead to enlargement of the extraocular muscles that can also cause strabismus or restriction of extraocular muscles. Optic neuropathy can be caused by benign intracranial hypertension or even advanced glaucoma. Proptosis can be caused by orbital tumors. CT or MR imaging can be useful in ruling out some of these other entities and should be performed on all patients suspected of having TED.

Management

Initially, management of TED is directed at managing the active phase and preventing long-term ophthalmic complications. Once in the inactive phase, attention is turned to correcting static strabismus and cosmetic disfigurement, if present. Treatment can be subdivided into medical management versus surgical management. Some patients with mild disease will have spontaneous improvement in their symptoms and require no further intervention. Others will require significant medical and surgical intervention before returning to a premorbid state. Reactivation of inflammation occurs in 5–10% of cases, and patients should be counseled accordingly.

TED is best managed as a collaborative effort, in particular with an endocrinologist. Other specialties that are frequently consulted in severe forms of the disease include radiation oncology and otolaryngology.

Medical Management

The mainstay of medical management in TED is lubrication of the ocular surface with artificial tears during the day and/or gels at nighttime. With proptosis and/or lid retraction, the inferior cornea becomes exposed, which can lead to symptomatic dryness and nocturnal lagophthalmos (incomplete closure of the eyelid). Elevation of the head of the bed and/or a reduction of dietary salt is recommended to help reduce orbital edema. More recently, a prospective trial has suggested a mild benefit of taking selenium, an oral antioxidant (200 mcg twice daily). If double vision is present, a temporary Fresnel prism lens can be applied to a spectacle lens to help the patient maintain single vision.

Coexisting thyroid abnormalities should be treated by an endocrinologist with a mind to avoid prolonged hypothyroidism. In patients treated with radioactive iodine (RAI), there is a small chance orbitopathy can worsen in the aftermath of treatment. In part, the provocative effect of RAI is the result of unrecognized, induced hypothyroidism and consequent elevation of TSH, which should be carefully monitored post-treatment. The added risk of RAI can be mitigated by the concurrent administration of prednisone (1/4 mg/kg daily for 6 weeks after RAI is administered).

In severe disease, oral or intravenous corticosteroids may be necessary to improve either unbearable orbital congestion or optic neuropathy. The dosing for prednisone typically starts at 1 mg/kg and is tapered slowly over several weeks, once a clinical response is appreciated. Corticosteroid therapy can be associated with a variety of adverse side effects. To reduce the duration and total dose of corticosteroid treatment, orbital radiotherapy is considered in cases of steroid-responsive optic neuropathy and rapidly progressive orbitopathy. While the mechanism behind radiotherapy is not well understood, it is thought that terminal differentiation of orbital fibroblasts is induced, which quells the local inflammatory response within the orbit. Terminal differentiation of fibroblasts is thought to limit glycosaminoglycan deposition, preadipocyte differentiation into fat cells, and lymphocyte migration to the orbit. Radiotherapy is also thought to decrease secretion of pro-inflammatory cytokines and to decrease adhesion of blood-borne lymphocytes to activated endothelial cells. Orbital radiotherapy, however, should be avoided in patients with diabetes or another vasculitic disease, as radiotherapy in this group can produce or worsen retinopathy.

Surgical Management

If possible, surgery in TED should be delayed until the inactive phase of the disease. The exceptions are cases of optic neuropathy which are not responsive to corticosteroids or patients in whom corticosteroids and orbital radiotherapy are contraindicated. In these patients, urgent bony decompression should be considered, to include either the medial orbital wall, lateral orbital wall, orbital floor, or a combination thereof. The goal of surgery is to create more space for the pathologically expanded orbital tissues to occupy, particularly in the crowded orbital apex.

More commonly, bone or fat decompression is considered in the inactive phase. The goal of treatment in the stable phase is to restore premorbid function and appearance, by reducing the volume of orbital fat or by increasing bony orbital space for the pathologically expanded soft tissues, thereby reducing proptosis. As described above, all orbital walls can be decompressed. We typically employ a graded approach to decompression that removes orbital fat in addition to one or more walls of decompression in order to achieve the desired degree of proptosis reduction, based on a preoperative analysis of the patient's premorbid appearance, as appreciated in old photos, MR or CT orbital imaging. Patients should be cautioned that double vision may worsen after a bony or fat decompression.

Strabismus surgery is offered to patients with eye misalignment and consequent double vision. When necessary, it is performed after bony or fat decompression. Surgery to correct upper eyelid retraction is the last aspect of the disease to be addressed surgically. The goal of surgery is to restore bilateral lid height and contour to the pre-disease state. With both strabismus and lid retraction surgery, reoperations are required in approximately 15% of cases due to the unpredictable nature of wound healing in TED.

Conclusion

The diagnosis and management of TED can be challenging for the clinician, given the diversity of clinical phenotypes. Treatment must be tailored to the severity and prognosis of the disease in each individual patient. All patients who smoke should be strongly encouraged to stop given that this is the most prominent modifiable risk factor. While most patients require only supportive measures, a significant minority requires medical and/or surgical intervention to reverse the disabling and vision-threatening features of the disease.

Suggested Reading

Bahn RS, Kazim M. Chapter 12: Thyroid eye disease. In: Fay A, Dolman PJ, editors. Diseases and disorders of the orbit and ocular adnexa. 1st ed: Elsevier; 2016. p. 219–34.

Kazim M. Chapter 8. The role of orbital radiotherapy in the management of thyroid related orbitopathy. In: Guthoff R, Katowitz JA, editors. Oculoplastics and orbit. 1st ed: Springer; 2006. p. 91–5.

Kazim M, Garrity JA. Orbital radiation therapy for thyroid eye disease. J Neuroophthalmol. 2012;32(2):172–6.

Rootman J, Dolman PJ. Chapter 8, Thyroid orbitopathy. In: Diseases of the orbit. A multidisciplinary approach: Lippincott Williams & Wilings; 2003.

Eyelid Lesions

Bryan J. Winn and Christine Zemsky

The presence of an eyelid lesion is a common patient complaint. Most are benign masses of limited clinical significance; however, some are potentially life-threatening and, to further complicate matters, may have subtle and underwhelming presentations. These facts and the proximity to the eye create significant anxiety among patients and clinicians alike. The following paragraphs are meant to introduce the clinician to the most common and most clinically important benign and malignant eyelid lesions in terms of demographics, risk factors, clinical presentation, work-up, treatment, and prognosis. The photographs, by and large, represent classic presentations. As with all disease entities, atypical presentations are not uncommon. Even seasoned clinicians at times may misdiagnose these eyelid lesions based on presentation and appearance alone, further stressing the importance of histopathologic confirmation of all excised tissues.

B. J. Winn, MD (✉)
Columbia University Irving Medical Center,
New York, NY, USA

Department of Ophthalmology, Edward S. Harkness
Eye Institute, Columbia University Vagelos College
of Physicians and Surgeons, New York, NY, USA
e-mail: bjw15@columbia.edu

C. Zemsky, BS
Department of Ophthalmology, Columbia University
Irving Medical Center, Edward S. Harkness Eye
Institute, New York, NY, USA

Approach to the Patient

History

The clinical course including the rapidity of onset, duration, growth, and any recent changes as well as associated symptoms and signs such as pain, swelling, erythema, itching, and bleeding often are critical to making the correct diagnosis. In addition, a personal history or strong family history of prior skin malignancy should be ascertained.

Examination

Inspection

Although most lid lesions are best visualized under magnification, it is often not required for a correct diagnosis to be made. Many lesions have hallmark features that allow for their identification. These will be discussed in more detail below. For the most part, benign lesions tend to have a more regular and organized shape, whereas malignant lesions tend to be irregular and often sclerotic. Malignant lesions may also show signs of ulceration, induration, or spontaneous hemorrhage, as well as evidence of an enriched blood supply, either in the form of a "feeder vessel" or multiple telangiectasias associated with the lesion. In the eyelid margin, benign lesions typically do not affect marginal architecture such as the lashes, meibomian gland orifices, and mucocutaneous junction, and only

© Springer Nature Switzerland AG 2019
D. S. Casper, G. A. Cioffi (eds.), *The Columbia Guide to Basic Elements of Eye Care*,
https://doi.org/10.1007/978-3-030-10886-1_30

cause focal displacement, pushing these structures to either side of the lesion. Malignant lesions, being infiltrative, frequently cause destruction and loss of normal margin architecture, the most common finding being loss of lashes in the area of the lesion. Inflammatory lesions, especially in the active phase, frequently demonstrate associated signs of inflammation such as swelling and erythema. The color of the lesion should be noted: yellow or yellow-orange color usually indicates the presence of lipid in the lesion, as can be seen in benign xanthelasma and malignant sebaceous cell carcinoma. The presence of pigmentation should also be noted: the appearance of a new, darkly pigmented lesion, or change in pigmentation of an existing lesion, especially with irregular boarders and destruction of eyelid margin architecture, must elicit a strong suspicion for malignant melanoma.

Palpation

It is critical to not only inspect the lesion but to palpate it and the surrounding eyelid, often using the contralateral side for comparison. Malignant and inflammatory lesions frequently demonstrate firmness and thickening of the eyelid beyond what is visible by inspection alone. Malignant lesions are often non-tender, in contrast with active, inflammatory lesions which commonly are tender to palpation. On occasion, the only sign of a malignant lesion such as a sebaceous cell carcinoma or morpheaform basal cell carcinoma may be palpable firmness of the eyelid. In addition, palpating lymph nodes associated with the eyelids, including the preauricular and submandibular nodes, is important in the setting of potentially malignant and certain infectious lesions. Enlarged nodes can alert the clinician to possible lymphatic spread of malignancy. Tender, palpable nodes can aid in the diagnosis of certain viral-related lesions, such as herpes simplex skin vesicles and dacryoadenitis secondary to Epstein-Barr virus.

Measurement

A flexible, millimeter ruler (as can frequently be found on a near-vision card) can be used to document the size of the lesion and the extent of any associated changes on the eyelid. Height, width, and depth, or outward extension from the lid, are noted, as well as the longest dimension of the lesion.

Photography

Digital photography, especially with a macro lens, is useful in documenting the characteristics of the lesion at a given point in time, and including a millimeter rule in the image is often helpful. Serial photographs can be used to detect changes during subsequent examination. In addition, photography is helpful at documenting the exact location of a lesion prior to excision or biopsy and helps in planning the best surgical approach. This is also helpful when a lesion is proven to be malignant on histopathologic evaluation, necessitating further treatment subsequent to wound healing; a photographic record of the preoperative lesion location greatly assists with further management.

Biopsy

In most cases, the eyelid lesion diagnosis is straightforward; however, on rare occasions, up to 2–5% of lesions without obvious suspicious characteristics may prove malignant on histopathologic examination. For this reason, we recommend histopathologic evaluation of all excised lesions when possible, with rare exceptions. Lesions which are incised and drained (such as eyelid abscesses and chalazia) are not typically biopsied unless there are underlying suspicious characteristics. However, culture may be warranted in certain situations.

Benign Lesions

Chalazion and Hordeolum

A chalazion is a sterile, chronic granuloma arising from an obstructed meibomian gland. The lesion usually presents as a subacutely expanding eyelid nodule, with or without associated discomfort. Meibomian glands are sebaceous glands oriented vertically throughout the tarsi. Therefore, a chalazion can arise anywhere along the vertical extent of the tarsus, from the eyelid margin to about 10 mm above the margin in the upper eyelid and to about 4–5 mm below the margin in the lower lid (Fig. 30.1). Occasionally, a chalazion may evolve from an infected, painful meibomian

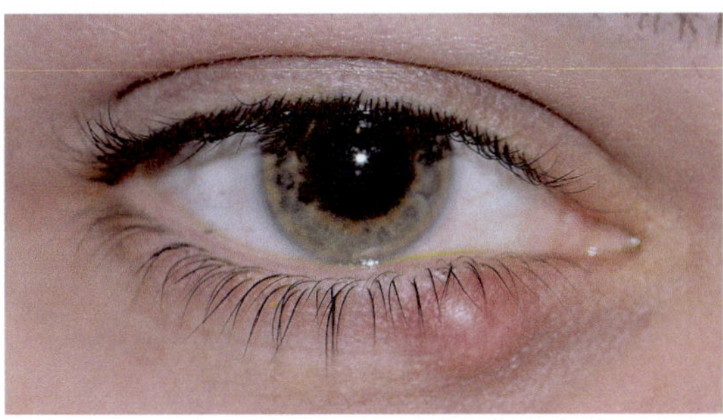

Fig. 30.1 Internal chalazion of the right lower lid. Note mild erythema associated with this round, intratarsal lesion

gland, known as a hordeolum, commonly referred to as a stye (see below).

Risk factors for development of chalazia and hordeola may include blepharitis, meibomian gland disease (MGD), ocular rosacea, floppy eyelid syndrome, chronic conjunctivitis, emotional stress, and lack of sleep.

Careful examination of the lesion at the slit lamp by an ophthalmologist can aid in diagnosis and allow for detection of more sinister lesions, such as basal cell or sebaceous cell carcinomas, which may masquerade as a recurrent or non-resolving chalazion.

The natural history of chalazia is that they tend to resolve spontaneously, although they can take weeks, to months, to years to fully disappear. On occasion, they may drain spontaneously through a meibomian gland orifice, the skin or the pretarsal conjunctiva. Warm compresses and massage can be used to help disimpact the obstructed meibomian gland and allow for a chalazion or hordeolum to resolve more rapidly. In the case of an infected hordeolum, especially if there are signs of associated eyelid cellulitis, an oral antibiotic that is appropriate for *Staphylococcus* species may be prescribed, such as a second-generation cephalosporin, clindamycin, or doxycycline. There is little evidence that topical antibiotics or antibiotic/steroid preparations have any significant role in the treatment of chalazia or hordeola.

If the patient is particularly symptomatic and chalazion resolution has stalled, the lesion can either be injected with a corticosteroid such as triamcinolone or undergo incision and curet-

tage with or without concurrent steroid injection by an ophthalmologist. Steroid injections carry a risk of secondary local atrophy and depigmentation of the skin, and the extremely rare, but devastating complication of visual loss secondary to embolic retinal artery occlusion. Recurrent, non-resolving, or otherwise atypical-appearing, or behaving, chalazia should undergo biopsy to rule out masquerading malignancy.

Subsequent chalazia may be prevented by incorporating eyelid hygiene maneuvers, such as warm compresses, into the patient's daily routine. However, care must be used in prescribing warm compresses in patients with signs of ocular rosacea, as heat may trigger further rosacea-related inflammation.

Eyelid Abscess

Eyelid abscesses can occur anywhere from the eyelid margin to the brow and develop from obstructed sebaceous glands or sweat glands, inflamed hair (lash or brow) follicles, or minor breaks in the skin. A hordeolum is a specific eyelid abscess associated with an obstructed meibomian gland. Minor lesions can be treated with warm compresses to encourage spontaneous drainage. Larger lesions, or ones associated with signs of preseptal cellulitis, frequently require incision and drainage by an ophthalmologist with concurrent systemic antibiotics with activity toward *Staphylococcus* and *Streptococcus* species, such as a second-generation cephalosporin. The contents of the abscess should be cultured and antibiotic sensitivities obtained. With the rise of community-acquired methicillin-resistant *Staphylococcus aureus* (MRSA), antibiotics with activity toward MRSA such as clindamycin, trimethoprim/sulfamethoxazole, or doxycycline may be considered as first-line agents in endemic areas.

Xanthelasma

Xanthelasmas are soft, yellow, plaque-like deposits of lipid-laden macrophages frequently found

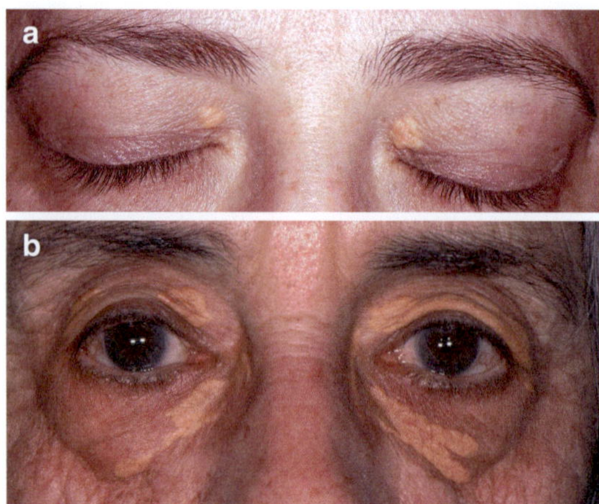

Fig. 30.2 (a) (mild) and (b) (advanced). Bilateral xanthelasma of the eyelids. Lesions are slightly raised and yellow in color. Xanthelasma are frequently bilateral, although often not completely symmetric, and are usually medial

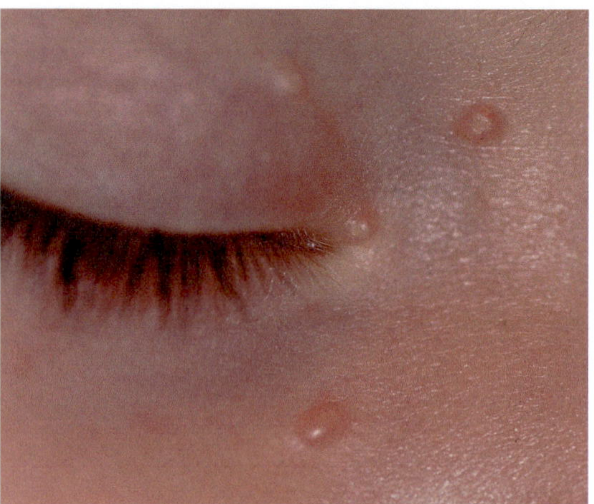

Fig. 30.3 Molluscum contagiosum. Multiple, umbilicated, non-erythematous lesions in the periocular region

bilaterally in the medial upper and lower eyelids. Their distinct appearance is pathognomonic, and biopsy is typically not needed for diagnosis (Fig. 30.2). Although benign, xanthelasma can be associated with a number of lipid abnormalities, including hyperlipidemia in up to 50% of cases. They can be seen in up to 75% of patients with familial hypercholesterolemia and 10% of patients with hyperapobetalipoproteinemia. Work-up with a serum lipid profile is therefore recommended in patients presenting with xanthelasma. Treatment for aesthetic concerns may be attempted by an oculoplastic surgeon or dermatologist and can include excision, carbon dioxide laser ablation, or trichloroacetic acid peel. However, recurrence is common.

Molluscum Contagiosum

Molluscum contagiosum is a nodular, centrally umbilicated lesion caused by infection with the poxvirus (Fig. 30.3). Viral spread is typically via direct physical contact or fomites. Lesions may be single or multiple. Occasionally, patients may have a concurrent follicular conjunctivitis associated with lesions that are close to the eyelid margin and able to shed virus particles into the

ocular fornix (see Fig. 9.7). Asymptomatic lesions may be observed and tend to resolve spontaneously. For symptomatic patients, excision, cryodestruction, thermal destruction, or curettage performed by an ophthalmologist can be curative. While the majority of patients with mollusca are immunocompetent, up to 20% of patients with human immunodeficiency virus (HIV) infection may develop these lesions. The appearance of a large number of molluscum lesions should suggest the possibility of an immunocompromised state.

Eyelid Cysts

Apocrine hidrocystomas are benign sweat gland cysts which frequently occur along the eyelid margin. The cysts are filled with clear liquid and transilluminate on examination (Fig. 30.4a, b). These lesions rarely cause symptoms and are typically removed by an ophthalmologist for aesthetic considerations. It is recommended that the cysts be excised in their entirety as residual embedded epithelium can lead to recurrence. Alternatively, these lesions may be marsupialized by excising the anterior 70% of the lesion and cauterizing the remaining posterior epithelium. The rare Schöpf-Schulz-Passarge syndrome is an autosomal recessive condition characterized by

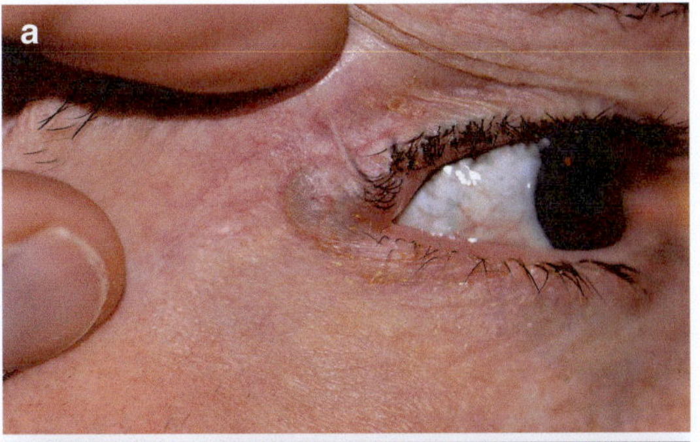

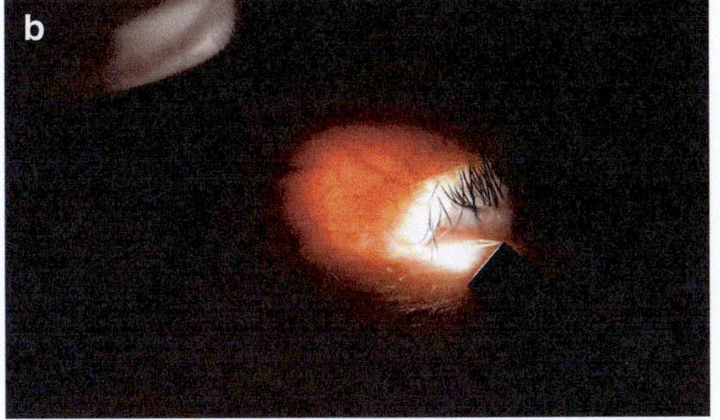

Fig. 30.4 (**a**) Round, clear fluid-filled apocrine hidrocystoma of the lateral canthus. Note that the lesion is subdermal. (**b**) Note how the hidrocystoma easily transilluminates, demonstrating the clear fluid contents

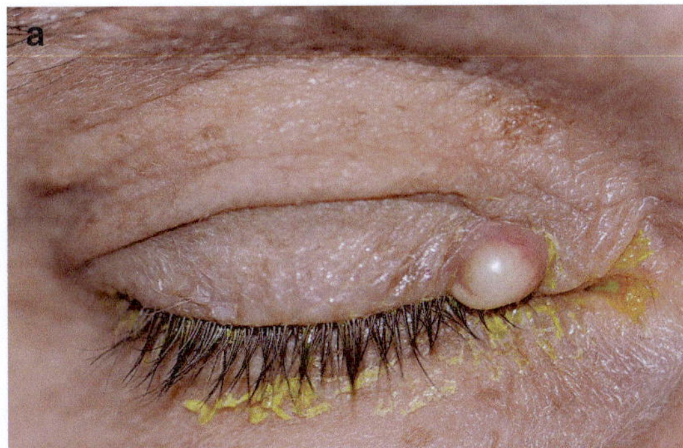

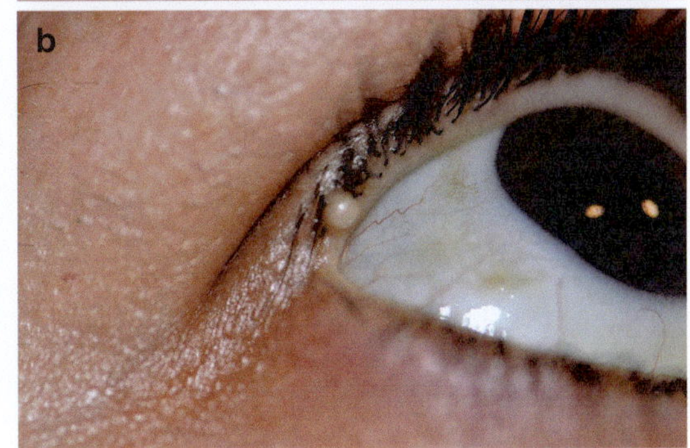

Fig. 30.5 (**a**) Epithelial inclusion cyst of the right upper lid margin. Note how the lesion is filled with white material. (**b**) Milia of the lateral upper eyelid margin

eyelid hidrocystomas, palmoplantar hyperkeratosis, hypotrichosis, and hypodontia.

Epithelial inclusion cysts, also known as epidermoid cysts, typically form after trauma or surgery. Epithelial structures, particularly the infundibula of hair follicles, become incorporated into the dermal plane, allowing for a proliferation of epidermal cells producing proteinaceous material (Fig. 30.5a). Inflammation and discomfort may result from leakage of the cyst's contents into the dermal plane. Complete surgical excision of the cyst, including the entire cyst wall is curative. Malignant transformation is rare and thought to be the result of chronic irritation and repetitive trauma to the epithelial lining of the cyst.

Milia are small, white, submillimeter, epidermal inclusion cysts often found along the eyelid margin, caused by keratin-plugged hair follicles (Fig. 30.5b). They may be treated for esthetic reasons by an ophthalmologist via incision of the lesion with a 20-guage needle and expression of its contents.

Seborrheic Keratosis

Seborrheic keratoses are the most common benign eyelid tumors of older individuals and increase with age. They are thought to arise from a clonal expansion of a mutated epidermal keratinocyte, and most are associated with mutations in the gene encoding tyrosine kinase receptor FGFR3. Sunlight may be a contributing factor to their development, although some cases demonstrate an autosomal dominant mode of inheritance. There is no sex predilection, and they are more common in less-pigmented individuals. On the eyelid, seborrheic keratoses have a greasy, crenulated, "stuck-on," and frequently pigmented, appearance (Fig. 30.6). Although the diagnosis can almost always be made by appearance alone, on rare occasions pigmented basal cell carcinomas can have similar features. Lesions with any atypical features or recent growth warrant excision with biopsy, which can be accomplished using a shave technique.

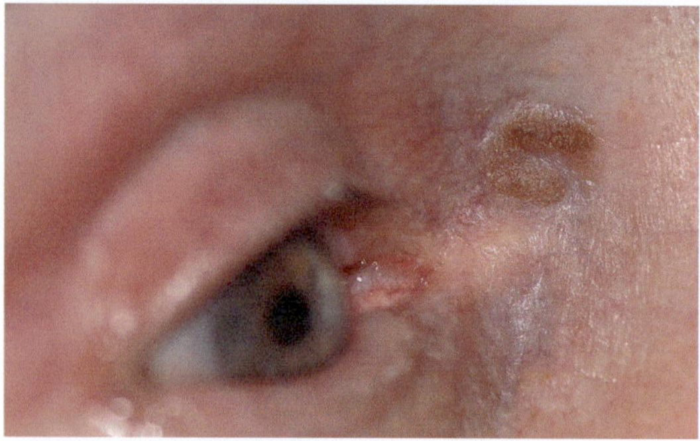

Fig. 30.6 Seborrheic keratosis of the right medial canthus. Note the "stuck-on," plaque-like quality of the lesion

Squamous Papilloma/Skin Tag

Squamous papillomas are the most common benign eyelid tumors and result from infection with the human papilloma virus. They may present as pedunculated lesions with a central vascular core, commonly referred to as skin tags, or may be sessile (Fig. 30.7a, b). Frequently, these lesions may be found on the eyelid margin with lashes growing through the lesion. Simple excision is usually curative, but care must be taken when excising these lesions from the eyelid margin, so as not to inadvertently excise nearby lash follicles. Recurrent lesions may be treated with serial intralesional interferon α-2b injections.

Acquired Hemangioma (Cherry Hemangioma)

Cherry hemangiomas are solitary, benign, vascular cutaneous lesions occurring in middle-age and older adults and are usually between 0.5 and 5 mm in size. Smaller lesions are typically bright red, while larger lesions may demonstrate a bluish hue (Fig. 30.8). As there is no malignant transformation potential, the lesions are frequently observed, although they may be excised if cosmetically unacceptable or if they exhibit suspicious characteristics.

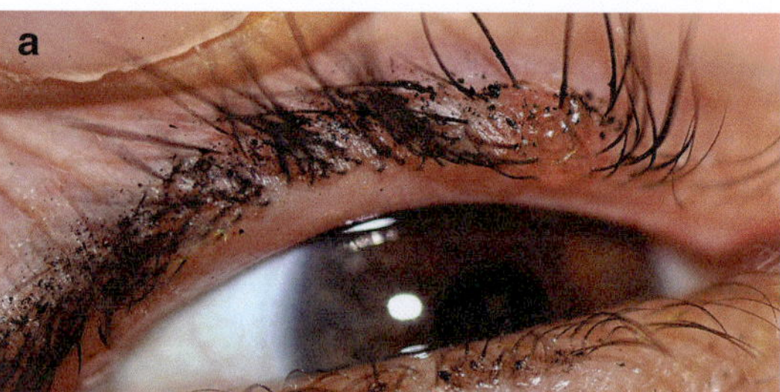
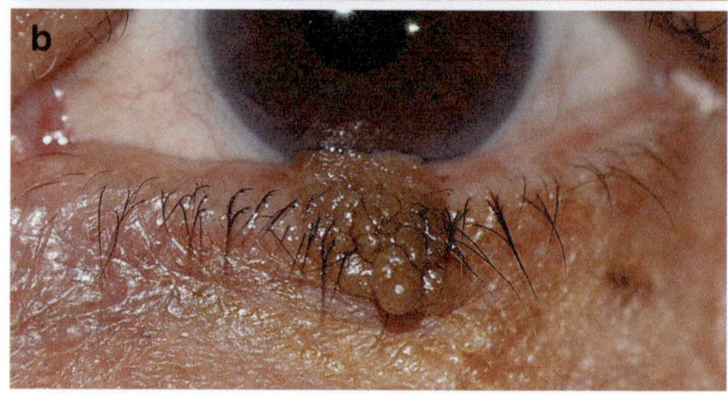

Fig. 30.7 Eyelid margin papillomas. (**a**) The lesion has a "cluster of grapes" or fimbriated appearance under magnification. There is no associated lash loss. (**b**) Pigmented eyelid margin papilloma

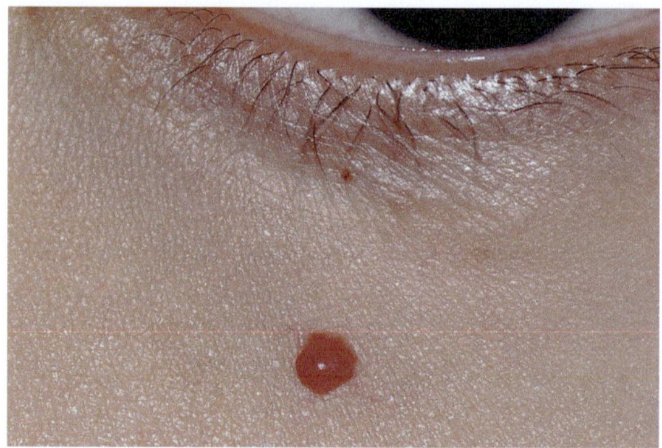

Fig. 30.8 Cherry hemangioma below the margin of the lower lid. Note the regular, round, red, homogeneous appearance

Capillary Hemangioma

Capillary hemangiomas, also referred to as superficial hemangiomas of infancy, are the most common periocular tumor seen in children, occurring in 1–2% with a 3:1 ratio of girls to boys (see Fig. 33.3). Hamartomas rather than true neoplasms, 30% of lesions are present at birth and 90% are present by 6 months of age. Capillary hemangiomas often increase in size initially and usually involute spontaneously by 7 years of age. The lesions are most commonly seen in the brow and upper eyelid and may involve cutaneous, subcutaneous, or orbital structures. Superficial lesions typically are bright red, nodular, and raised. Deeper, subcutaneous lesions are often blueish or purple in hue (See Fig 33.3). Orbital lesions may not demonstrate any superficial redness and may present only with proptosis or globe dystopia.

Lesions should be evaluated by ultrasound to determine depth and the presence of orbital extension. Orbital lesions should be further imaged with MR or CT to determine the full extent of the lesion. Lesions of the upper eyelid may cause ptosis and subsequent form-deprivation or astigmatic amblyopia. Orbital lesions may induce strabismus or result in optic nerve compression.

Treatment is reserved for hemangiomas which cause visual compromise, are associated with necrosis, or produce a severe cosmetic defect. Treatment typically consists of systemic beta-blockers, such as propranolol. Beta-blocker therapy is managed by pediatric ophthalmologists and dermatologists, as there are potential severe side effects of use in this population, including hypoglycemia and bronchospasm. Topical beta-blockers may be used for superficial lesions. Other treatment modalities, such as systemic corticosteroids, may have benefit in refractory cases. Intralesional steroid injection is frequently effective but carries a significant risk of central retinal artery occlusion. As these lesions are uncircumscribed, surgical excision carries a significant risk of hemorrhage.

Capillary hemangiomas may be associated with a number of systemic syndromes. Kasabach-Merritt syndrome is a potentially fatal coagulopathy resulting from platelet sequestration within large lesions. Maffucci syndrome consists of multiple cutaneous, visceral hemangiomas, and enchondromas. PHACES is a syndrome of **p**osterior fossa malformations, **h**emangiomas, **a**rterial anomalies, **c**oarctation of the aorta and **c**ardiac abnormalities, **e**ye abnormalities, **s**ternal clefting, and **s**upraumbilical raphe.

Melanocytic Nevus

Benign melanocytic nevi may be pigmented or nonpigmented. Congenital lesions typically appear within the first 6 months of life but may not be recognized until puberty or during pregnancy when they have a tendency to grow or darken. Nevi may develop in non-sun-exposed sites, and ultraviolet light exposure has been demonstrated to be an important factor for the development of acquired nevi.

Nevi are composed of nests of melanocytes and classified according to histologic location. Junctional nevi tend to be flat, presenting as brown-black macules. The nests reside at the tips of the rete ridges closely opposed to the dermal-epithelial junction. Compound nevi are elevated relative to the uninvolved adjacent skin and are typically lighter in color than junctional nevi (Fig. 30.9a, b). In compound nevi, nests are histologically at the

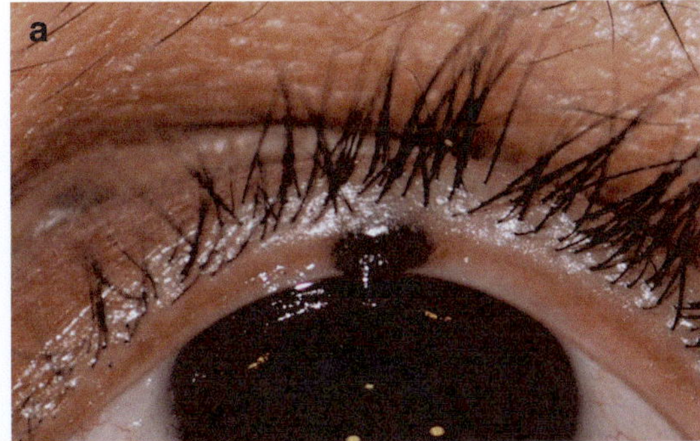

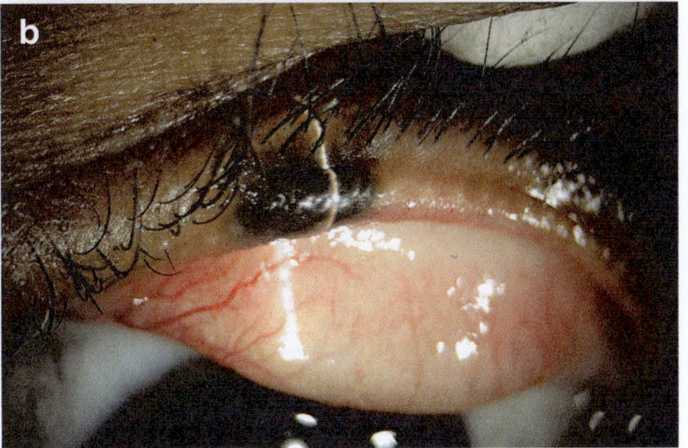

Fig. 30.9 (**a**) Small compound nevus of the upper eyelid margin. Note that the lesion is slightly elevated but small, round, and homogenous in color which are all reassuring characteristics. (**b**) Upper lid intradermal nevus

dermal-epidermal junction as well as within the dermis; intradermal nevi are made up of nests located completely within the dermis and frequently present as nonpigmented, fleshy nodules.

Malignant transformation of nevi may occur in approximately 5% of lesions. The mnemonic ABCDE can be helpful when evaluating for suspicious characteristics. *Asymmetry*, irregular *borders*, heterogeneous *color*, *diameter* greater than 6 mm, and *evolving* size, shape, or color should alert the practitioner to the possibility of malignancy and prompt a biopsy.

A "kissing nevus" is a unique form of compound nevus seen on opposing upper and lower lid margins. It is comprised of nests of melanocytes which migrated to the region between the 9th and 14th weeks of gestation, prior to embryonic lid division at week 24.

The Nevus of Ota is a high-risk lesion, typically seen in Blacks and Asians in which there is melanocytosis of the V1 and V2 dermatomal regions. Pigmentation may involve the skin, conjunctiva, sclera, tympanic membrane, or oral/nasal mucosa and typically is present before the first year of life, although may become apparent at puberty. Approximately 10% will develop glaucoma, and some experience ipsilateral sensorineural hearing loss. Melanoma may develop in patients with Nevus of Ota: uveal melanoma is most common, although it may manifest in the CNS, orbit, or skin. Asymptomatic patients are followed yearly with ophthalmic examinations and must be educated about the signs and symptoms of malignant transformation.

Actinic Keratosis

Actinic keratosis (AK), also known as solar keratosis, is a premalignant lesion in which there is a proliferation of atypical epidermal keratinocytes. It is highly associated with chronic sun exposure and sunburns. Other risk factors for development include fair skin color, advancing age, male sex, and chronic immunosuppression. Studies have shown that ultraviolet light protection can help prevent AKs by as much as 50%. The lesion usually appears as a red, scaly macule, papule, or plaque and at times may be associated with a

cutaneous horn. Patients may give a history of the lesion spontaneously disappearing or "falling off" only to reappear weeks to months later. Approximately 0.6% of AKs may transform into squamous cell carcinoma (SCC) over 1 year and as much as 2.4% over 4 years. However, up to 60% of cutaneous SCCs arise from pre-existing AKs.

On the eyelid, these lesions may be difficult to distinguish from SCC and atypical basal cell carcinoma. Pigmented AKs may be difficult to distinguish from lentigo maligna. Biopsy to rule out malignancy is recommended. Once biopsy confirms a diagnosis of AK, the lesions should be treated to avoid conversion to SCC. Typically, this can be accomplished by an oculoplastic surgeon. Liquid nitrogen cryotherapy is the most common treatment for AKs on the body, but this can prove difficult on the eyelid and may cause skin discoloration. Surgical excision or laser ablation is commonly performed. More recently, the use of topical 5-fluorouracil cream has been advocated, especially in cases of AKs that involve large portions of the eyelid margin (Fig. 30.10a, b).

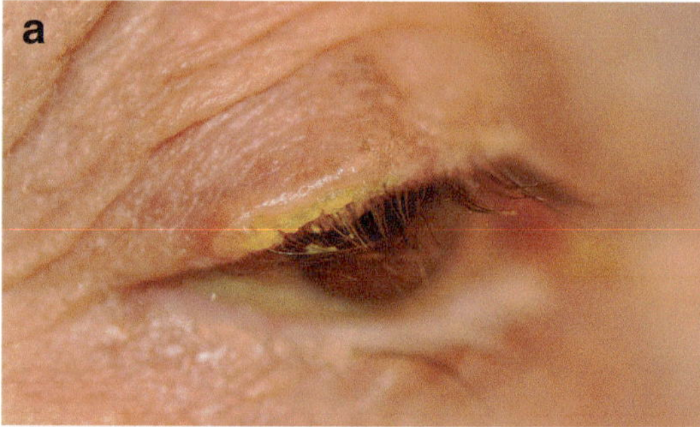
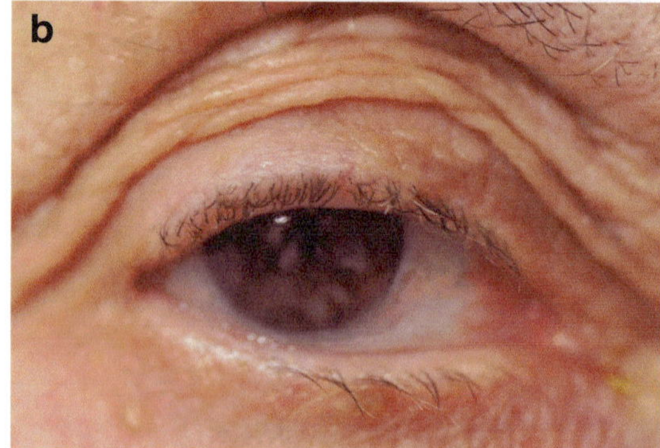

Fig. 30.10 (**a**) Large actinic keratosis of the right upper lid margin. (**b**) The same right upper lid margin actinic keratosis has completely regressed after a 2-week course of topical 5% 5-fluorouracil cream

Malignant Lesions

Basal Cell Carcinoma

Basal cell carcinoma (BCC) is the most common cutaneous malignancy of the eyelids and periocular region. They are most often found on the lower eyelid, followed by medial canthus, upper eyelid, and lateral canthus (Fig. 30.11a–d). Basal cell carcinomas are related to frequent and prolonged sun exposure and most commonly found in fair-skinned patients. Patients who develop multiple basal cell carcinomas, especially at a young age should be evaluated for nevoid basal cell carcinoma syndrome (Gorlin-Goltz or Gorlin syndrome) or xeroderma pigmentosum. Nevoid basal cell carcinoma syndrome (NBCCS) is a rare autosomal dominant condition related to a germline mutation. It is often associated with early development of multiple basal cell carcino-

mas, mandibular bone cysts, palmar and plantar pitting, craniofacial abnormalities and malformations, and early-onset medulloblastomas.

The nodular form of basal cell carcinoma is most common and typically involves a firm, solitary, slow-growing lesion with pearly edges and induration. It may be associated with telangiectasias and occasional ulceration. On the eyelid margin, there is often lash loss in the area of the lesion. The morpheaform type is less common, but often more difficult to diagnose. On the eyelid margin, these may present as a subtle thickening, often associated with lash loss and occasional outturning of the eyelid (ectropion). While these lesions rarely metastasize, they can be locally invasive and destructive.

Clinical suspicion should prompt a biopsy of the lesion by an oculoplastic surgeon. Once a diagnosis is conformed, lesions should be excised via Mohs micrographic surgical technique or under

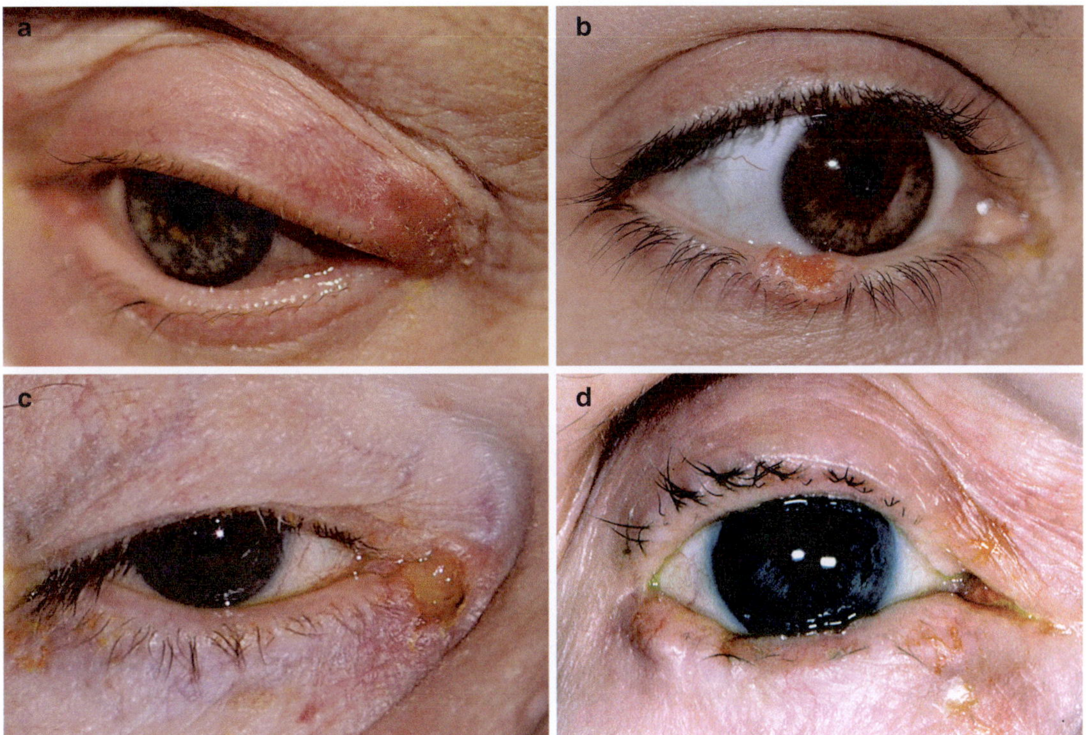

Fig. 30.11 (**a**) Nodular basal cell carcinoma of the lateral, left upper lid just above the margin. Note the pearly, rolled edges and central area of telangiectasis. (**b**) Nodular basal cell carcinoma of the lower lid margin. Note the disorganization of lash architecture and central area of ulceration. (**c**) Nodular basal cell carcinoma of the medial canthus. Lesions in this region are of particularly high risk as they can easily spread into the medial orbit. (**d**) Basal cell carcinoma of the lower lid margin. The lesion extends beyond the obvious nodule to incorporate the more medial areas associated with increased telangiectasis

frozen section control. The resulting eyelid and periocular defects are then repaired by an oculoplastic surgeon. Using these techniques, recurrence rates are less than 2%. The area of the lesion should be observed by an ophthalmologist or oculoplastic surgeon for at least 5 years for signs of recurrence.

Recurrent or neglected lesions in the periocular region, especially in the area of the medial canthus, have a high risk of invading into the orbit and requiring orbital exenteration in order to prevent invasion into the brain. External beam radiation can also be used as an adjunct to wide excision. Recently, chemotherapies aimed at the germline mutation malignancies, including vismodegib and sonidegib, have been approved for patients with metastatic basal cell carcinoma, and those who are not candidates for surgery, locally advanced disease in the setting of recurrence, and for patients with NBCCS. While these chemo-

therapies may be used for advanced disease in the area of the orbit, side effects frequently prevent long-term medication adherence.

Squamous Cell Carcinoma

Squamous cell carcinoma (SCC) accounts for up to 10% of malignant eyelid tumors and often arise from pre-existing actinic keratoses (AK). Like basal cell carcinoma, lesions are typically found on the lower eyelid and other more sun-exposed areas. Unlike basal cell carcinoma, they are more rapidly growing, and there is increased risk of spread to local lymph nodes and distant metastasis. Lesions have a varied appearance ranging from small erythematous patches resembling AKs to large, ulcerated lesions associated with hemorrhage (Fig. 30.12a). Lesions on the

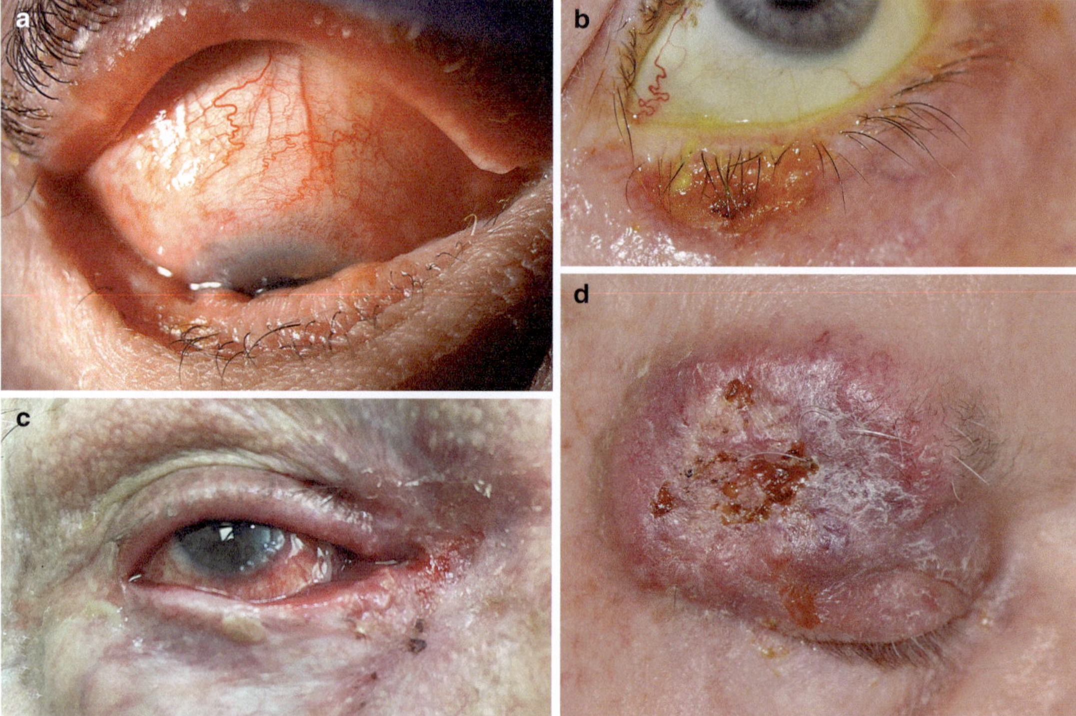

Fig. 30.12 (a) Squamous cell carcinoma of the middle right lower lid, showing early, nodular thickening, predominantly on the conjunctival surface (Courtesy of Brian P. Marr, MD). (b) Squamous cell carcinoma of the temporal right lower lid in a chronically immunosuppressed patient after lung transplantation. Note the central area of ulcer-

ation and hemorrhage. (c) Squamous cell carcinoma of the medial lower lid with early ulceration and secondary medial ectropion. (d) Large squamous cell carcinoma of the right brow region. At the time of this photograph, the patient had evidence of spread of the lesion into the right orbit requiring orbital exenteration to achieve a surgical cure eyelid margin are frequently associated with lash loss. The edges of the lesion may be well-circumscribed or ill-defined. Due to the varied appearance, incorrect clinical diagnosis may be as high as 50%.

Suspicious lesions should undergo incisional biopsy to confirm the diagnosis followed by either Mohs micrographic excision of the lesion or excision under standard frozen section control. These techniques have been shown to limit recurrence to less than 2%. Due to the more rapid growth and potential for spread, complete excision should be expedited.

Lesions may spread from the eyelid into the orbit and cavernous sinus via perineural invasion. Perineural invasion may exist in up to 15% of facial SCC, and those lesions with histologic evidence of invasion may benefit from postoperative radiation to prevent recurrence and distant spread. Orbital invasion may present with extraocular muscle restriction and may require exenteration to prevent extension into the brain (Fig. 30.12b).

Keratoacanthoma

Keratoacanthoma (KA) is a dome-shaped mass with a central crater (Fig. 30.13). The natural history of the lesion is typically one of rapid growth, followed by a period of stability and ultimately spontaneous involution after several weeks to several months. The vast majority are found in middle-to-older age, fair-skinned individuals. Other risk factors for development include ultraviolet radiation, trauma, smoking, human papillomavirus infection, and certain BRAF inhibitor chemotherapeutics including vemurafenib and dabrafenib. While most agree that the lesion arises from the follicular infundibulum, the pathophysiologic mechanism for development and resolution is poorly understood. Histologically, these lesions resemble squamous cell carcinoma, and there is debate as to whether this lesion is really a variant of SCC as there have been isolated reports of aggressive lesions with distant metastases. While the classic teaching had been that these lesions may be observed for spontaneous regression, most now advocate surgical management. As opposed to SCC and BCC, an excisional biopsy down to the layer of the subcutaneous fat, which permits evaluation of the entire lesional architecture, is critical for diagnosis. If there is evidence of the lesion beyond the biopsy borders, Mohs micrographic surgical excision or excision under frozen section control is typically recommended to clear residual lesion. However, there have been reports of KA successfully treated with intralesional injections of either 5-fluorouracil, methotrexate, or interferon α-2a.

Sebaceous Cell Carcinoma

Sebaceous cell carcinoma is the third most common malignant eyelid neoplasm, after basal cell carcinoma and squamous cell carcinoma. It is often described as a masquerade lesion, as its clinical presentation is often subtle and may be interpreted as that of more common, benign conditions leading to delayed diagnosis. The neoplasm arises from meibomian glands, Zeiss glands, or other sebaceous glands of the eyelid or caruncle.

Most patients are over age 50, with a median age of 72. Individuals with Muir-Torre syndrome, an autosomal dominant condition associated with sebaceous carcinoma and visceral malignancies such as colon, urethral, ovarian, and endometrial, may present at an earlier age.

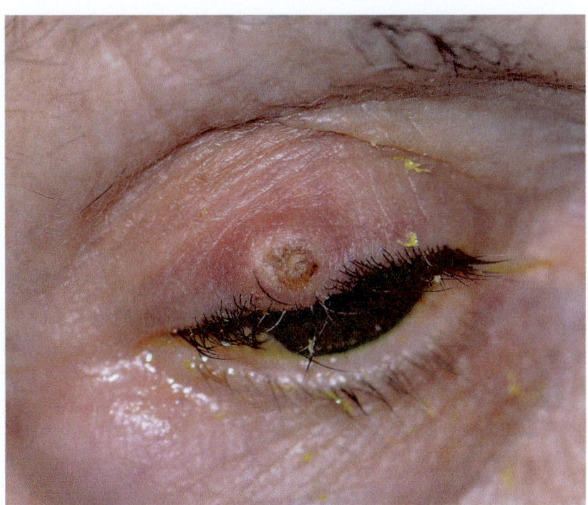

Fig. 30.13 Keratoacanthoma of the right upper lid with a large central crater. The onset of the lesion was rapid, suggesting the diagnosis

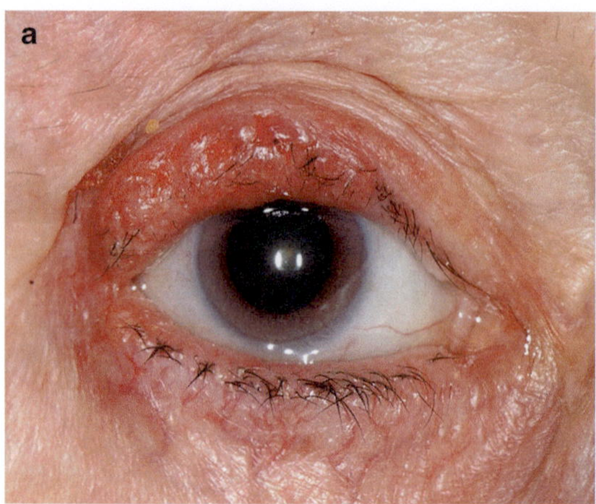

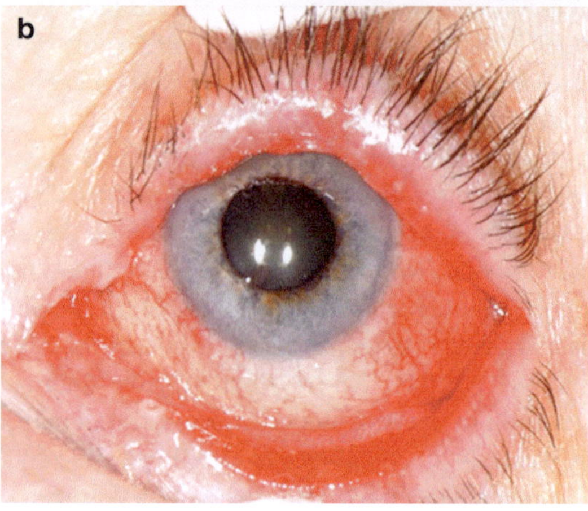

Fig. 30.14 (**a**) Sebaceous cell carcinoma. Note the diffuse thickening of the upper lid margin with lash loss. (**b**) Sebaceous cell carcinoma involving upper and lower lid margins as well as pagetoid spread on the conjunctiva. (Courtesy of Brian P. Marr, MD)

The typical presentation is that of a mildly inflamed, yellow, round, nodular lesion arising on the eyelid margin, initially mimicking the appearance of a chalazion. Another common presentation is that of unilateral diffuse, inflamed eyelid margin thickening, which may be initially misdiagnosed as blepharitis (Fig. 30.14a). Lesions most frequently occur on the upper eyelid as there are more meibomian glands in the upper eyelid than lower eyelid, and it is rare for lesions to be ulcerated. Often there is eyelash loss in the region. In up to 44–80% of cases, the tumor may also involve pretarsal and bulbar conjunctiva as well as cornea via direct extension or pagetoid spread. Multifocal origin of the tumor, including upper and lower lids, may occur (Fig. 30.14b). The lesion may spread to regional lymph nodes and may metastasize to distant sites, including the liver, lung, and bone.

Suspicious lesions, such as non-resolving chalazia or unilateral thickened eyelid, warrant biopsy. Due to the frequent intratarsal tumor location, shave biopsy of the skin will often be unrevealing, and full-thickness wedge excisional biopsy is recommended to confirm the diagnosis.

Once diagnosed, complete excision of the tumor with permanent section control and delayed closure is recommended. Concurrent map biopsies of the conjunctiva should be performed to rule out ocular surface involvement. This is best performed by an ocular oncologist or oculoplastic surgeon. Mohs surgery and frozen section control have also been employed for this lesion but remain controversial, as subtle intraepithelial spread may be difficult to interpret. Lesions involving a large portion of the ocular surface or orbit may require exenteration, although globe-sparing excision with concurrent cryotherapy and adjuvant topical chemotherapy is gaining favor among ocular oncologists. After the tumor is cleared, secondary reconstruction can be performed. Patients need to be followed for signs of local recurrence and should be encouraged to perform self-examination for regional lymph node involvement.

A metastasis rate up to 30% has been reported in the older literature. More recently, large multicenter tumor registries have demonstrated much lower rates. According to the National Cancer Institute Surveillance, Epidemiology, and End Results (SEER) database, 4.4% of ocular sebaceous cell carcinoma may demonstrate regional lymph node metastasis. This rate may be as high as 10% in poorly differentiated lesions, and less than 1% for well-differentiated tumors. Larger tumors (>10 mm) carry a higher risk of lymph node metastasis, and distant metastasis may occur. Sentinel lymph node biopsy may be beneficial in high-risk lesions. The relative survival rates for sebaceous cell carcinoma according to the SEER database are 92.72% at 5 years and 86.98% at 10 years.

Melanoma

While malignant melanoma accounts for less than 1% of all eyelid malignancies, it is responsible for over 2/3 of eyelid malignancy-related mortality. Peak incidence is age 50–80, and lesions typically arise on the lower eyelid, as in basal cell and squamous cell carcinoma. Risk factors include fair skin, sun or UV light exposure, positive family history, and the presence of congenital nevi. Normal melanocytes are thought to transform into melanomas via accumulations of a number of genetic mutations. Pathogenic mutations in the MAP kinase signal transduction pathway and loss of tumor suppressor gene functions add to pathogenesis. Cutaneous melanoma of the eyelid may be separated into three types: lentigo maligna (melanoma in situ), superficial spreading, and nodular (Fig. 30.15). Although superficial spreading is the most common type elsewhere in the body, lentigo maligna and the more aggressive nodular form are most commonly found on the eyelid.

Lentigo maligna (melanoma in situ) typically appear as flat, variably pigmented, ill-defined macules on sun-damaged skin of older, fair-skinned individuals. The risk of this lesion transforming to invasive, malignant melanoma is estimated at 2.2–4.7%. Histologically, the lesion is characterized by atypical, predominantly spindle-shaped melanocytes at the basal epidermis and may show evidence of pagetoid spread. Surgical excision, often with map biopsy, performed around the lesion, with 0.5–1.0 mm clear margins has been the standard treatment. In the periocular area, this can result in a large defect requiring oculoplastic repair. Due to this, some authors have advocated the use of Mohs micrographic surgery for melanoma in situ, as this may allow for more complete excision of this frequently ill-defined tumor. Concurrent use of immunohistochemical stains facilitate identification of tumor cells in Mohs surgery for melanoma in situ. Topical 5% imiquimod has also been recommended as a primary or adjunct therapy for periocular lentigo maligna by some authors.

The mnemonic ABCDE can be helpful when evaluating melanocytic lesions for suspicious characteristics. *A*symmetry, irregular *b*orders, heterogeneous *c*olor, *d*iameter greater than 6 mm, and *e*volving size, shape, or color should alert the practitioner to the possibility of malignant melanoma and prompt biopsy. The color of melanomas can range from dark brown or blue to light tan or white. Amelanotic melanomas can be particularly difficult to diagnose clinically. Because of this, most practitioners recommend biopsy of eyelid lesions with any suspicious characteristics, including any of the ABCDE criteria, ulceration, erythema, scaling, or irregular boarders. When melanoma is diagnosed histologically, characteristics including Breslow thickness, ulceration, and the number of mitotic figures should be documented in the pathology report.

Superficial spreading melanoma is histologically characterized by nests of epithelioid cells throughout the epidermis and, to a lesser extent, may demonstrate vertical growth into the dermis. In contrast, nodular melanoma is categorized by predominantly vertical growth of epithelioid cells into the dermis. Typically, lesions with greater vertical growth demonstrate higher numbers of mitotic figures and carry greater risk of metastatic spread.

Frozen section control has traditionally been thought to be not appropriate for superficial spreading and nodular melanomas. Mohs surgery with concurrent use of immunohistochemical stains is controversial for non-lentigo maligna melanoma. "Slow Mohs" micrographic surgical

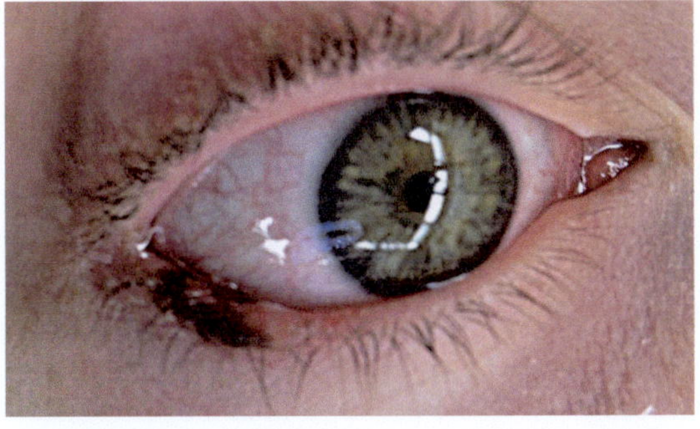

Fig. 30.15 Cutaneous melanoma on the lower lid margin. Note the irregular shape, sclerosis of the eyelid margin, and loss of lashes. (Courtesy of Brian P. Marr, MD)

excision of the lesion has been advocated. In "slow Mohs," the specimen is excised and oriented in the same manner as traditional Mohs surgery, but instead of frozen sections, permanent histologic evaluation is obtained between stages. While awaiting processing for permanent histology, the wound is left open and the eye patched, or a temporary tarsorrhaphy may be placed to prevent exposure keratitis.

While 1 cm margins are typically recommended elsewhere in the body, many oculoplastic surgeons advocate for 5 mm margins for thin melanomas (<0.75 mm) without other high-risk features. With thicker lesions, those with signs of ulceration, or those with >1 mitotic figure per high-power field, 1 cm margins are generally recommended. Sentinel lymph node (SLN) biopsy is also recommended for melanomas thicker than 1 mm or ones with any other high-risk characteristics (ulceration, mitotic figures). Although SNL biopsy has not been shown to confer benefit in terms of decreasing mortality risk, SLN is useful in terms of prognosis and determining therapeutic options. Any higher-risk lesions should prompt consultation with a medical oncologist to assess for signs of metastasis.

Merkel Cell Carcinoma

Merkel cell carcinoma (MCC) is a rare, highly aggressive, malignant neoplasm most often seen in elderly, Caucasian individuals (>95%) on sun-exposed areas. Fifty percent of MCCs arise in the head and neck region, with 5–10% in the periocular region, most often the upper eyelid. Immunosuppression, especially HIV infection and chronic lymphocytic leukemia, greatly increases risk of MCC development. Over 80% of MCC is associated with infection by the polyomavirus.

The lesion is thought to arise either from malignant transformation of the Merkel cell, which is an epithelial cell with neuroendocrine differentiation thought to facilitate the sensation of light touch and shape/texture discrimination, or a dermal pluripotent stem cell with similar electron microscopic and immunohistochemical characteristics to the Merkel cell.

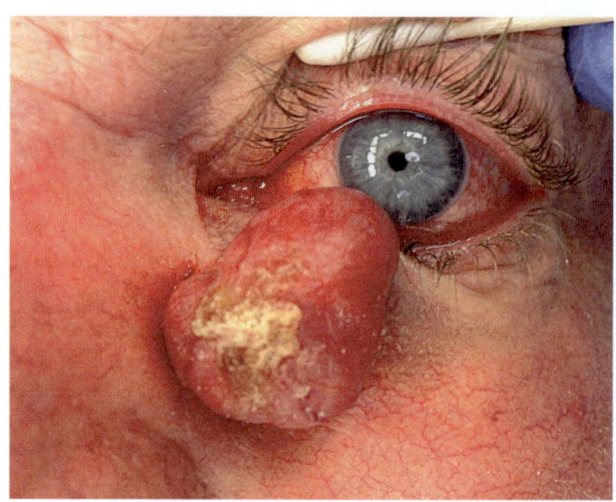

Fig. 30.16 Large Merkel cell carcinoma involving the left lower eyelid. (Courtesy of Brian P. Marr, MD)

MCC typically presents as a rapidly growing, red/purple solitary nodule on the eyelid margin, often with significant lash loss (Fig. 30.16). The lesion may show signs of ulceration and overlying telangiectasias. Lesions are frequently misdiagnosed as basal cell carcinoma, squamous cell carcinoma, keratoacanthoma, sebaceous cell carcinoma, or chalazion. Palpation of the preauricular, submandibular, and neck lymph nodes is important to assess for nodal spread.

Excisional or full-thickness incisional biopsy of the lesion is recommended. Given the difficulty of differentiating this lesion from sebaceous cell carcinoma using routine histopathologic examination, special immunohistochemical stains and electron microscopy can prove useful.

MCC spreads to local lymph nodes early in the disease course, with 22% of cases showing evidence of lymph node involvement at presentation, and up to 2/3 within 18 months of diagnosis. Five-year survival in patients without lymph node involvement is 97%. In contrast, lymph node positivity carries a poor prognosis with 5-year survival dropping to 52%.

MCC is treated with wide local excision. Classically, 2.5–3 cm margins are recommended. However, on the eyelid, this is impractical and would involve the globe in most circumstances. Good success with Mohs micrographic surgery and 5 mm margins has been reported. Due to the high predilection for nodal spread, sentinel lymph node biopsy is recommended for detecting metastasis and helping with disease staging and prognosis. The use of adjuvant chemotherapy and radiation may be potentially beneficial but is controversial. A multidisciplinary team involving an oculoplastic surgeon, head and neck surgeon, medical oncologist, and radiation oncologist is recommended for optimal management.

Kaposi Sarcoma

Kaposi sarcoma (KS), first reported in 1872, is an endothelial and vascular smooth muscle cell neoplasm. The "classic" form of the disease typically occurs in elderly men of Mediterranean or Ashkenazi Jewish origin and usually consists of slow-growing purple or red cutaneous macules, plaques, or nodules, which often arise on the hands and feet. In some patients, the lesions will involve visceral and mucosal structures. Other risk factors for classic KS include topical steroid use and a history of asthma or atopy. Three other clinical forms of KS have been described: the endemic (African or lymphadenopathic) form; the transplant-related or immunocompromised form; and the epidemic, or AIDS-related form. The African endemic form may present with indolent, cutaneous lesions in elderly men in the same manner as the "classic" form or with aggressive and often rapidly fatal lymphatic involvement in young children. Transplant-related KS is due to systemic immunosuppression and often resembles that of classic KS but frequently involves the visceral cavity. AIDS-related KS is the most aggressive form, often presenting with lesions involving the skin, mucous membranes, lymphatics, and viscera simultaneously.

Histologically, KS is characterized by a proliferation of spindle cells, often in a directional streaming pattern, around vascular channels with a surrounding mix of endothelial cells, fibroblasts, lymphocytes, and plasma cells. KS has been linked to the human herpesvirus-8, which is highly endemic in central and southern Africa and, to a lesser extent, in Mediterranean areas. While KS appears to be necessary for the development of

KS, additional cofactors are required for tumor development, such as immunosuppression.

Ocular involvement of KS is rare but when present is typically in the setting of AIDS (epidemic form), often presenting as eyelid or conjunctival lesions in the setting of multicentric disease.

The most widely accepted staging system for AIDS-related KS was developed by the AIDS Clinical Trial Group of the National Institute of Health and separates patients into those with good or poor prognosis based on three parameters: extent of tumor, immune status, and severity of systemic illness. Patients with KS limited to the skin and CD4 count >200 have a more favorable status. In contrast, patients with KS involving visceral or oral cavities, CD4 count <200, history of opportunistic infections, and/or B symptoms (fever, weight loss, night sweats, diarrhea >2 weeks) have a less favorable prognosis.

Patients diagnosed with KS should be managed with an ocular oncologist, medical oncologist, and infectious disease specialist as KS of the ocular adnexa can at times be the first clinical sign of AIDS. Physical examination, including attention to the lower extremities, face, and oral mucosa, should be performed. Chest X-ray is useful for detecting pulmonary lesions, and testing stool for occult blood can screen for gastrointestinal involvement. CD4 count and HIV viral load are critical for staging and prognosis.

In general, treatment consists of prevention of disease progression, and symptom palliation, including reducing psychological stress. In AIDS-related KS, anti-retroviral therapy has been shown to significantly decrease the incidence and severity of KS. In the periocular region, most tumors have an indolent course and may not require treatment. The goal of local treatment in this area would be to relieve symptoms and preserve vision. Indications for treatment include corneal breakdown, discomfort, eyelid malposition, and unacceptable cosmetic appearance. Local therapies include surgical excision, cryotherapy, topical and intralesional interferon α-2a and 2b, and radiation therapy. Systemic therapy is typically reserved for patients with advanced, multicentric disease, especially with evidence of rapid disease progression. Currently, pegylated liposomal doxorubicin is recommended as the first-line systemic treatment for KS. Paclitaxel, bleomycin, vinblastine, vincristine, and etoposide have also been used successfully. Agents directed against PDGF, VEGF, and the mTOR pathway are currently being investigated for KS.

Suggested Reading

Actis AG, Actis G, De Sanctis U, Fea A, Rolle T, Grignolo FM. Eyelid benign and malignant tumors: issues in classification, excision and reconstruction. Minerva Chir. 2013;68(6 Suppl 1):11–25.

Allen RC. Surgical management of periocular cancers: high- and low-risk features drive treatment. Curr Oncol Rep. 2017 Sep;19(9):57.

Campbell AA, Grob SR, Freitag SK. Controversies in sentinel lymph node biopsy for ocular neoplasms. Int Ophthalmol Clin. 2015 Fall;55(4):73–9.

Dekmezian MS, Cohen PR, Sami M, Tschen JA. Malignancies of the eyelid: a review of primary and metastatic cancers. Int J Dermatol. 2013;52(8):903–26; quiz 922–3, 926

Deprez M, Uffer S. Clinicopathological features of eyelid skin tumors. A retrospective study of 5504 cases and review of literature. Am J Dermatopathol. 2009;31(3):256–62.

Ho VH, Ross MI, Prieto VG, Khaleeq A, Kim S, Esmaeli B. Sentinel lymph node biopsy for sebaceous cell carcinoma and melanoma of the ocular adnexa. Arch Otolaryngol Head Neck Surg. 2007;133(8):820–6.

Silverman N, Shinder R. What's new in eyelid tumors. Asia Pac J Ophthalmol (Phila). 2017;6(2):143–52.

Slutsky JB, Jones EC. Periocular cutaneous malignancies: a review of the literature. Dermatol Surg. 2012;38(4):552–69.

Yin VT, Merritt HA, Sniegowski M, Esmaeli B. Eyelid and ocular surface carcinoma: diagnosis and management. Clin Dermatol. 2015;33(2):159–69.

Lora Dagi Glass

The upper and lower eyelid structures are similar and analogous, yet distinct, each with a complex anatomy that allows the lids to retain form and function. Anatomic pathology of any cause can disrupt eyelid position, stability, and movement, thus allowing for a range of symptoms including tearing (epiphora), disruption in vision, conjunctival injection, keratopathy, or in extreme cases, corneal perforation. This chapter will briefly review eyelid anatomy, followed by an anatomically based discussion of the etiology and treatment of five common eyelid malpositions – ectropion, entropion, epiblepharon, ptosis, and retraction – as well as a brief review of trichiatic eyelashes.

Anatomy

Both the upper and lower eyelids can be divided into an "anterior lamella," comprised of skin and orbicularis oculi muscle, and a "posterior lamella," comprised of tarsus, septum, fat pads, retractor muscles, and conjunctiva.

The anterior lamellae are perfectly mirrored in the upper and lower eyelids, with the exception of the upper eyelid crease, which is formed by

L. Dagi Glass, MD (✉)
Columbia University Irving Medical Center,
New York, NY, USA

Department of Ophthalmology, Edward S. Harkness
Eye Institute, Columbia University Vagelos College
of Physicians and Surgeons, New York, NY, USA
e-mail: ld2514@cumc.columbia.edu

adhesions between the skin, orbital septum and levator aponeurosis.

The posterior lamellae of the upper and lower eyelids remain analogous but differ in certain fundamental ways. For the purposes of this chapter, we will focus on the tarsal plates and eyelid retractors. The septal and conjunctival layers remain symmetric.

Eyelashes arise long the lid margin just anterior to the tarsus and exit along the anterior margin. The tarsal plate, comprised of dense connective tissue and meibomian glands, is approximately triple the height centrally in the upper eyelid compared to the lower; both are anchored to the medial and lateral canthal tendons.

Two upper eyelid and two lower eyelid muscles act as lid retractors: the levator palpebrae superioris muscle and Müller's muscle in the upper lid and the capsulopalpebral fascia and inferior tarsal muscle in the lower. Of note, the levator muscle has a long, nonmuscular, aponeurotic section that inserts over the anterior surface of the tarsal plate and the posterior skin surface as well. The capsulopalpebral fascia arises from the inferior rectus muscle and wraps around the inferior oblique prior to inserting on the inferior tarsal plate. The levator muscle is innervated by cranial nerve III (oculomotor), whereas Müller's and the inferior tarsal muscles are sympathetically innervated via the superior cervical ganglion. Figure 31.1 shows a schematic sagittal view of transected upper and lower eyelids, highlighting the lid retractors and protractors.

© Springer Nature Switzerland AG 2019
D. S. Casper, G. A. Cioffi (eds.), *The Columbia Guide to Basic Elements of Eye Care*,
https://doi.org/10.1007/978-3-030-10886-1_31

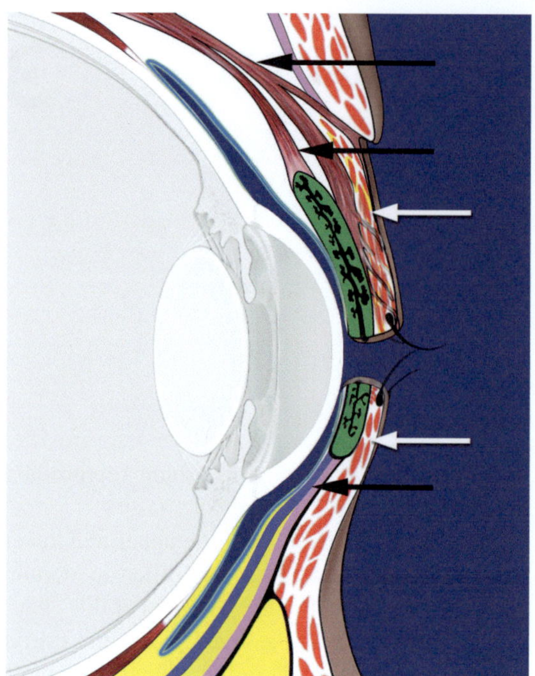

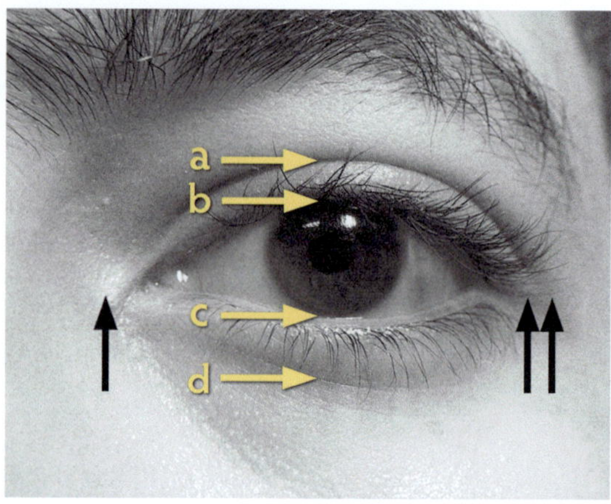

Fig. 31.2 Photograph of a left eye, showing normal anatomy. Single arrow, region of medial canthus; double arrows, lateral canthus. The upper lid fold is seen at (a), the lower lid fold at (d). Centrally, the upper lid margin normally falls below the upper limbus, as seen in (b), and the lower lid margin is typically located at the inferior limbal border, as seen in (c)

Fig. 31.1 A schematic sagittal section through the anterior globe and eyelids. Protractor muscles (the orbicularis) are indicated by the white arrows. Retractor muscles (the levator aponeurosis complex and associated sympathetic Müller's muscle in the upper lid, and the fused capsulopalpebral fascia and orbital septum in the lower) are indicated by the black arrows

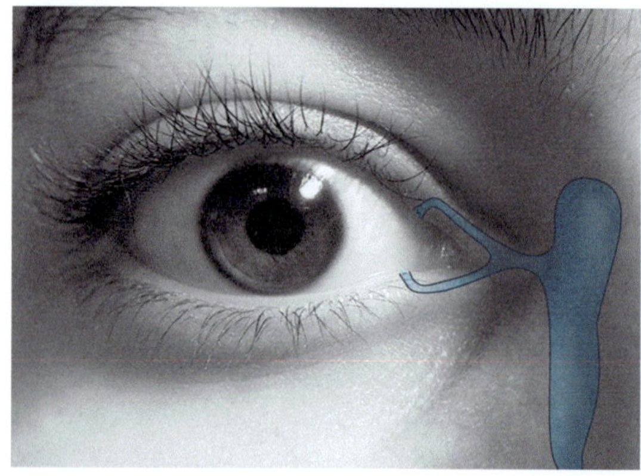

Fig. 31.3 Tear drainage showing the upper and lower lid puncta and canaliculus leading to nasolacrimal canal drainage system

The eyelids are arranged like a hammock, firmly attached medially and laterally at the canthi. Equal anterior and posterior forces maintain the lids in their normal vertical positions, closely apposed to the anterior surface of the eye, without outward or inward rotation (Fig. 31.2). These equivalent forces, as will be described below, depend on normal anatomy and constitution of muscle, skin, tarsal plate, and conjunctival layers. Abnormalities of opposing forces can lead to unequal traction on anterior or posterior lamellae, resulting in lid misdirection.

Importantly, the symmetrically placed upper and lower lid puncta and their associated canalicular drainage systems are found along the medial eyelid (Fig. 31.3).

Lid Malpositions

Ectropion

Presentation

An eyelid with ectropion leans away from the globe. The patient may present with complaints of a droopy lower lid with abnormal appearance, tearing, lower eyelid redness and irritation, a red and uncomfortable eye, and eye dryness. Most symptoms develop from chronic corneal exposure.

Examination

Examination may show a range of ectropic lid changes ranging from mild lower lid laxity to severe, nearly complete lower eyelid eversion (Fig. 31.4a, b). The entire lower lid may be involved, or the area of ectropion may be limited. In medial eyelid ectropion, for example, punctal eversion may cause impaired tear drainage and resultant epiphora. The eyelid margin may appear inflamed, with keratinization of the conjunctiva in cases of longstanding eversion. Depending on the severity, there may be pooling of tears, conjunctival injection, and exposure keratopathy.

Anatomic Correlation

Ectropion may be classified by cause: involutional changes, palsy, cicatricial pathology, or mechanical disturbance. Involutional ectropion is age-related laxity of the medial and/or lateral canthal tendons. Paralytic ectropion is due to imbalance in forces of the lower eyelid musculature due to facial nerve palsy affecting the orbicularis muscle. Cicatricial changes to the anterior lamellae, such as after trauma, may cause a relative stiffness and contracture, pulling the eyelid outward. Finally, the weight of an external eyelid mass may cause ectropion.

Treatment Options

Treatment for lower eyelid ectropion relies upon an understanding of the anatomic disturbance in the individual patient: what is the underlying etiology, and is the ectropion medially based, laterally based, or diffuse? Eyelid masses causing ectropion need treatment first and foremost addressing the mass itself; this is addressed in Chap. 30.

All cases of ectropion may find some relief with lubrication, which mitigates chronic corneal desiccation secondary to exposure.

Laterally based and mild diffuse ectropion may be repaired via a surgical reinsertion of the lateral canthal tendon to its origin on the lateral orbital wall. Both the lateral canthal strip and quick strip procedures attempt to recreate this tendinous attachment. Severe ectropion may also require the addition of retractor reinsertion surgery.

Medially based ectropion is more difficult to repair due to the fragile nature of the canalicular system. Typical procedures create a relative shortening of the medial posterior lamellae via excision of conjunctival and retractor tissue inferior to the punctum, or one can expose and carefully plicate the medial canthal tendon. These procedures are at times combined with laterally based or wedge procedures.

If the underlying pathology has not yet been identified, paralytic ectropion requires a work-up for facial nerve palsy. In addition to the repair procedures discussed above, these patients may

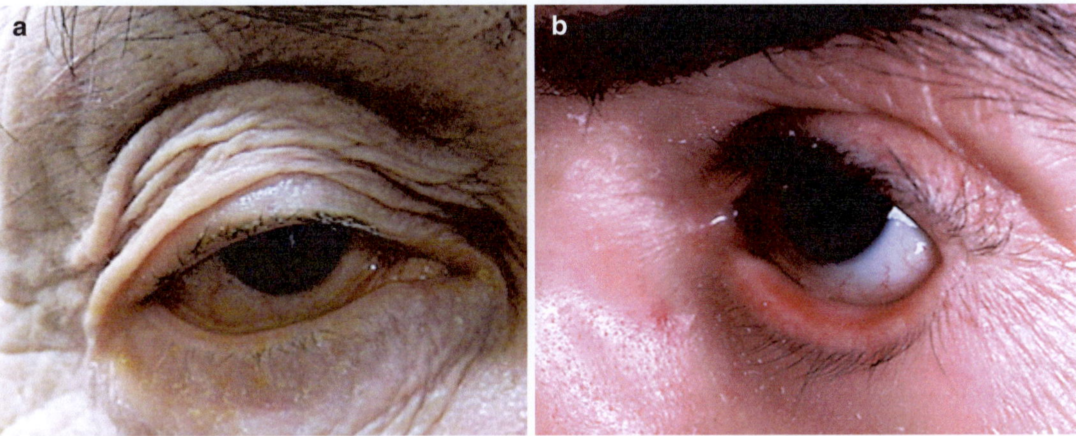

Fig. 31.4 (**a**) Upper eyelid ptosis and eyelid ectropion, predominantly lateral. (**b**) Severe ectropion, predominantly medial, with eversion of the punctum, which typically results in chronic epiphora

require tarsorrhaphy and midface reanimation procedures that are beyond the scope of this book.

Cicatricial ectropion may be managed either medically or surgically, depending on the underlying condition. If dermatitis is the culprit, whether due to atopy, glaucoma drops, or another reaction, medical treatment of the underlying dermatitis and removal of any culprit source may completely resolve the issue. However, in cases of scarring, a skin graft may be needed to augment the vertical height of the anterior lamellae, typically combined with a lateral canthal tendon procedure.

Entropion

Presentation

An eyelid with entropion curves abnormally toward the globe, with eyelash-globe touch. The patient may present with tearing, discomfort, and a red eye, and severe cases may exhibit keratitis related to mechanical irritation from the inturned lashes, with secondary infection after epithelial disruption.

Examination

Examination may show overt entropion with nearly complete "hiding" of the eyelashes as they curl inward (Fig. 31.5). Alternatively, the eyelid may at first appear completely normal, with entropion only induced when the patient is asked to squeeze the eyelids shut (and even then, potentially only during the actual movement, with quick resolution upon eyelid opening). The eye may appear injected. The cornea may show abrasions secondary to eyelash rub.

Anatomic Correlation

Entropion may be due to involutional changes, orbicularis muscle spasm, or cicatricial pathology of the posterior lamella. Involutional changes are thought to be caused by some combination of horizontal eyelid laxity due to canthal tendon disinsertion, lower eyelid retractor disinsertion, and orbicularis oculi muscle override. The orbicularis muscle can also go into spasm, causing "spastic" entropion. Finally, conjunctival or other posteri-

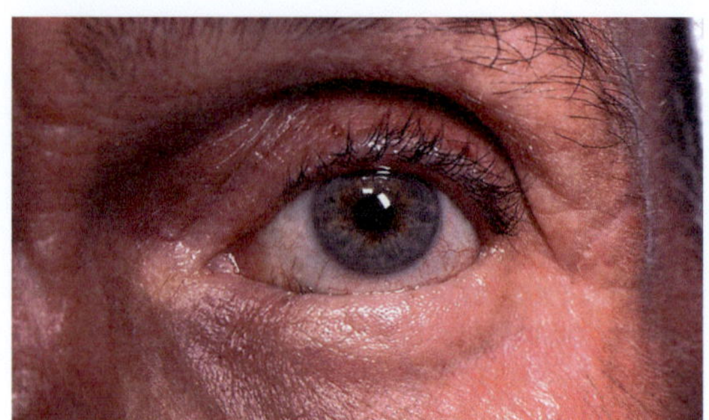

Fig. 31.5 Lower lid entropion

orly based scarring, such as that seen in trachoma, can cause relative posterior lamellar shortening and resultant entropion.

Treatment Options

All symptomatic eyes should be lubricated as a temporizing measure. Additionally, a bandage contact lens may protect the cornea from lash-induced de-epithelialization. An inferiorly directed, piece of tape strategically placed along the lateral lower lid may help evert the eyelid until appropriate surgical intervention can take place. Botulinum toxin has been used successfully to treat spastic entropion, allowing for a relative but temporary palsy of the overly active orbicularis muscle.

Surgical intervention must take the anatomic pathology into account. Should a procedure need to take place urgently, a temporizing procedure employs sutures to evert the eyelid margin (e.g., a Quickert procedure), though treatment with this procedure alone is not considered definitive.

Horizontal eyelid laxity may be treated with a combination procedure involving lateral canthal tendon tightening, retractor muscle reinsertion from an anterior or posterior approach, and potentially excision of a strip of orbicularis muscle along the length of a subciliary incision to decrease orbicularis override. Retractor muscle reinsertion from an anterior approach has the added benefit of producing anterior scarring, which further pulls lashes away from the globe.

Posterior cicatrix is a more challenging pathology, often requiring insertion of a spacer graft to directly address the vertical tissue imbalance.

Multiple materials have been promoted, including mucous membrane grafts. At times, rotation of the eyelid margin away from the globe is required, in which case a tarsal fracture with marginal rotation may be performed.

Epiblepharon

Presentation
Epiblepharon refers to overriding of the anterior lamella past the lower eyelid margin. The patient is typically a young Asian and often completely asymptomatic. However, some patients do complain of eye irritation.

Examination
Examination shows upwardly overriding skin. The eyelashes are typically displaced in a more upright position (Fig. 31.6). In some cases, overt eyelash-globe touch may occur. It is unusual for keratopathy to occur, but there are cases in which the eyelashes may abrade the cornea.

Anatomic Correlation
Epiblepharon is actually due to both skin and orbicularis override. This is quite common in Asian children, who typically "outgrow" the pathology over the course of their childhood as facial anatomy matures.

Treatment Options
Most epiblepharon does not require treatment. Symptomatic epiblepharon will likely do well with lubrication. In the rare case of corneal abrasion or continued symptoms despite maturation, epiblepharon may be surgically corrected with a subciliary resection of excess orbicularis combined with a conservative excision of excess skin.

Ptosis (Upper, Lower)

Presentation
Ptosis may refer to both the upper and lower lids. In both cases, the ptotic eyelid approaches the pupil in primary gaze: the upper eyelid is lower,

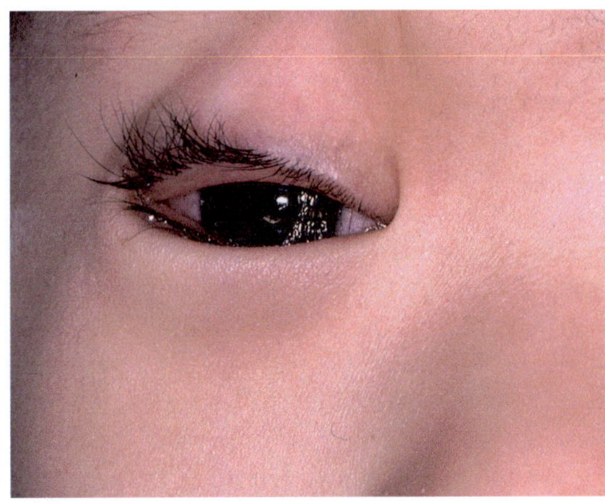

Fig. 31.6 Epiblepharon

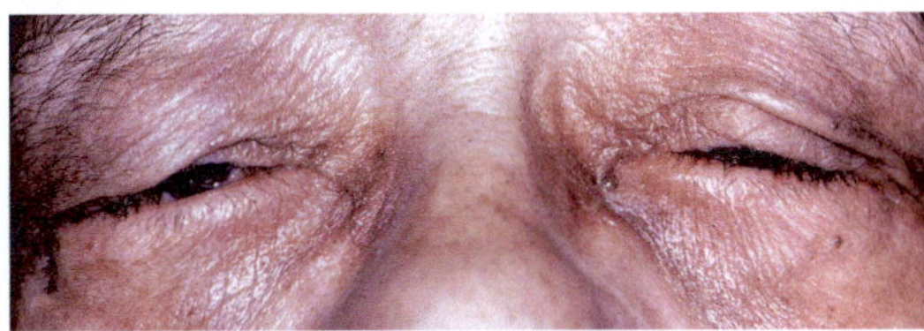

Fig. 31.7 Bilateral upper eyelid ptosis and dermatochalasis

and the lower eyelid is higher, than baseline. The patient may complain of droopy eyelids or eyelid asymmetry, blocked fields of vision, a view of the eyelashes in the field of vision, or the need to lift the eyelid to see. The patient may have had botulinum toxin injection in the months prior to presentation.

Examination
A ptotic upper eyelid appears low (Fig. 31.7; normal lid positions seen in Fig. 31.2). The eyelids may be symmetrically ptotic, or one may be more ptotic than the other. The less ptotic eyelid may demonstrate pseudoretraction as the jointly innervated eyelids attempt to elevate. The patient may be actively recruiting the frontalis muscle to raise the eyelid/s, which will result in an elevated eyebrow on the affected side. The skin crease may be elevated or effaced, the superior sulcus may be more pronounced than normal, and the levator function may be intact or reduced. The pupil may be relatively miotic, or dilated, compared to the non-ptotic side.

A ptotic lower lid sits above the inferior limbus.

Additional ancillary testing and imaging may be warranted depending on the physician's exam findings, as described below.

Anatomic Correlation

As is evident by the number of potential examination findings, there are multiple causes of upper eyelid ptosis. Broadly speaking, these are involutional, traumatic, myogenic, and neurogenic.

Involutional ptosis is related to levator aponeurosis disinsertion from the tarsus, typically due to normal aging. Traumatic disinsertion and even iatrogenic disruption are possible.

Myogenic ptosis is typically congenital in nature, due to levator dysgenesis. It may vary in severity, and a mild case may go undiagnosed until adulthood. Other inheritable syndromes, such as oculopharyngeal dystrophy, may also impact levator function. Chronic progressive external ophthalmoplegia (CPEO), a progressive mitochondrial disorder, may cause both ptosis and strabismus. CPEO may occur as an isolated finding, or in association with other systemic conditions such as Kearns-Sayre syndrome, which would require further cardiac and neurologic evaluations.

Neurogenic ptosis can be due to sympathetic disarray, such as Horner's syndrome or third nerve palsy. A third nerve palsy may be segmental (particularly if orbital), involving the superior branch innervating the levator and superior rectus muscles, or complete, as in the case of third nerve cerebral aneurysmal compression. A dilated pupil is concerning for aneurysmal compression. A combination of upper and lower eyelid ptosis, particularly with an ipsilateral miotic pupil, is concerning for Horner's syndrome involving the sympathetically innervated Müller's and inferior tarsal muscles; if confirmed, this warrants a medical workup. Myasthenia gravis is an autoimmune disease that produces antibody against acetylcholine receptors found in the neuromuscular junction and can cause varying ptosis with or without strabismus. Botulinum toxin can cause ptosis via iatrogenic palsy.

Enophthalmos due to anophthalmos or phthisis can cause a relative ptosis due to lack of underlying orbital volume. Inflammatory, infectious, or traumatic orbital or periocular pathology may cause eyelid edema with secondary mechanical ptosis; once the mechanical ptosis is relieved, there may be a secondary levator disinsertion, which in and of itself will cause additional ptosis secondary to a completely different mechanism.

Treatment Options

After the underlying etiology of a ptosis has been identified, and other pressing concerns such as infection, mass, or aneurysm have been ruled out or treated as appropriate, there remain three major approaches to upper eyelid ptosis repair: the anterior approach (modification/repair of the levator muscle), the posterior approach (modification/repair of Müller's muscle and/or tarsus), and the frontalis approach. Lower eyelid ptosis is not typically repaired, and botulinum-related ptosis should self-resolve within 3–4 months of injection. Traumatic ptosis may take months to spontaneously resolve and is typically not considered a surgical problem for at least 6 months.

Advancement of the levator aponeurosis, which "tightens" the retractor system, is typically performed for disinserted levator muscles, as in the case of involutional or traumatic ptosis. However, levator advancement or even resection (i.e., shortening of the muscle, leading to enhanced functioning) may also be performed in some myogenic cases of congenital ptosis.

A conjunctivomüllerectomy may be performed from the posterior approach, similar to the classic Fasanella-Servat procedure, in which tarsus is excised in addition to conjunctiva and Müller's muscle, thereby shortening the vertical height and enhancing retractor function (Fig. 31.8a–f). These procedures work even if the underlying etiology is not specifically due to a Müller's pathology. In-office topical phenylephrine testing helps determine which patients may benefit from a conjunctivomüllerectomy procedure.

A frontalis sling is helpful in all cases of limited levator function, although if one has enough levator function to attempt a levator or Müller's procedure, the latter are preferred. In a frontalis

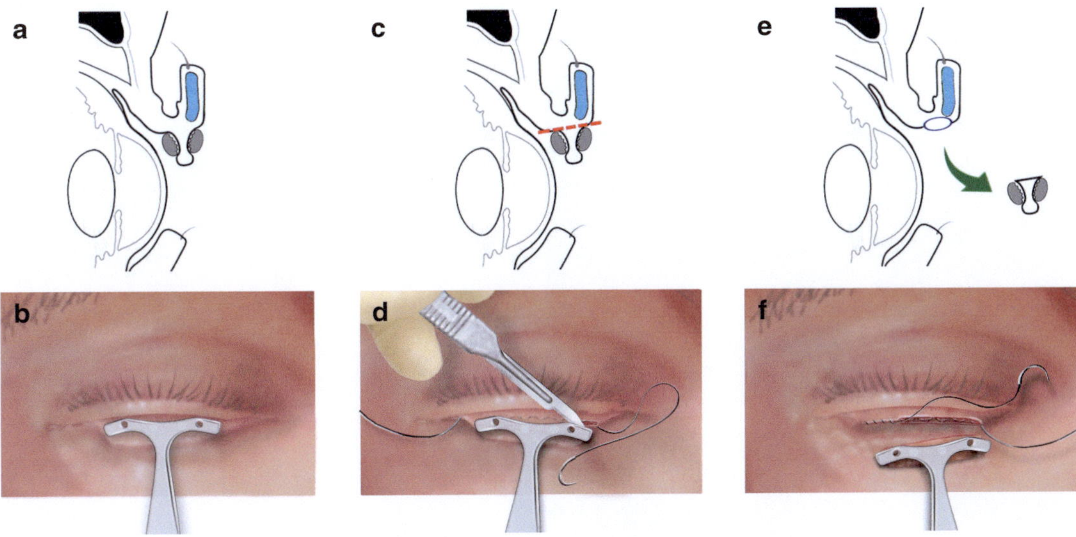

Fig. 31.8 (**a–f**) Conjunctivomüllerectomy technique: (**a, c, e**) demonstrate the sagittal anatomic view of surgical figures (**b, d, f**). A wedge of tissue is removed, foreshortening lid, thereby lessening ptosis

sling procedure, the levator muscle is bypassed by autogenous, allogeneic, or man-made material that is fixed to the tarsus and the frontalis muscle. By contracting the frontalis muscle, the patient can lift the eyelid. Of note, this treatment will not work in cases of frontalis palsy.

Retraction (Upper, Lower)

Presentation
Retraction of the upper, lower, or both eyelids refers to abnormally increased opening of the eyelid. Patients may complain of a "staring" or startled appearance, eyelid asymmetry, and chronic dryness manifesting as a red, uncomfortable eye.

Examination
Examination shows an upper eyelid that is abnormally elevated (at the upper limbus or higher), and/or a lower eyelid that is too retracted (below the lower limbus) (Fig. 31.9a–c; see normal aperture in Fig. 31.2). One can consider any visible sclera above or below the limbus (referred to as superior or inferior "scleral show") in primary gaze to be evidence of retraction. Associated findings may include eyelid asymmetry, eyelid lag in downgaze, lagophthalmos, proptosis, stra-

bismus, injection, and exposure keratopathy. It is important to distinguish true lid retraction from pseudoretraction, which is a compensatory action which attempts to correct abnormal elevation of a contralateral, ptotic eyelid.

Additional ancillary testing and imaging may be warranted depending on the exam findings.

Anatomic Correlation
Retraction may be due to underlying bone structure, with so-called "shallow" orbits, or with relatively large globes, as is seen in high myopia. A facial nerve palsy can cause retraction due to orbicularis (protraction) palsy with unrestrained retractor muscle action. Retraction may be due to traumatic tissue loss, with shortened vertical lid height, as well as iatrogenic shortening as in the case of overly aggressive upper or lower eyelid blepharoplasty. Strabismus surgery involving recession of the inferior rectus muscle may cause unintended lower eyelid retraction due to the capsulopalpebral fascia's inherent connection to the rectus muscle.

The most common cause of eyelid retraction is thyroid eye disease, which results in fibrotic scarring of all components of the eyelid (see Chap. 29). Additionally, proptosis in the setting of thyroid eye disease may cause a secondary retraction, particularly in the lower lid. Thyroid-related

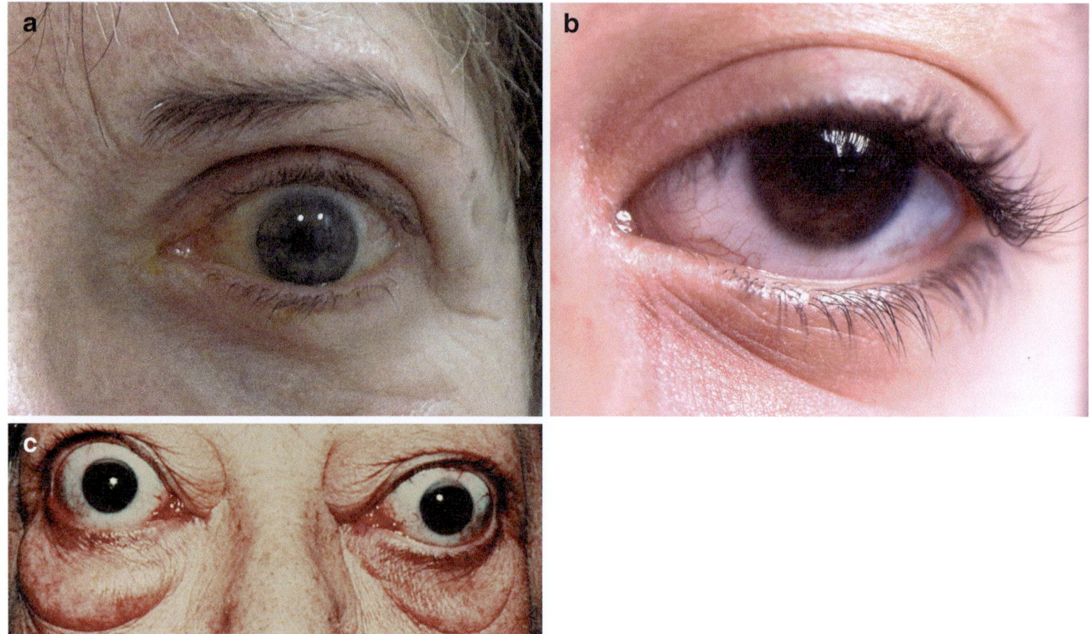

Fig. 31.9 (**a**) Upper eyelid retraction. (**b**) Lower lid retraction. (**c**) Retraction of all four lids, demonstrating bilateral scleral show, in thyroid disease

overaction of the sympathetically controlled lid muscles will further add to lid retraction and the typical appearance of a classic "thyroid stare."

Treatment Options

Patients with familial, or baseline, retraction need not be treated if they are asymptomatic, and the corneas are in good condition, without evidence of the effects of chronic exposure. Most patients with symptomatic retraction will benefit from lubrication until the retraction is repaired. Patients with thyroid eye disease typically should not undergo surgical retraction repair until their disease has stabilized, and any planned decompression or strabismus surgery has been performed.

In patients with upper eyelid retraction due to palsy, a gold or platinum weight may be surgically placed beneath skin and orbicularis, over the tarsal plate, to literally weigh the upper lid down to a lower position; the desired lid height is controlled by the choice of weight. Other causes of upper eyelid retraction typically require a blepharotomy (i.e., a surgical release of one or more of the retractor lamellae) to produce lid recession.

Mild lower lid retraction may benefit from a lateral tarsorrhaphy, where the palpebral fissure is purposely reduced by surgical apposition of the lids. However, most lower eyelid retraction repair typically requires a spacer graft, which adds tissue vertically. This may be an anterior, full-thickness skin graft, such as after a lower lid blepharoplasty with skin excision, or a posteriorly based mucous membrane or other spacer graft, as used in patients with thyroid eye disease.

Injectables have also been used in the temporary treatment of both upper and lower eyelid retraction. For example, hyaluronic acid can be used to lower the upper lid or raise the lower lid. Botulinum toxin can be used to purposefully induce a relative ptosis.

Trichiasis

Presentation

Trichiasis refers to abnormally growing eyelashes. Patients may complain of irritation or pain, eye redness, and tearing.

Examination

Examination shows a variable number of erratically growing eyelashes, exiting the lid margin in an inappropriate location or direction (Fig. 31.10). This is different than eyelash malposition due to entropion, in which the eyelashes remain parallel to each other, but the margin itself is inverted. In symptomatic trichiasis, eyelashes typically touch the globe, eventually causing corneal abrasion. Examination may demonstrate an underlying cause, such as scars from past trauma or surgery, inflammation as in cases of severe blepharitis or Stevens-Johnson syndrome, or infection with secondary conjunctival scarring, as seen in trachoma.

Anatomic Correlation

Eyelash follicles may be disorganized, with lashes exiting the margin in abnormal directions.

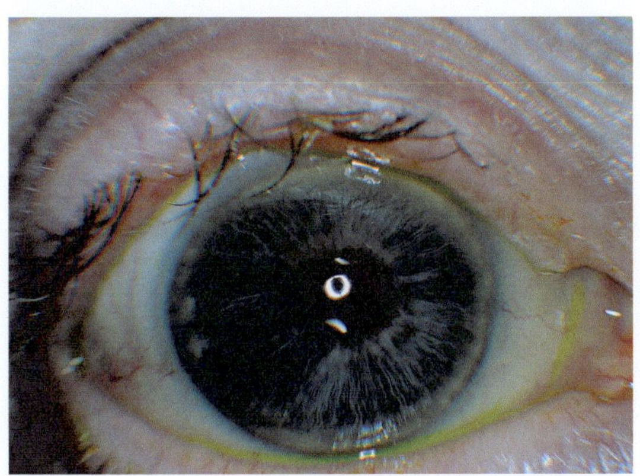

Fig. 31.10 Upper eyelid trichiasis

Treatment Options

Trichiasis need not be treated if it is asymptomatic and does not cause corneal damage. Should trichiasis warrant treatment, a small number of lashes may be repeatedly removed with epilation. Hyfrecation may be effective after several rounds, and cryotherapy may be beneficial, though secondary eyelid notching is possible.

Surgical realignment of the lid margin for treatment of trichiasis may allow for a single procedural cure, obviating multiple visits for epilation or hyfrecation. A small, discrete group of trichiatic lashes can be permanently excised using a wedge excision. More diffuse trichiasis may require tarsal fracture and marginal rotation or more extensive surgical excision of eyelash follicles.

Suggested Reading

AAO Basic and Clinical Science Course: Orbit, Eyelids and Lacrimal System.

AAO Website: The Oculofacial Plastic Surgery Education Center   http://www.aao.org/oculoplastics-center/oculoplastics-education-center.

Callahan MA, Callahan A. Ophthalmic plastic and orbital surgery. Birmingham: Aesculapius Publishing Company; 1979.

Tenzel RR. Orbit and Oculoplastics. In: Podos SM, Yanoff M, editors. Textbook of ophthalmology, vol. 4. New York: Gower Medical Publishing; 1993.

Orbital Infections and Inflammations

Michelle M. Maeng and Bryan J. Winn

Orbital inflammatory disease encompasses a large collection of entities which can be grouped into infectious and noninfectious inflammations. Infectious causes can be bacterial, fungal, or viral. Noninfectious causes may be autoimmune, vasculitic, granulomatous, inflammatory, drug-related, and idiopathic. Orbital inflammation can be vision and life-threatening and is often intimidating and challenging to the clinician. The paragraphs below divide orbital inflammation into infectious and noninfectious categories and provide the clinician with a framework for accurate diagnostic work-up and management.

M. M. Maeng, MD
Department of Ophthalmology, Edward S. Harkness
Eye Institute, Columbia University Vagelos College
of Physicians and Surgeons, New York, NY, USA
e-mail: mmm2412@cumc.columbia.edu

B. J. Winn, MD (✉)
Columbia University Irving Medical Center,
New York, NY, USA

Department of Ophthalmology, Edward S. Harkness
Eye Institute, Columbia University Vagelos College
of Physicians and Surgeons, New York, NY, USA
e-mail: bjw15@columbia.edu

Infectious Orbital Inflammation

Preseptal and Orbital Bacterial Cellulitis

Relevant Anatomy

The orbit is a pear-shaped structure containing the eye, extraocular muscles, cranial nerves II through VI, lacrimal gland, lacrimal sac, and orbital fat. The anterior border of the orbit is the orbital septum, a thin multilayered sheet of connective tissue separating the superficial eyelids from the deeper orbit. It fuses with the periosteum and periorbita at the *arcus marginalis* circumferentially along the orbital rim. The thin bony orbital walls separate the orbit from the frontal sinus and brain superiorly, ethmoid sinuses medially, maxillary sinus inferiorly, and temporalis fossa laterally. The periorbita is the extension of the periosteum posterior to the *arcus marginalis* and lines the internal aspect of the orbital walls. The periorbita is loosely adherent to bone posterior to the *arcus marginalis*, which allows for orbital subperiosteal abscesses (SPAs) to develop adjacent to areas of infected paranasal sinuses. Space-occupying orbital lesions will often cause the eye to protrude outward; if the lesions are extensive or rapidly enlarging, compression of adjacent structures such as the optic nerve may occur, possibly producing irreversible visual loss.

© Springer Nature Switzerland AG 2019
D. S. Casper, G. A. Cioffi (eds.), *The Columbia Guide to Basic Elements of Eye Care*,
https://doi.org/10.1007/978-3-030-10886-1_32

Pathophysiology

Preseptal cellulitis is an infection of the eyelid and periorbital structures anterior to the orbital septum. Common causes of preseptal cellulitis include sinusitis, folliculitis, hordeolum, upper respiratory infection, otitis media, lid abscess, dacryocystitis, trauma, foreign body, insect bites, animal bites, and, rarely, bacteremic seeding in infants from *Streptococcus pneumonia*, *Streptococcus pyogenes*, *or Haemophilus influenzae.*

Blood cultures for preseptal cellulitis are almost always negative and often technically difficult to obtain. Of those with positive cultures, 60–77% of cultures may include *Staphylococcus* species and *Streptococcus* species. With the onset of antimicrobial resistance, community-acquired methicillin-resistant *Staphylococcus aureus* (CA-MRSA) is also playing an increasing role. In one report of adults presenting to emergency departments in 2004 with skin and soft tissue infections, 59% of infections were caused by MRSA and 97% of cases of MRSA were caused by CA-MRSA. Less common pathogens include *Haemophilus influenzae* (less prominent now with vaccinations), *Klebsiella pneumoniae*, anaerobes, and skin flora/contaminants.

Preseptal cellulitis is often difficult to distinguish from orbital cellulitis, which refers to infection involving deeper orbital structures posterior to the septum, which can be of bacterial or fungal origin. Orbital cellulitis is much less common than preseptal cellulitis, 6–13% vs. 87–94%, respectively, and, like preseptal cellulitis, is most often seen in children. Studies have shown that orbital cellulitis can be sight-threatening in up to 11% of cases and life-threatening in 1–2%.

The most common cause of orbital cellulitis is adjacent bacterial sinusitis (86–98%). With sinuses flanking two-thirds of the bony orbit (Fig. 32.1), infections can easily invade orbit via contiguous spread. In particular, the orbit and ethmoid sinus are separated by a paper-thin medial orbital wall (the lamina papyracea), which contains perforations for blood vessels and nerves as well as natural fenestrations called Zuckerkandl's dehiscences. This configuration is believed to be the reason that the most common precipitating site resulting in postseptal cellulitis is the region of the ethmoid sinuses. Other causes of orbital cellulitis include bacterial infections of the teeth, middle ear, or face; orbital trauma with fracture or foreign body; fungal rhinosinusitis; dacryocystitis; an infected mucocele that erodes into the orbit; endophthalmitis; ophthalmic surgery; or injections to induce retrobulbar/peribulbar transcutaneous anesthesia.

Blood cultures are positive in orbital cellulitis in 33% of children and 5% of adults. When positive, the growth is usually polymicrobial, especially in adult patients. *Staphylococcus* and *Streptococcus* species are the most common pathogens, leading with *Streptococcus anginosus* (15%), *Staphylococcus aureus* (9%), *group A beta-hemolytic Streptococcus* (6%), and *Streptococcus pneumonia* (4%). Other less common culprits include anaerobic bacteria, *Pseudomonas aeruginosa*, *Eikenella corrodens*, and *Haemophilus influenza*. Fungal species including *Mucor*, *Rhizopus*, and *Aspergillus* may cause a life-threatening cerebro-sino-orbital cellulitis in immunosuppressed patients. Fungal orbital infections are further addressed in a separate section below.

Clinical Presentation

Preseptal cellulitis presents chiefly with eyelid swelling. Eyelid erythema and eye pain/tenderness may or may not be evident. Patients will have no pain with eye movements, proptosis, ophthalmoplegia, diplopia, or visual impairment. Chemosis (conjunctival edema) is rarely found; fever and leukocytosis may be present.

In contrast, orbital cellulitis presents with eyelid swelling, with or without erythema, and restricted extraocular motility. Patients may complain of deep orbital pain or pain on attempted eye movement, diplopia, and vision impairment. Proptosis is usually evident, but presentation may be subtle. Chemosis may be present, and fever and leukocytosis are commonly found. In severe cases, signs of optic neuropathy may be evident, including a relative afferent pupillary defect and decreased color vision. Corneal and facial numbness may be a sign of an infiltrative and potentially ischemic process (Fig. 32.2).

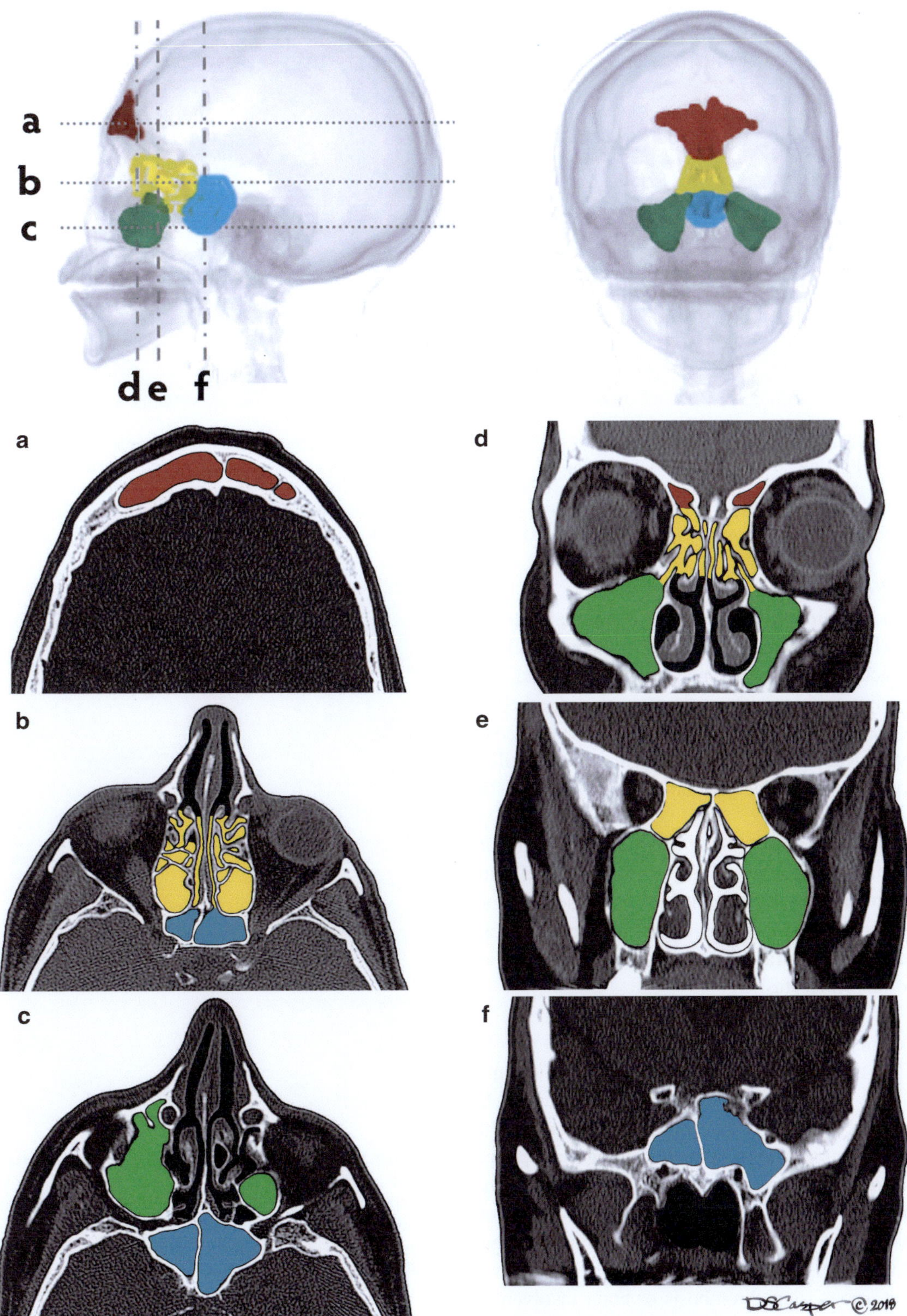

Fig. 32.1 Paranasal sinuses and the orbit. (**a–f**) CT images demonstrate the relationship between the frontal (red), ethmoid (yellow), maxillary (green), and sphenoid (blue) sinuses and the orbit. Infection may spread from any of the sinuses to the orbit through the thin, bony, orbital walls

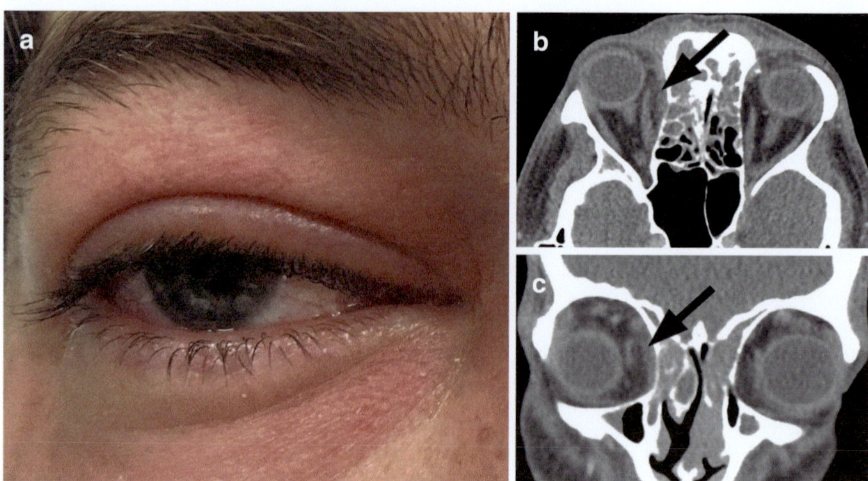

Fig. 32.2 (**a**) Clinical photograph of a patient with orbital cellulitis. From the photograph alone, it would be impossible to differentiate preseptal from orbital cellulitis. This patient also had fever, pain with eye movements, and limitation of adduction of the eye. (**b**) Axial orbital CT demonstrated ethmoid sinusitis with a small subperiosteal abscess along the medial orbital wall. (**c**) Coronal orbital CT showing subperiosteal abscess. Arrows indicate the small subperiosteal abscesses in both CT images

Differential Diagnosis

The differential diagnosis for preseptal cellulitis includes orbital cellulitis, chalazion, allergic reaction, erysipelas, necrotizing fasciitis, viral conjunctivitis with secondary eyelid swelling, cavernous sinus thrombosis, varicella zoster virus, insect bite, angioedema, trauma, maxillary osteomyelitis, dacryoadenitis, and dacryocystitis (Fig. 32.3).

The differential diagnosis for bacterial orbital cellulitis includes fungal sino-orbital cellulitis, acute orbital inflammation (orbital pseudotumor, see below), cavernous sinus thrombosis, sickle cell-related infarction of the sphenoid bone, and orbital metastasis.

Work-Up

The diagnosis of preseptal cellulitis can often be made clinically. However, contrast-enhanced CT scan of the orbits and sinuses is recommended if the presentation is atypical or concerning for postseptal involvement. Imaging can also be considered when patients are not responding to appropriate antibiotic therapy after 24–48 h. Magnetic resonance imaging (MRI) can be helpful when there is a suspicion for cavernous sinus thrombosis or brain involvement. Magnetic resonance venography (MRV) should be ordered when cavernous sinus thrombosis is in

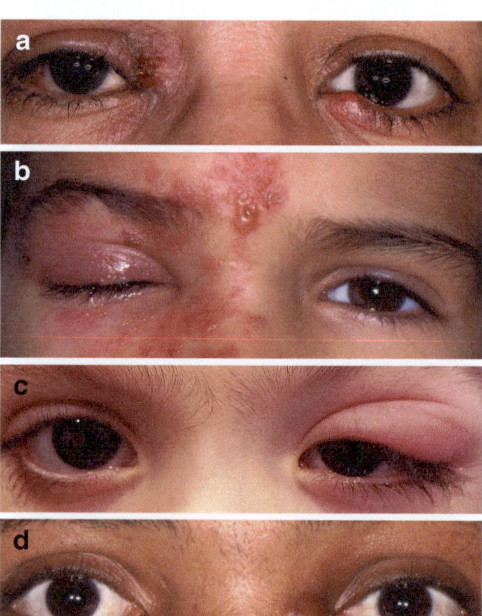

Fig. 32.3 (**a**) Inflamed hordeola/chalazia of the right upper and left lower lid. (**b**) Herpes zoster of the V1 distribution on the right. Note that the lesions do not cross the midline. This patient is at risk for intraocular inflammation and requires a full ophthalmic examination including dilated fundus examination. (**c**) Left dacryoadenitis. Note the S-shaped deformity of the left upper lid indicating inflammation of the lacrimal gland (Courtesy of Peter Michalos, MD). (**d**) Left dacryocystitis. Note the dilated lacrimal sac (dacryocystocele)

question. Blood cultures are usually obtained if the patient is febrile or if orbital cellulitis is suspected, although these are usually of low yield.

Any patient who is suspected of having orbital cellulitis should be evaluated by an ophthalmologist and otolaryngologist.

Management

Treatment of preseptal cellulitis includes broad-spectrum antibacterial coverage. With the high incidence of CA-MRSA, the recommended antibiotic regimen has evolved to include coverage for this entity. CA-MRSA is typically sensitive to clindamycin, trimethoprim-sulfamethoxazole (TMP-SMX), and doxycycline. TMP-SMX and doxycycline are not reliably effective for *group A Streptococcus* coverage and doxycycline is not safe for use in children or pregnant women. Therefore, the recommendation for coverage of the most common pathogens, including CA-MRSA, is clindamycin monotherapy or dual therapy with trimethoprim-sulfamethoxazole and amoxicillin, amoxicillin-clavulanic acid, or cefpodoxime.

For adults and children >1 year old with preseptal cellulitis and without signs of toxicity, oral antibiotics for 7–10 days are preferred with close outpatient follow-up. Admission for intravenous antibiotics and monitoring should be considered for neonates, toxic-appearing patients, severely ill patients, and those suspected of having orbital cellulitis.

Patients diagnosed with orbital cellulitis are admitted for intravenous broad-spectrum therapy with activity against *S. aureus* (including MRSA), *Streptococci* species, and *gram-negative bacilli*. The antibiotic regimen of choice is vancomycin plus either ampicillin-sulbactam, piperacillin-tazobactam, or ceftriaxone. If ceftriaxone is employed and there is concern for intracranial extension, metronidazole is added for anaerobic coverage. If the patient is penicillin allergic, vancomycin plus ciprofloxacin or vancomycin plus levofloxacin can be utilized. Once the patient shows signs of clinical improvement, the therapy regimen can be bridged to oral, with total duration of treatment typically lasting 2–4 weeks.

Complications

The prognosis for preseptal cellulitis is generally good. Complications can arise with delay or inadequate treatment, leading to orbital cellulitis, with subsequent development of subperiosteal abscess, orbital abscess, or cavernous sinus thrombosis. Orbital extension can lead to central nervous system involvement, with resulting meningitis and abscesses of the brain, extradural or subdural spaces. Necrotizing fasciitis is a rare complication caused by *beta-hemolytic Streptococcus*, presenting as a rapidly progressive cellulitis.

Complications of orbital cellulitis include orbital/subperiosteal abscess (15–59%); intracranial extension (4%); and, rarely, meningitis; cavernous sinus thrombosis; brain, subdural, or epidural abscess; vision loss; and death.

Subperiosteal abscesses (SPAs) usually present along the medial orbital wall (see Fig. 32.2). For medial SPAs, if the patient is otherwise healthy and older than 1 year, but less than 9 years old, the patient can often be treated with intravenous antibiotics alone. If the SPA is atypical, greater than 1 cm in diameter, and non-medial, or the patient is outside the age range above, incision and drainage of the abscess and concurrent endoscopic sinus surgery performed by an oculoplastic surgeon and otolaryngologist are usually required (Fig. 32.4).

Cavernous sinus thrombosis should be suspected if signs of orbital inflammation also occur in the contralateral eye. Cavernous sinus thrombosis can lead to multiple cranial nerve palsies and permanent vision loss and can facilitate extension of the infection to the brain. Hallmarks of cavernous sinus thrombosis include loss of corneal sensation, limited extraocular movements, ptosis, and chemosis. Vision loss or relative afferent pupillary defect may be present. On CT scan, a dilated superior ophthalmic vein can be seen. MRI may also reveal widening of the cavernous sinus. This is an emergency and should prompt immediate evaluation by an oculoplastic surgeon and otolaryngologist with surgical treatment of the underlying sinusitis. Anticoagulation to treat the thrombosis is controversial but may be beneficial in certain cases (Fig. 32.5).

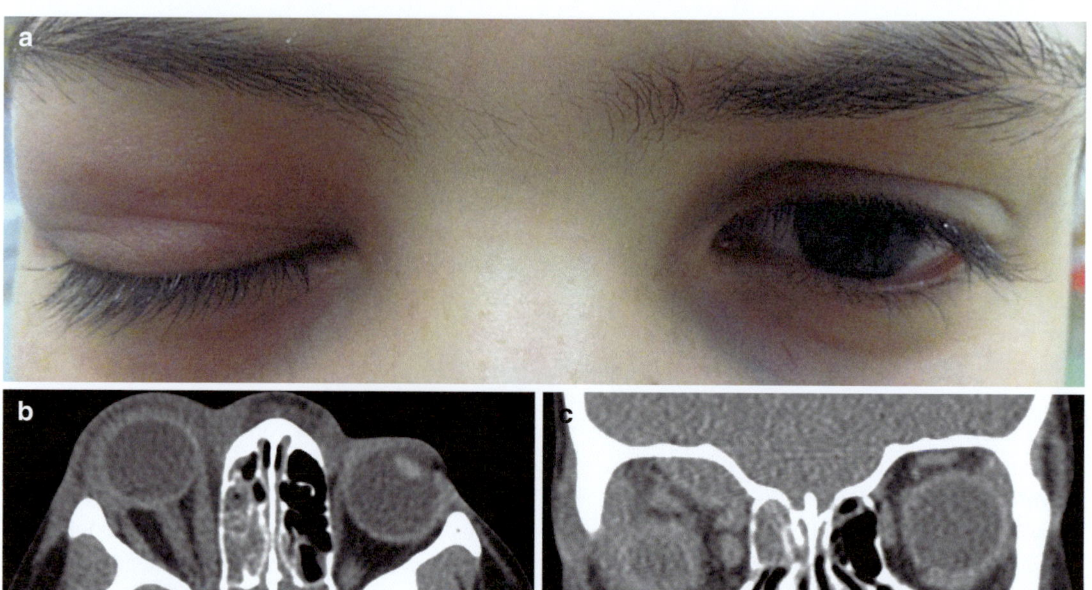

Fig. 32.4 Nonmedial subperiosteal abscesses. (**a**) Clinical photograph of a patient with right orbital cellulitis. (**b**) The axial CT demonstrated ethmoid sinusitis. (**c**) Coronal CT demonstrated a superior subperiosteal abscess which required drainage via anterior orbitotomy with concurrent endoscopic sinus surgery

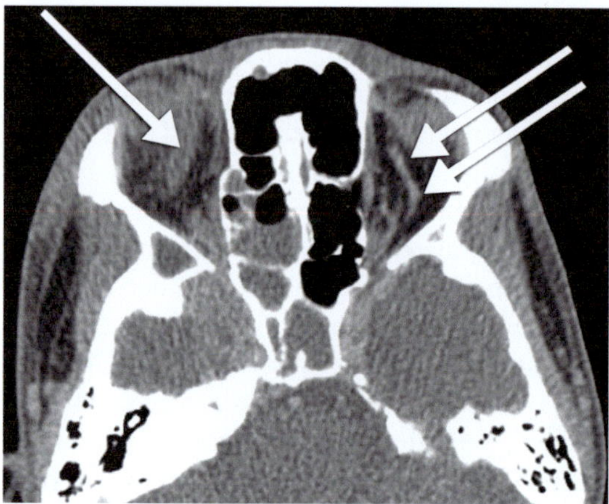

Fig. 32.5 Axial CT demonstrating a dilated superior ophthalmic vein on the right (arrow) in the setting of cavernous sinus thrombosis. The normal ophthalmic vein is seen on the left (double arrows). Notice the opacification of the posterior ethmoid and sphenoid sinus predisposing to direct extension of infection to the cavernous sinus

Fungal Sino-orbital Infection

Fungal sino-orbital infections are among the most serious, life-threatening conditions encountered by the ophthalmologist. The most important elements to successful treatment of this condition are a high level of suspicion and early initiation of treatment.

The most common fungal orbital infections are mucormycosis and invasive aspergillosis. Mucormycosis is most commonly caused by *Rhizopus oryzae*, followed by *Absidia corymbifera*, *Mucor ramosissimus*, *Rhizomucor pusillus*, and *Apophysomyces elegans*. Invasive aspergillosis is caused by *Aspergillus fumigatus*, *Aspergillus flavus*, and *Aspergillus niger*. In diabetic and immunocompromised patients, inhaled fungal spores can infect the paranasal sinus mucosa (see Fig. 22.12). Spread to adjacent structures, including the orbit and brain, typically occurs via an invasive, ischemic vasculitis.

Presentation

Patients with mucormycosis may present with fever, acute sinusitis, nasal congestion and discharge, headache, and sinus pain. Signs of orbital involvement may include periorbital edema, chemosis, ptosis, ophthalmoplegia, numbness and loss of corneal sensation, proptosis, and acute vision loss. Extension to the cavernous sinus can

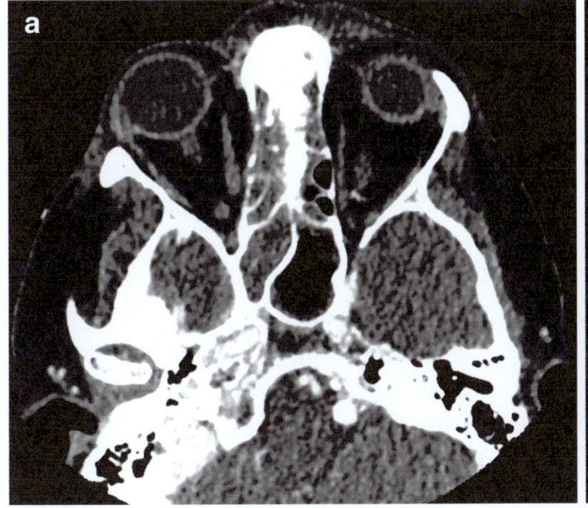
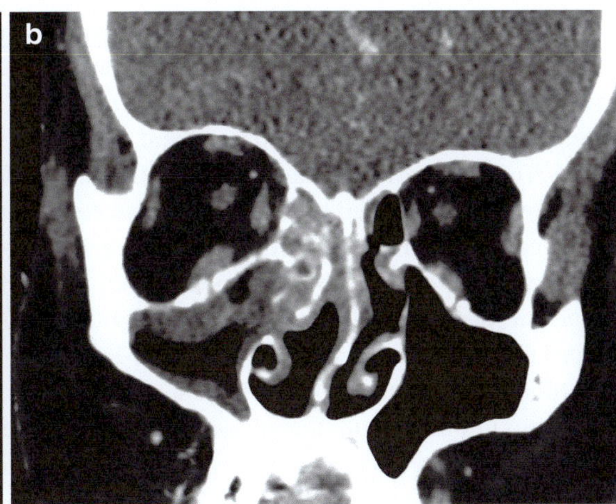

Fig. 32.6 Mucormycosis. (**a**) Axial CT and (**b**) coronal CT. A 45-year-old with past medical history of lung transplantation on chronic immunosuppression presented with sinusitis refractory to oral and intravenous antibiotics and new right periorbital edema. CT demonstrated predominantly right pansinusitis and with minimal orbital involvement. Intravenous antifungals were added including liposomal amphotericin. A decision was made to place an indwelling catheter in the inferomedial orbit to irrigate the orbital tissues with 1–1.5 mL of liposomal amphotericin at a concentration of 3.5 mg/cc for 3 days, after which the periorbital inflammation markedly diminished

result in cranial nerve palsies, cerebral venous sinus thrombosis, and invasion into the carotid artery. Spread of infection to the brain can cause fungal meningitis, obtundation, and, eventually, death. Additional signs of spread beyond the sinuses can include necrosis of the palate, perinasal swelling, as well as erythema or cyanosis of the periorbital skin. While the classic black palatal eschar is pathognomonic for invasive fungal disease, it is a very late sign (Fig. 32.6).

Invasive aspergillosis may also present with proptosis, pain, cranial neuropathies, and acute loss of vision. However, the presentation can be variable and can often mimic other conditions such as bacterial orbital cellulitis, acute orbital inflammation, giant-cell arteritis, and sino-orbital malignancies.

While mucormycosis is most commonly seen in patients with diabetic ketoacidosis or hematologic malignancies, invasive aspergillosis is more commonly seen in neutropenic patients, classically in patients with solid organ and bone marrow transplants as well as patient on high-dose corticosteroid treatment. On occasion, invasive aspergillosis can even be seen in immunocompetent patients. Other risk factors for fungal sino-orbital disease include chronic renal failure, hemodialysis, deferoxamine iron chelation, AIDS, intravenous drug use, trauma, burns, and malnutrition. The mortality rate is high for both sino-orbital invasive *aspergillosis* (~30%) and mucormycosis (>50%).

Work-Up

Work-up includes imaging of the head, orbits, and paranasal sinuses with computed tomography (CT) and magnetic resonance imaging (MRI) both with and without contrast to evaluate for sinus disease and assess involvement of nearby structures, such as the orbit, cavernous sinus, and brain. Given the predisposing immunosuppression, the extent of sinus disease may be underwhelming in comparison to the clinical picture. CT imaging will often show bone erosion as well as allow for the differentiation between air, hemorrhage, and mycetoma. Fungal disease on MRI will often be hypointense on both T1 and T2 sequences, as opposed to bacterial infections and neoplasms which are hyperintense on T2. Images may show lack of contrast enhancement in areas of ischemic vasculitis and necrosis. Diagnosis involves a high clinical index of suspicion, especially in patients with associated risk factors. If suspicion is high, systemic antifungal therapy with liposomal amphotericin B should not be delayed while awaiting confirmatory data.

Fungal 1,3-beta-D-glucan and *Aspergillus* galactomannan assays may detect the presence of invasive Aspergillus but do not detect mucormycetes. Enzyme-linked immunosorbent assay (ELISA), immunoblots, and immunodiffusion tests can also be utilized but have varied success. While cultures can be difficult to obtain, an endonasal examination can be performed to look for tissue necrosis and collect specimens. Calcofluor white and methenamine silver are especially helpful stains to detect fungal elements. In addition to traditional culture techniques, polymerase chain reaction (PCR) on histologic specimens and matrix-assisted laser desorption ionization-time of flight (MALDI-TOF) mass spectrometry can be useful diagnostic tests. Patients in more advanced stages of immunosuppression, as reflected by a CD4 count less than 200 cells/µL or absolute neutrophil count (ANC) less than 600 cells/µL, are at higher risk of infection with invasive fungal sinusitis, especially in the pediatric population. The definitive diagnosis includes sinus surgery with debridement and biopsy with frozen section confirmation of fungal elements.

Treatment

Proper management of invasive sino-orbital infection begins with early diagnosis. It is critical for the physician to suspect fungal disease when assessing patients with signs of orbital cellulitis and sinusitis in any patient who is immunocompromised. Studies have shown that early initiation of treatment with systemic antifungals, rapid reversal of the underlying immunocompromised state, and surgical debridement of involved tissues lead to better outcomes. These cases are best managed with a team-based approach at a tertiary care center, involving infectious disease specialists, otolaryngologists, and ophthalmologists.

Antifungal therapy should begin with intravenous liposomal amphotericin B. It is the first-line treatment for mucormycosis and is also effective for invasive aspergillosis. Posaconazole can be used as adjunctive therapy with amphotericin or as a single agent in patients who are amphotericin intolerant. Caspofungin is a newer drug in the echinocandin class of antifungals and has been shown to increase survival in patients with mucormycosis when used in combination with amphotericin. In addition to systemic therapy, local amphotericin may also be delivered directly into the orbit through an indwelling catheter. Once a diagnosis of invasive sino-orbital aspergillosis is made, systemic therapy can be changed to voriconazole, which has the best efficacy for *Aspergillus* and lowest side effect profile among antifungals.

Surgical debridement of all involved necrotic tissue, which may necessitate complete orbital exenteration in the most severe cases, is required to clear the infection and halt progression.

Prognosis

Mortality rates from invasive fungal sino-orbital infections have been reported as high as 70% in some studies. Aspergillosis typically carries a better prognosis than mucormycosis. Early initiation of treatment, when infection is confined to the sinuses, and successful reversal of immunosuppression, most easily accomplished in cases of diabetic ketoacidosis, are associated with better outcomes. Prognosis is particularly poor for patients with brain, cavernous sinus, or carotid artery involvement or for those in whom immunosuppression cannot be corrected.

Infectious Dacryoadenitis

Pathophysiology

Dacryoadenitis refers to the acute or chronic inflammation of the lacrimal gland. The etiology is thought to be idiopathic, viral, or bacterial. Viral causes can include mumps, Epstein-Barr virus, cytomegalovirus, influenza, varicella zoster, and others. Bacterial cases are rare but have been associated with staphylococci, *Haemophilus*, pneumococci, streptococci, Pseudomonas, diphtheroids, and *Micrococcus*. Eyelid laxity, as in the case of floppy eyelid syndrome, may predispose individuals to bacterial dacryoadenitis.

Presentation

Acute disease presents with rapid-onset unilateral redness and pain, especially with palpa-

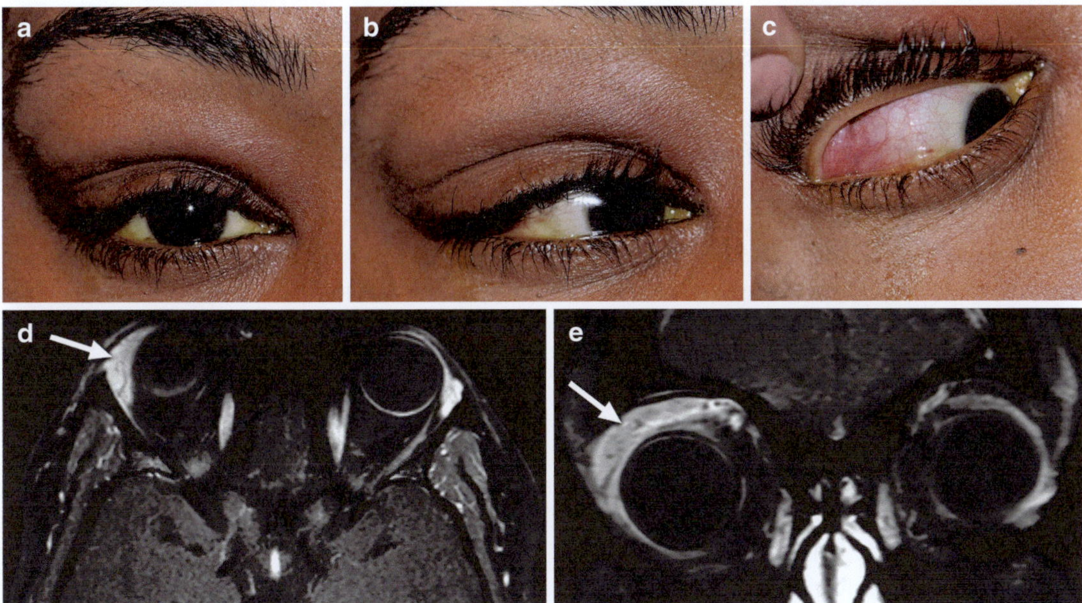

Fig. 32.7 (**a–e**) A 34-year-old woman presented with pain, localized to the right superior-lateral orbit and an S-shaped deformity of the eyelid. The patient was treated elsewhere with topical antibiotic-steroid drops, with worsening symptoms. Her exam was otherwise normal. Imaging showed mild thickening of the preseptal soft tis-sues laterally, enlargement of the right lacrimal gland (white arrows), and some infiltration of the extraconal fat in the superior and lateral orbit. Examination and imaging are consistent with acute dacryoadenitis; a swollen preauricular lymph node on the ipsilateral side suggested a viral etiology. She responded to oral prednisone therapy

tion. Inflammation over the lateral third of the upper eyelid clinically leads to the characteristic S-shaped eyelid deformity and ptosis. Lacrimal secretions may be either increased or decreased; discharge may also be reported. Ipsilateral preauricular lymphadenopathy typically indicates a viral etiology. Patients also may present with ipsilateral temporal conjunctival chemosis, fever, and leukocytosis (Fig. 32.7).

Work-Up

After a thorough history and physical exam, further work-up can be obtained with imaging. Contrast-enhanced CT of the orbit is preferred to MRI for better assessment of adjacent bony anatomy. Imaging will show enlargement of the lacrimal gland and involvement of adjacent soft tissue without bony erosion. Bony erosion suggests malignant neoplasm rather than dacryoadenitis. In such cases when tumor needs to be excluded, a biopsy is indicated for a more definitive diagnosis.

Treatment

In the case of viral dacryoadenitis, supportive management is recommended with cold compresses and nonnarcotic analgesics as needed. Systemic corticosteroids may be added. When suspecting a bacterial etiology, broad-spectrum antibiotic coverage can be initiated with amoxicillin/clavulanate or cephalexin. When the specific etiology remains unclear, a trial of oral antibiotics can be pursued with reexamination in 24 h for further management.

Lyme-Associated Orbital Inflammation

A rare cause of orbital inflammation, *B. burgdorferi*, can lead to subacute orbital inflammation. A number of cases of extraocular muscle involvement (myositis) have been reported in the literature. Cases may present painlessly and include findings such as ptosis, proptosis, and papillitis. Lyme antibody testing may only be positive after

6 weeks of infection. Treatment may include oral doxycycline or intravenous ceftriaxone.

Noninfectious Orbital Inflammation

Differentiating noninfectious orbital inflammation from orbital cellulitis can be difficult, as many of the clinical signs and symptoms overlap, including proptosis, eyelid and periocular edema, pain, chemosis, diplopia, and vision loss. Unlike orbital cellulitis, orbital inflammation is typically not associated with fever, leukocytosis, or acute sinusitis. A comprehensive history, complete ocular and orbital examination, laboratory testing, and orbital imaging are often necessary to come to a correct diagnosis and management plan.

The differential diagnosis of noninfectious orbital inflammation includes specific, named inflammatory entities such as: sarcoidosis, IgG4-related disease, granulomatosis with polyangiitis (formerly known as Wegener's granulomatosis), and thyroid eye disease, as well as idiopathic, non-granulomatous orbital inflammation, also known as orbital pseudotumor (an older terminology utilized prior to the availability of current imaging modalities, when a neoplastic process was presumed, but not identified on surgical exploration). In addition, orbital inflammation may occur in response to a neoplastic process, especially metastasis. Rare causes of inflammation include reactions to medications such as bisphosphonates and edema secondary to sphenoid wing infarction in sickle cell disease. Chronic cocaine use can lead to a destructive sino-orbital inflammation which may mimic that seen in granulomatosis with polyangiitis.

Nonspecific Orbital Inflammation and Approach to the Inflamed Orbit

As with most diagnostic challenges, much of the necessary information required to come to an accurate assessment can be obtained via a thorough history. Of particular importance are timing of onset and the presence or absence of pain. Most cases of typical acute nonspecific orbital inflammation (NSOI) are associated with rapid onset within a day or two and severe pain. In that sense, it may be difficult to differentiate it from orbital cellulitis; however, patients with NSOI will typically be otherwise well-appearing, without fever or other constitutional symptoms. Insidious onset and lack of pain should point toward atypical inflammation, such as sarcoid or sclerosing orbital inflammation, or may suggest a neoplastic process. A personal or strong family history of autoinflammatory disease is frequently found in patients with NSOI including Crohn's disease, systemic lupus erythematosis, rheumatoid arthritis, type 1 diabetes mellitus, and HLA-B27 disease. A review of systems should include trouble breathing/asthma symptoms (sarcoid); glomerulonephritis and sinusitis (granulomatosis with polyangiitis); anxiety, palpitations, heat/cold intolerance, and weight loss (thyroid eye disease); sickle cell disease (sickle cell-related orbital inflammation); cocaine use (cocaine-related sinoorbitopathy); bisphosphonate use (bisphosphonate-related orbital inflammation); and retroperitoneal fibrosis/pancreatitis/cholangitis/hydronephrosis (IgG4-related disease and sclerosing orbital inflammation).

A complete ophthalmic examination follows the history. In severe cases of orbital inflammation, visual acuity, pupil function, and intraocular pressure may be affected. As with orbital infections, eyelid and periorbital edema will likely be present in most cases of orbital inflammation. Other signs may include eyelid retraction (common in thyroid eye disease), ptosis (common in non-thyroid-related inflammation), an S-shaped deformity of the eyelid suggesting lacrimal gland enlargement and inflammation (dacryoadenitis; see Fig. 32.6), loss of the superior sulcus, or frank proptosis. Extraocular movements may be limited or associated with pain. In thyroid eye disease (TED), extraocular muscles may become enlarged and stiff, often associated with restriction of the enlarged muscle. Imaging reveals sparing of the muscle tendon as it inserts on the globe in TED. In non-thyroid-related orbital myositis, enlarged muscles are typically weak rather than tight, producing the opposite effect. In over 50% of patients with NSOI myositis, the extraocular muscle tendons may be thickened.

Most cases of adult NSOI are unilateral. Bilateral presentations of orbital inflammation should suggest a systemic process such as sarcoid, TED, granulomatosis with polyangiitis, IgG-4 related disease, or multifocal fibrosclerosis.

Laboratory testing includes a complete blood count, erythrocyte sedimentation rate (ESR), C-reactive protein (CRP), Lyme antibodies, thyroid function tests, and thyroid-related antibodies including the thyroid-stimulating immunoglobulin (TSI), angiotensin-converting enzyme (ACE), antineutrophil cytoplasmic antibodies (ANCAs), rapid plasma reagin (RPR), antinuclear antibodies (ANA), rheumatoid factor, quantiferon-TB gold, and serum IgG4 levels.

Orbital imaging consisting of contrast-enhanced high-resolution computed tomography (CT) or magnetic resonance imaging (MRI) should be obtained. CT is typically adequate for diagnostic purposes and is superior for imaging bony structures and demonstrating contrast between orbital fat, extraocular muscles, paranasal sinuses, and areas of inflammation. MRI has advantages in terms of soft tissue structures as well as imaging the orbital apex, cavernous sinus, and superior orbital fissure. With both CT and MRI, there will be marked, often feathery, contrast enhancement in areas of active inflammation (Fig. 32.8). Diffusion-weighted MRI may be helpful in distinguishing between orbital cellulitis, inflammation, and lymphoproliferative processes.

Orbital inflammation is often categorized by the anatomic location of the inflammatory process. These patterns of inflammation can often help the clinician narrow the differential diagnosis. Inflammation may be diffuse or localized to a specific area or tissue in the orbit, such as the lacrimal gland (dacryoadenitis), extraocular muscle(s) (myositis), sclera (scleritis), or optic nerve sheath (perineuritis). The diffuse form involves more than one tissue and often includes orbital fat. It may have a predominantly anterior, posterior, medial, or lateral focus.

If serologic testing and imaging are nondiagnostic and the presentation is "typical" (i.e., painful with rapid onset), a presumptive diagnosis of nonspecific orbital inflammation is made. There currently is no consensus whether to treat empirically with corticosteroids or obtain a biopsy prior to initiation of treatment. Those who favor biopsy cite that lacrimal gland biopsies in the setting of orbital inflammation often reveal a specific entity, enabling initiation of more precise treatment. In addition, lacrimal gland and anterior orbital biop-

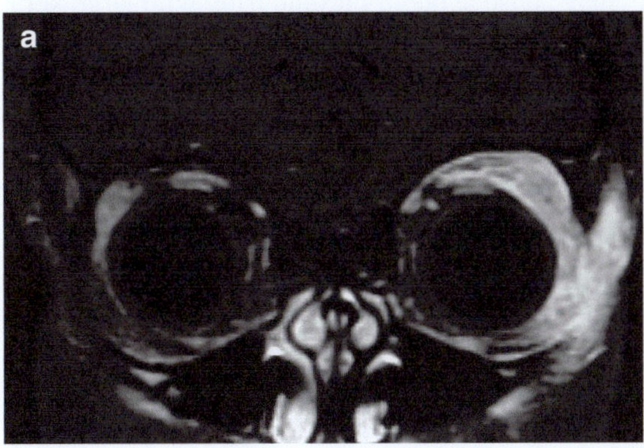
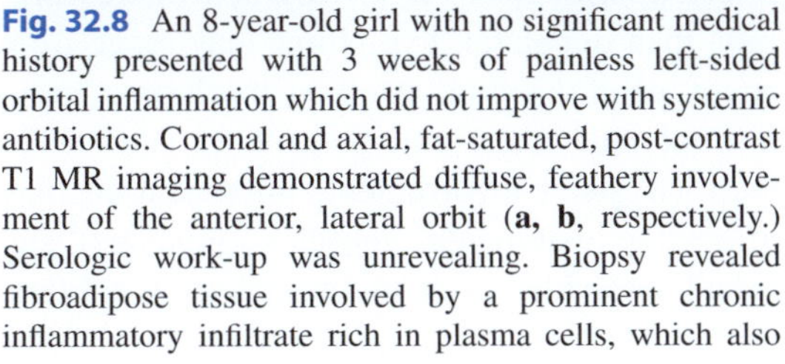
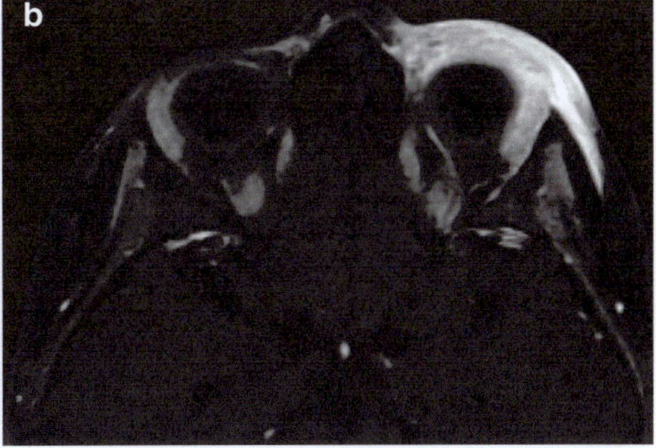

Fig. 32.8 An 8-year-old girl with no significant medical history presented with 3 weeks of painless left-sided orbital inflammation which did not improve with systemic antibiotics. Coronal and axial, fat-saturated, post-contrast T1 MR imaging demonstrated diffuse, feathery involvement of the anterior, lateral orbit (**a, b**, respectively.) Serologic work-up was unrevealing. Biopsy revealed fibroadipose tissue involved by a prominent chronic inflammatory infiltrate rich in plasma cells, which also involved the fibrous septa and adipose tissue of the lacrimal gland. No granulomatous inflammation or vasculitis was identified, and trichrome stains were negative for interstitial fibrosis. Special stains for organisms (gram, GMS, and AFB) were negative. There were only sparse IgG4-positive cells. A c-kit immunostain was negative, excluding a mast cell process. A diagnosis of nonspecific orbital inflammation was made, and the patient responded well to a long taper of prednisone

sies carry a low risk of morbidity. Virtually all agree that atypical, unusual, and bilateral presentations should be biopsied as they are more likely to be associated with a systemic inflammatory process or malignancy. Exceptions include orbital myositis and orbital apex syndrome, given the morbidity associated with biopsy. In these cases, empiric steroids should be administered and biopsy only pursued upon treatment failure.

Oral prednisone is typically instituted and tapered slowly once the inflammation is resolved. Most cases of NSOI respond exquisitely well to steroids, with dramatic improvement over 12–24 h. In cases of poor response to steroids, the diagnosis must come back into question, and repeat biopsy (or initial biopsy if steroids were started empirically) should be performed. For recurrent episodes of NSOI, orbital radiation or biologic agents may be considered.

There is a sclerosing form of nonspecific orbital inflammation which often presents in a chronic or subacute fashion without pain, with extraocular dysmotility, mass effect, and vision loss. Many believe this is a distinct clinical entity separate from NSOI. Biopsy is required in these cases as the presentation can be mimicked by metastatic or contiguous carcinoma, infiltrating lymphoid lesion, chronic fungal infection, sarcoid, or a primary orbital neoplasm. The histopathology of sclerosing orbital inflammation (also called sclerosing orbital pseudotumor) demonstrates a sparse inflammatory infiltrate within dense fibrosis. This fibrosclerosis can tether orbital tissues, causing restrictive strabismus as well as cause mass-like compression of the optic nerve. A number of these cases are associated with systemic multifocal fibrosclerosis, in which case patients have a collection of similar areas of mass-like fibrosclerosis infiltrating or encasing organs such as the kidney and ureters (retroperitoneal fibrosis), liver and gall bladder (sclerosing cholangitis), great vessels and airway (mediastinal fibrosis), and thyroid gland (Riedel's thyroiditis). Work-up should include imaging of the orbit; imaging of the chest, abdomen, and pelvis to look for multifocal fibrosclerosis; liver function tests; and kidney function tests. Winn and Rootman found that most cases of multifocal fibrosclerosis in the setting of sclerosing orbital

inflammation had significantly elevated erythrocyte sedimentation rates and bilateral orbital disease. Many of these cases are now being recognized as a sclerosing form of IgG-4 related disease.

Treatment of sclerosing orbital inflammation can be frustrating as it generally responds poorly to corticosteroids or radiation. Some authors have had more success with chemotherapeutics and biologics such as cyclophosphamide, infliximab, and rituximab.

Specific Orbital Inflammatory Conditions

Sarcoidosis

Sarcoidosis is an idiopathic, multisystem disorder characterized by noncaseating, granulomatous inflammation. It is most commonly seen in women between the ages of 20 and 50 years and more often affects individuals of African and Scandinavian decent. In systemic sarcoidosis, 90–95% of patients have lung involvement, 50% have thoracic/hilar lymph node enlargement, 30% have skin lesions, and 25–50% have associated ophthalmic manifestations.

In the anterior segment of the eye, sarcoidosis may cause acute or chronic iritis with large keratoprecipitates on the endothelial surface of the cornea (see Fig. 27.4). In the posterior segment, it may manifest as vitritis, vasculitis, granulomatous choroiditis, and/or optic nerve infiltration. Patchy venous sheathing and cellular infiltrates around retinal vessels are classic findings.

Orbital involvement is less common than intraocular involvement, and only about a quarter of those with intraocular involvement have concurrent orbital disease. In the orbit, the lacrimal glands (dacryoadenitis) are most commonly affected, with bilateral involvement more common than unilateral. Symptoms may range from acute, painful orbital swelling to chronic, painless lacrimal gland enlargement. In addition to lacrimal gland involvement, inflammation may affect the extraocular muscles (myositis) and sclera (scleritis) or may present as a solitary, often palpable anterior orbital mass. Cases with extra-lacrimal gland involvement are almost

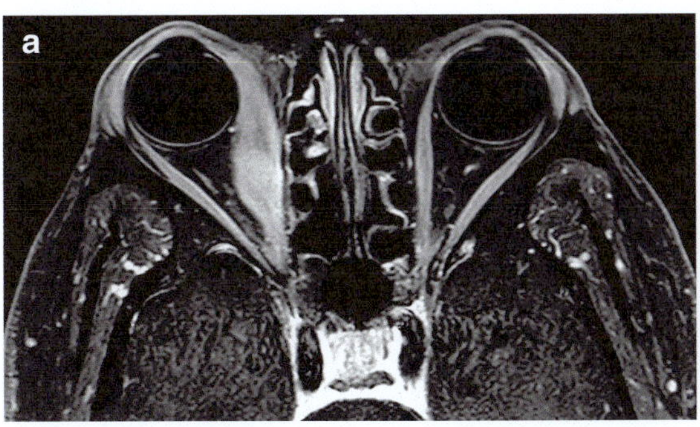

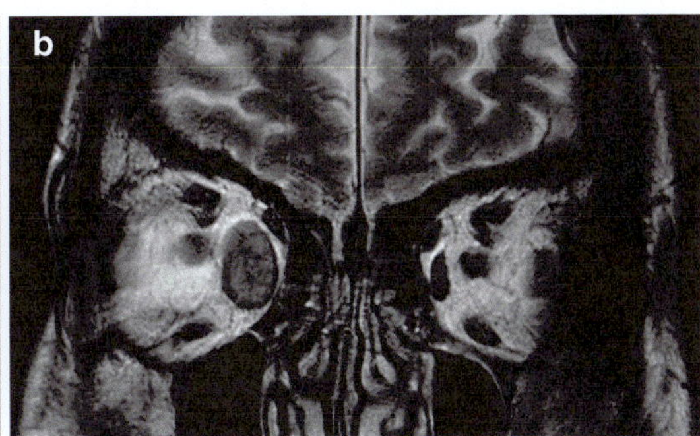

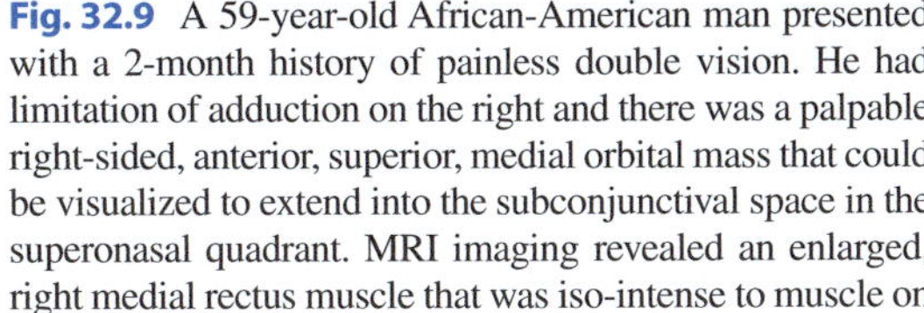

Fig. 32.9 A 59-year-old African-American man presented with a 2-month history of painless double vision. He had limitation of adduction on the right and there was a palpable right-sided, anterior, superior, medial orbital mass that could be visualized to extend into the subconjunctival space in the superonasal quadrant. MRI imaging revealed an enlarged, right medial rectus muscle that was iso-intense to muscle on T1 (**a**), minimally hyperintense on T2 (**b**), and only very modestly contrast enhancing. The lesion involved the tendon of the medial rectus muscle (**a**). Biopsy revealed non-necrotizing granulomatous inflammation. Systemic work-up for sarcoidosis was otherwise unremarkable. A diagnosis of orbital sarcoidosis was made, and the patient responded well to an oral prednisone taper without recurrence for 12 months

always unilateral. When there is orbital disease but without any evidence of systemic involvement, this is termed "orbital sarcoidosis" (Fig. 32.9).

The differential diagnosis includes lymphoma, metastasis, sclerosing orbital inflammation, and IgG4-related disease. The history should include racial/ethnic background, constitutional symptoms, cancer history, ocular history, and respiratory symptoms. A family history of autoimmune disease may be present.

The serologic workup for sarcoid is often unremarkable. Laboratory testing may include a serum angiotensin-converting enzyme (ACE). ACE is produced by the epithelial cells surrounding the inflammatory granulomas associated with the disease. ACE may be elevated in 60–90% of patients with active sarcoidosis. However, there are a number of non-sarcoid conditions, including diabetes mellitus, osteoarthritis, and hyperthyroidism, as well as other orbital conditions such as orbital lymphoma and idiopathic orbital inflammation, in which ACE levels may be elevated. Because of this, the utility of serum ACE levels has been called into question for making the diagnosis of orbital sarcoid. That said, it can be helpful creating a complete picture when used alongside of the clinical history, imaging, and histopathology. The differential diagnosis can also include syphilis, histoplasmosis, leprosy, and atypical fungal infections.

Additional testing with pulmonary function tests, chest X-ray, and gallium scan may be helpful in confirming systemic sarcoidosis. Chest X-ray or CT may demonstrate hilar infiltrates when there is systemic involvement.

Biopsy is critical for confirming the diagnosis and should be attempted when possible. Lacrimal gland is often involved and should be included in the sample as well as any obviously suspicious areas of conjunctiva – random conjunctival biopsies typically have minimal yield. Histopathology demonstrates noncaseating granulomas.

Treatment begins with oral steroids on a very slow taper. Recurrences may occur and require treatment with steroid-sparing immunosuppressive agents such as methotrexate, azathioprine, leflunomide, or tumor necrosis factor-alpha inhibitors.

Granulomatosis with Polyangiitis (Wegener's Granulomatosis)

Granulomatosis with polyangiitis (GPA) is a necrotizing granulomatous vasculitis which may affect any organ system. While GPA most frequently affects older individuals, the disease may occur at any age. It is found equally in men and women and is most commonly seen in Caucasian individuals. The systemic form of the disease manifests as sinus involvement with bony erosion, necrotic lesions of the respiratory tract, glomerulonephritis, and small vessel necrotizing vasculitis. The orbit and lacrimal outflow system may become involved by direct extension from the paranasal sinuses. Patients may also present with scleritis, corneal ulceration, uveitis, retinal vasculitis, and optic neuropathy.

Extraocular symptoms include fatigue, fever, weight loss, arthralgias, rhinosinusitis, cough, shortness of breath, and urinary dysfunction. Pain, diplopia, and vision loss are typical ocular symptoms. Examination may reveal proptosis, extraocular dysmotility, nasolacrimal duct obstruction, and ocular inflammation. While CT imaging will reveal bony erosion of the sinuses and nose, MRI may be more helpful in the diagnosis as the fibrosclerotic inflammation will be hypointense on T2-weighted imaging, in contrast to T2-hyperintensity typically seen in active inflammation. Antineutrophil cytoplasmic antibodies (ANCAs) are positive in up to 96% of patients with systemic involvement; its positivity, coupled with prototypical clinical findings, may be enough to confirm a diagnosis. While tissue confirmation is preferred, treatment should not be held back in cases where a biopsy cannot be performed in a safe and timely manner. Histopathologic examination of involved tissues reveals granulomatous inflammation involving small- and medium-sized arterioles, necrosis, and fibrosis.

Limited GPA, without respiratory or renal involvement, may manifest as isolated orbital inflammation which is more often unilateral than bilateral. These cases may be more difficult to diagnose as ANCAs may be negative in one-third of cases and biopsy may lack evidence of vasculitis or necrotizing granulomas. The differential diagnosis of limited orbital GPA includes cocaine-associated orbitopathy, sclerosing orbital inflammation, nonspecific orbital inflammation, sarcoidosis, histiocytosis, and metastasis.

Untreated systemic GPA has up to a 90% 2-year mortality. Treatment in the acute setting is critical and consists of corticosteroids combined with cyclophosphamide or rituximab. Management of GPA involving the eye or orbit is best done with a multidisciplinary team consisting of ophthalmologist, rheumatologist, nephrologist, pulmonologist, and otolaryngologist.

Cocaine-Related Orbital Inflammation

Long-term intranasal cocaine use can lead to chronic, sclerosing orbital inflammation. Findings often include limitation of abduction due to spread of inflammation beyond the sinuses into the medial orbit. Concurrent optic neuropathy has also been reported. Imaging may reveal loss of the nasal septum, destruction of the sinuses, and loss of portions of the medial orbital wall. The differential diagnosis includes malignancy and granulomatosis with polyangiitis. Biopsy reveals chronic inflammation without granulomas or vasculitis. Inflammation typically responds to oral steroids, although muscle restriction and optic neuropathy may not reverse. Rituximab has been used with success in refractory cases or in patients with steroid intolerance (Fig. 32.10).

Bisphosphonate-Induced Orbital Inflammation

Bisphosphonates are a class of medication used to treat osteoporosis, osteolytic bone tumors, skeletal metastatic disease, and Paget's disease. A handful of cases in the literature have now cited bisphosphonates, especially the aminobisphosphonates, such as pamidronate, alendronate, and zoledronate, as a rare cause of acute orbital inflammation. Most cases have been associated with intravenous infusions of zoledronate, marketed as Zometa and Reclast. The orbital inflammation is of acute onset and may present with diffuse involvement or as myositis. Inflammation responds rapidly to steroids. Although patients typically have no long-term sequelae, there have been cases reported of permanent vision loss due to an associated ischemic optic neuropathy.

Sickle Cell Orbitopathy

Patients in sickle cell crisis may develop infarcts of the greater wing of the sphenoid bone causing acute inflammation, orbital compartment syndrome, and hemorrhagic and exudative subperiosteal collections along the lateral orbital wall. Clinically, this manifests as pain, proptosis, extraocular dysmotility, chemosis, and frequently compressive optic neuropathy. The patients are often children or young adults. The presentation can mimic that of orbital cellulitis. MR imaging

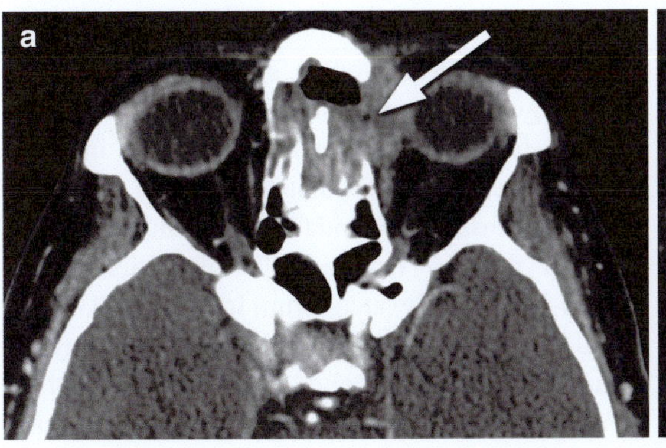 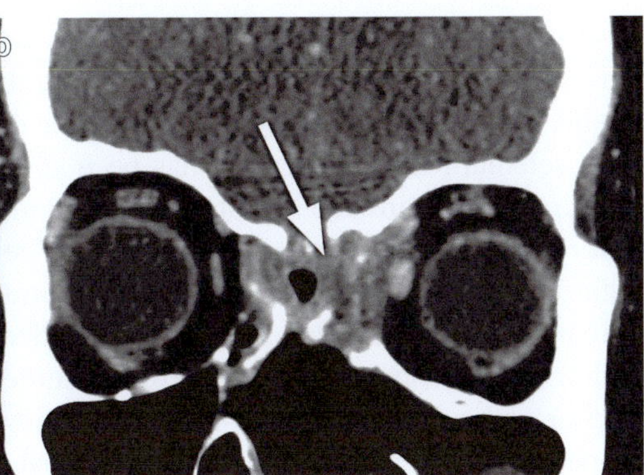

Fig. 32.10 (**a**, **b**) A 53-year-old woman with a history of cocaine use presented with 2 weeks of double vision. The patient had significant limitation of abduction and upgaze on the left. She reported 12 months of epistaxis and symptoms of chronic sinusitis. MRI 8 months prior showed chronic inflammation in the left ethmoid sinuses and loss of the nasal septum. CT imaging at presentation revealed an ill-defined mass extending from the ethmoid sinuses into the medial orbit, eroding the medial orbital wall, and involving the medial rectus muscle (white arrows). ANCAs and the remainder of the rheumatologic workup were negative. Biopsy revealed tissue infiltrated by a polymorphous infiltrate composed predominantly of lymphocytes, histiocytes, and plasma cells. No well-formed granuloma or necrotizing granuloma was appreciated. There were few perivascular lymphoid aggregates, but no true vasculitis or ischemic necrosis. The patient could not tolerate corticosteroids due to psychosis and eventually responded well to rituximab

reveals infarction of the greater wing of the sphenoid and an absence of sinusitis. Patients typically respond well to intravenous corticosteroids. Treatment should be started rapidly in cases of optic nerve dysfunction. If cellulitis cannot be ruled out, treatment should include intravenous antibiotics along with corticosteroids.

Thyroid Eye Disease

Far and away the most common orbital inflammatory condition is thyroid eye disease (TED) also known as Graves' ophthalmopathy (see Chap. 29). As an entire chapter of this book is devoted to this condition, its inclusion here will be brief. Six times more common in women than men, TED usually presents with bilateral, often asymmetric, subacute-to-chronic-onset orbital inflammation. Eyelid retraction, proptosis, and restricted eye movements are commonly found. The orbit may demonstrate varying amounts of inflammatory signs such as eyelid edema and redness, conjunctival chemosis and injection, and caruncular edema. Patients may complain of a dull retro-ocular ache, especially with eye movements. In severe cases, enlarged extraocular muscles and hypertrophied orbital fat can cause a compressive optic neuropathy, leading to vision loss if not addressed early. In addition, eyelid retraction and lid lag can lead to severe exposure keratitis which may also require urgent intervention. Orbital imaging typically reveals enlargement of the extraocular muscle bodies, sparing the tendons, with the medial and inferior recti being most involved, as well as an increase in orbital fat.

Patients with TED may have an established diagnosis of hyper- or, less commonly, hypothyroidism. Frequently, patients have the simultaneous onset of TED and a dysthyroid state, although in some cases orbital inflammation may precede any thyroid abnormality. Often patients will have abnormal thyroid function tests as well as elevated thyroid-related antibodies, especially thyroid-stimulating immunoglobulin (TSI). Smoking can greatly exacerbate the severity of TED and should be avoided by all with TED. Hyper- and hypothyroid states (as compared with the euthyroid state) have been shown to be associated with worsening TED and should be addressed by the patient's endocrinologist.

The active phase of TED is self-limited, usually ranging from 12 to 24 months, with longer durations reported among smokers. Many clinicians believe that the amount of inflammation during this active phase directly influences the severity of the disease. Because of this, most strive to drive the inflammation down during this period. In patients with mild-moderate, active disease, selenium supplementation has been shown to decrease the signs and symptoms of inflammation. In addition, topical ocular lubricants help with dry eye symptoms related to eyelid retraction, proptosis, and resultant exposure. In patients with more inflammation, corticosteroid treatment with or without orbital radiation has been shown to decrease inflammation and may ultimately reduce long-term morbidity. Kazim and colleagues found that external beam radiation with concurrent corticosteroids was associated with a sixfold reduction in the need for subsequent orbital decompression surgery versus steroids alone. More recently a number of biologic agents have shown promise in reducing inflammation associated with steroid-refractive TED, including rituximab, an anti-CD20 monoclonal antibody; tocilizumab, an IL-6 receptor antibody; and teprotumumab, an anti-IGF-1 receptor antibody.

Surgery for TED often consists of orbital decompression, followed by strabismus surgery and ultimately eyelid retraction repair. Not all patients will require rehabilitative surgery and not every patient who undergoes surgery requires all three types. When possible, surgical interventions are delayed until the active, inflammatory phase has completed and the condition is said to enter the quiescent phase. On occasion, usually due to vision-threatening compressive optic neuropathy or severe exposure keratitis, surgery is performed more urgently.

TED should be managed by an orbital surgeon and endocrinologist. At times, the clinical team will include a rheumatologist when considering biologic and chemotherapeutic agents to decrease inflammation, a radiation oncologist to administer orbital radiation, and a thyroid surgeon when thyroidectomy is indicated. Close communication by all members of the team is critical for optimal outcomes.

IgG4-Related Orbital Inflammation

IgG4-related disease (IgG4-RD) is a relatively newly recognized clinical entity of chronic tumor-like inflammation and fibrosis which may be present in a number of organ systems including the orbit. IgG4-RD lesions share a common histopathologic feature of a lymphoplasmacytic infiltrate with an enriched population (>40%) of IgG4-positive plasma cells and fibrosis arranged in a storiform pattern. Up to 60% of patients with IgG4-RD have elevated serum IgG4 as well. While IgG4-RD was first recognized in autoimmune pancreatitis, the number of organ systems in which this type of inflammation is recognized continues to increase. It is estimated that 5–20% of orbital inflammatory cases are IgG4-RD. Retrospective histopathologic reviews have determined that up to 50% of cases previously diagnosed as orbital lymphoid hyperplasia, 50% of previously diagnosed sclerosing orbital inflammation, and 24% of cases previously diagnosed as nonspecific orbital inflammation (NSOI) would be reclassified as IgG4-related orbital disease (IgG4-ROD). It is now believed that the majority of cases of Mikulicz's disease (lacrimal, parotid, and submandibular gland enlargement) and retroperitoneal fibrosis syndrome (frequently causing periaortitis and hydronephrosis) are, in fact, IgG4-RD.

In the orbit, the most common site of inflammation is the lacrimal gland, followed by trigeminal nerve (often seen radiographically as enlargement of the infraorbital nerve/canal), extraocular muscles, orbital fat, eyelid, nasolacrimal duct, and sclera. Bilateral orbital involvement is most common.

Although IgG4-RD predominantly affects older males, most studies of IgG4-ROD have a somewhat younger age (average 55 years) and no sex predilection. Patients with IgG4-ROD do have a higher risk of developing subsequent lymphomas. The etiology of the condition is unclear but thought to be related to immune dysfunction. A large number of patients have a prior history of asthma and allergy.

A consensus agreement on the histopathologic features required to make the diagnosis of IgG4-RD has been difficult to reach. However, most use the convention of >40% positive IgG4 plasma cells with >10 IgG4+ cells/high power field.

Cases of IgG4-ROD should be managed by a multidisciplinary team including an ophthalmologist and rheumatologist. Liver and kidney function tests are critical as IgG4-RD lesions can silently encase organs and cause dysfunction. Imaging of the chest, abdomen, and pelvis with MRI with contrast can detect lesions in these regions. More recently, fluorodeoxyglucose (FDG) PET/CT has been found to be helpful in detecting extraorbital disease and in determining response to therapy.

Most IgG4-RD responds well to corticosteroids, in contrast to sclerosing orbital inflammation, which typically requires chemotherapeutic or biologic agents to halt progression. In cases of recurrent or resistant disease, biologic agents such as rituximab have been shown to be useful.

Suggested Reading

Amrith S, Hosdurga Pai V, Ling WW. Periorbital necrotizing fasciitis – a review. Acta Ophthalmol. 2013;91(7):596–603.

Dagi Glass LR, Freitag SK. Orbital inflammation: corticosteroids first. Surv Ophthalmol. 2016;61(5):670–3.

Derzko-Dzulynsky L. IgG4-related disease in the eye and ocular adnexa. Curr Opin Ophthalmol. 2017;28(6):617–22.

Kalin-Hajdu E, Hirabayashi KE, Vagefi MR, Kersten RC. Invasive fungal sinusitis: treatment of the orbit. Curr Opin Ophthalmol. 2017;28(5):522–33.

Mombaerts I, Rose GE, Garrity JA. Orbital inflammation: biopsy first. Surv Ophthalmol. 2016;61(5):664–9.

Pirbhai A, Rajak SN, Goold LA, Cunneen TS, Wilcsek G, Martin P, Leibovitch I, Selva D. Bisphosphonate-induced orbital inflammation: a case series and review. Orbit. 2015;34(6):331–5.

Siemerink MJ, Freling NJM, Saeed P. Chronic orbital inflammatory disease and optic neuropathy associated with long-term intranasal cocaine abuse: 2 cases and literature review. Orbit. 2017;36(5):350–5.

Smith A, Thimmappa V, Shepherd B, Ray M, Sheyn A, Thompson J. Invasive fungal sinusitis in the pediatric population: systematic review with quantitative synthesis of the literature. Int J Pediatr Otorhinolaryngol. 2016;90:231–5.

Sokol JA, Baron E, Lantos G, Kazim M. Orbital compression syndrome in sickle cell disease. Ophthal Plast Reconstr Surg. 2008;24(3):181–4.

33

Kristen E. Dunbar and Michael Kazim

The orbit is the bony compartment that contains the eye and its surrounding structures. In addition to the eye, it is comprised of densely packed fat, muscle, blood vessels, lacrimal tissue, and nerves. As with other parts of the body, a genetic defect or overgrowth of any of these tissues can create a space-occupying malformation or lesion. These lesions can affect the health of the eye, and depending on the size, location, and rate of growth, orbital masses may cause deterioration in visual acuity, proptosis, alterations in appearance, ptosis, and restriction of extraocular movements, with or without diplopia. If malignant, orbital tumors can metastasize and ultimately be fatal. It is important to perform a comprehensive ophthalmic examination for correct detection, diagnosis, and early treatment of orbital lesions.

Orbital Examination

Any orbital exam includes a complete history and physical examination. Important screening questions for orbital lesions include changes in appearance, globe displacement, the presence of

double vision, and duration and progression of symptoms. The presence of pain, changes in overlying skin, the rate of growth, and the age of occurrence are other questions that can give clues to whether a lesion might be malignant or benign.

It is often helpful to ask for an old photograph to detect subtle changes that might have otherwise gone unnoticed by the patient and their family. An abrupt change in refractive error (i.e., hyperopia) can be a sign of axial compression causing a shift in the focal point. A history of medical conditions such as cancer, previous orbital disease, radiation, or trauma can also provide clues for diagnosis.

Every ophthalmologic examination begins with visual acuity, intraocular pressure, extraocular movements, pupillary examination, and confrontational visual field examination. These ophthalmic vital signs are also helpful in orbital examination. Additional useful testing includes periocular palpation, resistance to retropulsion, Hertel exophthalmometry (Fig. 33.1), and Valsalva testing.

It is important with any orbital lesion to rule out a compressive optic neuropathy. The presence or absence of optic neuropathy can significantly change management of a lesion. Specialized types of visual field examination (including Humphrey and Goldmann visual fields; see Chap. 18) can help pick up small field defects that might not be detectable on confrontational visual fields. Color vision testing with Ishihara or Hardy-Rand-Rittler (HRR) plates

K. E. Dunbar, MD (✉)
Department of Ophthalmology, New York University
Langone Medical Center, New York, NY, USA

M. Kazim, MD
Edward S. Harkness Eye Institute, Columbia
University Vagelos College of Physicians
and Surgeons, New York, NY, USA

© Springer Nature Switzerland AG 2019
D. S. Casper, G. A. Cioffi (eds.), *The Columbia Guide to Basic Elements of Eye Care*,
https://doi.org/10.1007/978-3-030-10886-1_33

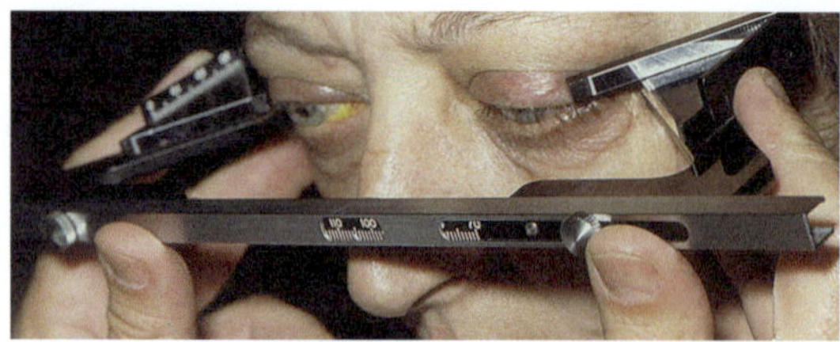

Fig. 33.1 Exophthalmometer

may also aid in documenting and diagnosing the degree of optic neuropathy. Optical coherence tomography (OCT) can help diagnose more subtle swelling of the optic nerve or longstanding optic nerve atrophy from optic nerve compression that may be missed on a dilated fundus exam. After evaluation of the above testing, the appropriate type(s) of imaging (i.e., ultrasound, MRI, MRA, MRV, or CT with or without contrast) can be ordered.

Common Pediatric Tumors of the Orbit

Benign Orbital Masses

Dermoid Cyst

Dermoid cysts are a type of choristoma characterized by normal tissue(s) found at an abnormal site. They are commonly found in children and considered to be benign cystic lesions. Although they are considered a congenital malformation, dermoids characteristically enlarge slowly and symmetrically leading to their ultimate discovery months to years after birth. Their cysts are lined by keratinized epithelium with dermal appendages including sweat glands, fat, hair, bone, or even teeth.

On examination, dermoid cysts are typically smooth, rubbery in texture, and round. Their most common location is the frontozygomatic suture at the temporal part of the brow. Some dermoids, however, can extend posteriorly through the suture in a dumbbell-type fashion into the orbit (Fig. 33.2). When an external dermoid is identified in this location, CT scan is commonly performed to rule out this posterior growth pattern to assist in surgical planning.

Imaging characteristically shows a circumscribed lesion that is cystic in appearance. Internal fat attenuation and calcification are common. Depending on the age of the child, bony remodeling can also be seen around the lesion.

Given the proximity to the brow, dermoid cysts are most commonly treated with complete excision through an incision within the lid crease. Care must be taken to remove the entire lesion in one piece without rupture: violation of the capsule can result in release of keratin and oil tissue into the surrounding tissue, thereby inciting an inflammatory reaction.

Capillary Hemangioma

Capillary hemangiomas are the most common type of benign orbital neoplasm. They result from an abnormal proliferation of endothelial cells. As seen in Fig. 33.3, they are often identified by parents or practitioners as a soft, reddish, or deeper bluish, non-tender lesion just beneath the skin. Slow and progressive enlargement in size is often noted over the first year; however, after that time, many spontaneously involute, with 75% completely resolving after 4–5 years.

Risk factors for capillary hemangiomas include prenatal chorionic villus sampling and premature birth. While diagnosis can only be confirmed histopathologically, the clinical appearance, behavior, and MRI features make biopsy unnecessary in most cases. Findings on MRI include fine intralesional vascular channels with high blood flow.

Although most lesions resolve on their own, some can cause permanent ophthalmologic issues if not treated. Those that put pressure directly on the globe can cause astigmatism or ptosis, which often results in visual obscuration, which places a child at risk for development of amblyopia if not treated in an expeditious manner. Lesions around the neck that can lead to airway obstruction would be another indication for treatment.

The mainstay of treatment for symptomatic capillary hemangioma is oral propranolol. Alternate treatment options include injection of

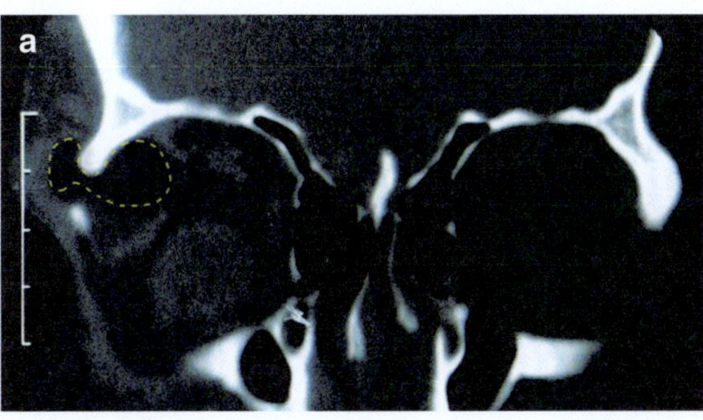 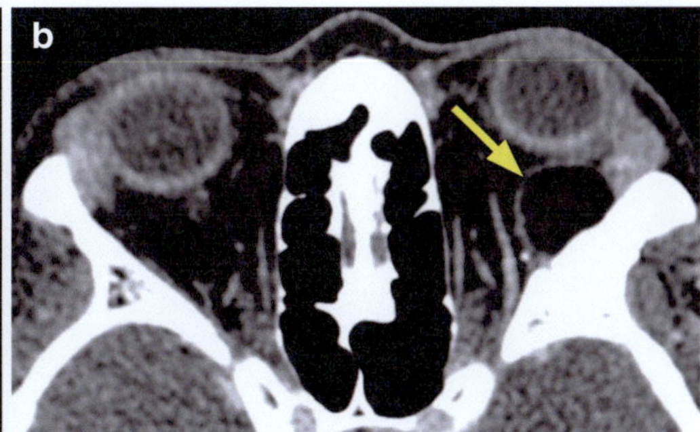

Fig. 33.2 (**a**) Coronal CT scan of a "dumbbell" dermoid piercing the lateral orbital wall, outlined in dashed yellow. (**b**) CT scan of a 22 × 18 mm encapsulated dermoid (yellow arrow) along the left lateral wall of the orbit

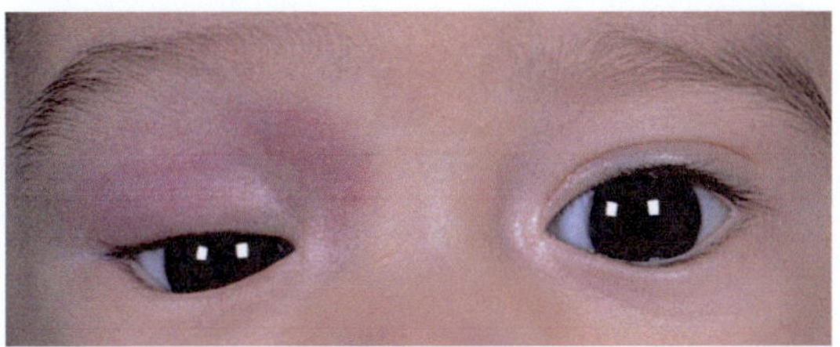

Fig. 33.3 A 4-month-old boy with capillary hemangioma on the right upper eyelid

steroids and or B-blockers, topical timolol gel, excision, or pulsed dye laser, depending on the particular clinical features.

Kasabach-Merritt syndrome is associated with multiple capillary hemangiomas. In these patients, lesions trap platelets which can lead to a life-threatening thrombocytopenia. Patients with multiple large lesions, hepatomegaly, or other unexplained symptoms need baseline blood testing and further evaluation with a specialist.

Lymphatic Malformations/ Lymphangioma (Combined Venous Lymphatic Malformations)

Lymphatic malformations, previously known as lymphangiomas, are hemodynamically isolated lesions comprising approximately 1–3% of orbital tumors. They are classified as a congenital malformation and typically present at a young age.

As with other orbital lesions, lymphatic malformations can present with ptosis, restriction of extraocular movements, and decreased vision.

More unique to these lesions is sudden proptosis caused by an acute bleed into their cyst-like cavities. Acute bleeds are characteristically associated with pain and, if superficial, can give the skin a bluish appearance. Respiratory infections have been associated with a usually transient increase in lesion size.

CT imaging of a lymphatic malformation is consistent with other cystic masses. MRI shows "grapelike" blood-filled cystic lesions which demonstrate fluid layering after an acute hemorrhage.

Treatment depends on the location, extent of the lesion, and presence of compressive optic neuropathy. A complete excision with surgery can be difficult given its infiltrative nature and lesions often recur after excision. Initial injection with an intralesional sclerosing agent or needle drainage of lesions can be employed therapeutically.

Optic Nerve Glioma

Optic nerve gliomas are benign, slow-growing tumors primarily found in children. Approximately one third of these tumors are associated with neurofibromatosis type 1 (von Recklinghausen disease). Presentation is typically in the first decade of life with gradual, painless ipsilateral proptosis. Depending on the size of the lesion, there may be associated decreased vision, an afferent pupillary defect, and optic nerve swelling or pallor.

On CT and MRI imaging, optic nerve gliomas classically present as a "fusiform enlargement"

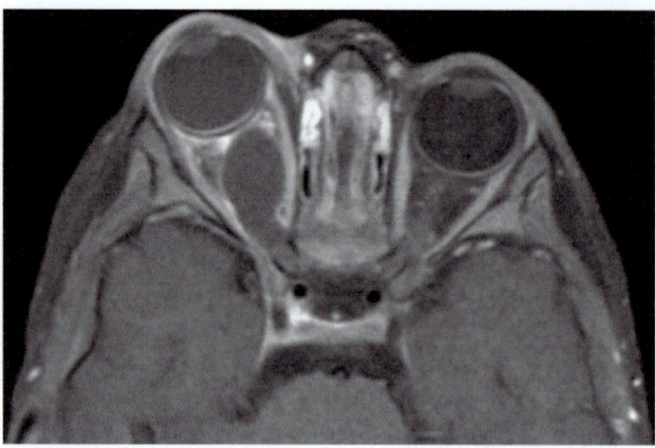

Fig. 33.4 MRI T1 axial image with fat suppression shows hypointensity with fusiform enlargement of the optic nerve

of the optic nerve (Fig. 33.4). These lesions can be unilateral or bilateral, with or without chiasmal involvement.

Better outcomes are associated with unilaterality, association with neurofibromatosis type 1, prechiasmal lesions, and lack of other ocular findings (i.e., optic nerve atrophy or visual field deficits). The treatment protocol typically depends on the degree of optic nerve damage present at the time of evaluation. Those without vision changes can be observed; however, in the case of rapid growth or advanced optic nerve damage, surgical excision is often preformed. Radiation and chemotherapy have also been shown to be effective for those that cannot be completely resected.

Glioblastomas are the malignant counterpart of optic nerve gliomas. They are more commonly found in older adults and appear more commonly in males. They classically present with retro-orbital pain and optic nerve head edema and hemorrhage. These highly malignant lesions are treated with high-dose radiation and chemotherapy. Unfortunately, despite aggressive treatment, most patients die within 6–12 months of diagnosis.

Malignant Lesions

Rhabdomyosarcoma

Rhabdomyosarcoma is the most common soft tissue orbital malignancy in children. It is a particularly aggressive lesion with poorly defined margins and frequent invasion of adjacent structures including bone, sinuses, and soft tissues. Metastases to lungs, bone, and neck are common.

Rhabdomyosarcoma commonly presents in the first decade of life with an average age of presentation of 6–8 years. There are four subtypes of rhabdomyosarcoma each of which distinctly affects prognosis and treatment. *Embryonal* is the most common subtype and is typically found in the superonasal orbit. *Alveolar* rhabdomyosarcoma, which is usually found in older patients, is uncommon; however, it carries the worst prognosis. The *pleomorphic* subtype has the best prognosis with a mean survival rate of 97%. Finally, the *botryoid* subtype is a variant of embryonal that originates in the sinuses or conjunctiva and subsequently invades the orbit.

Symptoms of rhabdomyosarcoma include chemosis, proptosis, downward and outward globe displacement (Fig. 33.5a), darkening of the eyelid skin, strabismus, and ptosis. Biopsy is required to confirm the diagnosis, suspected based on imaging studies. CT often shows a well-circumscribed mass with bony erosion or invasion of the sinuses (Fig. 33.5b). MRI is useful to rule out intracranial extension.

Treatment is determined based on the extent of the lesion. Most often an incisional or excisional biopsy is performed, accompanied by radiation and chemotherapy. Chest imaging, bone marrow biopsy, and lumbar puncture are also recommended to check for metastatic spread.

Metastatic Lesions

When evaluating an orbital lesion, one must always be cognizant of the possibility that this is not the primary site of the tumor. The most common orbital metastases in children are neuroblastoma, leukemia, and Ewing's sarcoma. Less commonly Wilms' tumor and other types of sarcoma have been reported in the orbit as well. In these cases, it is important to determine the extent of the systemic disease and establish a treatment plan accordingly.

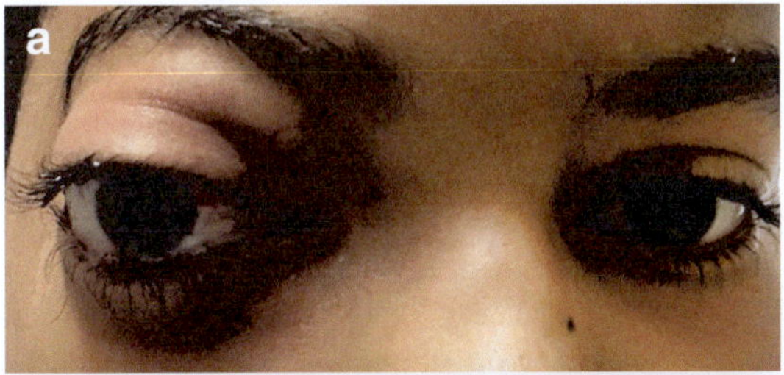

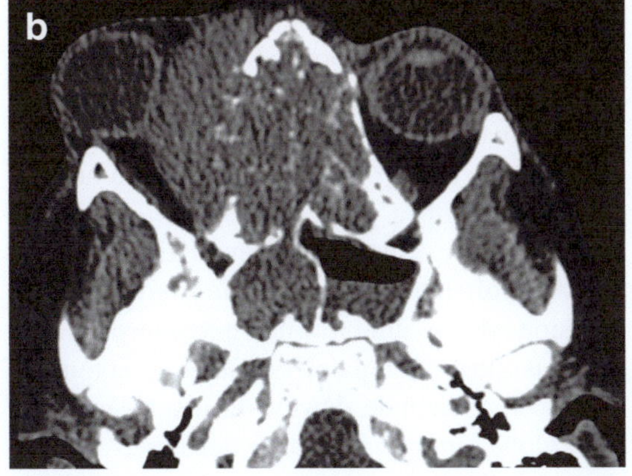

Fig. 33.5 (a) A 12-year-old with right eye pain, diminished eye movements, diplopia, proptosis, and downward displacement of the globe. Biopsy was positive for rhabdomyosarcoma, alveolar type. (b) Axial CT scan shows a rhabdomyosarcoma, alveolar type centered in the ethmoid sinuses with extensive bony destruction of the right orbital floor, paranasal sinuses, and right nasolacrimal duct

Common Adult Tumors of the Orbit

Benign Orbital Masses

Cavernous Hemangiomas

Cavernous hemangiomas are the most common benign lesion found in the adult orbit, comprising approximately 10% of all orbital tumors (Fig. 33.6a, b). Often, they present with progressive, painless proptosis, diplopia, or decreased vision in the second through fourth decades of life. There is a female preponderance in the literature. Interestingly, the size of the lesions has been association with fluctuation of hormone levels (e.g., increased tumor size during pregnancy).

The lesion is comprised of a collection of blood vessels surrounded by a fibrous pseudocapsule. MRI demonstrates an enhancing signal

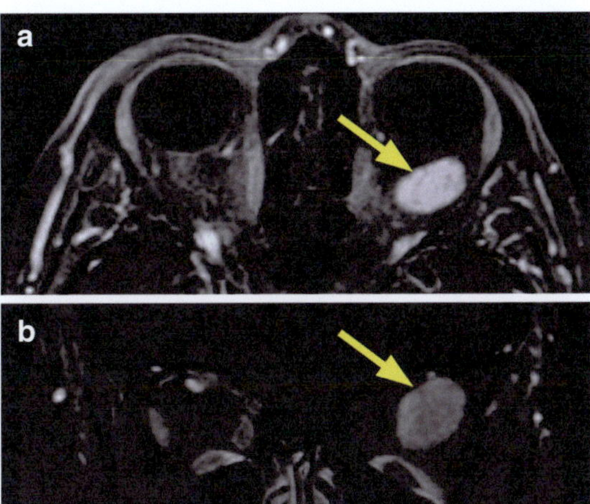

Fig. 33.6 Axial (a) and coronal (b) images of a cavernous hemangioma (yellow arrows) in a 42-year old woman who noticed blurring and diplopia on left lateral gaze

with slow flow of blood through microchannels. Depending on the location of the lesion and degree of symptoms, surgical excision and observation are the primary treatment options.

Neurofibromas

Neurofibromas are soft, encapsulated lesions comprised of Schwann cells. Plexiform neurofibromas, the most common subtype of neurofibromas, are associated with neurofibromatosis type 1. These lesions typically present in the lateral eyelid resulting in an S-shaped contour. They are commonly described as resembling "a bag of worms" on palpation. Treatment typically involves surgical excision; however, sometimes the extensive vascularization and infiltration can make complete excision without recurrence difficult.

Meningiomas

Meningiomas arise from the cap cells of arachnoid villi. They can arise intracranially from the optic nerve or de novo from orbital soft tissues. Presentation can vary depending on their origin. For example, lesions arising from the optic nerve sheath often present with unilateral decreased vision and optic nerve edema or atrophy. Those affecting the sphenoid are more likely to be associated with proptosis or non-axial displacement (Fig. 33.7).

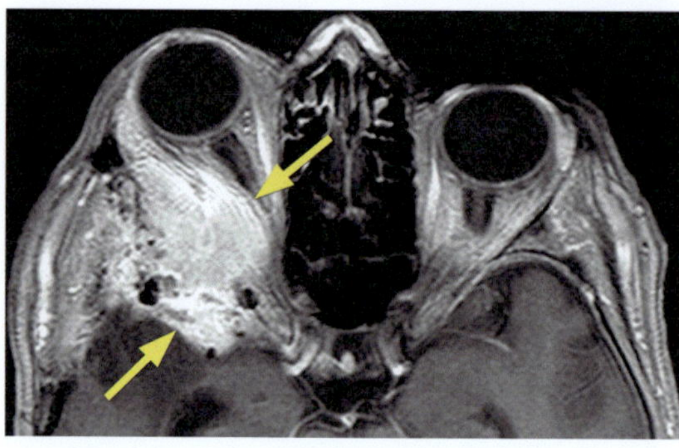

Fig. 33.7 Axial CT of large sphenoid wing meningioma, producing proptosis and optic nerve compression

As with many lesions, treatment varies based on the location, symptoms, and degree of optic nerve compromise. Optic nerve meningiomas are observed for progressive optic nerve dysfunction, at which time treatment with orbital radiotherapy has been shown to stabilize vision, as opposed to surgical intervention, which more commonly leads to vision loss. In the case of sphenoid wing meningiomas invading the orbit and producing compressive optic neuropathy, surgical debulking through a transcranial approach, followed, in selected cases, by orbital radiotherapy, is preferred.

Malignant Orbital Masses

Pleomorphic Adenoma

Pleomorphic adenomas (also referred to as benign mixed tumors) are tumors of the lacrimal gland. They are typically slow growing and most commonly present with painless, unilateral proptosis and downward and inward displacement of the globe. On exam, resistance to retropulsion and the palpation of an enlarged, mobile mass just under the orbital rim are common findings.

CT imaging shows diffuse enlargement of the lacrimal gland and expansion of the lacrimal bony fossa. MR imaging often shows a nodular well-demarcated mass with moderate enhancement.

Complete excision is the treatment of choice; if the lesion is not completely excised, there is potential for recurrence or malignant transformation.

The rate of malignant transformation is approximately 10% in the first 20 years and 20% by 30 years.

Adenoid Cystic Carcinoma

It is important to differentiate pleomorphic adenoma from adenoid cystic carcinoma (ACC) as the treatment and prognosis is very different. ACC is the most common malignant epithelial tumor of the lacrimal gland. The mean age of presentation is older than that typically seen with pleomorphic adenomas, with a peak incidence in the fourth decade of life. Another differentiating factor is that ACC often presents with pain from perineural invasion of the tumor, while pleomorphic adenoma is most often painless. Other symptoms of both lesions include downward displacement of the globe, proptosis, and decreased vision. Adenoid cystic carcinomas have a much more rapid growth phase than pleomorphic adenomas and consequently have a much worse prognosis.

Since this tumor lacks a capsule, it can easily extend deep into the posterior orbit. On MRI imaging, perineural invasion is commonly noted. Lesions are often hypointense on T1 imaging and slightly hyperintense on T2.

Treatment is controversial. Surgical excision with clear margins and adjunctive conventional stereotactic radiotherapy is most commonly employed, with chemotherapy used for metastases. Alternative treatment includes intra-arterial chemotherapy followed by orbital exenteration and proton beam radiation. Despite aggressive treatment, the prognosis is poor, with the majority of patients expiring by 15 years of age.

Orbital Metastases

Unlike children, where distant tumors more commonly metastasize to the orbit, tumors in adults more often metastasize to the choroid. While any cancer can potentially metastasize to the orbit, adult carcinomas have an increased incidence of metastases over sarcomas. The opposite is true in childhood metastases. The most common metastatic orbital lesions in adults are prostate, breast, and lung carcinomas.

Breast carcinoma is the most common metastasis in women. While most breast metastases cause proptosis, bony destruction, and pain, scirrhous breast cancer can cause enophthalmos, which is an uncommon presenting sign in orbital lesions. Prostate cancer is the most common metastatic lesion in men. It typically produces lytic bone lesions. Treatment is either systemic chemo/hormonal therapy or radiotherapy.

Conclusion

A wide variety of tumors can present in the orbit. Treatment varies based on the type of lesion, current (or potential for) visual compromise, and cosmetic deformity. It is important for every patient to receive a complete ophthalmologic examination and appropriate imaging or biopsy in order to determine proper management.

Suggested Reading

Chung E, Smirniotopoulos J, Specht C, Schroeder J, Cube R. Pediatric orbit tumors and tumorlike lesions: nonosseous lesions of the extraocular orbit. Radiographics. 2007;27(6):1777–99.

Lai T, Prabhakaran VC, Malhotra R, Selva D. Pleomorphic adenoma of the lacrimal gland: is there a role for biopsy? Eye (Lond). 2009;23(1):2–6.

Nguyen J, Fay A. Pharmacologic therapy for periocular infantile hemangiomas: a review of the literature. Semin Ophthalmol. 2009;24:178–84.

Orbit, eyelids and lacrimal system, section 7. Basic and clinical science course, AAO, 2011–2012.

Robert-Boire V, Rosca L, Samson Y, Ospina LH, Perreault S. Clinical presentation and outcome of patients with optic pathway glioma. Pediatr Neurol. 2017;75:55–60.

Rootman J. Diseases of the orbit. A multidisciplinary approach. 2nd ed. Philadelphia: Lippincott; 2003.

Tang D, Zhao H, Song G. A follow-up survey of lacrimal gland surgery of pleomorphic adenoma. Chin J Ophthalmol. 1997;33:354–6.

Wasserman BN, Medow NB, Homa-Palladino M, Hoehn ME. Treatment of periocular capillary hemangiomas. J AAPOS. 2004;8:175–81.

Orbital Trauma

34

Peter Michalos

Orbital trauma may cause significant vision impairment, deformity, and collateral ocular and tear duct dysfunction. Typical sources of orbital trauma include falls, sports-related injuries, motor vehicle accidents, industrial accidents, interpersonal altercations, and other forms of assault. Orbital trauma is often accompanied by injury to the eye itself, in addition to adnexal structures such as the lids and tear drainage system. It is critical to obtain a detailed history of how the trauma occurred and to perform a complete physical exam, as other injuries can be missed elsewhere on the body, particularly adjacent intracranial trauma which could prove devastating if undetected.

An understanding of orbital anatomy is critical for the diagnosis and treatment of potentially vision-threatening injuries. Orbital anatomy is reviewed in Chap. 1, but some key points will be reiterated here. The orbits are bilateral, symmetrical cavities situated in the upper skull, each approximately 30 ml in volume, housing the eyes and associated structures. A mosaic of bones make up the four walls or "house of the orbit." The posteriorly located orbital apex can be thought of as a "fifth side" or back wall, for consideration of the approach to trauma.

The outside, or lateral wall, is made up of the greater wing of the sphenoid and zygomatic bones. The inside, or medial wall, is made of the thin ethmoid bone, lacrimal bone, and maxilla. The "roof," or superior wall, is comprised of frontal bone and sphenoid. The "floor" of the orbit consists of maxillary bone, a small contribution of the palatine bone and the zygomatic.

Residing within the bony orbit are the eye; retrobulbar fascia and fat; extraocular muscles; cranial nerves II, III, IV, V, and VI; blood vessels; the lacrimal gland; tear ducts; lacrimal sac; ligaments; the ciliary ganglion; and autonomic and ciliary nerves.

The optic nerve has its own foramen, the optic canal, which also transmits the ophthalmic artery and sympathetic fibers. The majority of other neurovascular structures which support the globe are carried via the superior orbital fissure, with some lesser structures passing through the inferior orbital fissure. The structural integrity of the orbital canals, fissures, and foramen is critical for the integrative functioning of the eye.

The orbit can be thought of as a five-sided protective cave for the eye, where the only opening is the exposed and vulnerable anterior aperture,

P. Michalos, MD (✉)
Department of Ophthalmology, Edward S. Harkness
Eye Institute, Columbia University Vagelos College
of Physicians and Surgeons, New York, NY, USA

© Springer Nature Switzerland AG 2019
D. S. Casper, G. A. Cioffi (eds.), *The Columbia Guide to Basic Elements of Eye Care*,
https://doi.org/10.1007/978-3-030-10886-1_34

which contains the unprotected front surface of the globe, and the adjacent, movable lids. Although this bony housing affords excellent armor for the orbital contents, the anterior and anterolateral globe's sole protection is the delicate lids. Furthermore, the "cave" configuration contributes to the typical pattern of post-traumatic orbital anomaly seen after trauma: if there is significant retrobulbar hemorrhage or edema present within the confined space, the globe is forced to protrude outwards (proptosis), via the only available aperture. This same mechanism underlies the proptosis which occurs with the presence of intraorbital abscesses, tumor masses, and the like, as an increase in intraorbital volume will almost invariably result in anterior displacement of the eye.

Orbital Trauma Evaluation

Blunt Trauma

Approximately 2.5 million cases of blunt orbital trauma occur in the USA per year. The amount of force per unit area that strikes the orbit will result in varying amounts of injury and damage ranging from predominantly external laceration and bruising of the skin and lids to deeper, potentially more severe injuries to the tear duct apparatus, bones surrounding the orbit, optic nerve and other orbital structures, including the globe, the periorbital sinuses, and intracranial contents, including the anterior frontal and temporal lobes, and neurovascular structures traversing the cavernous sinus to connect the orbital apex and middle cranial fossa.

Evaluation of orbital trauma requires a complete eye exam whenever possible. Documented vision that is best connected at near and far is the ideal goal. In cases of associated, life-threatening, or other severe concomitant trauma, this may be impossible, as the patient frequently has other comorbidities and may be unconscious, intubated, or in need of immediate surgical intervention for associated injuries. The eyelids may be swollen shut after orbital trauma, preventing a proper eye exam to evaluate collateral damage to the eye. Whenever possible, assessment of extraocular muscle functioning is critical to identify diplopia, which can be a sign of an orbital floor fracture with or without muscle entrapment, or direct injury to intracranial nerves III, IV, or VI.

Fortunately, modern high-speed CT scans are able to provide vast amounts of information on the integrity of orbital bones and globe in minutes. HRCT (high-resolution CT) with thin sections to include coronal and sagittal reconstruction is the study of choice for optimal evaluation. Axial and coronal scans offer the best views, while newer 3D reformatting options, available at many institutions, can greatly aid both diagnosis and treatment planning. When the presence of an intraorbital or intraocular metallic foreign body is suspected by history or exam, MRI is contraindicated, as additional trauma can be introduced by magnetic-induced movement of certain metallic foreign bodies.

Plain film studies are used less and less, as radiation levels associated with high-speed scans of the orbit have lessened. The actionable data obtained from axial and coronal CT scans is far greater than any which plain film has to offer.

Orbital B-scans may have value for quick screening of the eye and orbit when the lids are tightly swollen and possibly injured after trauma. Muscle trauma, vitreous hemorrhage, retinal detachments, and foreign bodies can be seen quickly through closed lids with a good quality B-scan ultrasound. Such a study must be performed by an examiner well-versed in this technique, as any excessive pressure exerted on an occult ruptured globe can have devastating consequences.

Summary of Types of Orbital and Associated Fractures

Both zygomaticomaxillary complex (also known as "tripod" fractures, which typically occur after a blow to the cheek) and Le Fort types II and III fractures may result in disruption of orbital walls. More commonly seen, however, are fractures localized to the medial wall (lamina papyracea) and/or floor, which are the thinnest and therefore the most easily fractured orbital walls. Such injuries are usually a result of direct trauma to the front of the orbit, with resultant rapid compression of orbital walls and intraocular contents. These are commonly referred to as blowout fractures; as these thin walls separate the orbit from the ethmoid and maxillary sinus, respectively, pathogens residing in the sinuses may traverse the fractured barrier, resulting in orbital cellulitis (Fig. 34.1). Other sequelae of blowout fractures may include entrapment of an extraocular muscle body (typically the inferior rectus, with floor fracture), resulting in vertical diplopia or limitation of eye movements, orbital hemorrhage with resultant proptosis (see above), or air within the orbit or lids, which originated in the adjacent sinus(es) (so-called "orbital emphysema"). Although blowout fractures frequently require no intervention other than antibiotic and decongestant administration, complicated fractures with muscle entrapments may require surgical intervention. Fractures of the lateral wall and/or roof will often require a combined approach with facial plastic surgeons or neurosurgeons (Fig. 34.2).

Both zygomaticomaxillary complex and Le Fort fractures usually require management by facial plastic surgeons or dental trauma specialists, with assistance from ophthalmic surgeons as needed for orbital complications.

Penetrating Trauma

Penetrating trauma is another form of potentially devastating orbital insult, usually resulting from sharp objects such as knives and high-velocity bullets, shrapnel, and explosions. The use of high-speed power tools is also a common cause of penetrating orbital injuries, as metallic, wooden, or other fragments are flung at high velocities, and, in the absence of proper eye protective safety wear, may penetrate deep into the

orbital tissues, often lacerating the globe as well. A rise in terrorism, wars, and escalating urban violence have unfortunately brought more cases of penetrating orbital trauma to emergency care centers. Often a combination of blunt and penetrating trauma is found to coexist (Fig. 34.3).

Orbital Hemorrhage and Apex Syndrome

Orbital hemorrhage and apex syndrome may occur from blunt or penetrating orbital trauma from presumed tears of thin walls of orbital vessels or bony fracture edges. Blood may be found in intra- or extraconal locations, including within the orbital or canalicular optic nerve sheath. In orbital apex syndrome, the presence of hemorrhage and edema at the apex leads to compression of the neurovascular structures that interconnect the posterior orbit and anterior middle cranial fossa.

The location and amount of blood present, as well as the duration of the hemorrhage within the orbit, will affect the clinical presentation. CT imaging is very helpful to identify the site of blood and is of tremendous use for surgical planning, if needed. Some of the complications of orbital hemorrhage include vein or artery occlusion, visual loss, proptosis, motility disturbances, or afferent pupillary defects or dangerous eye pressure elevations. Depending on the amount of bleeding and associated edema, orbital apex syndrome typically presents with acute proptosis, ophthalmoplegia, visual loss, chemosis, pain, and ptosis.

Lid and Lacrimal Canalicular Disruption

Any lid laceration, particularly if located in the nasal one-third of the lid, must raise suspicion of accompanying trauma to the lacrimal excretory system, including the punctae, canaliculi, and common canaliculus and nasolacrimal duct and

Fig. 34.1 Schematic of the extent of zygomaticomaxillary and Le Fort fractures, types II and III, all of which may involve the inferior, and to some extent lateral, orbit. Zygomaticomaxillary fractures occur due to a blow to the cheek, while Le Fort injuries are a result of midfacial trauma which involves the pterygoid plates and results in pterygomaxillary bony separation. Note that Le Fort types II and III involve disruption of the orbital walls (type I injuries are confined to the maxillary region and do not result in orbital disruption). (Modified with permission from Casper DS, Trokel SL, Chi TL. Orbital disease: imaging and analysis. New York: Thieme Medical Publishers Inc.; 1993.)

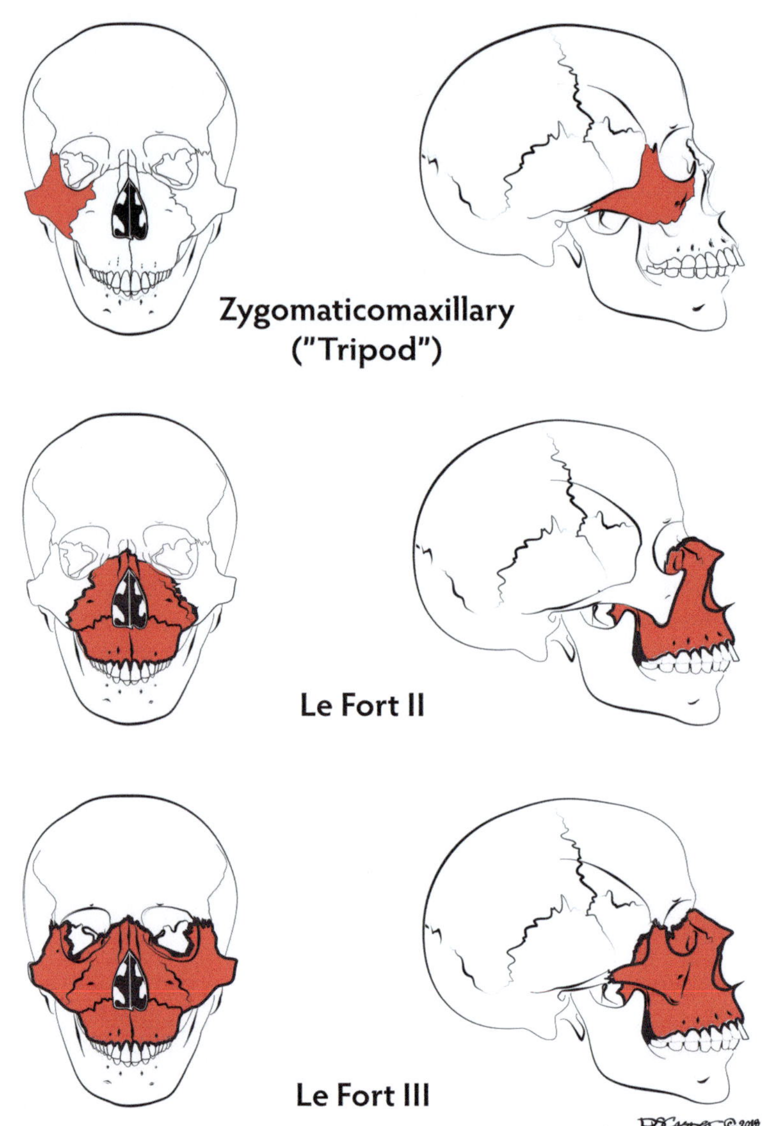

canal. Canalicular lacerations will not spontaneously recanalize, and if not properly repaired, the tear egress route will be obliterated. These injuries require stenting performed by an ophthalmologist to avoid a lifetime of tearing. These repairs are complex and require meticulous technique, usually utilizing an operating microscope and specialized stenting instruments. Injuries which involve significant loss of lid tissue require complex reconstructive procedures to recreate a lid structure that will, as closely as possible, resemble and function as a normal lid would (Fig. 34.4).

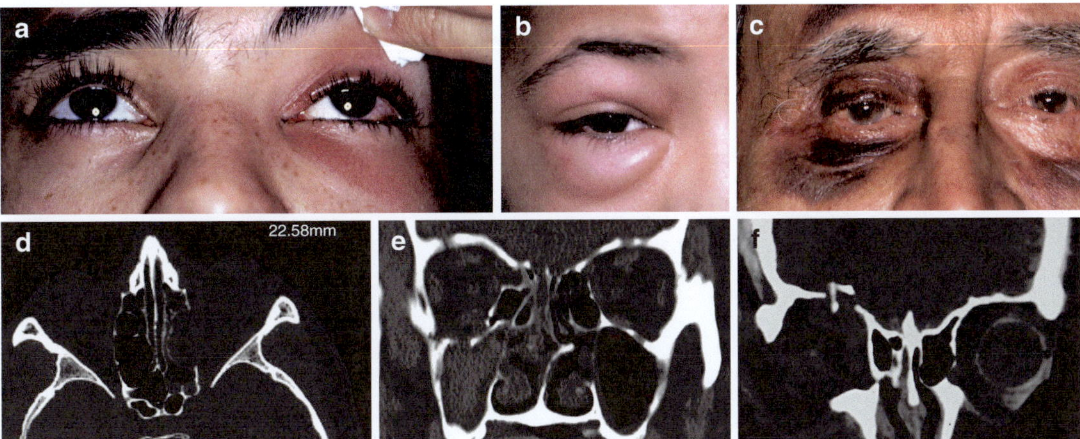

Fig. 34.2 (**a–c**) Clinical examples of orbital wall fractures. (**a**) A child with a small floor fracture which showed mild erythema and some restriction of movement which cleared spontaneously over time. (**b**) Another child with a small medial wall fracture that showed significant upper and lower lid ecchymosis after sneezing. (**c**) A man with periorbital and forehead ecchymosis after floor fracture with some mild globe ptosis noted. (**d–f**) Imaging studies after orbital trauma. (**a**) Axial CT showing a large medial wall fracture with bulging of orbital contents into the adjacent ethmoid; (**b**) a fracture of the orbital floor, showing opacification of the maxillary sinus from hemorrhage and orbital contents displaced within. Also, note the small dark profile just above the floor, representing sinus air which has entered the orbit through the bony defect (orbital emphysema). A small fracture of the ipsilateral medial wall is seen superiorly, as well. (**a**, **c**) "Trapdoor" roof fracture, much less commonly seen than medial and floor fractures, due to the thicker bony structure found superiorly. In a case such as this, cerebrospinal fluid may leak into the orbit

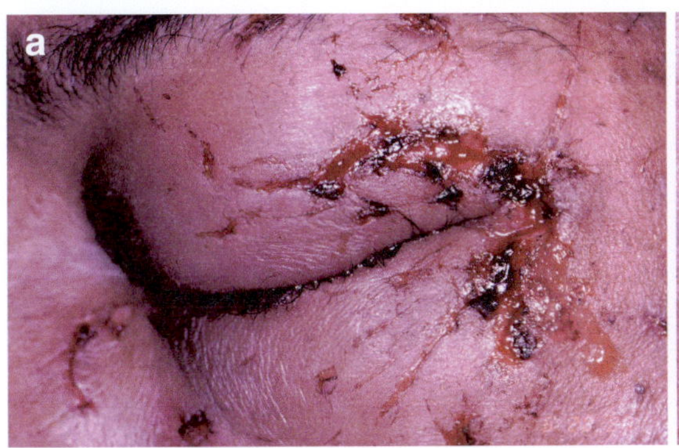

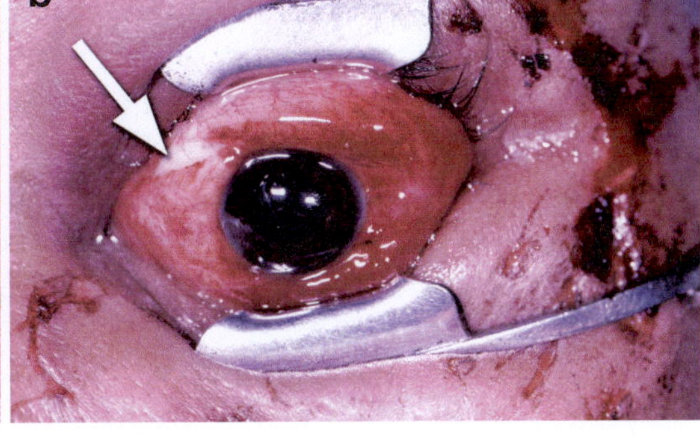

Fig. 34.3 (**a**, **b**) A temporal lid laceration which appeared small and superficial on external exam. Upon examination of the globe, however, a small medial conjunctival laceration was noted (arrow) with chemosis and conjunctival hemorrhage temporally. On exploration in the operating room, an occult globe laceration was found as well

Conclusions

There are many etiologies of orbital trauma which require prompt evaluation, imaging, and treatment. The goals of treatment are restoring and preserving acuity, eyelid functionality, binocular vision, and lacrimal system and tear duct integrity.

A multidisciplinary approach by specialists in ophthalmology, otolaryngology, neurosurgery, and plastic surgery is usually required to maximize the potential for restoration of orbital integrity and health. The use of improved microsutures, the binocular operating microscope, and micro titanium screws and plates has all contributed to vast improvements in the treatment of orbital trauma.

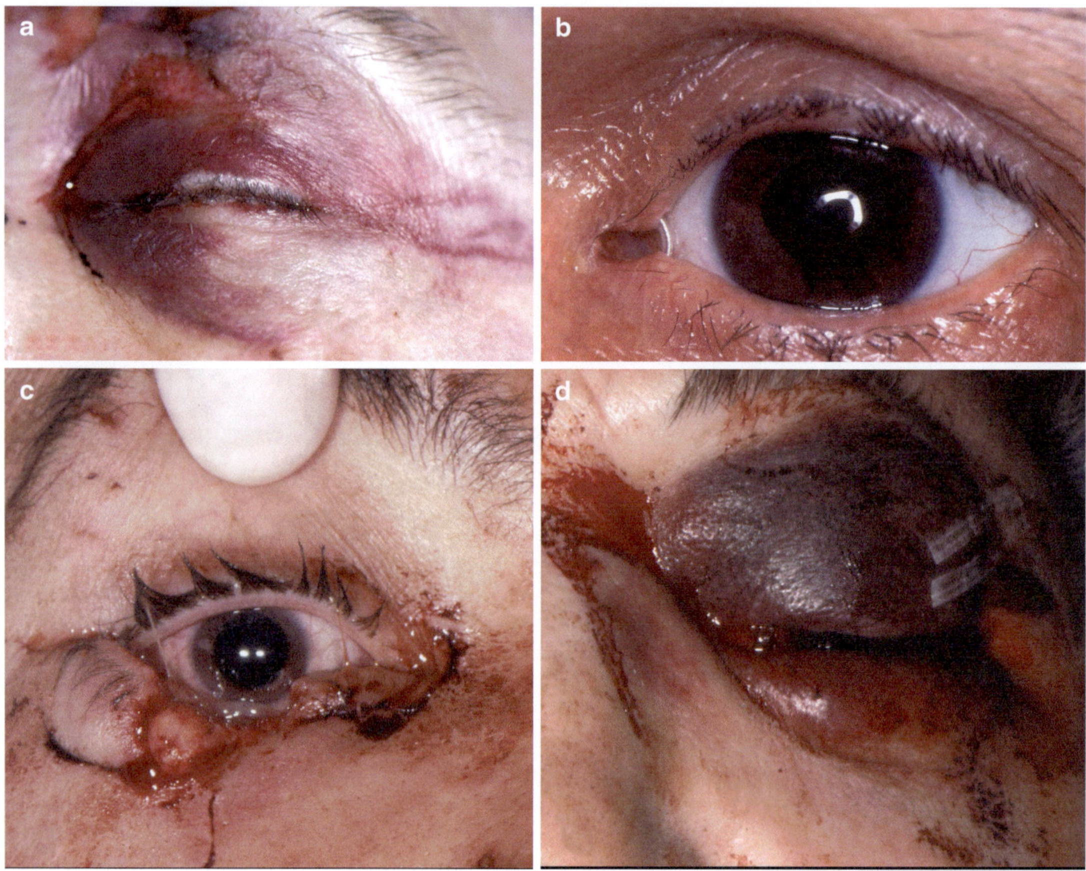

Fig. 34.4 Examples of lid lacerations. (**a**) A relatively small medial lid laceration which involved the canalicular drainage system and required stenting; a silicon tube stent is seen present in (**b**). Canalicular stenting tubes are usually left in place for a period of months to permit sufficient recanalization of a normal tear excretory route to the phar- ynx. (**c**) Shows a large, medial lid laceration that involved loss of tissue, but did not involve the excretory apparatus. Similarly, (**d**) shows trauma which caused significant upper and lower lid edema and ecchymosis, with temporal upper lid laceration, but no trauma to the canalicular system

Non-ophthalmologists should familiarize themselves with the vocabulary of the eye and orbit to be able to accurately describe traumatic injuries to consultants on the telephone. Such conversations should include an accurate history of how, when, and where the trauma occurred, and if child or spousal abuse is suspected, appropriate protocols must be followed, and scrupulous documentation maintained throughout. Periocular and non-orbital lacerations must be measured and documented as well and, if possible, photographed with a ruler included in the image for reference purposes. Increasing pain or decreasing sensation must also be documented and addressed. If an occult foreign body is suspected, a careful examination of the surrounding skin must be made looking for entrance wounds, and appropriate imaging performed if required. Finally, the suspicion for concomitant globe injury must always be high and, if suspected, requires urgent ophthalmic consultation. A small metallic foreign body seen, on plain X-ray or CT, located in the posterior orbit may well have passed through the eye on its course. If missed, such injuries will usually result in loss of vision and medicolegal action.

Suggested Reading

Casper DS, Trokel SL, Chi TL. Orbital disease: imaging and analysis. New York: Thieme Medical Publishers Inc.; 1993.

Fay A, Dolman PJ. Disease and disorders of the orbit and ocular adnexa. Edinburgh: Elsevier; 2016.

Holck DEE, Ng JD. Evaluation and treatment of orbital fractures: a multidisciplinary approach. Philadelphia: Saunders; 2006.

Nikolaenko VP, Astakhov YS, editors. Orbital fractures: a physicians manual. Berlin: Springer; 2015.

Rootman J. Diseases of the orbit. Philadelphia: Lippincott, Williams & Wilkins; 2002.

Welkoborsky H, Wiechens B, Hinni ML. Interdisciplinary management of orbital diseases: textbook and Atlas. Stuttgart: Thieme Publishing Group; 2017.

Headache

35

Nailyn Rasool

Headache is one of the most common conditions for which adults seek medical attention. According to the World Health Organization, approximately 50% of the adult population globally has experienced a headache at least once over the past year, and it is one of the highest causes worldwide for disability.

Patients frequently assume that their headaches are of ophthalmic origin, and this is usually not correct. The majority of headaches do not have an ocular etiology, but certainly this must be ruled out, particularly in patients who have persistent unexplained pain, those who are certain that their discomfort is related to visual activities, and those with associated complaints, such as weight loss, visual changes, jaw claudication, or vertigo.

The International Classification of Headache Disorders (ICHD) is the current, globally accepted classification of headache disorders containing explicit criteria for the diagnosis of multiple types of headache (Table 35.1). By understanding which type of headache the patient is suffering from, the clinician is then better equipped to provide counseling, determine which diagnostic tests (if any) should be performed, and offer the best treatment regimen.

Table 35.1 Headache classification: Adapted from International Classification of Headache Disorders, 3rd Edition

Part 1: Primary headache disorders
Migraine
Tension-type headache (TTH)
Trigeminal autonomic cephalalgias (TAC)
Other primary headache disorders
Part 2: The secondary headaches
Headache attributed to trauma or injury to the head and/or neck
Headache attributed to cranial or cervical vascular disorder
Headache attributed to nonvascular intracranial disorder
Headache attributed to a substance or its withdrawal
Headache attributed to disorder of homeostasis
Headache or facial pain attributed to disorder of the cranium, neck, eyes, ears, nose, sinuses, teeth, mouth, or other facial or cervical structures
Headache attributed to psychiatric disorder
Part 3: Painful cranial neuropathies, other facial pains, and other headaches
Painful lesions of the cranial nerves and other facial pain
Other headache disorders

Primary Versus Secondary Headaches

Headaches can be broadly categorized into primary and secondary headaches. Primary headaches have no known underlying cause and

N. Rasool, MD (✉)
Department of Ophthalmology, University of California, San Francisco, San Francisco, CA, USA

© Springer Nature Switzerland AG 2019
D. S. Casper, G. A. Cioffi (eds.), *The Columbia Guide to Basic Elements of Eye Care*,
https://doi.org/10.1007/978-3-030-10886-1_35

include headaches such as migraine, tension-type headaches, trigeminal autonomic cephalalgias, and other primary headache disorders (activity-induced, cough-induced, cold-induced, and many others). Secondary headaches are a result of another condition such as trauma, cervical or intracranial structural disorders, vascular disorders, inflammatory diseases, medication or substance use or withdrawal.

Headache Evaluation

The key to determining the underlying etiology of a patient's headache is a thorough clinical history. Mandatory information includes a description of the headache – onset, type of pain (stabbing/throbbing/squeezing), inciting factors, aggravating factors, alleviating factors, severity, and location. The examiner should determine if an aura precedes the headache, if there are any autonomic features as part of the presentation, and if the patient has tried medications previously. The age of onset of the headache, and family and personal history of headaches, is important. A detailed social history, medication and substance use list should also be obtained.

The examination begins with an assessment of the patient's overall appearance and stability, including their level of consciousness, comfort or discomfort, and ability to comprehend and express themselves. In addition, a general neurological examination including an assessment of their cranial nerves, motor and sensory system, speech and gait is important. Specific to the ophthalmologist, ptosis, pupillary examination, optic nerve assessment, and eye movements should be reviewed. Lastly, scalp tenderness, prominent vessels on the head and neck, and temporomandibular joint tenderness and stiffness should be assessed.

Red Flags

Worrisome features in the headache evaluation include:

- Sudden onset "thunderclap" headache or the worst headache of one's life
- New onset headache (particularly in older patients)
- Abnormality in the physical examination, including neurologic changes, optic nerve swelling, and altered mental status
- Scalp tenderness and prominent temporal arteries
- Triggers including cough, Valsalva maneuver, and exertion
- Pregnancy-related or postpartum headache
- Systemic illness (fevers, joint pain, rash, diaphoresis, neck stiffness)
- Immunocompromised patients or patients with a history of cancer
- Headaches worsening upon lying flat
- Headaches that awaken the patient from sleep

Diagnostic Testing

The most common headache, migraine, does not require further imaging or laboratory testing. These patients typically have completely normal physical examinations and a long-standing history of headache that is unchanged.

Should the patient have concerning features in the history or physical examination, or "red flags," the patient should undergo appropriate neuroimaging and laboratory testing. If one suspects a more concerning headache, consultation with a neuro-ophthalmologist, neurologist, or referral to an emergency room for appropriate imaging and work-up, is the most appropriate next step.

Treatment

Treatment of headache primarily depends upon the underlying etiology. For patients with primary headache disorders in which there is no identifiable cause, infrequent and mild symptoms are often managed conservatively with lifestyle modification and infrequent non-opioid analgesics and abortive medications. More frequent and debilitating headaches may require daily preventative medication to reduce the burden of the symptoms on the patient. Secondary headaches often require treatment of the underlying etiology, whether it be structural, vascular, infectious, or inflammatory to achieve improvement or relief from the headache.

Primary Headache Disorders

Migraine

Migraine affects 12% of individuals per year, most commonly those in their second and third decades of life. It has a strong female predominance with women being affected three times more readily than men.

There are two major subtypes of migraine headache: migraine with aura and migraine without aura. Migraine without aura is the most common subtype and often occurs with greater frequency and intensity (Table 35.2). In migraine with aura, the aura experience is a set of reversible neurologic symptoms that classically develop gradually and then subside, often followed by a typical migraine headache. The aura may consist of visual symptoms (either positive photopsias or negative features such as loss of vision or scotomas), sensory symptoms, or speech disturbances. Auras may include multiple sensory experiences; however if this occurs, they usually propagate gradually over 5 min each and in succession over 5 min lasting a total of 60 min. Rarely, patients may have motor (hemiplegic migraine) or brain-

stem symptoms as a manifestation of their aura, but one must be careful to ensure this is not the manifestation of a more severe type of headache, stroke or other neurologic condition. The pathophysiology of migraine aura is based upon cortical spreading depression, whereby over the course of approximately 20 min, a wave of electrophysiological hyperactivity is followed by a wave of inhibition, resulting in initial vasoconstriction and subsequent vasodilation of cortical arterioles.

The headache in patients who experience aura typically occurs either during or within 60 min following the aura. The features of the head pain are consistent with the criteria for migraine without aura. This includes moderate to severe attacks that last between 4 and 72 h, are typically unilateral (60%), pulsatile, aggravated by activity and often associated with nausea, vomiting, photophobia, and phonophobia.

In the so-called ophthalmic, ocular, retinal, or acephalgic migraine, an aura is experienced as a waxing and waning visual distortion that may include scotomas and photopsias, typically lasting 20 min, and subsequently resolving without headache development. The theory is that this limited phenomenon is due to a vasoconstriction phase as with classic migraine, but, for unclear reasons, it is not followed by the arteriolar vasodilation that results in the pain typical of classic migraines.

Treatment of migraine ultimately begins with appropriate diagnosis of the headache disorder and education of the patient. The physician must ensure that the patient does not have a coincident medication overuse headache which can occur if the patient uses analgesic medications greater than three to four times per week or greater than 10 days per month. Conservative management begins with realistic goal setting of decreasing headache frequency and intensity, as a complete cure may not be possible. This includes keeping a headache diary, whereby the patient can identify triggers, aggravating, precipitating, and alleviating factors.

Classes of medication that can be used to treat migraine include non-specific analgesics (nonsteroidal anti-inflammatory drugs), such as acetaminophen and other simple analgesics. Abortive medications such as ergot derivatives and triptans (e.g., 5-hydroxytryptamine receptor 5-HT $_{1B/1D}$

Table 35.2 International classification of headache disorders ICHD-3 (beta) migraine without aura

A. At least five headache attacks fulfilling criteria B–D
B. Attacks last 4–72 h
C. With at least two of the following characteristics
1. Unilateral location
2. Pulsating quality
3. Moderate or severe pain intensity
4. Aggravation by or causing avoidance of routine physical activity
D. At least one of the following during headache
1. Nausea and/or vomiting
2. Photophobia and phonophobia
E. Not better accounted for by another ICHD-3 diagnosis

receptor agonists) are employed early when the headache begins. However, they promote vasoconstriction and should not be used in patients with vascular disease (including coronary artery or cerebrovascular disease), and in patients on vasoactive medications. Triptans are relatively contraindicated in patients who smoke, take serotonin derivative medications or hormone replacements as the vasoconstrictive effects can be compounded and lead to stroke or myocardial infarction. Lastly, for patients experiencing migraine pain frequently resulting in common use of analgesic medications and impairment to their quality of life, prophylactic medications should be highly considered. Prophylactic migraine medications are taken daily to prevent the development of migraine and should be trialed for approximately 3 months for their full effect to be realized. These medications include oral beta-blockers, anticonvulsants, calcium channel blockers, antidepressants, and botulinum toxin injections. Migraine medications should be managed by the patient's neurologist or primary care physician, as they may have serious systemic side effects.

As this book goes to press, the FDA has just approved a new potentially promising migraine prophylactic medication for patients with severe, disabling attacks. Erenumab-aooe (marketed as Aimovig) blocks activity of a molecule involved in migraine attacks, calcitonin gene-related peptide (CGRP), by targeting its receptor. The medication is administered as an injection once per month.

Tension-Type Headache

Tension-type headache is the most common headache with a lifetime prevalence of up to 78% in the general population (Table 35.3). It is most common in patients in their fourth to fifth decades of life but can be seen in patients of all ages. Similar to migraine, it has a female predominance.

Tension-type headaches are typically mild to moderate in severity and bilateral. The pain is dull and often described as a squeezing "band around the head." Symptoms can last hours to days and are not associated with constitutional or neurological symptoms. Tension headaches are subdivided by frequency: infrequent, frequent, and chronic. Infrequent tension-type headache is

Table 35.3 International classification of headache disorders ICHD-3 (beta) infrequent episodic tension-type headache

A. <1 day per month
B. 30 min to 7 days duration
C. At least two of the following
  1. Bilateral location
  2. Pressing or tightening (non-pulsating) quality
  3. Mild or moderate intensity
  4. Not aggravated by routine physical activity
D. Both of
  1. No nausea or vomiting
  2. No more than one of photophobia or phonophobia

the most common and often experienced by almost every person at some point during their lives. Palpation of the pericranial muscles is quite helpful as a diagnostic maneuver, as patients with tension headache often have increased myofascial sensitivity in the head.

Treatment of tension-type headache begins with conservative management – keeping a headache diary, avoiding triggers, and preventing medication overuse. Nonpharmacologic therapy may include relaxation exercises, hot/cold packs, and postural changes. Simple analgesics are usually sufficient to treat tension headaches including aspirin and acetaminophen, and caffeine has also demonstrated some benefit. Opioids or sedatives should be avoided. Should the patient suffer from frequent or chronic tension-type headaches, preventative medications may be considered in conjunction with the patient's primary care physician or neurologist. These may include amitriptyline, selective serotonin reuptake inhibitors (SSRIs), mirtazapine, and venlafaxine.

Trigeminal Autonomic Cephalalgias

The trigeminal autonomic cephalalgias (TAC) are a group of uncommon primary headache disorders which are characterized by recurrent short-lasting episodes of unilateral headache with cranial autonomic symptoms. The autonomic symptoms associated with this group of disorders include ptosis, miosis, conjunctival injection, lacrimation, facial flushing, facial sweating, nasal congestion, and rhinorrhea typically ipsilateral to the headache. The TAC disorders are subdivided based upon duration of the attack and frequency of recurrence and include the following: cluster headache, paroxysmal hemicrania, hemicrania continua, short-lasting unilateral neuralgiform headache with conjunctival injection and tearing (SUNCT), and short-lasting unilateral neuralgiform headache attacks with autonomic features (SUNA).

Intracranial lesions, particularly in the pituitary, have been reported to present as TACs and therefore some advocate performing an MRI with attention to the pituitary gland in patients that present with TAC syndromes.

The pathophysiology of the TAC syndromes is based upon activation of the hypothalamus with subsequent involvement of the trigeminovascular and cranial parasympathetic pathways. Activation of the trigeminal nucleus via the ophthalmic branch of the trigeminal nerve results in increased levels of CGRP in the blood and excitation of the superior salivatory nucleus, thereby activating the cranial parasympathetic system (often via the sphenopalatine ganglion).

Clinical Syndromes

Cluster Headache

Cluster headache is a very uncommon headache syndrome; however, it is the most common of the trigeminal autonomic cephalalgias. It is characterized by extremely severe unilateral headaches often maximal behind the eye, lasting 15–180 min with at least one autonomic symptom ipsilateral to the pain or a sense of agitation. It can occur from one to eight times per day causing significant restlessness in patients and is approximately three times more common in men than women. Cluster headache can be episodic or chronic. The most common presentation is the episodic form whereby attacks occur daily for weeks followed by remission for months or years. Although patients typically experience their attacks in the spring or autumn, the reasons for this predilection are unknown. Chronic cluster headache is defined as attacks which occur for more than 1 year without a remission lasting more than 1 month.

Treatment of cluster headache consists of acute and preventative treatment. Treatment of acute attacks includes the administration of 100% oxygen through a high-flow mask at a rate of 12–15 L/min, which has been reported to provide relief in up to two-thirds of patients. The effect is often seen to begin approximately 20 min after the initiation of treatment. In addition, one of the most effective abortive treatments is the administration of triptans (5-HT $_{1B/1D}$ receptor agonists) preferably subcutaneously (sumatriptan) or intranasally (zolmitriptan, sumatriptan). Lastly, intranasal lidocaine, ipsilateral to the headache, has also been reported to provide pain relief. Short-term treatments that can be used during a cluster include short courses of corticosteroids or occipital nerve blocks. Preventative therapies include calcium channel blockers, lithium, and topiramate – all of which are used daily to prevent the occurrence of cluster attacks.

Paroxysmal Hemicrania

Paroxysmal hemicranias is similar to cluster headache in that both are short, unilateral headaches with ipsilateral, cranial autonomic symptoms which can be both episodic and chronic. However, paroxysmal hemicrania occurs more frequently than cluster with a shorter duration of attacks (and specifically less propensity for nocturnal attacks). This TAC occurs for approximately 2–30 min at a time and attacks occur greater than five times per day. Attacks may be triggered by mechanical stimuli such as head bending or applying pressure to the C2 root or occipital nerve. In contrast to cluster headache, there is no sex predilection. Paroxysmal hemicrania is characterized by complete response to indomethacin – often at a dose of 150 mg daily which can be gradually titrated up as needed. If indomethacin cannot be tolerated, acetylsalicylic acid, celecoxib, acetazolamide, topiramate, and verapamil have demonstrated some benefit.

Hemicrania Continua

Hemicrania continua is a unilateral headache of mild-to-moderate intensity which is constant and unremitting. Exacerbations of the pain occur almost daily, lasting anywhere from 30 min to 3 days. It is typically during these more painful flares that cranial autonomic symptoms present. In addition, features more typical of migraine, including photophobia, phonophobia, and nausea, are often present. Similar to paroxysmal hemicrania, hemicrania continua is very responsive to treatment with indomethacin but often requires higher doses.

Short-Lasting Unilateral Neuralgiform Headache Attacks

SUNCT and SUNA are the rare TACs and are characterized by extremely short, severe headache attacks lasting seconds. The pain is typically characterized as stabbing or lancinating and is unilateral. Attacks can be a single stab, a series of stabs, or recurrent stabs over minutes. The episode can last anywhere from 1 s to 10 min and may occur up to 100 times per day. SUNCT is associated with conjunctival injection and tearing, and SUNA is associated with other autonomic features. Intracranial lesions, particularly in the posterior fossa or sella, may present with these attacks, and therefore all patients who present with SUNCT or SUNA should have an MRI. Treatment includes the following: lamotrigine (first line), topiramate, gabapentin, and short-term IV lidocaine to induce remission. These medications must be taken chronically to prevent recurrent attacks.

Idiopathic Intracranial Hypertension

Idiopathic intracranial hypertension (IIH), (previously referred to as pseudotumor cerebri) is a term used to describe elevated intracranial pressure with normal brain parenchyma, without ventriculomegaly, a mass lesion or underlying infection or malignancy. The typical patient with idiopathic intracranial hypertension is an obese adolescent or adult female patient of childbearing age. Upon further questioning, many of these patients may have incurred recent weight gain prior to the development of their symptoms. Despite the common association with obese young women, the disease can affect pre-pubertal patients of both sexes more equally.

Patients who do not fit this demographic and are slim and/or male should undergo further investigation to determine if there is an alternate underlying etiology of their symptoms. Medications that can result in elevated intracranial pressure include steroids (or steroid withdrawal), synthetic growth hormone, tetracycline derivatives, and vitamin A or retinoic acid compounds. Anemia, venous sinus thrombosis, dural arteriovenous malformations, Addison's disease, and lupus may also result in a similar clinical picture and must be considered and ruled-out.

The presenting features of IIH most commonly include a new or worsening headache (in over 90% of patients), which may increase upon lying flat or be associated with neck pain or stiffness. Approximately three quarters of patients have transient visual obscurations during which they either lose vision or their vision "sparkles" briefly when they change position. Pulsatile tinnitus is also a classic feature of this condition. Upon ophthalmologic examination, the patient typically presents with optic nerve swelling, with vessel obscuration and loss of spontaneous venous pulsations (See Fig. 36.2c). Depending upon the degree of optic nerve swelling, the patient may have subnormal visual acuity, a relative afferent pupillary defect, affected color vision, and an enlarged blind spot (or additional visual field loss should optic nerve function be significantly compromised) upon visual testing. Other cranial nerve abnormalities, most commonly an abducens nerve palsy, may be present.

All patients with suspected papilledema should undergo magnetic resonance imaging (MRI) and MR venogram to rule out a mass lesion and venous sinus thrombosis. If these studies prove normal, the patient should undergo lumbar puncture for opening pressure determination and to analyze cerebrospinal fluid constituents to ensure they are normal and the optic nerve swelling is not secondary to other underlying etiologies.

Neuroimaging features of IIH include an empty sella, flattening of the posterior aspect of the globes, distension of the perioptic subarachnoid space with distension of the optic nerve sheath, and often transverse venous sinus stenosis.

Treatment of IIH is usually conservative and medical, but can be surgical. Weight loss is a critical component of disease treatment in patients that are overweight. Patients need to lose approximately 5–10% of their body weight in order to have an improvement in their disease process and symptoms. As weight loss cannot be achieved immediately, patients must concurrently be started on CSF pressure-lowering medications to protect the optic nerve from further damage. This is most commonly acetazolamide, the dose of which can be adjusted dependent upon severity of the papilledema and visual dysfunction. Topiramate is a possible alternative or addition to acetazolamide treatment. Should the patient have severe visual dysfunction secondary to IIH, discussions between ophthalmology, neurology, and neurosurgery should be undertaken to determine whether the patient requires a lumbar drain, shunt, or optic nerve sheath fenestration. Each of these procedures is invasive, with potentially severe complications (including visual loss) and should be managed by a highly specialized multidisciplinary team.

Table 35.4 Modified Dandy Criteria: Diagnostic criteria for idiopathic intracranial hypertension

(a) Papilledema
(b) Normal neurological examination, except for cranial nerve abnormalities
(c) Neuroimaging: normal brain parenchyma without evidence of hydrocephalus, mass, or structural lesion and no abnormal meningeal enhancement on MRI, with head without gadolinium, and no venous sinus thrombosis demonstrated on MR venogram
(d) Normal CSF composition
(e) Elevated lumbar puncture opening pressure (>250 cm H20 in adults) in the lateral decubitus position

Giant Cell Arteritis

Giant cell arteritis (GCA), otherwise known as temporal arteritis, is the most common systemic vasculitis among North Americans. It affects large- and medium-sized blood vessels, with a predisposition for the cranial arteries, and can have devastating visual and neurologic complications. GCA typically affects individuals older than 50 years of age, with an even higher incidence in patients greater than 70 years of age. It is most common in patients of Northern European and Scandinavian descent with a lower incidence in patients of other ethnic backgrounds.

Patients presenting with giant cell arteritis typically complain of a new, moderate-to-severe headache, often unilateral in presentation. The headache is often continuous, and there can be tenderness to palpation of the temples, (in the areas of the temporal arteries), at times with prominence of the temporal arteries and decreased palpable pulsation of the temporal arteries. Patients also often present with jaw claudication which can be elicited by inquiring whether they have experienced discomfort with chewing food. Scalp tenderness, general malaise, myalgias, fatigue, and recent weight loss are additional prominent symptoms which may be part of the symptom constellation. Visual symptoms may include transient monocular vision loss, permanent loss of vision, and double vision. Visual loss is typically severe, of rapid onset and irreversible (See Fig. 36.11).

Laboratory testing that is helpful in diagnosis of the condition includes an elevated erythrocyte sedimentation rate (ESR), C-reactive protein (CRP), and a thrombocytosis. Additionally, patients may have a normocytic anemia. The gold standard for diagnosis of GCA is a temporal artery biopsy (TAB). Given that the vasculitis presents with "skip lesions" in the vessel, it is recommended that the length of the temporal artery biopsy is at least 1.5 to 2.0 cm to increase the diagnostic yield and prevent the possibility that a negative biopsy is secondary to the presence of normal skip lesions. Surgeons differ whether they perform initial unilateral TAB or bilateral TAB; bilateral procedures have been reported to increase diagnostic sensitivity up to 12.7% in comparison to unilateral biopsies. Histopathology of involved tissue shows transmural inflammation of the artery and disruption of the internal elastic lamina. Multinucleated giant cells may be seen but are not necessary for the diagnosis.

Imaging of the temporal arteries and cranial arteries has been recently used to diagnose the presence of vasculitis. Temporal artery high-resolution Doppler ultrasound has been demonstrated to identify vasculitis with the presence of a concentric hypoechogenic mural thickening (halo) of the vessel. Additionally, others have used MRI to look at mural contrast enhancement of the temporal arteries and cranial vessels, although differing results with both these modalities (related to the sensitivity of these diagnostic techniques) necessitate continued reliance on the gold standard. As GCA is a systemic disease and some of the most devastating complications can result from inflammation of the aorta and more proximal vascular branches, positron emission tomography (PET) can be used to demonstrate the presence of vasculitis in these more central structures. Central vascular imaging should be considered, particularly in patients with atypical presentations such as fever of unknown origin, anorexia, and diffuse myalgias.

Urgent and aggressive management of GCA is of the utmost importance to prevent devastating neurologic complications, including blindness and stroke. Corticosteroids are the cornerstone of treatment of GCA, and early institution of steroids upon the suspicion of the presence of GCA dramatically reduces the frequency of severe visual ischemic complications. The initial dose of

prednisone can range from 1 mg/kg/day to 1000 mg of intravenous solumedrol dependent upon the patient's medical comorbidities and severity of disease (those with visual symptoms often receive higher initial doses). Should the patient be started upon IV solumedrol, within 1–3 days they are tapered to oral prednisone and gradually furthered tapered off medications over the course of months, ensuring their symptoms and inflammatory markers do not flare.

Steroid-sparing agents such as methotrexate have been used with some success in patients intolerant of long-term steroid therapy. More recently, tocilizumab, a monoclonal antibody directed at interleukin-6, has demonstrated promising results in the management of GCA and as an effective steroid-sparing agent. Management of patients on such medications should be done in conjunction with a rheumatologist.

Suggested Reading

Bendtsen L, Jensen R. Tension-Type Headache. Neurol Clin. 2009;27(2):525–35.

Headache Classification Committee of the International Headache Society (IHS) The International Classification of Headache Disorders, 3rd edition. Cephalalgia. 2018;38(1):1–211.

Rizzoli P, Mullally WJ. Headache. Am J Med. 2018;131(1):17–24.

Jay GW, Barkin RL. Primary headache disorders part I-migraine and the trigeminal autonomic cephalalgias. Dis Mon. 2017;63(11):308–38.

Bruce BB, Biousse V, Newman NJ. Update on idiopathic intracranial hypertension. Am J Ophthalmol. 2011;152(2):163–9.

Puledda F, Messina R, Goadsby PJ. An update on migraine: current understanding and future directions. J Neurol. 2017;264(9):2031–9.

Newman LC. Trigeminal autonomic cephalalgias. CONTINUUM: Lifelong Learning in Neurology. 21:1041–57.

Stone JH, Tuckwell K, Dimonaco S, Klearman M, Aringer M, Blockmans D, Brouwer E, Cid MC, Dasgupta B, Rech J, Salvarani C, Schett G, Schulze-Koops H, Spiera R, Unizony SH, Collinson N. Trial of tocilizumab in giant-cell arteritis. N Engl J Med. 2017;377(4):317–28.

Solomon CG, Weyand CM, Goronzy JJ. Giant-cell arteritis and polymyalgia rheumatica. N Engl J Med. 2014;371(1):50–7.

Table 35.5 American College of Rheumatology criteria for the diagnosis of giant cell arteritis (1990)

1. Age at disease onset >50 years
2. New headache
3. Temporal artery abnormality such as tenderness to palpation or decreased pulsation
4. Elevated erythrocyte sedimentation rate >50 mm/h
5. Abnormal artery biopsy demonstrating vasuclitis characteritized by mononuclear cell infiltration or granulomatous inflammation, usually with multinucleated giant cells

Larissa K. Ghadiali and Jeffrey G. Odel

Optic neuropathy, or damage to the optic nerve, is diagnosed by characteristic visual field loss, color vision deficit, decreased brightness sense, afferent pupillary defect, nerve fiber layer dropout, optic nerve pallor, or optic nerve swelling. Optical coherence tomography (OCT) can demonstrate optic neuropathy by exhibiting decreased nerve fiber layer thickness, ganglion cell layer complex loss, or nerve fiber layer swelling. OCT can also show normal outer retinal structure and thereby aid in localizing the problem to the optic nerve. Visual field loss in optic neuropathy reflects the nerve fiber course thru the retina. Cecocentral visual field loss, as seen in nutritional optic neuropathy, autosomal dominant optic neuropathy, ethambutol toxicity, and optic neuritis, reflects damage to the so-called papillomacular bundle and is accompanied by decreased color vision (as measured by color plates, e.g., AO/HRR color plates) and decreased central acuity. In optic neuropathy accompanied by cecocentral visual field loss, color vision loss is markedly decreased compared to visual acuity. Arcuate and altitudinal visual field loss, as in non-arteritic ischemic optic neuropathy (NAION), optic nerve head drusen, and glaucoma produce color vision loss in the area of the visual field loss but may spare color vision as tested by color plates. Patients with unilateral optic neuropathy, particularly involving the central visual field, will notice ipsilateral decreased color saturation and brightness sense. With unilateral or markedly asymmetric optic neuropathy, an ipsilateral relative afferent pupillary defect (RAPD) will be present; with bilateral optic neuropathy, however, an RAPD may not be seen. Careful examination of the fundus may reveal congenital anomalies of the disc as in optic nerve hypoplasia, a tilted optic disc, optic disc pit, optic disc coloboma, the papillorenal syndrome, or the morning glory syndrome. Optic disc pallor (atrophy) may be seen in various patterns such as generalized, temporal, band, or altitudinal. The optic disc may appear simply swollen or swollen with hemorrhages, macular star exudates, cilioretinal artery occlusions, cotton wool spots, optociliary shunt vessels (meningioma), or telangiectatic vessels (Leber's disease) (Figs. 36.1 and 36.2).

An approach to the diagnosis of optic neuropathy may be simplified by categorizing the various presentations as shown here and detailed in Table 36.1:

L. K. Ghadiali, MD
Department of Ophthalmology, Loyola University
Medical Center, Maywood, IL, USA

J. G. Odel, MD (✉)
Columbia University Irving Medical Center,
New York, NY, USA

Department of Ophthalmology, Edward S. Harkness
Eye Institute, Columbia University Vagelos College
of Physicians and Surgeons, New York, NY, USA
e-mail: jgo1@cumc.columbia.edu

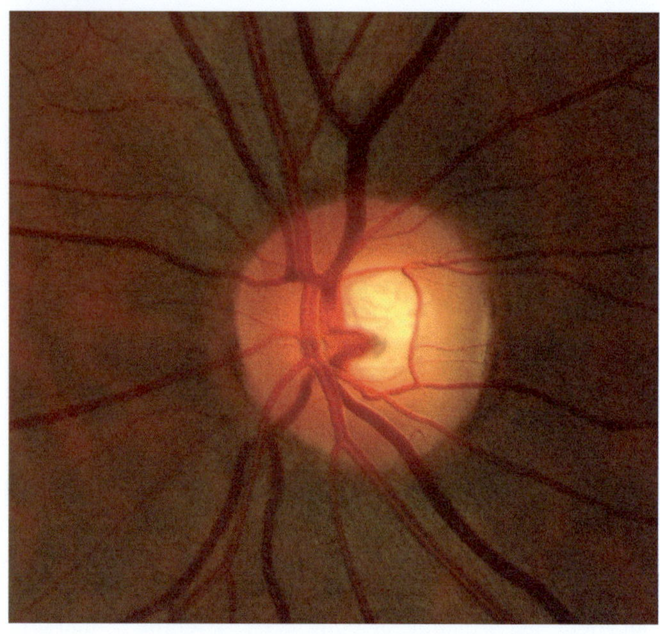

Fig. 36.1 The normal optic nerve head. The neuroretinal rim is pink with a cup-to-disc ratio of 0.3. The optic disc margins are sharp. There is no edema and there are no hemorrhages

- Acute unilateral optic neuropathy with disc swelling
- Acute unilateral optic neuropathy without disc swelling
- Chronic progressive unilateral optic neuropathy with disc swelling
- Chronic progressive unilateral optic neuropathy without disc swelling
- Sequential optic neuropathy
- Bilateral slowly progressive optic neuropathy
- Sudden bilateral retrobulbar optic neuropathy

The more common optic neuropathies are examined in the section "Categorization of the Optic Neuropathies."

Evaluation of the Patient with Suspected Optic Neuropathy

History

The history is paramount in assessing patients with possible optic neuropathy. Patient demographics, particularly age and gender, may provide significant clues to the diagnosis.

Time Course

Sudden visual loss is typically due to ischemic, traumatic, demyelinating, or inflammatory events. Leber's hereditary optic neuropathy may also present with sudden visual loss. Gradual vision loss is more characteristic of compressive, toxic, nutritional, infiltrative, and most hereditary optic neuropathies. Glaucoma, the most common type of optic neuropathy worldwide, also presents with gradual vision loss.

Age

Children are more commonly affected by congenital, hereditary, post-viral, postvaccination, and traumatic optic nerve disorders. Young adults commonly present with demyelinating optic neuropathy, NAION is more commonly encountered in middle aged patients, and arteritic anterior ischemic optic neuropathy (AION) is typically seen in the elderly population. Compressive conditions can occur at any age.

Associated Symptoms

Demyelinating optic neuritis is associated with *eye pain in 90% of cases*, particularly pain on eye movement. *Uhthoff's phenomenon*, an exacerbation of neurological symptoms which occurs with

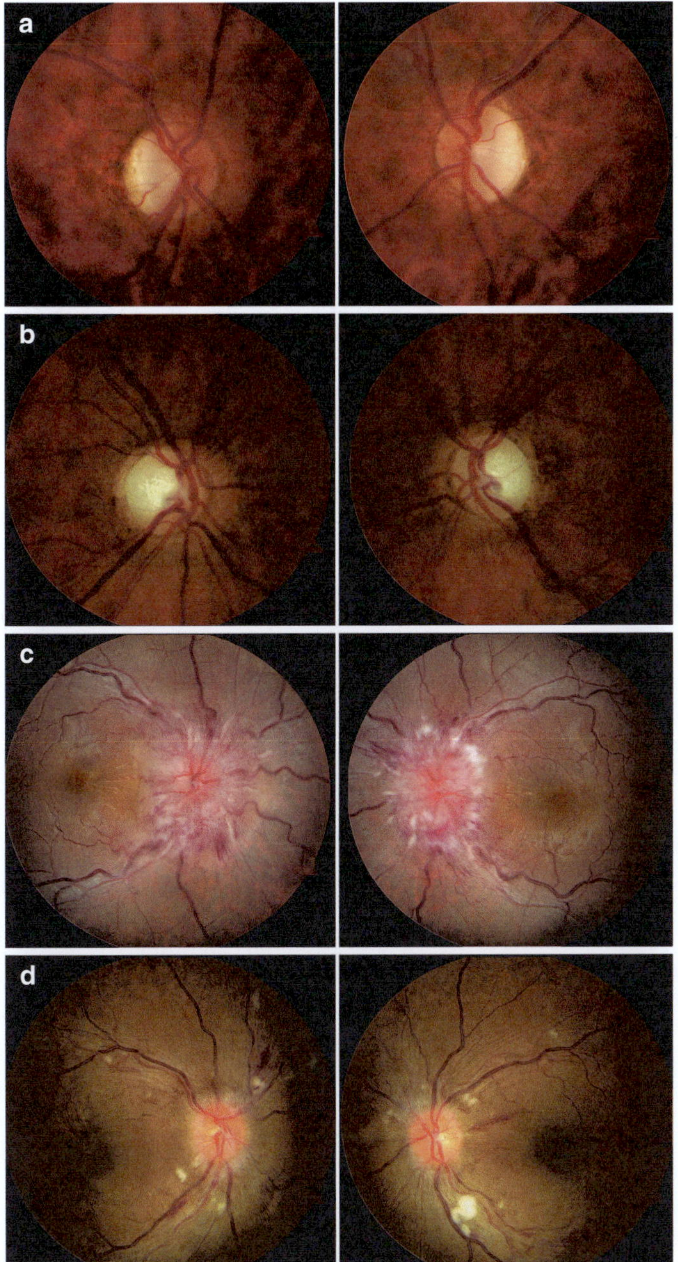

Fig. 36.2 (**a**) Autosomal dominant optic atrophy. The neuroretinal rim is pale temporally, and the optic disc margins are sharp. The retinal blood vessels are attenuated. (**b**) Optic atrophy in Wolfram syndrome. The neuroretinal rim is diffusely pale and the optic disc margins are sharp. The blood vessels are attenuated. (**c**) Idiopathic intracranial hypertension. Bilateral papilledema is seen. The optic discs are hyperemic, and the optic disc margins are blurred with obscuration of the blood vessels. Flame-shaped retinal nerve fiber layer hemorrhages are seen in both eyes, and the retinal veins are dilated and tortuous. The cup-to-disc ratio cannot be determined. (**d**) Hypertensive retinopathy. The retinal arteries are constricted. Retinal hemorrhages, hard exudates, cotton wool spots, and retinal edema are seen

Table 36.1 Approach to the diagnosis of optic neuropathy

1. Acute unilateral optic neuropathy with disc swelling
   - (a) Optic neuritis – papillitis
     - (i) Multiple sclerosis
     - (ii) Post-viral optic neuritis
     - (iii) Syphilitic optic neuritis
     - (iv) Paraneoplastic optic neuritis
     - (v) Autoimmune optic neuritis
     - (vi) Sarcoidosis
     - (vii) Neuroretinitis
     - (viii) Nematode
   - (b) Ischemic optic neuropathy
     - (i) Non-arteritic anterior ischemic optic neuropathy
     - (ii) Arteritic anterior ischemic optic neuropathy
     - (iii) Post general surgery anterior ischemic optic neuropathy (AION)
     - (iv) Post cataract surgery AION
     - (v) Optic disc drusen-related AION
     - (vi) Diabetic papillopathy
     - (vii) Drug-related anterior ischemic optic neuropathy
   - (c) Infiltrative optic neuropathy
     - (i) Sarcoidosis
     - (ii) Lymphoma
     - (iii) Optic nerve glioma
     - (iv) Polyneuropathy, organomegaly, endocrinopathy, monoclonal gammopathy, and skin changes (POEMS) syndrome
     - (v) Langerhans cell disorders
2. Acute unilateral optic neuropathy without disc swelling
   - (a) Demyelinating
     - (i) Multiple sclerosis
     - (ii) Neuromyelitis optica
     - (iii) Autoimmune
     - (iv) Paraneoplastic
   - (b) Acute compressive retrobulbar neuropathy
     - (i) Pituitary apoplexy
     - (ii) Mucocele
     - (iii) Aneurysm
   - (c) Posterior ischemic optic neuropathy
     - (i) Arteritic
     - (ii) Post-general surgery
     - (iii) Idiopathic
3. Chronic progressive unilateral optic neuropathy with disc swelling
   - (a) Optic nerve sheath meningioma
   - (b) Sarcoidosis
   - (c) Thyroid eye disease
   - (d) Orbital tumors
   - (e) Hemangioma
4. Chronic progressive unilateral optic neuropathy without disc swelling
   - (a) Intracranial meningioma

Table 36.1 (continued)

   - (b) Optic canal meningioma
   - (c) Pituitary adenoma
   - (d) Intracranial aneurysm
5. Sequential optic neuropathy
   - (a) Leber's hereditary optic neuropathy (LHON) acute
   - (b) NAION acute
   - (c) Foster-Kennedy syndrome progressive
   - (d) Sequential demyelinating optic neuritis acute
6. Bilateral slowly progressive optic neuropathy
   - (a) Nutritional amblyopia
   - (b) Vitamin B12 deficiency
   - (c) Ethambutol
   - (d) Compressive
   - (e) Papilledema
   - (f) Glaucoma
7. Sudden bilateral retrobulbar optic neuropathy
   - (a) Postsurgical
   - (b) Optic neuritis
   - (c) Pituitary apoplexy
   - (d) Chiasmal apoplexy – AVM of chiasm

increased body temperature, suggests a demyelinating etiology.

Patients with giant cell arteritis (GCA) may present with *transient visual loss* (amaurosis fugax), *diplopia*, *headache*, *temporal tenderness*, and *jaw claudication*. Many also experience systemic signs of inflammation, such as fevers, chills, weight loss, and polymyalgia rheumatica (PMR) symptoms.

Clinical symptoms of elevated intracranial pressure (ICP) include headache (typically worse on recumbent positioning), *horizontal binocular diplopia* (secondary to cranial nerve six palsy), *transient visual loss*, and *pulsatile tinnitus* (rhythmic whooshing sound in the ears).

Review of Medications

Certain medications may lead to optic neuropathy. Examples include ethambutol, linezolid, amiodarone, isoniazid, cimetidine, vincristine, methotrexate, tacrolimus, and cyclosporine.

Nutritional Status

Alcoholics, patients consuming idiosyncratic diets, and patients with poor GI absorption secondary to intestinal surgery or disease may suffer from poor nutrition and nutritional amblyopia.

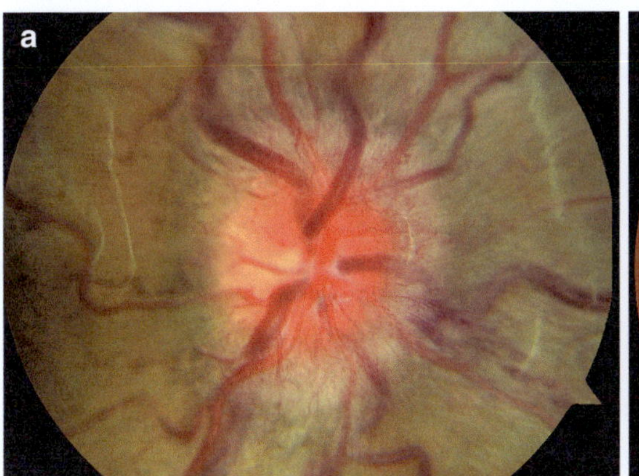 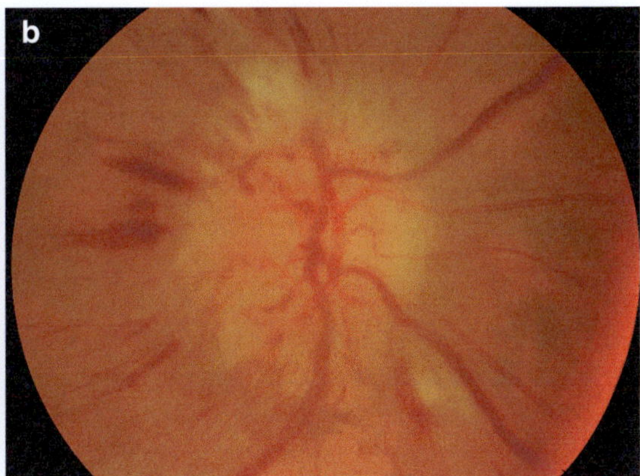

Fig. 36.3 (**a**) Diabetic papillopathy. The optic disc is hyperemic, and the optic disc margins are blurred with obscuration of the retinal blood vessels. The cup-to-disc ratio cannot be determined, and the retinal vessels are dilated and tortuous. (**b**) Non-arteritic ischemic optic neuropathy. The optic disc is hyperemic, and the optic disc margins are blurred with obscuration of the retinal blood vessels. Flame-shaped hemorrhages are seen. The cup-to-disc ratio cannot be determined, and the retinal blood vessels are attenuated

Deficiency of multiple B vitamins should be evaluated in such cases.

Vascular Risk Factors

Hypertension, hypercholesterolemia, and diabetes may put patients at higher risk of suffering from diabetic papillopathy or NAION (Fig. 36.3a, b).

History of Malignancy

A history of malignancy raises the suspicion of metastatic or infiltrative disease of the afferent visual pathway. Carcinomatous meningitis or metastatic lesions compressing or infiltrating the optic nerves or chiasm may result in optic neuropathy. Paraneoplastic optic neuropathies should also be considered.

Family History

Obtaining a careful family history of vision loss can provide clues to hereditary optic neuropathies and glaucoma.

Exposure to Pets

A scratch or a bite from a cat, particularly a kitten, may transmit *Bartonella henselae*, the organism responsible for cat scratch fever, which may cause neuroretinitis. Children who accidentally ingest dog, cat, or fox feces or adults who eat uncooked meat or raw vegetables may develop a nematode optic neuritis from *Toxocara* species.

Physical Examination

Visual Acuity

Visual acuity should be tested with the patient's prescription glasses. Visual acuity may be variably affected in optic neuropathy.

Color Vision

Color vision may be assessed using the Hardy-Rand-Rittler (HRR) color plates which are more sensitive for acquired dyschromatopsia than are Ishihara color plates. Alternatively, red desaturation is assessed by having the patient view a red object with each eye separately and asking them to identify any desaturation of the red color. Color vision is affected in most acquired optic neuropathies. It is relatively spared in ischemic optic neuropathy and glaucoma. Retinal pathology may be associated with color vision abnormalities as well. However, retinal pathologies affecting color vision usually impact visual acuity to a lesser degree than optic neuropathies affecting color vision.

Pupils

The direct pupillary response may be sluggish in optic neuropathy. If only one eye is affected by optic neuropathy, a relative afferent pupillary defect (RAPD) may be detected by the swinging flashlight test. However, when both eyes are affected by optic neuropathy, the swinging flash-light test may not reveal an RAPD.

Fundus Examination

A direct ophthalmoscope, indirect ophthalmo-scope, or slit lamp may be used to assess the appearance of the optic nerve and fundus. The optic nerve is examined for color, contour, cup/disc ratio, and circumference. The vitreous, mac-ula, vasculature, and peripheral fundus are exam-ined for vitreous cells, subtle macular changes, emboli, retinal vascular sheathing, snow banking, and retinitis.

Color

A normal healthy optic nerve head is orange/pink in appearance (see Fig. 36.1). Pallor of the optic nerve head is an indication of axonal death (Fig. 36.4). Following axonal injury, it typically takes 3–4 weeks for the optic nerve to become pale in appearance. Temporal pallor in particular is indicative of damage to the papil-lomacular bundle and correlates with cecocen-tral scotomas.

A normal optic nerve head has sharp borders between the outer rim of the optic nerve head and the surrounding retina. Blurred optic disc mar-gins suggest optic disc edema, though optic disc drusen may have a similar appearance. Optic disc edema may be diffuse or segmental.

Cup/Disc Ratio

The disc of the optic nerve is the visible distal portion of the optic nerve head after it passes through the scleral opening or lamina cribrosa. The cup is the pale excavated center of the optic nerve head and corresponds to the absence of neuroretinal tissue. The cup/disc (C/D) ratio can be estimated based on the vertical diameter of the cup and disc. A normal C/D ratio is smaller than 0.4. Larger C/D ratios are suspicious for glau-coma particularly if there is asymmetry of the C/D ratio between the two eyes (Fig. 36.5).

Size

The normal optic nerve head is approximately 1500 µm in vertical diameter. Optic disc size should be considered when evaluating patients for glaucoma and ischemic optic neuropathy.

Characteristic Appearance of the Disc in Common Optic Neuropathies

NAION

When seen early, this condition commonly pres-ents with a *swollen* and *hyperemic* optic nerve head, typically with splinter hemorrhages at the disc margin. The retinal arteries are focally nar-rowed near the disc. Over the course of several days, the hyperemic swelling turns to pallid swelling. The swelling, hyperemia, and pallor are frequently segmental. A *small C/D ratio* and small optic nerve head predispose patients to this condition. A small C/D ratio in the unaffected eye is supportive of NAION.

Arteritic Anterior Ischemic Optic Neuropathy AION/GCA

A chalk white or *pale swollen* optic nerve head with *cotton wool spots and/or cilioretinal artery occlusion* suggests GCA. Additional findings include choroidal ischemia and delayed choroi-dal filling on fluorescein angiography. A normal or large C/D ratio in the unaffected eye is sup-portive of AION rather than NAION.

Optic Neuritis

Two-thirds of adult cases of optic neuritis present in a retrobulbar fashion, displaying no clinical abnormalities of the optic nerve head. One third of patients present with optic disc swelling. In childhood, most optic neuritis presents with optic disc swelling. In patients suspected of demyelin-ating optic neuritis, the contralateral fundus should be carefully inspected for optic disc pallor or nerve fiber layer thinning with red-free light indicating prior subclinical optic neuritis.

Uveitis

Passive optic disc edema may occur secondary to uveitis. In syphilis, sarcoid, Behçet's disease, Toxoplasmosis, and Chikungunya virus uveitis may accompany optic neuritis.

Optic Disc Drusen (Pseudopapilledema)

Deposits of extracellular protein (optic disc dru-sen) that progressively calcifies in the optic nerve head may cause optic nerve head elevation and the appearance of optic disc edema. Unlike true

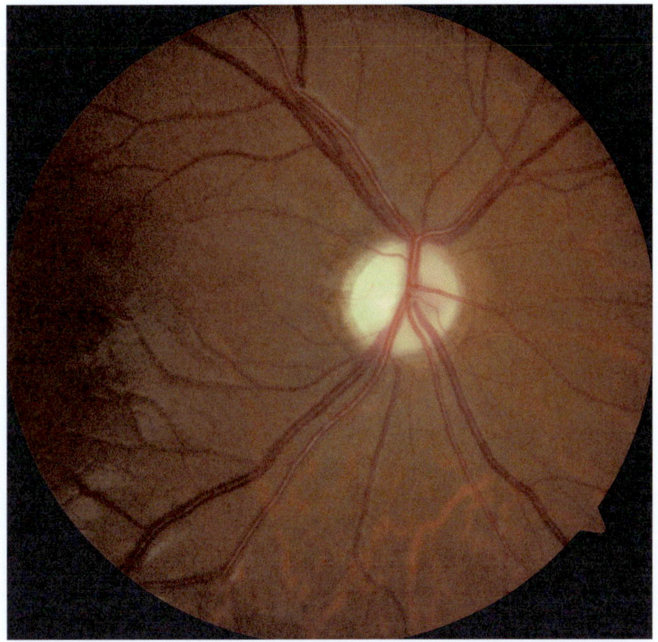

Fig. 36.4 Optic disc pallor. The optic nerve head is pale and optic disc margins are sharp. The cup-to-disc ratio cannot be determined. The retinal blood vessels are attenuated

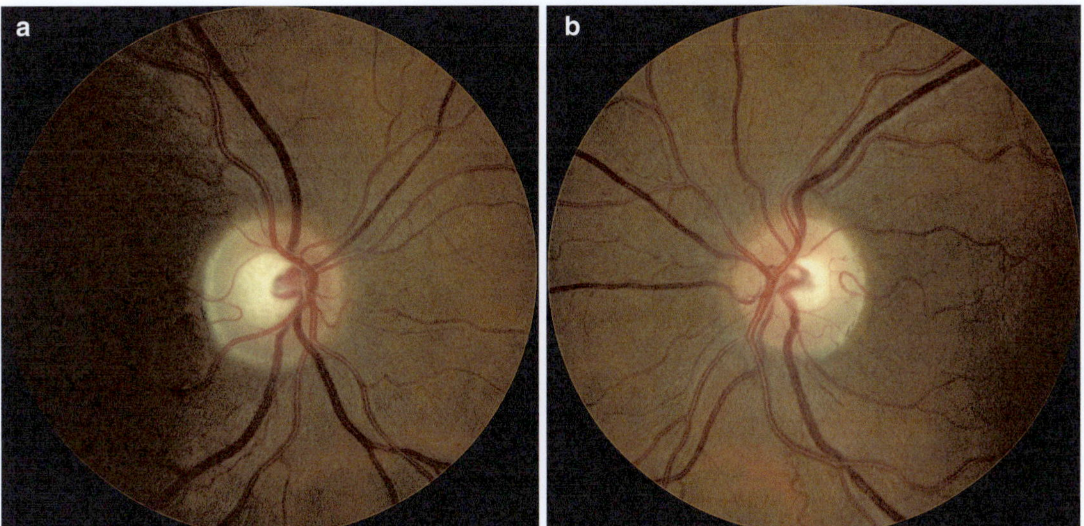

Fig. 36.5 (**a, b**) Cup-to-disc asymmetry. The cup-to-disc ratio is 0.55 in the right eye and 0.25 in the left eye. Cup-to-disc asymmetry is suspicious for glaucoma

disc edema, optic disc drusen will not cause obscuration of the peripapillary retina vessels (Fig. 36.6). Ultrasound, CT scan, autofluorescence, and OCT can help distinguish pseudopapilledema caused by optic disc drusen from true optic disc edema. As the patient gets older, the drusen may erupt thru the disc surface where they appear as small spherules.

Optic Disc Pallor

Disc pallor indicates longevity of optic nerve damage (at least 3–4 weeks) (Fig. 36.4).

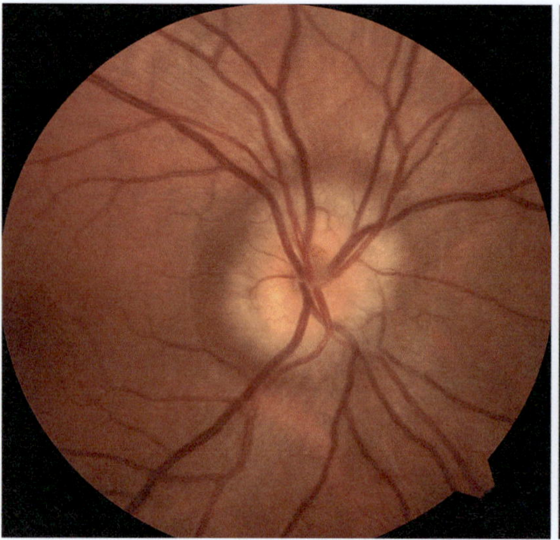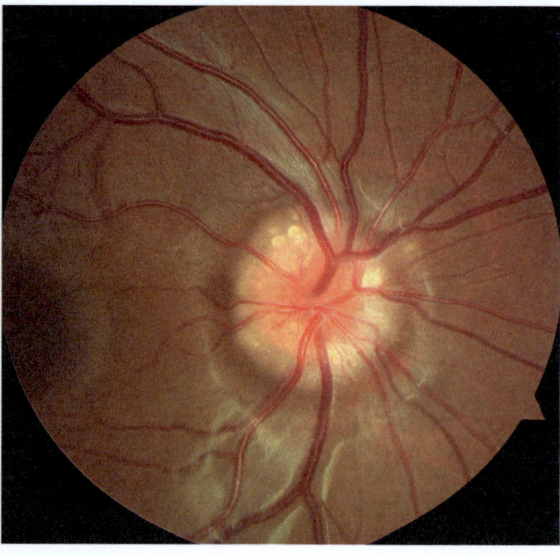

Fig. 36.6 Optic disc drusen. Hyaline bodies deposit in the optic nerve causing optic nerve head elevation. There is early bifurcation of the retinal blood vessels and the vessels are not obscured. The drusen may be buried (seen in **a**) or visible (seen in **b**)

Temporal Pallor

Temporal pallor indicates damage to the papillo-macular fibers, which correlates with cecocentral scotomas on visual field testing and poor visual acuity (see Fig. 36.2b). Examples of conditions leading to temporal pallor include toxic/nutritional, hereditary, and inflammatory optic neuropathies.

Sectoral Pallor

Sectoral pallor indicates localized damage and may be seen in NAION.

Pseudo-Foster-Kennedy Syndrome

In Pseudo-Foster-Kennedy syndrome, one optic nerve head is *pale* and the other is *swollen*. This condition mimics the *Foster-Kennedy syndrome* in which a large frontal lobe tumor causes chronic compression and optic atrophy of one optic nerve (seen as pallor) and elevated intracranial pressure (seen as optic disc edema in the contralateral eye). Pseudo-Foster-Kennedy syndrome is frequently seen in sequential NAION, in which a previous NAION has resulted in optic nerve pallor in one eye and an acute NAION causes optic disc edema in the contralateral eye.

Pallor with Cupping

Disc pallor with cupping may be seen in patients with previous AION, compressive optic neuropathy, hereditary optic neuropathy, or methanol poisoning (Fig. 36.7).

Visual Field Testing (Also See Chap. 18)

Optic neuropathy is associated with visual field defects, which can be assessed by using confrontation visual field testing. The defects may be confirmed and better defined by automated perimetry using Humphrey visual field, Octopus perimetry, or manual Goldmann visual field testing (Fig. 36.8).

Visual Field Patterns in Optic Neuropathy

Certain patterns of visual field loss are more characteristic of optic nerve lesions than lesions of the retina or lesions posterior to the optic nerves. These defects correspond anatomically to the reti-

Fig. 36.7 Optic disc pallor with cupping. The optic nerve has a cup-to-disc ratio of 0.8 with pallor of the neuroretinal rim. The optic disc margins are sharp. This type of cupping may be seen in conditions such as resolved arteritic ischemic optic neuropathy, compressive optic neuropathy, hereditary optic neuropathy, or methanol poisoning

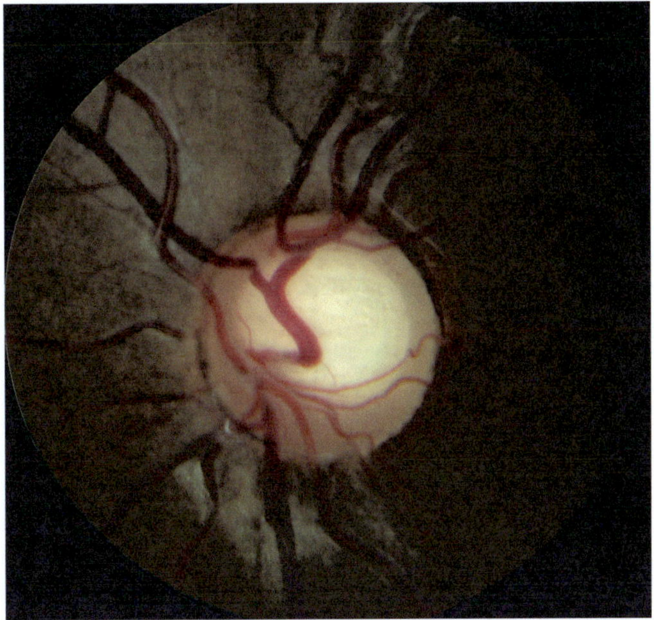

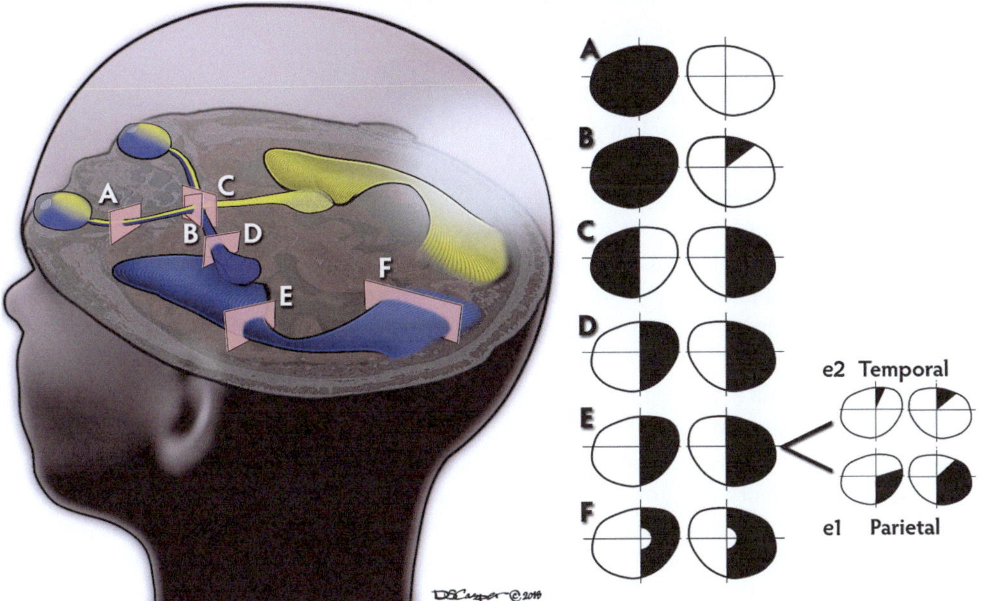

Fig. 36.8 Common visual field defects by anatomical location along the visual pathway (note: the visual field defects have been simplified for illustrative purposes). (**a**) Optic nerve lesion resulting in monocular visual field defect. (**b**) Junctional scotoma (ipsilateral monocular scotoma with contralateral superotemporal defect) due to anterior chiasmal lesions affecting the ipsilateral optic nerve and contralateral inferonasal fibers located in Wilbrand's knee. (**c**) Chiasmal lesion resulting in bitemporal hemianopia. (**d**) Optic tract lesion resulting in a contralateral homonymous hemianopia. (**e**) Parietotemporal lesion resulting in contralateral homonymous hemianopia. (**e1**) Parietal lobe lesion resulting in contralateral homonymous inferior defect. (**e2**) Temporal lobe lesion resulting in contralateral homonymous superior quadrant defect ("pie in the sky"). (**f**) Occipital lobe lesion resulting in contralateral homonymous hemianopia with macular sparing

nal nerve fiber layer and most commonly respect the *horizontal meridian* (See Figs. 15.9 and 15.10).

Cecocentral scotomas extend from fixation temporally toward the blind spot (15° temporal to fixation). This defect corresponds anatomically to the papillomacular nerve fiber bundle, the area between the macula and optic nerve head, and is more commonly seen in hereditary, toxic, nutritional, and inflammatory optic neuropathies.

Aruate scotomas extend nasally from the area of the blind spot and are limited to the superior or inferior hemifield. This defect corresponds anatomically to hemispheric nerve fiber layer defects and is commonly associated with glaucoma, optic nerve head drusen, and NAION. Glaucomatous field defects typically have a predilection for the superior hemifield, while NAION has a predilection for the inferior hemifield.

A *nasal step* is a peripheral contraction or scotoma that is located in the nasal field and extends along the horizontal meridian. This defect corresponds anatomically to a temporal nerve fiber layer defect in the arcuate bundles, which end at the horizontal retinal raphe. A nasal step is commonly seen in glaucoma.

A *temporal wedge* scotoma extends from a temporal area to the blind spot within a hemifield. This defect corresponds anatomically to nasal retinal nerve fibers entering the optic nerve and may be seen in glaucoma or in nasal optic nerve hypoplasia.

An *altitudinal* scotoma is limited to one hemifield and corresponds anatomically to the nerve fiber layer within the opposite hemifield. This type of scotoma also occurs as a consequence of the horizontal retinal raphe and commonly occurs in glaucoma and ischemic optic neuropathy. Glaucomatous altitudinal defects typically have a predilection for the superior hemifield, while ischemic optic neuropathies show a predilection for the inferior hemifield.

Enlargement of the normal blind spot can be seen in any type of disc swelling such as papilledema, papillitis, disc edema from compression or infiltration, vein occlusion, or congenital anomaly of the disc. Acquired disorders of the outer retina such as the acute idiopathic blind spot enlargement syndrome and the multiple evanescent white dot syndrome (see Chap. 27) can also enlarge the blind spot.

Visual Field Patterns Not Consistent with Optic Neuropathy

A generalized decrease in field sensitivity suggests media opacities such as corneal, lenticular, or vitreous opacities. Ring scotomas are seen in retinal dystrophies, while central scotomas that are not connected to the blind spot are most frequently caused by retinal damage. Defects respecting the vertical meridian are caused by lesions anatomically located at or posterior to the optic chiasm. Respect for the vertical meridian implies the defect abuts the vertical meridian and stops there abruptly, like a step or step-off (i.e., the defect does not slope toward or slope over the vertical meridian).

The location and pattern of visual field defects may provide very accurate information as to the pathologic location (Fig. 36.8).

Bitemporal Hemianopia

Defects which are bitemporal in location, respecting the vertical meridian, indicate chiasmal involvement and are typically compressive or infiltrative in origin. Bitemporal visual field defects always require neuroimaging.

Junctional Scotoma

The junctional scotoma of Traquair is a unilateral superotemporal scotoma. This scotoma is typically seen in conjunction with a contralateral central or cecocentral scotoma in the setting of a compressive lesion on the inferonasal aspect of the optic nerve at its junction with the chiasm. In patients presenting with a cecocentral or central scotoma in one eye, it is imperative to inspect the other eye for an upper temporal defect (indicating a chiasmal lesion rather than an isolated optic neuropathy). Neuroimaging is required in such cases.

Homonymous Hemianopia

Homonymous hemianopias are visual field defects located on the same side of the vertical meridian in each eye and anatomically correlate to lesions posterior to the optic chiasm: the optic tract, geniculate body, the geniculo-calcarine pathway, or occipital lobe. For example, in a right hemianopic defect, both the right and left eyes will exhibit a right-sided visual field defect (caused by a left-sided lesion). All homonymous hemianopic visual field defects require neuroimaging.

Categorization of Common Optic Neuropathies

Acute Unilateral Optic Neuropathy with Disc Swelling

Optic Neuritis/Papillitis

Multiple Sclerosis/Neuromyelitis Optica
See section on acute unilateral optic neuropathy without disc swelling.

Post-Viral Optic Neuritis
Optic neuritis in the pediatric population frequently occurs following a viral illness such as measles, mumps, varicella, pertussis, or mononucleosis. Postvaccination optic neuritis may also occur in children. Post-viral and postvaccination optic neuritis is frequently bilateral and tends to be associated with a significant decrease in visual acuity, dyschromatopsia, and ocular pain. Prognosis for recovery is typically very good. Scanning of the brain, spinal tap, and search for viral etiology is indicated.

Syphilitic Optic Neuritis
Ocular involvement by syphilis may involve any part of the eye and more frequently occurs in secondary and tertiary syphilis. Syphilitic optic neuritis frequently presents with acute or subacute visual loss, optic disc edema, and blind spot enlargement on visual field testing. It may be accompanied by retinitis, retinal vasculitis, or uveitis. Visual prognosis is good if treatment (IV penicillin G with or without adjuvant corticosteroid treatment) is initiated promptly.

Sarcoidosis
Systemic sarcoidosis may result in anterior uveitis, posterior uveitis, retinal vascular sheathing (candle wax dripping), and optic neuropathy. In sarcoid disc infiltration, the nerve head takes on a "lumpy-bumpy" appearance, and blood vessels of the optic nerve may be infiltrated, causing sarcoid vasculitis. Sarcoid can also infiltrate the retrobulbar nerve and optic nerve meninges. Optic nerve involvement is frequently subacute but may also be chronic progressive. Sarcoidosis-related optic nerve involvement may also be due to passive disc edema from sarcoid uveitis or papilledema. In the majority of cases, simultaneous inflammation of other ocular structures does not occur. Visual field loss is frequently in the distribution of the papillomacular bundle, but other optic nerve-related visual field defects may be seen as well. Optic nerve involvement may be unilateral or bilateral; when sarcoidosis involves the chiasm, bitemporal visual field loss is typical. Treatment with high-dose corticosteroids or stronger immunosuppression may be required.

Neuroretinitis
Neuroretinitis is an inflammation of the optic nerve and neural retina, which presents with decreased visual acuity, central or cecocentral scotomas, optic disc edema, and a macular star (see Fig. 27.2). The pathophysiology is believed to be inflammation of optic disc vasculature leading to leakage of exudate into the peripapillary retina. The macular star pattern likely results from the lipid-rich component of the exudate penetrating into the outer plexiform layer of the macula. The aqueous fluid portion collects below the neurosensory retina and can be visualized on OCT.

The underlying cause of neuroretinitis may be infectious or idiopathic. Infectious neuroretinitis is usually due to *Bartonella*, following a cat scratch or bite, and may be accompanied by lymphadenopathy, headache, fever, and fatigue. Other infectious etiologies which may cause neuroretinitis include syphilis, Lyme disease, Rocky Mountain spotted fever, toxoplasmosis, toxocariasis, histoplasmosis, and leptospirosis. Visual acuity is often diminished to the 20/200 range in the acute phase due to macular edema; however, prognosis is typically good.

Ischemic Optic Neuropathy

Non-arteritic Anterior Ischemic Optic Neuropathy

Non-arteritic anterior ischemic optic neuropathy (NAION) is the second most common cause of optic neuropathy in older adults (after glaucoma). Its pathophysiology is incompletely understood. Age of onset is usually after age 45, although rare cases have been seen in children and young adults. There is no sex predilection. NAION is more common in Caucasians than African Americans, likely reflecting larger optic disc cup sizes in more pigmented individuals, which may offer some degree of protection.

Ocular Complaints

Patients with NAION complain of acute-to-subacute vision loss in one eye, typically noted upon awakening. Pain with globe motion is typically not seen in NAION, although some patients complain of a mild ache. Vision and visual fields may worsen over subsequent days to weeks, and blurring or clouding in a particular area of the visual field is often described, most frequently inferiorly.

Evaluation of a Patient with Suspected NAION

Physical Exam

Visual acuity is variably affected though typically it is in the 20/50–20/100 range but may also be better. Visual acuity in NAION is generally better than that seen in the arteritic form.

VF defects may include any optic neuropathy-type defect. Inferior altitudinal defects are most common, followed by superior altitudinal loss.

Color vision generally correlates with visual acuity but tends to be affected to a lesser degree than in demyelinating optic neuropathy.

Pupillary reaction is typically sluggish in the affected eye. If only one eye is affected, an RAPD will be seen.

Optic disc appearance in acute NAION is characterized by edema (sometimes segmental), hyperemia, disc hemorrhages, and arteriolar narrowing. The presence of pallid edema, cotton wool spots, or cilioretinal artery occlusion should raise suspicion for giant cell arteritis. Both the affected and unaffected eye are frequently found to have a small optic nerve head and small C/D ratio (Fig. 36.9).

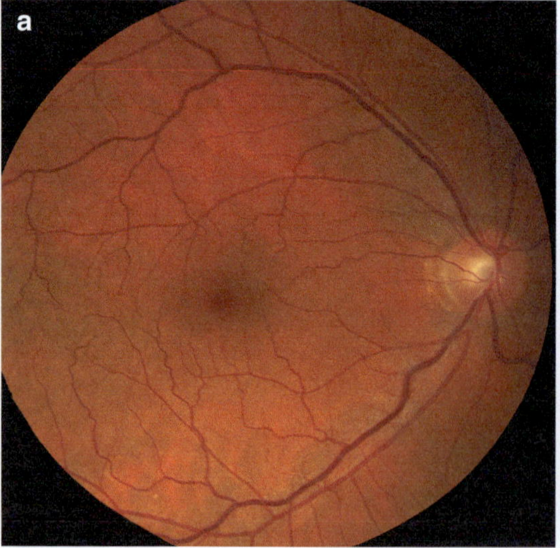
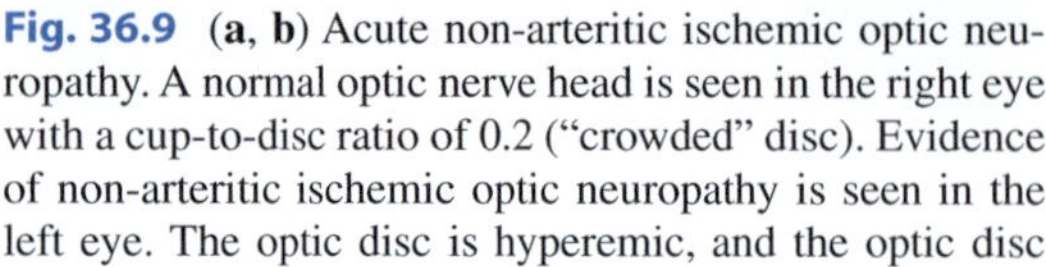
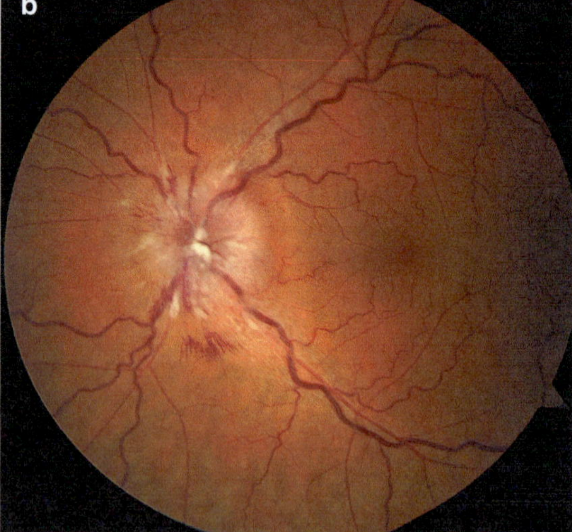

Fig. 36.9 (**a**, **b**) Acute non-arteritic ischemic optic neuropathy. A normal optic nerve head is seen in the right eye with a cup-to-disc ratio of 0.2 ("crowded" disc). Evidence of non-arteritic ischemic optic neuropathy is seen in the left eye. The optic disc is hyperemic, and the optic disc margins are blurred with obscuration of the retinal blood vessels and cotton wool spots. Flame-shaped hemorrhages are seen superonasally and inferiorly. The cup-to-disc ratio cannot be determined, and the retinal blood vessels are tortuous

Risk Factors for NAION

The pathophysiology of NAION is poorly understood, but a number of risk factors have been identified.

A "crowded" disc, characterized by a small optic nerve head and small C/D ratio, is found in almost all cases of NAION. It is believed that crowding of nerve fibers at the lamina cribrosa predisposes the nerve fibers to ischemic events (Fig. 36.10).

Nocturnal Hypotension

There is disagreement as to whether NAION is associated with nocturnal hypotension. Given the possibility, physicians may recommend that patients at risk take antihypertensive medications during the day rather than at night.

Additional Risk Factors

Hyper- or hypotension, diabetes mellitus, hyperlipidemia, anemia, obstructive sleep apnea, hyperhomocysteinemia, coagulopathies, migraine, smoking, optic disc drusen, cataract extraction, and certain medications (e.g., interferon alpha, phosphodiesterase five inhibitors, amiodarone) have all been implicated as possible NAION risk factors.

Risk of NAION to the Contralateral Eye

After a unilateral episode of NAION, the fellow eye has a 15–20% risk of subsequently developing NAION. This risk may increase to 50% if the eye undergoes cataract surgery.

Diagnosis of NAION

The diagnosis of NAION is made clinically, based on history, clinical course, and physical examination. Many other optic neuropathies can be ruled out on this basis. CBC, ESR, CRP, ACE, and RPR/FTA-ABS are obtained, but neuroimaging is necessary only in atypical presentations. Evaluation of modifiable risk factors, such as hypertension, hyperlipidemia, diabetes, and obstructive sleep apnea is indicated in all cases of NAION.

Treatment

No effective treatment has been found for NAION. Left untreated, most cases remain stable after the first few weeks, although improvement or worsening may be seen. Optic nerve head

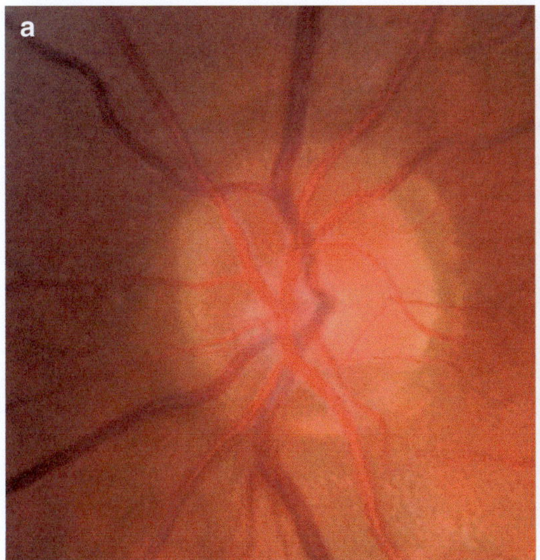
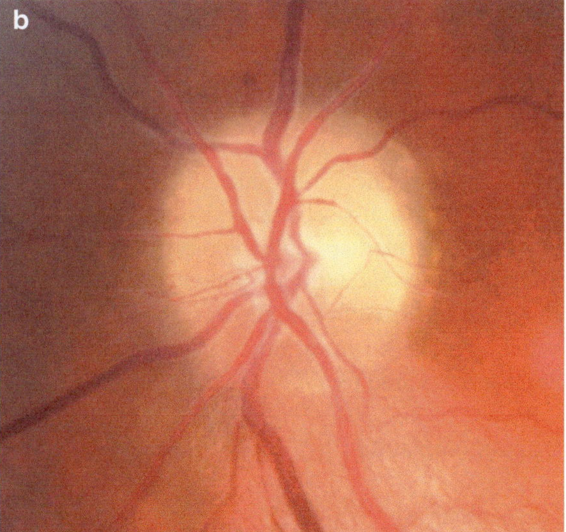

Fig. 36.10 (**a**) A "crowded" disc with a small cup-to-disc ratio is seen prior to an episode of NAION. The neuroretinal rim is pink and the disc margins are sharp. (**b**) The same eye after an episode of NAION. Sectoral pallor of the superior neuroretinal rim is seen. The disc margins are sharp

swelling resolves and pallor develops over a period of weeks.

Arteritic Anterior Ischemic Optic Neuropathy

Arteritic anterior ischemic optic neuropathy is a dreaded complication of giant cell arteritis (GCA) also known as temporal arteritis. GCA is a vision and life-threatening inflammatory condition of medium and large-sized blood vessels. It is critical to recognize the clinical signs and symptoms of GCA in order to establish the diagnosis and rapidly initiate treatment to prevent end-organ damage. Permanent visual loss from arteritic anterior ischemic optic neuropathy is the most common ocular manifestation of GCA. Any ocular manifestation of GCA is considered a medical emergency and should prompt immediate workup and treatment. If left untreated, monocular AION will progress to binocular in 25–50% of patients within 1–14 days.

Giant Cell Arteritis (GCA)

GCA is a systemic vasculitis which affects primarily large and medium-sized arteries. It is a disease of the elderly, occurring primarily in patients older than 50 with incidence rates increasing with each passing decade. The median age of onset is 75 years and women are more commonly affected.

Polymyalgia Rheumatica (PMR)

PMR is another inflammatory condition of the elderly, which presents with muscle stiffness and pain in the pelvic girdle and shoulders. Like GCA, PMR is also characterized by elevated inflammatory markers and overlapping clinical findings. Over one-third of patients with GCA also have PMR. Both conditions respond to systemic steroids; however, much higher treatment doses are required for GCA control.

Ocular Complaints

Loss of Vision

The most common visual complaint in patients with GCA is *loss of vision*. Vision loss in GCA is secondary to ischemia due to reduced perfusion of the optic nerve, choroid, or retina. Vision loss may be transient (also referred to as amaurosis fugax) or permanent. More than half of patients with amaurosis fugax secondary to GCA go on to develop permanent visual loss in an average of 8.5 days. Therefore, amaurosis fugax in a patient with suspected GCA is a medical emergency and should be immediately identified and treated aggressively. Clues that can help distinguish transient vision loss secondary to GCA from other causes of amaurosis fugax include short duration of vision loss (1–2 min), alternation between eyes, vision loss associated with postural changes, and vision loss associated with photopsias.

Diplopia

Diplopia is the second most common ocular manifestation of GCA. Pathophysiological mechanisms for diplopia in GCA include ischemic cranial and brain stem neuropathies and ischemia of the extraocular muscles.

Systemic Complaints

Patients with GCA commonly complain of bilateral headache and craniofacial pain including scalp tenderness, fevers, chills, weight loss, myalgias, fatigue, odontogenic pain, or audiovestibular symptoms. Jaw claudication is the most specific symptom and is due to maxillary artery ischemia. However, this symptom is present in less than half of patients. Less common manifestations include stroke, dementia, psychosis, spinal cord infarctions, seizures, subarachnoid hemorrhage, peripheral neuropathy, myocardial infarction, cardiomyopathy, aortic valve insufficiency, and bowel infarction.

Evaluation of a Patient with Suspected AION

Physical Exam

Visual acuity is typically poor (counting finger range or worse).

VF defects are usually globally depressed, though any optic neuropathy-type VF defects may be seen.

Color vision is often profoundly decreased.

Pupillary reaction is sluggish in the affected eye. If only one eye is affected, an RAPD will be seen.

Optic disc appearance is consistent with pallid optic disc edema. Cilioretinal artery occlusions

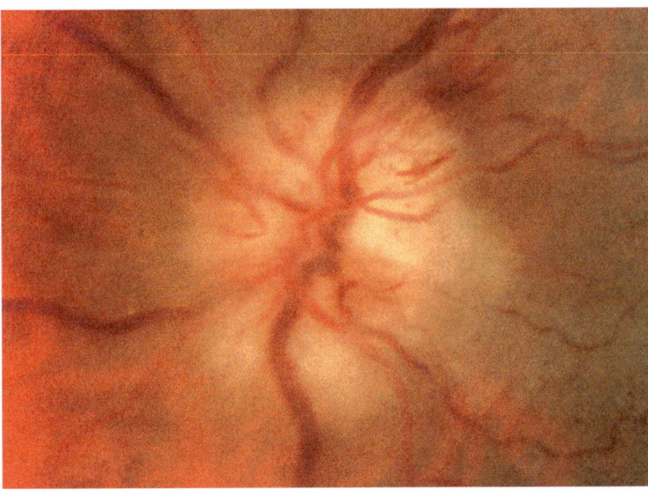

Fig. 36.11 Giant cell arteritis/arteritic ischemic optic neuropathy. The optic disc is pale, and the optic disc margins are blurred with obscuration of the retinal blood vessels. Flame-shaped hemorrhages are seen superotemporally. The cup-to-disc ratio cannot be determined

are pathognomonic for AION. Cotton wool spots or central retinal artery occlusions may be seen. A normal or large-sized cup in the opposite eye (i.e., no evidence of a "crowded disc") is supportive of arteritic rather than non-arteric ischemic optic neuropathy (Fig. 36.11).

Diagnosis of GCA

In 1990, the American College of Rheumatology set forth a classification system for the diagnosis of GCA. In order to make a diagnosis of GCA, the patient must fulfill three out of the following five criteria:

- Age greater than 50 years at disease onset
- New onset of localized headache
- Temporal artery tenderness or decreased temporal artery pulsation
- Elevated erythrocyte sedimentation rate greater than or equal to 50 mm/h
- Temporal artery biopsy sample showing necrotizing arteritis

Other factors taken into account included jaw or tongue claudication and scalp tenderness.

Occult GCA

Occult GCA is a term used to describe patients who do not have symptoms of systemic inflammation but display end-organ damage (such as AION). Such patients may be missed with the classification system above, as they lack systemic symptoms.

Laboratory Studies

The standard laboratory workup for GCA includes erythrocyte sedimentation rate (ESR), C-reactive protein (CRP), and platelet count.

Although ESR may be helpful in the diagnosis of GCA, numerous factors other than GCA may elevate the ESR and should be taken into account including increasing age, female gender, pregnancy, anemia, inflammatory disorders, infarctions, connective tissue disorders, trauma, hypercholesterolemia, and malignancy. Factors that lower ESR include polycythemia, hereditary spherocytosis, and impaired hepatic protein synthesis. While ESR is a useful marker in the diagnosis of GCA, values may be normal in 7–20% of affected patients.

CRP is an inflammatory marker insensitive to age, gender, and hematologic factors and appears to have a higher sensitivity and specificity for GCA. When suspicion for GCA exists, both ESR and CRP are indicated, as the combined sensitivity of detecting GCA has been reported to be over 99%.

Thrombocytosis may be present in approximately half of patients.

Temporal artery biopsy (TAB) is currently the gold standard of diagnosis of GCA and may be performed by vascular surgeons, neurosurgeons, or ophthalmologists. Practitioners differ in their preference of unilateral vs. bilateral biopsy. Characteristic pathological findings on TAB include panarteritis with lymphocyte and macrophage infiltration, disruption of the internal elastic lamina, and thickening of the intima. When a diagnosis of GCA is suspected, it is prudent to treat patients with steroids immediately and arrange for a temporal artery biopsy shortly thereafter. Histopathological acute changes may be seen for 4–6 weeks after initiating steroid treatment. However, even patients on chronic treatment with inactive or healed arteritis may display histopathological changes. We prefer bilateral simultaneous temporal artery biopsies.

Treatment of GCA

Patients with GCA without end-organ damage should be treated with high-dose oral prednisone or IV methylprednisolone for (3 days before switching to high-dose oral prednisone) immediately, in order to suppress inflammation and prevent life-threatening and vision-threatening complications. With visual loss or amaurosis fugax thought to be secondary to GCA, we prefer to start with IV methylprednisolone and switch to high-dose oral prednisone in 3–5 days. Within days of initiation of treatment, systemic symptoms of GCA recede. There is disagreement among neuro-ophthalmologists regarding the decision to treat AION with oral steroids or IV steroids. Currently, no randomized controlled trials address this issue, and retrospective studies have demonstrated inconsistent results. Due to the risk of dangerous systemic complications from high-dose IV steroids and the fragility of the elderly patient population, many practitioners recommend initiating therapy with IV solumedrol in an inpatient setting. Once systemic symptoms of GCA have abated, visual symptoms have stabilized, and the inflammatory markers are low, GCA is considered to be controlled. This may take several weeks, after which a prolonged steroid taper is begun.

While undergoing treatment for GCA, patients must be monitored and treated for complications arising from systemic steroids including osteoporosis, peptic ulcer disease, hypertension, and diabetes.

Post General Surgery Anterior Ischemic Optic Neuropathy

Ischemic optic neuropathy with disc swelling may occur immediately following surgical cases under general anesthesia and is thought to be due to ischemia of the optic nerve head (supplied via the short posterior ciliary arteries). Its incidence is highest following coronary artery bypass grafting (CABG), followed by spinal surgery. Patients present with sudden, painless visual loss, often with inferior altitudinal visual field defects. Risk factors are believed to include intraoperative blood loss, hypotension, administration of vasoconstrictive agents, large volumes of intraoperative crystalloid resuscitation, prolonged length of surgery, and systemic peripheral vascular disease. Some advocate immediately correcting postoperative anemia in the setting of ischemic optic neuropathy.

Post Cataract Surgery AION
See section on NAION above.

Optic Disc Drusen-Related AION
Optic nerve head drusen (ONHD) are acellular calcific deposits within the optic nerve head that develop in childhood and worsen throughout adult life. When superficial, they can be easily visualized on fundus examination. However, when buried deep within the substance of the nerve, they are difficult to see and may be mistaken for optic disc edema (pseudo-disc edema) (see Fig. 36.6). ONHD are associated with anomalous vasculature of the optic nerve and small C/D ratios. Unlike true disc edema, there is no obscuration of the retinal vessels exiting the optic nerve. The majority of patients with ONHD are asymptomatic; however, transient visual obscurations and chronic visual field defects may occur. In some patients, buried drusen lead to NAION, retinal vascular occlusions, sub-retinal disc hemorrhages, and peripapillary choroidal neovascularization. B-scan echography is the most sensitive measure of detecting ONHD (Fig. 36.12). However, CT scan, fundus autofluorescence,

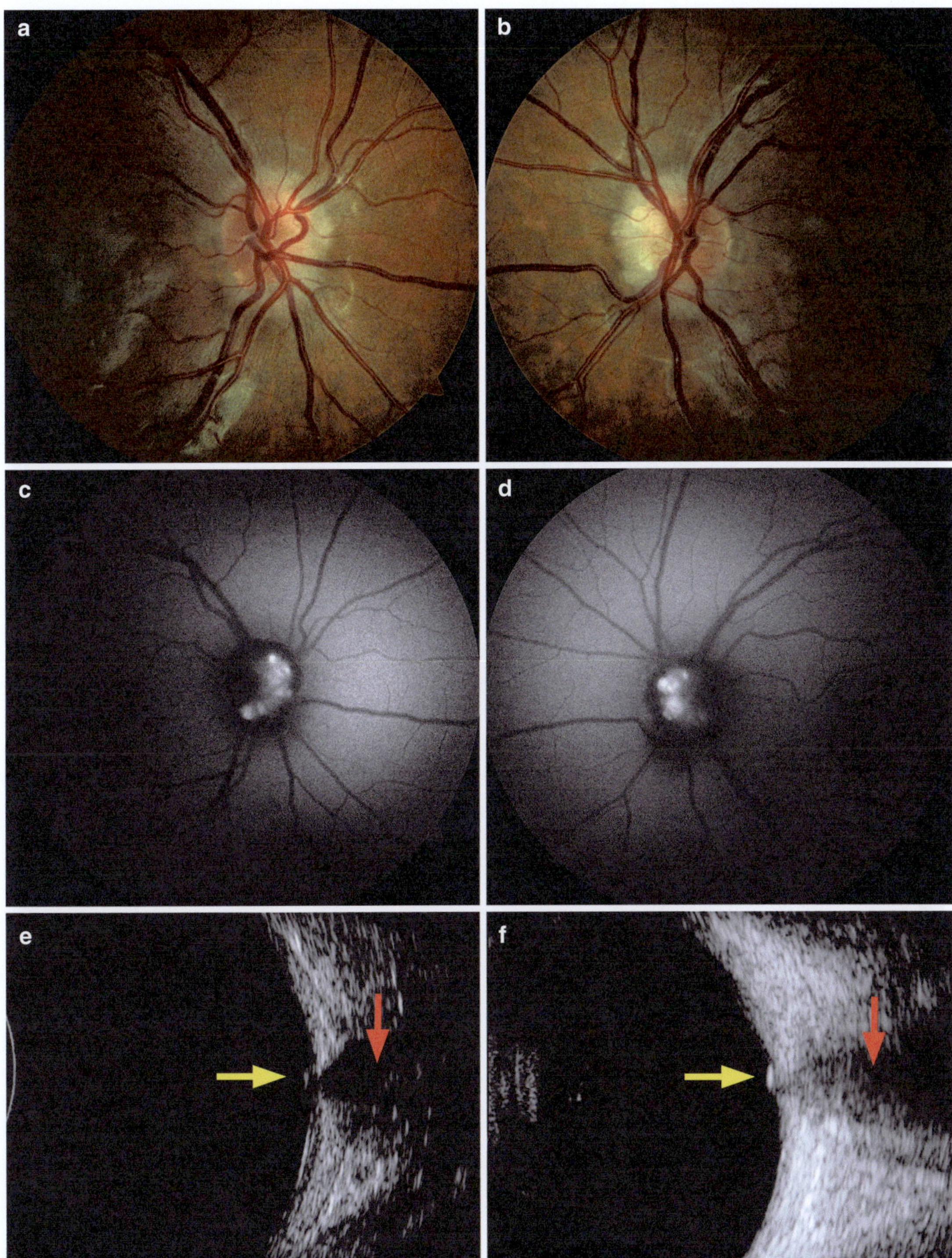

Fig. 36.12 Optic disc drusen. Hyaline bodies located within the optic nerve causing optic nerve head elevation. There is early bifurcation of the retinal blood vessels and the vessels are not obscured. Drusen may be buried, as seen in (**a**), giving the appearance of optic disc edema (pseudo-disc edema), or visible, as seen in (**b–d**). Right and left optic nerves seen in autofluorescence images reveal optic disc drusen correlating to areas of hyperauto-fluorescence (**c**, **d**). Drusen seen on B-scan ultrasound of the right (**e**) and left (**f**) eye, revealing hyperechoic areas within the optic nerve heads consistent with optic disc drusen. Yellow arrows, drusen; red arrows, optic nerve

fluorescein angiography, and OCT can aid in the diagnosis as well. There is currently no treatment for ONHD.

Diabetic Papillopathy

Diabetic papillopathy may occur in type 1 and type 2 diabetics and may be a clinical variant of NAION. Patients present with unilateral or bilateral, acute optic disc edema and vision loss. On exam, the small discs vessels are highly telangiectatic. Visual acuity and visual field loss tend to be less severe than in classical NAION, and visual prognosis is good (Fig. 36.13a–f).

Infiltrative Optic Neuropathy

Primary and, less commonly, secondary malignancies may infiltrate the optic nerve and cause loss of vision. Primary malignancies include optic gliomas, gangliogliomas, capillary hemangiomas, cavernous hemangioblastomas, and malignant teratoid medulloepitheliomas. Secondary malignancies include metastatic carcinoma, lymphoma, and leukemia. Depending on the location of the infiltration of the optic nerve (optic nerve head, orbital, intracanalicular, or intracranial) and the extent of the optic neuropathy, patients may have optic disc edema or pallor on exam. Visual acuity, visual fields, color vision, and pupils may be variably affected. Neuroimaging and lumbar puncture may aid in diagnosis. Optic nerve biopsy may be required in cases in which a diagnosis cannot otherwise be identified.

Sarcoidosis

See section on sarcoidosis.

Optic Nerve Glioma

Optic nerve gliomas are generally benign, low-grade pilocytic astrocytomas (WHO grade 1) affecting children. Malignant optic gliomas are very rare and present as either anaplastic astrocytomas (WHO Grade 3) or glioblastoma multiforme (WHO grade 4) in adults. Optic nerve gliomas of childhood are frequently associated with neurofibromatosis type 1. These hamartomas of the optic nerve may be very slow growing or rapidly progressive (causing proptosis and loss of vision). Management options include observation, chemotherapy, resection, and radiation.

Optic nerve gliomas of adulthood are rapidly progressive and fatal. Chemotherapy and radiation have been shown to prolong survival, but blindness and death generally occur within 1–2 years.

Acute Unilateral Optic Neuropathy Without Disc Swelling

Demyelinating Optic Neuritis

Multiple Sclerosis

Demyelinating optic neuritis (ON) is the most common optic neuropathy affecting young adults (Fig. 36.14). ON is commonly seen in multiple sclerosis (MS) with 38–50% of patients affected by ON during the course of their illness. ON is the presenting feature of MS in 15–20% of patients, making its recognition by the primary care physician critical. Women are more commonly affected than men, and it is uncommon for both eyes to be affected simultaneously.

Ocular Complaints ON is a clinical diagnosis. Patients with optic neuritis complain of subacute vision loss or blurring of vision in one eye. Ocular ache, tenderness, or pain on eye movement occurs in up to 90% of patients and is a sensitive but not specific sign of ON. Patients may complain of worsening vision with elevations of body temperature, for example, when taking a hot shower, exercising, or in warm weather (Uhthoff's phenomenon). Patients may also complain of perceiving flashing lights with eye movement (phosphenes).

Systemic Complaints A careful history of neurological symptoms should be taken as symptoms such as numbness, tingling, clumsiness, and weakness are suggestive of MS.

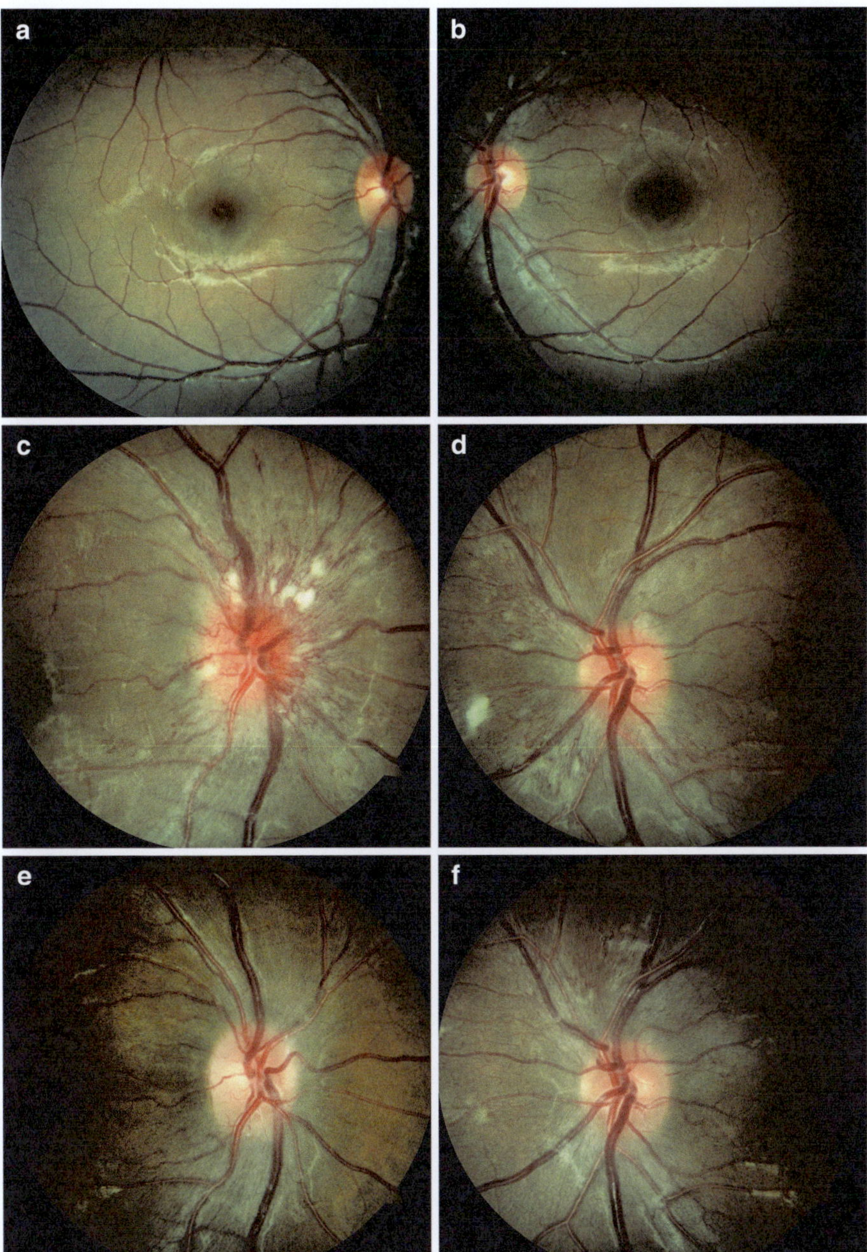

Fig. 36.13 (**a**) Normal right optic nerve head. The neuroretinal rim is pink and the cup-to-disc ratio is 0.2. The optic disc margins are sharp. (**b**) Normal left optic nerve head. The neuroretinal rim is pink and the cup-to-disc ratio is 0.2. The optic disc margins are sharp. (**c–f**) A patient with bilateral diabetic papillopathy. (**c**) Diabetic papillopathy of the right eye. The optic nerve head is hyperemic, and the optic disc margins are blurred with obscuration of the retinal blood vessels. The cup-to-disc ratio cannot be determined, and the retinal vessels are dilated. Cotton wool spots are seen superiorly and temporally. (**d**) Diabetic papillopathy of the left eye. The optic nerve head is hyperemic, and the optic disc margins are blurred with obscuration of the retinal blood vessels. Cotton wool spots are seen nasally. (**e**) Post-diabetic papillopathy of the right eye. The neuroretinal rim is slightly pale and the cup-to-disc ratio is 0.3. The optic disc margins are sharp. (**f**) Post-diabetic papillopathy of the left eye. The neuroretinal rim is slightly pale and the cup-to-disc ratio is 0.2. The optic disc margins are sharp

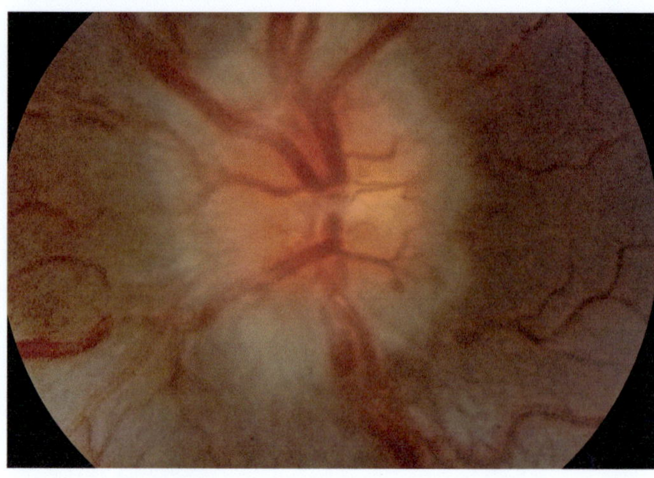

Fig. 36.14 Optic neuritis in multiple sclerosis. The optic disc is hyperemic, and the optic disc margins are blurred with obscuration of the retinal blood vessels. The cup-to-disc ratio cannot be determined, and the retinal blood vessels are dilated. Only one-third of patients with optic neuritis present with optic disc edema, while two-thirds present with retrobulbar optic neuritis

Evaluation of a Patient with Suspected ON/MS

Physical Exam

Visual acuity is variably affected, ranging from 20/20 to no light perception (NLP).

VF defects may include diffuse depression, cecocentral defects, arcuate defects, or combinations of the above.

Color vision is often profoundly and disproportionately affected compared to visual acuity. It is not unusual for patients to see none of the HRR color test plates in the setting of 20/20–20/30 vision.

Pupillary reaction is typically sluggish in the affected eye. If only one eye is affected, an RAPD will be present.

Optic disc appearance is unremarkable in two-thirds of patients (retrobulbar ON) and characterized by disc edema in one-third of patients. The retinal veins may be sheathed due to periphlebitis (Rucker's sign), and there may be pars planitis.

Diagnosis of MS

MRI Orbits with Fat Suppression

MRI of the orbits with fat suppression with and without gadolinium may show optic nerve enhancement but is generally not necessary in order to make a diagnosis.

MRI Brain

MRI of the brain with and without gadolinium should be performed in cases of suspected ON in order to assess the risk of developing MS. The best predictor of developing MS after an episode of ON is the presence of typical white matter lesions on MRI. Early initiation of immunomodulatory therapy may significantly reduce the patient's lifetime morbidity from MS, making early diagnosis critical.

Lumbar Puncture

Lumbar puncture may be useful in the diagnosis but is no longer routinely part of the investigation of MS. The presence of oligoclonal bands and intrathecal IgG production is supportive of MS.

Treatment of MS

The mainstay of ON treatment is based on the Optic Neuritis Treatment Trial (ONTT), a randomized, placebo-controlled clinical trial which compared IV steroids, oral steroids, and placebo. The study concluded that visual recovery was faster with IV steroids vs. placebo. However, there was no difference in final visual acuity. Recovery of vision occurs within weeks and is usually substantial (20/40 or greater). Oral steroids showed no benefit in the speed of recovery or final visual outcome. Based on the results from the ONTT, patients with ON are generally treated with 1 g IV methylprednisolone daily for 3 days followed by an oral prednisone taper over the next 11 days. Oral prednisone alone is not recommended.

Rates of Development of MS

The best predictor of development of MS in patients with optic neuritis is the presence of white matter lesions on brain MRI. Additional risk factors for developing MS include younger age, female sex, Caucasian race, and evidence of periphlebitis on fundus exam. Factors associated with a lower risk of development of MS include isolated optic neuritis without prior episodes of ON or neurologic events, male gender, disc edema, peripapillary hemorrhages, macular exudates, lack of pain, and NLP vision. When encountering lower-risk patients, other etiologies should be investigated.

Neuromyelitis Optica

Neuromyelitis optica (NMO), also known as Devic's disease, is an immune-mediated chronic inflammatory disease of the central nervous system. It was formerly considered a variant of MS but is now considered a distinct clinical entity. NMO involves optic neuritis and transverse or ascending myelitis extending over three or more vertebral segments. Women are more commonly affected than men, and patients are on average 10 years older than MS patients. The clinical course of NMO is frequently relapsing, and brain lesions have a characteristic pattern on MRI.

Ocular Complaints

Patients experience painful subacute loss of vision as in ON/MS. Binocular vision loss is more common in NMO.

Systemic Complaints

Patients may have brainstem symptoms, neuropathic pain, and painful tonic spasms.

Evaluation of a Patient with Suspected ON Associated with Neuromyelitis Optica

Physical Exam
Visual acuity is variably affected, ranging from 20/20 to no light perception (NLP).

VF defects may include diffuse depression, central or cecocentral defects, or localized visual field defects.
Color vision is often profoundly and disproportionately affected compared to visual acuity.
Pupillary reaction is typically sluggish in the affected eye. If both eyes are affected, no RAPD will be seen.
Optic disc appearance is more likely to be consistent with optic disc edema than in ON/MS.

Diagnosis

MRI of the brain and spinal cord with and without contrast should be performed to evaluate for transverse myelitis and brain lesions characteristic for NMO. Laboratory workup generally includes anti-myelin oligodendrocyte glycoprotein (MOG), anti-NMO antibodies, CBC, coagulation serologies, BMP, ESR, blood glucose, B12, folic acid, connective tissue disorder antibodies, urinalysis and sediment, Treponema pallidum particle agglutination assay, paraneoplastic antibodies (CV2/CRMP5, anti-Hu), copper levels, and zinc levels. Cerebrospinal fluid studies include cell count, cytology, protein, lactate, albumin CSF/serum ratio, IgG, IgA, IgM CSF/serum ratio, oligoclonal bands, measles, rubella, and varicella zoster virus.

Acute treatment is generally methylprednisolone followed by an oral taper of prednisone. Long-term immunosuppression is required to help prevent the natural relapsing course, which can lead to devastating neurological consequences. The mainstays of chronic treatment are azathioprine and rituximab.

Acute Compressive Retrobulbar Neuropathy

Pituitary Apoplexy

Pituitary apoplexy is a life-threatening condition, in which a pituitary tumor either hemorrhages or outgrows its blood supply and necroses. Symptoms include sudden onset of headache, nausea, altered level of consciousness, loss of vision, or double vision. Loss of vision may occur due to sudden compression of the optic nerves or chiasm. Compression of the cavernous sinus and cranial nerves III, IV, V, and VI may occur. Sequelae of pituitary apoplexy include subarachnoid hemorrhage and endocrine abnormalities. Endocrine abnormalities, particularly adrenal insufficiency, must be addressed immediately. Extravasation of blood into the subarachnoid space may result in altered level of consciousness, vasospasm, and secondary stroke. Pituitary apoplexy is a neurosurgical emergency.

Posterior Ischemic Optic Neuropathy

Arteritic Posterior Ischemic Optic Neuropathy

See section on arteritic AION.

Post-general Surgery Ischemic Optic Neuropathy

Posterior ischemic optic neuropathy (PION) is less common than AION following general anesthesia surgical cases. PION is thought to be due to ischemia of the intraorbital optic nerve, supplied by pial blood vessels. The incidence of PION is highest following prone spinal surgeries and radical neck dissections. PION may also occur following CABG. Patients present with sudden, painless, perioperative visual loss without optic disc edema (optic disc pallor occurs 4–6 weeks following the acute event). Contrast-enhanced orbital MRI usually reveals restricted diffusion and/or contrast enhancement. PION is likely multifactorial, and risk factors are believed to include intraoperative-prone or head-dependent positioning, surgery lasting longer than 5 hours, anemia, hypotension, increased venous pressure, increased cerebrospinal fluid pressure, crystalloid replacement instead of colloid replacement, and mechanical ocular compression. There is no definitive treatment for PION, but patients have improved following blood transfusion, high-dose corticosteroids, and vasopressors. Visual prognosis following PION is guarded.

Chronic Progressive Unilateral Optic Neuropathy with Disc Swelling

Optic Nerve Sheath Meningioma

Optic nerve sheath meningiomas (ONSM) are rare, benign tumors of the anterior visual pathway. The majority of ONSM originate in the orbit, with the minority originating from within the bony optic canal. Presentation is generally unilateral. Patients present in middle age and woman are more frequently affected than men. ONSM in the pediatric population is rare (4–7% of ONSM), is frequently associated with neurofibromatosis 2, and shows no sex predilection. Clinical presentation is characterized by slowly progressive painless visual loss, visual field defects, and color desaturation. Headaches occur in up to half of patients. On examination, patients may exhibit combined optic disc edema and pallor, while optociliary shunt vessels are seen in approximately one-third of patients (Fig. 36.15). Orbital signs such as proptosis, chemosis, limitations of extraocular motility, and orbital pain may also occur. Diagnosis is made based on imaging, with gadolinium-enhanced orbital MRI being the gold standard. CT scans may aid in the diagnosis through identification of calcifications within the tumor. Treatment options include careful monitoring, surgical resection, radiation therapy, and combined surgery and radiation. Advances in radiation therapy have made this treatment option safer, more effective, and more widely used in recent years.

Sarcoidosis

See section on sarcoidosis.

Thyroid Eye Disease (See Also Chap. 29)

Thyroid eye disease (TED) is an autoimmune orbital inflammation, which most frequently occurs in the setting of autoimmune hyperthyroidism (though it may also occur in hypothyroid or euthyroid states). Clinical signs of TED

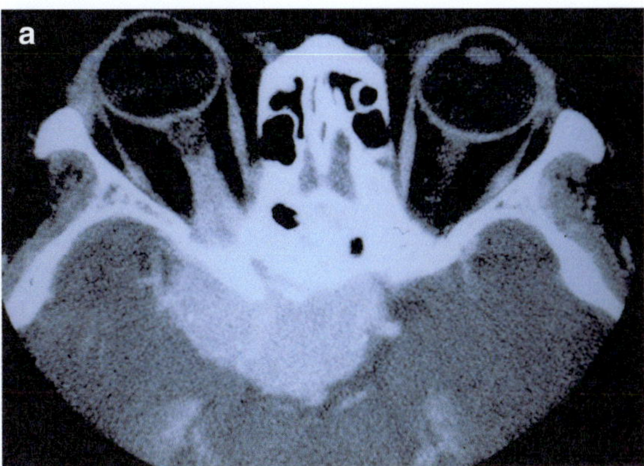

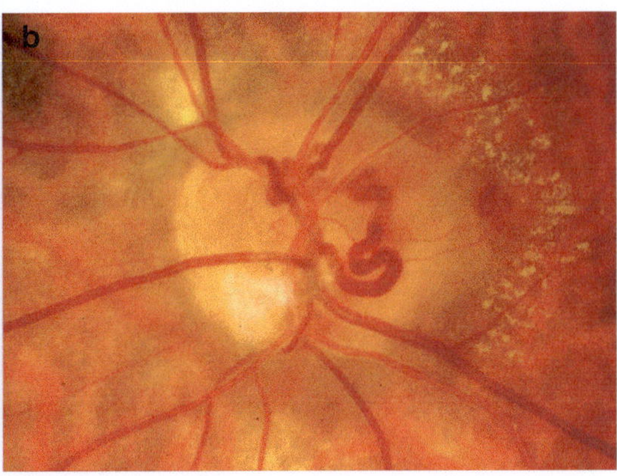

Fig. 36.15 (**a**) Axial contrast-enhanced orbital CT scan revealing medial sphenoid ridge meningioma extending down the optic nerve sheath into the orbit (tram-tracking). (**b**) Fundus photograph revealing optociliary shunt vessels and exudate from chronic central retinal venous insufficiency

include exophthalmos, eyelid retraction, conjunctival injection, chemosis, restrictive strabismus, periocular edema, and eyelid lag on downgaze. Patients may experience blurry vision, double vision, eye burning, and pain on eye movement and may notice that their eyes appear to protrude. Optic neuropathy is a sight-threatening complication of TED and is an ocular emergency. Diagnosis of optic neuropathy includes orbital imaging (MRI and CT) to evaluate for compression of the optic nerve by enlarged extraocular muscles at the orbital apex, visual field testing, color vision evaluation, and OCT. In cases of progressive optic neuropathy not responsive to the usual medical treatments, surgical orbital decompression may be necessary.

Orbital Tumors

See Chap. 34.

Chronic Progressive Unilateral Optic Neuropathy Without Disc Swelling

Intracranial Meningioma

Intracranial meningiomas may cause compression of the intracranial portion of the optic nerve leading to painless, progressive loss of vision.

Optic Canal Meningioma

See section on optic nerve sheath meningioma.

Pituitary Adenoma

Pituitary adenomas (PA) are the most common parachiasmal tumors. Nonsecretory PA are frequently undiagnosed until visual loss is experienced. Prolactinomas may cause impotence in males and infertility in females. *Other secretory adenomas may manifest themselves as acromegaly or Cushing's disease.* Visual loss is frequently bilateral, gradually progressive, and asymmetric. The visual field defects in PA are usually greatest above as they compress the anterior visual pathway from below. PA may compress the optic nerve(s), chiasm, optic tract, or combinations of the above, depending on the position of the chiasm and the extension pattern of the tumor. Thus, PA may cause cecocentral/central defects if compressing the optic nerve, a junctional scotoma of Traquair if compressing the nasal optic nerve at its junction with the chiasm (see above, under Visual Field Testing), bitemporal hemianopsia with pure chiasmal compression, and homonymous hemianopsia with compression of the optic tract. In bitemporal hemianopsia, the optic discs may exhibit band or bow-tie atrophy (Fig. 36.16), i.e., the temporal and nasal portions of the discs are pale. Unlike PA, craniopharyngiomas compress

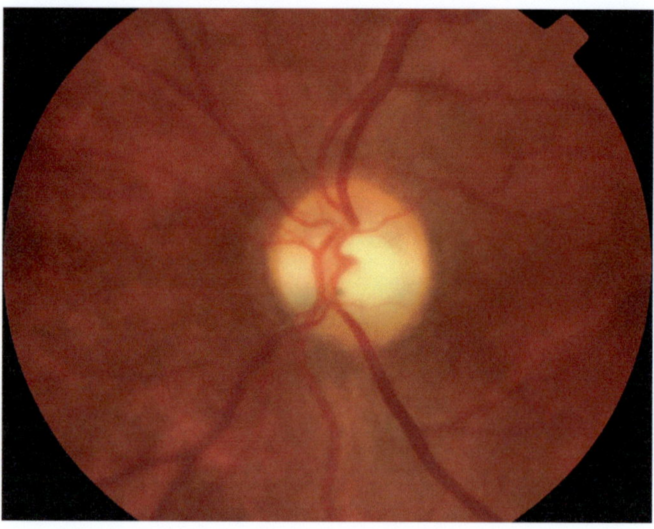

Fig. 36.16 Bow-tie atrophy. The neuroretinal rim of the left eye is pale nasally (left) and temporally (right) due to nerve fiber layer atrophy of the nasal retina. The optic disc margins are sharp and there are no hemorrhages

the anterior visual pathway from above, producing visual field defects greatest below.

Autosomal Dominant Optic Atrophy

Autosomal dominant optic atrophy (ADOA) is the most common of the hereditary optic neuropathies. Large cup-to-disc ratios may be seen and have been referred to as dominant pseudoglaucoma. Visual loss generally begins within the first decade of life and is progressive. Visual acuity typically remains at 20/200 or better. Visual field testing may reveal cecocentral scotomas due to loss of the papillomacular bundle. The genetic etiology entails a mutation in the OPA1 gene which encodes a mitochondrial-targeted protein. There is currently no approved treatment for ADOA, and goals of care include genetic counseling and low vision therapy.

Sequential Optic Neuropathy

Leber's Hereditary Optic Neuropathy (LHON)

LHON is transmitted by mitochondrial inheritance. Males are more frequently affected than females. Vision loss typically presents in adolescence and young adulthood but may occur later in life. Vision loss is subacute, painless, and frequently sequential (occurring simultaneously or separated by days to months). Visual acuity is typically markedly reduced, and visual field testing reveals scotomas due to loss of the papillomacular fiber bundle. The triad of microtelangiectatic changes of the peripapillary retinal capillaries, thickening of the peripapillary nerve fiber layer, and absence of staining on fluorescein angiography is highly suggestive of LHON. These changes may be seen prior to visual loss. The pathophysiology of LHON involves damage to retinal ganglion cells. There is currently no approved treatment for LHON, and goals of care include genetic counseling and low vision therapy. Trials which involve introducing normal copies of the abnormal mitochondrial DNA by viral vectors are ongoing. Certain forms of LHON may be associated with neurological or cardiac disorders, and EKG and neurologic consultation is therefore advised.

Sequential Demyelinating Optic Neuritis

See section on Multiple Sclerosis and Neuromyelitis Optica.

Bilateral Slowly Progressive Optic Neuropathy

Deficiency and Toxic Optic Neuropathies

Deficiency and toxic optic neuropathies are generally bilateral and symmetric. Due to the symmetric involvement of both optic nerves, a relative afferent pupillary defect is not seen. Cecocentral visual field defects are usually seen, though occasionally purely central defects may be demonstrated with automated perimetry. However, in our opinion, if studied at the tangent screen, a subtle nucleus of depression can be found between fixation and the blind spot. An exception to cecocentral defects is ethambutol toxicity, which may exhibit defects with a bitemporal character. Color vision loss, as measured by HRR color plates, is markedly depressed in excess of visual acuity. The onset is usually gradual and progressive, though some patients report an acute-to-subacute presentation. Pain is extremely uncommon, though in deficiency states that are accompanied by keratopathy some corneal pain may be experienced. The discs usually exhibit temporal pallor from dropout of the papillomacular bundle, though if seen acutely, these entities may rarely exhibit subtle disc edema and even small disc border splinter hemorrhages. Treatment involves discontinuation of the offending agent or supplying the missing vitamins in a bioavailable form. It is important to rule out outer retina problems such as cone dystrophies, occult macular dystrophies, and paraneoplastic and toxic retinopathies via spectral domain and swept source OCT of the macula or multifocal electroretinography. Hereditary optic neuropathies may rarely be confused with toxic or deficiency states and family history and genetic testing may aid in distinguishing these entities. Diagnosis of paraneoplastic etiologies may require blood testing for antibodies to antigens such as collapsin response-mediator protein-5-IgG (CRMP-5-IgG).

Nutritional Amblyopia

Optic neuropathy secondary to poor nutrition, particularly the absence of fresh green vegetables, is referred to as nutritional amblyopia. It occurs in two settings:

- Epidemic nutritional amblyopia (Strachan's syndrome), as occurred in British and American prisoners of the Japanese during World War II or the 1992–1993 Cuban epidemic after the collapse of the Soviet Union. After approximately 4 months of severe nutritional deficiency, patients may experience a superficial keratopathy followed by loss of color vision and acuity, sensorineural hearing loss, and peripheral neuropathy. Not every affected individual gets all the elements of the syndrome. The exact deficiency is unclear, but multiple B vitamin deficiency is suspected.
- The second type are individual or isolated cases secondary to poor nutrition, formerly called tobacco-alcohol amblyopia. Neither alcohol nor tobacco abuse is necessarily involved; if good nutrition or vitamin supplementation is given, the condition will not develop or will resolve, in spite of alcohol or tobacco use. However, alcohol and cigar use may be risk factors that predispose certain individuals to develop optic neuropathy in the setting of poor nutrition. Most patients present with slowly progressive bilateral painless loss of color vision, decreased visual acuity, and cecocentral scotomas. Some patients report acute-to-subacute loss of vision. Inability to identify the color of traffic lights is a frequent first symptom. Temporal disc pallor and dropout of the nerve fiber layer in the papillomacular bundle are observed and can be confirmed on OCT testing.

If caught early and treated with a diet rich in green vegetables, multiple B vitamin supplementation, and abstinence from alcohol (in cases of heavy alcohol use), most patients will experience some recovery.

Vitamin B12 Deficiency

B12 deficiency may present with slowly progressive painless loss of visual acuity, loss of color vision, cecocentral scotomas, and optic atrophy. The optic nerve changes may occur prior to the development of macrocytic anemia, myelopathy, and neuropsychiatric symptoms. In addition to classic pernicious anemia, B12 deficiency may be caused by veganism, abdominal surgery, disease or bacterial overgrowth of the stomach or ileum, tapeworms, nitrous oxide exposure, antacids, and oral hypoglycemic agents. Treatment consists of supplementation with parenteral and oral vitamin B12, with the duration of treatment depending on the etiology of the deficiency.

Ethambutol Optic Neuropathy

Up to 1% of patients using ethambutol at World Health Organization recommended doses (primarily for tuberculosis infection) may develop ethambutol optic neuropathy, a dose-dependent toxic optic neuropathy. Effects may be seen as early as 1 month after starting treatment but generally occur after 6 months. Patients generally present with painless loss of acuity, loss of color vision, and cecocentral scotomas. However, visual field defects may also include some bitemporal loss, as experimental studies in primates have shown that ethambutol causes an axonal neuropathy which may affect the chiasm. There are reports of generalized constriction of the visual fields due to ethambutol optic neuropathy as well. Treatment consists of discontinuation of ethambutol. Some authorities suggest zinc supplementation. It may take up to 1 or 2 years for recovery to take place, with some patients experiencing permanent damage.

Other Toxic Optic Neuropathies

Linezolid is an antibiotic used chronically for osteomyelitis and can present with acuity loss, dyschromatopsia, cecocentral scotomas, and temporal disc pallor. Chloramphenicol toxicity may also present similarly. Both of these optic neuropathies may improve over the course of months with discontinuation of the drug. Cobalt/chromium metallosis with loss of vision and hearing, cardiomyopathy, and rash may occur following the placement of a cobalt/chromium hip implant following a failed ceramic implant. Ceramic debris left behind from the prior failed ceramic head grinds down the cobalt/chromium implant, releasing elemental cobalt and chromium into the joint space and the circulation. Initially, the metallosis is toxic to the optic nerve and later affects the outer retina as well. Early recognition with removal of the cobalt/chromium implant and washout of the metallosis from the joint space may result in recovery. This rare conditional may be screened for by plain X-rays of the joint space which reveals a metallic shadow. Tumor necrosis factor alpha inhibitors may cause demyelinization with optic neuritis syndrome. Amiodarone, PDE-5 inhibitors, and cyclosporine have been implicated in cases of NAION.

Compressive Optic Neuropathy

Compressive optic neuropathies are characterized by slow, progressive vision loss and may be caused by intraorbital or intracranial mass lesions. Patterns of visual field loss may aid in identifying the location of the lesion, but neuroimaging is always necessary. Intraorbital causes include optic nerve sheath meningiomas, orbital tumors, and extraocular muscle enlargement in thyroid eye disease. Chiasmal lesions include meningiomas, pituitary tumors, and craniopharyngiomas. Benign and malignant intracranial lesions may cause compression of the intracranial optic nerve. Depending on the cause of compression, visual loss may be unilateral or bilateral.

Papilledema and Post-Papilledema Optic Atrophy

The term "papilledema" is frequently incorrectly used to describe any optic disc edema. Papilledema refers to optic disc swelling secondary to elevated intracranial pressure (Figs. 36.17 and 36.18). Disc swelling in papilledema is usually bilateral but may be unilateral. When papilledema is seen on exam, evaluation of the underlying cause should be performed immediately. Patients may present with headache, neck pain, loss of vision, double vision (from CN VI palsy), transient visual obscurations, and pulsatile tinnitus. In addition to optic disc edema, which is due to backup of axoplasmic transport onto the neuroretinal junction, fundus exam reveals disc hyperemia which represents telangiectasia of the fine capillaries of the disc, venous engorgement, loss of spontaneous venous pulsations, disc hemorrhages, and retinal and/or choroidal folds. Visual field defects may include blind spot enlargement, central defects, and arcuate scotomas. Frequently, acetazolamide is used to lower intracranial pressure, but treatment is largely dependent on the underlying cause.

The field defects in papilledema start as enlarged blind spots and then involve nasal loss with arcuate defects which, with chronicity, encroach on fixation leaving only a temporal island of vision before all vision is lost.

Without treatment, papilledema develops into post-papilledema optic atrophy with pallor and gliosis of the disc, sheathing and narrowing of the retinal vessels, and hard exudates in the macula.

Glaucoma

See Chap. 16.

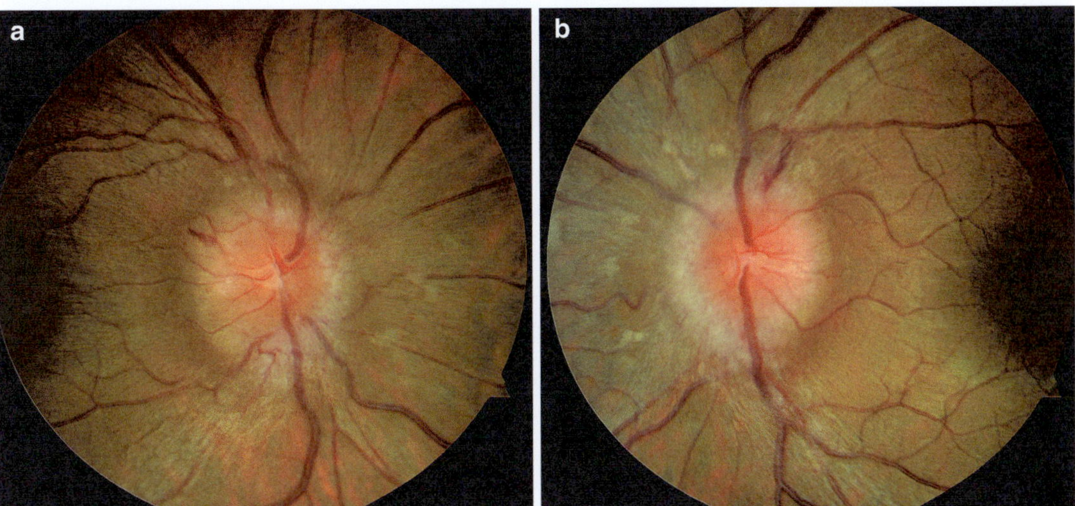

Fig. 36.17 (**a**, **b**) Bilateral papilledema. The optic discs are hyperemic, and the optic disc margins are blurred with obscuration of the retinal blood vessels. The cup-to-disc ratio cannot be determined

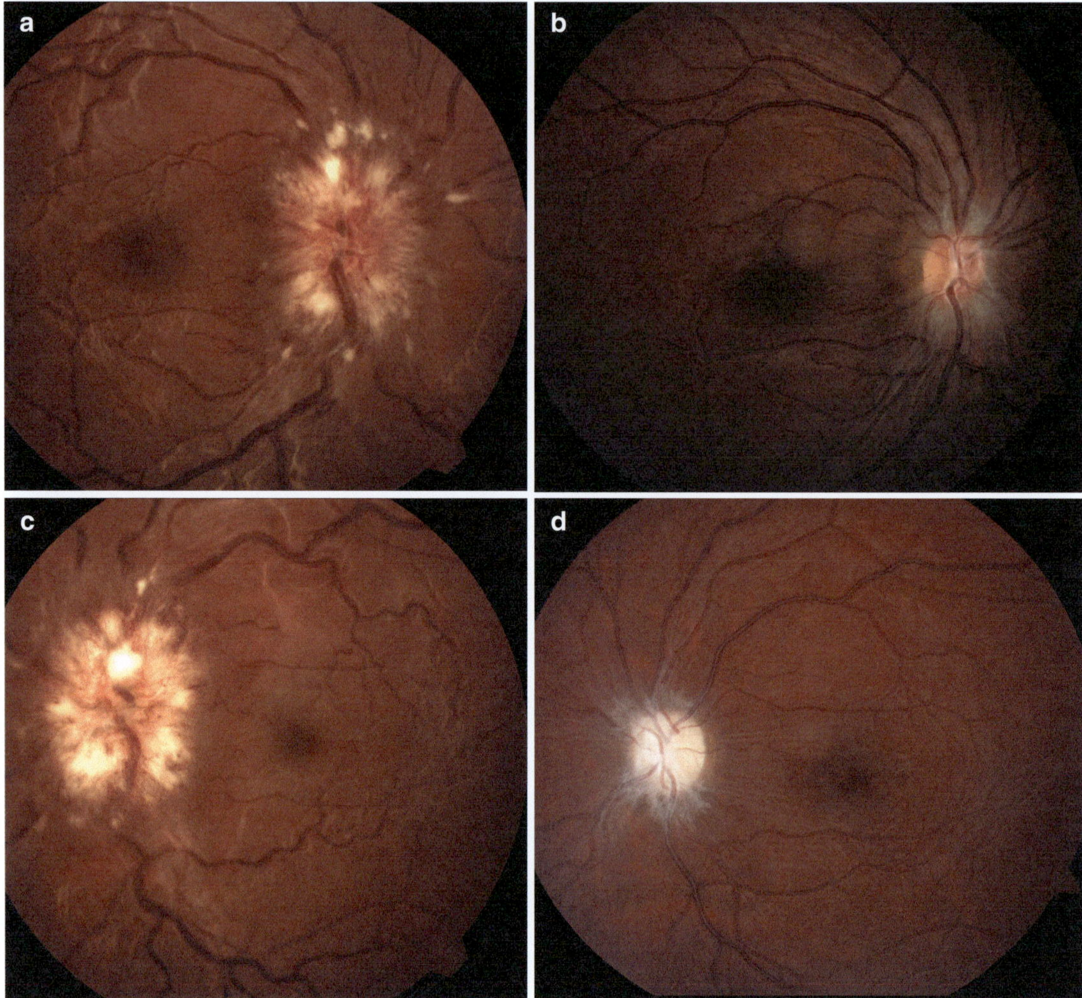

Fig. 36.18 (**a**) Acute papilledema of the right eye. The optic disc is hyperemic and swollen with blurring of the optic disc margin, disc hemorrhages, and cotton wool spots. The cup-to-disc ratio cannot be determined, and the retinal blood vessels are dilated. (**b**) Late stage papilledema of the right eye. The optic disc is slightly pale and swollen with some blurring of the optic disc margin and gliosis of the nerve fiber layer. There are no disc hemorrhages or cotton wool spots. (**c**) Acute papill-edema left eye. The optic disc is hyperemic and swollen with blurring of the optic disc margin, disc hemor-rhages, and cotton wool spots. The cup-to-disc ratio cannot be determined, and the retinal blood vessels are dilated. (**d**) Late stage papilledema of the left eye. The left optic disc shows marked pallor and is mildly swol-len with mild blurring of the optic disc margin and glio-sis of the nerve fiber layer. There are no disc hemorrhages or cotton wool spots

Sudden Bilateral Retrobulbar Optic Neuropathy

Postsurgical Optic Neuropathy

See section on posterior ischemic optic neuropathy.

Optic Neuritis

See section on optic neuritis.

Pituitary Apoplexy

See section on pituitary apoplexy.

Suggested Reading

Arnold AC. Evolving management of optic neuritis and multiple sclerosis. Am J Ophthalmol. 2005;139(6):1101–8.

Biousse V, Newman NJ. Ischemic optic neuropathies. N Engl J Med. 2015;372(25):2428–36.

Chamberlain PD, Sadaka A, Berry S, Lee AG. Ethambutol optic neuropathy. Curr Opin Ophthalmol. 2017;28(6):545–51.

Eddleman CS, Liu JK. Optic nerve sheath meningioma: current diagnosis and treatment. Neurosurg Focus. 2007;23(5):E4.

Hayreh SS. Ischemic optic neuropathies. New York: Springer; 2011. 456p

Hayreh SS, Zimmerman B. Management of giant cell arteritis. Our 27-year clinical study: new light on old controversies. Ophthalmologica. 2003;217(4):239–59.

Kawasaki A, Purvin V. Giant cell arteritis: an updated review. Acta Ophthalmol. 2009;87(1):13–32.

Lam BL, Morais CG Jr, Pasol J. Drusen of the optic disc. Curr Neurol Neurosci Rep. 2008;8(5):404–8.

Lessell S. Nutritional amblyopia. J Neuroophthalmol. 1998;18(2):106–11.

Miller NR, Arnold AC. Current concepts in the diagnosis, pathogenesis and management of nonarteritic anterior ischaemic optic neuropathy. Eye (Lond). 2015;29(1):65–79.

Miller NR, Subramanian P, Patel V. Walsh & Hoyt's clinical neuro-ophthalmology: the essentials. 3rd ed. Philadelphia: Lippincott Williams & Williams; 2015. 600p

Purvin V, Kawasaki A. Common neuro-ophthalmic pitfalls: case-based teaching. New York: Cambridge University Press; 2009. 234p

Diplopia

37

Linus D. Sun

Double vision is a common neuro-ophthalmic symptom for which the underlying etiology can vary from benignly simple to emergent; the difficulty of identification of the problem may also vary, from straightforward to diagnostically challenging. This chapter provides an overview of the approach to the patient with double vision from the perspective of an internist, and we will cover common and some less common diagnoses which will be in the differential diagnosis for the neuro-ophthalmologist. Anatomic locations for the diplopia pathologies can span the anterior surface of the eye to the occipital cortex. In the past, strabismus was described as underaction or overaction of the extraocular muscles. However, to avoid bias of incorrectly assigning the underlying mechanism, we follow modern practice to describe pathologic movements of the eyes rather than specific muscle actions if the diagnosis is not known. For details on the neuroanatomical pathways that may cause double vision, primary source and review articles are referenced at the end of this chapter.

A thorough history is often enough to make a diagnosis, and the exam is performed for confirmation. Initial questions asked are summarized in Table 37.1. A flow chart outlining thought process for diplopia diagnosis is summarized in the diagram in Fig. 37.1. Initial studies frequently needed for the workup of double vision are in Table 37.2. After initial workup is completed, referral to a specialist may be required.

A review of systems includes the following:

- What is the past medical history/current diagnoses?
- How is the patient's overall general health? Has there been any unplanned weight loss recently?
- Is there a history of diabetes, vasculopathy, and clotting disorder?
- Medication reconciliation, particularly recent changes or additions (e.g., lamotrigine)?
- Are there any neurological signs/symptoms: headache, nausea, vertigo, imbalance, ataxia, unstable/jumping vision, facial weakness or drooping of the lids (better in morning or after a nap?), difficulty with daily activities (e.g., getting objects off tall shelves, rising from chair), and frequent aspiration of liquids?
- Are there any signs of systemic inflammatory disease? Does the patient experience fever or chills, soreness of the neck or shoulders, or jaw claudication?
- History of smoking, other substances/ exposures?
- History of sexually transmitted diseases?
- Living in Lyme endemic areas?

L. D. Sun, MD, PhD (✉)
Department of Ophthalmology, Edward S. Harkness Eye Institute, Columbia University Vagelos College of Physicians and Surgeons, New York, NY, USA
e-mail: ls2747@cumc.columbia.edu

© Springer Nature Switzerland AG 2019
D. S. Casper, G. A. Cioffi (eds.), *The Columbia Guide to Basic Elements of Eye Care*,
https://doi.org/10.1007/978-3-030-10886-1_37

Table 37.1 Initial questions asked of patients with a chief complaint of "double vision"

Question	Rationale
"Does it go away when you close one eye?"	To distinguish monocular vs. binocular diplopia
If answer is "no" then monocular diplopia:	
Do your eyes feel dry or irritated? Any recent eye trauma/surgery?	To screen for corneal surface or tear film pathology
Does the double vision go away when looking through a pinhole?	A rapid test to confirm an optical cause for double vision
Testing with Amsler grid: "Do you see any distortions, missing, or doubling of the lines?"	To rule out retinal surface abnormalities, e.g., macular degeneration, detachments, foveal drusen, inflammation, edema, or epiretinal membrane
Any history of topiramate, zonisamide, or trazodone usage?	Medications associated with monocular diplopia
Timing:	
When did you first notice it? Did it appear suddenly or gradually? Is there any specific activity which causes the diplopia? Is it constant or intermittent? If episodic how long do the episodes last?	Duration and rapidity of onset. Traumatic cranial nerve palsies often appear rapidly, are constant and unchanging initially, improving later in the course of syndrome
	Ocular neuromyotonia is very rare but distinctive where EOMs contract involuntarily lasting for seconds to minutes several times per hour
Do you notice it more in the morning or evening?	Myasthenia gravis patients have worsening symptoms later in the day and when fatigued. Thyroid eye disease (Graves' Orbitopathy) is often worse in the morning
If binocular diplopia:	
"Is the double vision primarily horizontal (side-by-side), vertical (one right on top of the other), or at a diagonal?"	Sixth nerve palsies have horizontal diplopia; fourth and third nerve palsies have vertical/oblique palsies
If horizontal: Is it worse on left or right gaze?	If YES, eyes are incomitant, meaning they are not yoked with equal movement: this helps to lateralize the lesion. For horizontal diplopia caused by a 6th nerve palsy, diplopia is worse with gaze in the ipsilateral direction.
If vertical component exists, ask: "Any recent head injury? Is it worse on left and downward gaze? Is it worse when you tilt your head to the right? Least when you look up and to the right?"	If yes to all, suggests a traumatic right 4th nerve palsy. If no trauma, possibly a decompensated congenital 4th nerve palsy. If NO to any and eyes are comitant (move equally together): could be a long-standing strabismus or possibly a new skew deviation due to a brainstem lesion. Reversing vertical double vision on up versus down gaze suggests reduced action of the muscles to the oculomotor nerve (CN3).
Do movie theaters/opera/dark environments worsen the double vision?	This indicates a decompensation of divergence (ability to fuse eyes to targets at distance) where mechanisms may vary.
Is the double vision worse at near or far?	Screening for vergence disorders: does the patient have difficulty converging to a near target (suggesting a convergence insufficiency that is congenital, or due to concussion, Parkinson's Disease, or progressive supranuclear palsy). Or far target suggesting a divergence insufficiency/esotropia. Possible mechanisms include sagging eye syndrome in older patients or Arnold Chiari Malformation in younger patients)
Do you or any family members have a childhood history of a "lazy eye", wearing an eye patch, doing eye exercises (pencil pushups), or history of strabismus surgery?	Screening for history and treatment for amblyopia (also called "squint") or a family history of congenital strabismus (e.g. Duane's syndrome)
Medications history: botulinum injections? Use of lamotrigine?	Medications associated with binocular diplopia

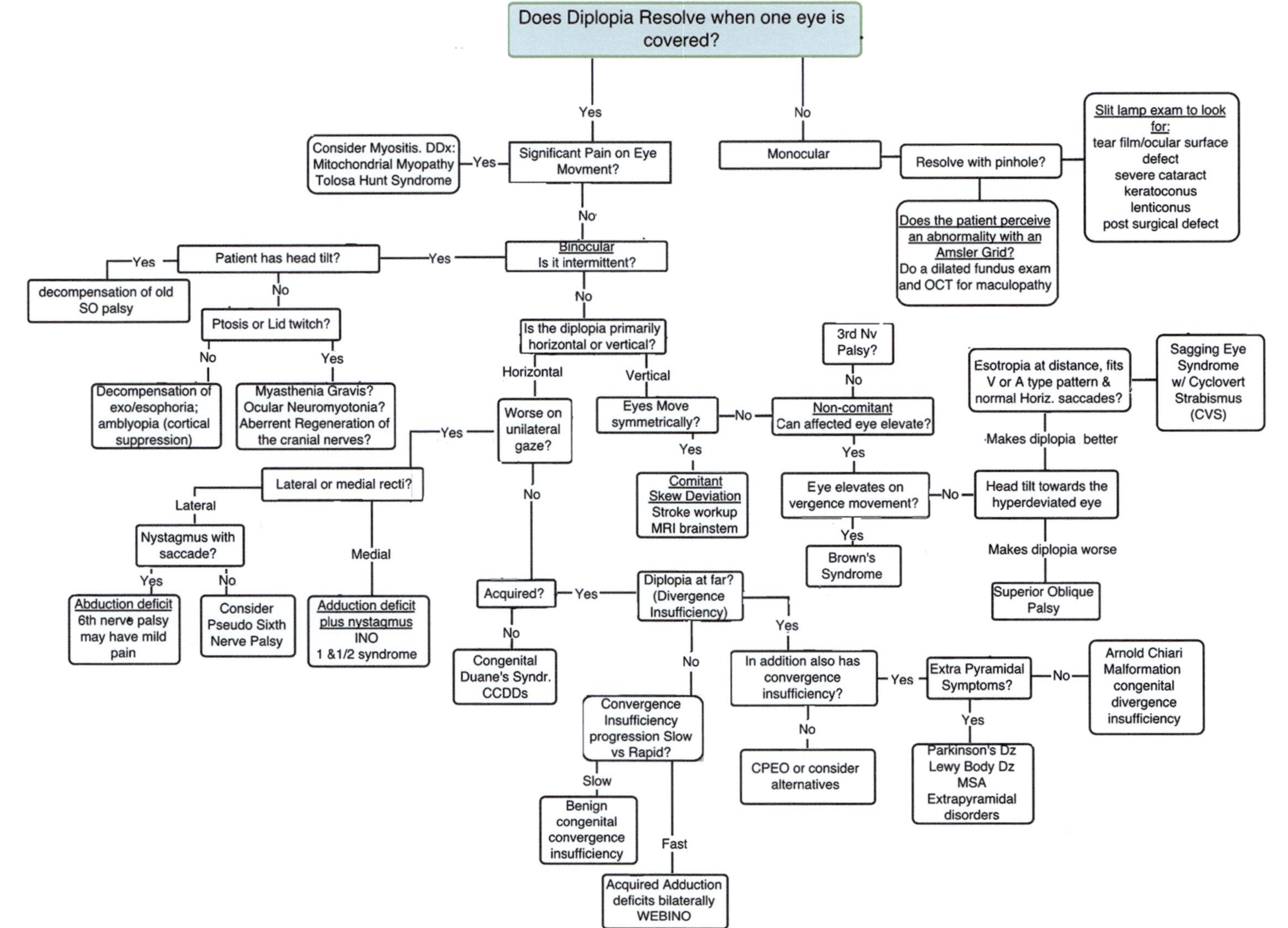

Fig. 37.1 A flow chart outlining example thought process for diplopia diagnosis

Table 37.2 Studies often ordered for a double vision consultation

Basal metabolic panel/complete blood count with differential (BMP/CBC)
T3/T4/TSH
Thyroid-stimulating immunoglobulin (TSI), thyroperoxidase antibody (TPO-Ab). Less commonly, thyroglobulin antibody (TgAb), and anti-microsomal antibody
Acetylcholine receptor antibodies (binding, blocking, modulating), muscle-specific kinase antibody (MuSK). If negative, repeat and add low-density lipoprotein receptor-related protein 4 (LRP4). Less commonly, titin and agrin antibodies
Erythrocyte sedimentation rate/C-reactive protein (ESR/CRP)
Serum Lyme testing: EIA/IFA for screening first. If EIA/IFA is equivocal or positive and <30 days from initial symptoms/rash: order IgM/IgG western blot. If >30 days: IgM western blot only. If EIA/IFA is negative, ID consulatation for convalescent phase serum screening.
Serum ACE level
B12/folate – especially if there are visual complaints
Fluorescent treponemal antibody absorption (FTA-ABS) test; may order rapid plasma reagin (RPR) and venereal disease research laboratory (VDRL) if unavailable
Lumbar puncture for elevated pressure/infectious/cytology especially if fundus exam is abnormal where optic discs margins appear blurred
High-resolution MRI with and without contrast of the orbits, employing fast imaging and steady-state acquisition (FIESTA, balanced FFE, or trueFISP sequencing) for imaging of the skull base and cranial nerves (3 Tesla magnet preferred). CT scan of orbits for EOM entrapment or evaluation of thyroid eye disease if no MRI available

Physical Examination

The patient is examined with their best corrected acuity. Clinical maneuvers are often mastered during neuro-ophthalmology, strabismus fellowships or learned at workshops. The typical equipment utilized in a diplopia workup is seen in Fig. 37.2:

1. Physical occluder to block vision from one eye
2. Maddox Wing for testing near horizontal, vertical, and cycloversion phorias
3. Fixation target on a wall at distance (>10 ft)
4. A near target to hold in one hand

5. Amsler grid
6. Pinhole (for testing monocular diplopia)
7. Optokinetic nystagmus (OKN) strip (a strip of cloth with alternating bars of white and red)
8. Prism set or prism bars
9. A meter-long ruler or stick for testing inconjugate cycloversion of a fourth nerve palsy
10. A direct ophthalmoscope
11. Neurological hammer
12. Hardy-Rand-Rittler (HRR) color plates

Examination for Binocular Double Vision

Evaluation of binocular diplopia requires a full ocular motility exam. The patient is directed to look in all directions of gaze at targets in distance and near. Saccades are elicited by having the patient gaze back and forth between outstretched hands and central gaze (back to the nose of the examiner). Particular attention is given to dynamic overshoot or undershoot of saccades, indicating a cerebellar lesion. Smooth pursuit is tested with a slowly moving high-contrast target (~10°/s). As a diagnosis is being formulated, Particular Close attention is given to eyelid position, symmetry of facial strength, and sensation in V1–V3 distribution, to light touch, pin prick and temperature. Injury to the facial nerve after a Bell's palsy is tested by asking the patient to pucker their lips (a "wink" in the periocular orbicularis muscles will be seen on exam in cases of aberrant regeneration). Optokinetic nystagmus testing (using the OKN flag) is very helpful for repeated testing for weakness in extraocular muscle action.

Emergencies vs. Emergent Causes of Double Vision

When approaching a case of binocular double vision, the immediate concern is whether the diplopia represents an acute central nervous system emergency (e.g., a potentially life-threatening stroke of the brainstem) or a non-emergency, but

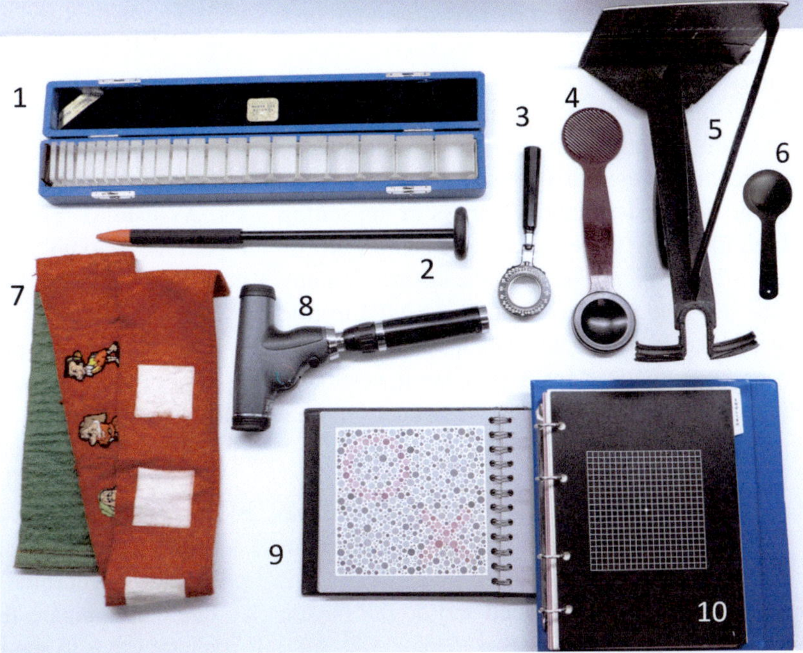

Fig. 37.2 The typical equipment utilized by a neuro-ophthalmologist in a diplopia workup: (1) prism set, (2) Queens Square neurological hammer, (3) Risley prism, (4) Occluder-Maddox Rod combination, (5) Maddox Wing, (6) pinhole, (7) OKN strip with multiple colors (pediatric and adult), (8) direct ophthalmoscope, (9) HRR color plates, and (10) Hamblin Amsler Chart Manual

newly emergent peripheral cause (e.g., cranial nerve palsy, decompensating congenital strabismus, etc.). If the patient's story is acute, occurring within hours, and/or the patient has new additional neurological symptoms (weakness, dizziness or headache), they warrant referral to the emergency room for evaluation and treatment (e.g., urgent imaging or consideration of IV tissue plasminogen activator). Evaluation of non-emergencies (e.g. chronic double vision) may be pursued as an outpatient. If an acute presentation occurs in the setting of an intermittent chronic condition, diagnosis may be challenging, even for the experienced neuro-ophthalmologist.

Key Signs of New-Onset Double Vision That Warrant Acute Referral

A new permanent vertical misalignment is worrisome when misalignment of the eyes is comitant (i.e., is roughly equal in all directions of gaze with alternate cover testing). If the misalignment is intermittent and is elicited by monocular viewing only (via cover-uncover testing) rather than a permanent misalignment during binocular viewing, it is called a phoria. Central brainstem lesions that produce vertical misalignment are called skew deviations, but not all vertical misalignments are due to central lesions (see evaluation of fourth nerve palsy vs. skew deviation below).

Additional neurological symptoms that accompany double vision that are especially worrisome:

(a) Unilateral *weakness in face, arm, or leg* indicates disruption to the corticospinal tract pathway.
(b) Unilateral *ataxia/discoordination* indicates unilateral cerebellar damage to either the cerebellar cortex or its input/output pathways.
(c) *Gait disturbance* not caused by loss of stereopsis.
(d) *Unilateral hearing loss* in one ear and facial weakness suggest a lesion in the cerebello-pontine angle or anterior inferior cerebellar artery stroke.
(e) Any *new severe headache* that accompanies diplopia, especially if the patient describes "the worst headache of my life," may indicate a bleeding aneurysm affecting brainstem structures or elevated intracranial pressure. This may be accompanied by bilateral papilledema and sixth cranial nerve palsies.

Dizziness in setting of skew deviation may be a worrisome finding that requires urgent evaluation. A combination of certain signs, however, is *reassuring* for a non-emergency. If covering one eye of the patient results in relief of a feeling of disorientation, then dizziness may be caused by loss of stereopsis. Acute dizziness in the setting of the following three signs is *not* acutely worrisome. These signs, when present, are actually more sensitive and specific than an MRI to rule out a stroke. If present, the patient may be worked up as an outpatient for a peripheral vestibular injury, and emergency evaluation is unnecessary:

(1) Head Impulse Testing is positive in one direction or there is a history of gentamicin causing inner ear damage.
(2) Patient's eyes are aligned and do *not* have a skew deviation.
(3) Patient has non-direction changing nystagmus and follows Alexander's Law: the fast phase of the nystagmus is always in same direction for different directions of gaze, suggesting a benign peripheral lesion. The amplitude is expected to increase with gaze towards the side of the healthy ear and be reduced or eliminated entirely with gaze towards the lesioned ear. High-speed video applications on modern smartphones are very useful to document non-direction changing vs direction changing nystagmus (the fast phase reverses due to central lesions) and oculomotor syndromes. (For HIPAA concerns, utilizing the patient's phone is often the best option.)

Diplopia with Anisocoria or Ptosis

An acute third nerve palsy from a rapidly expanding compressive lesion (e.g., posterior communicating artery aneurysm) will have a constellation of three ipsilateral signs:

- mydriasis (a large non-reactive pupil)
- ptosis
- oculomotor paresis

A resulting subtle vertical diplopia will reverse in up-gaze vs down-gaze, which can be revealed with the Maddox rod and hand-held light source. These patients should be sent to the emergency room for evaluation (see entry below on oculomotor nerve palsies). If other cranial nerves are involved (III, IV, V1, V2, VI), cavernous sinus pathology is probable (e.g., infection, thrombosis, AV-fistula). The faster the onset the more urgent the workup. Non-emergencies with emergent histories include:

- Diabetes causing an emergent (but non-emergency) microvascular third nerve palsy which spares the pupil, which remains reactive to light and accommodation; in other words, the pupils will be equal.
- If the ptosis is on same side as the smaller pupil, the patient must be evaluated for a Horner's syndrome. If the anisocoria >1mm, one can compare the patient's eyes with old photographs to see if the anisocoria is, in fact, new.

For the exam, in a completely dark setting, pupils are illuminated from below with a pen light. Room lights are turned on and off to test for dilation lag. If significant dilation lag occurs in the smaller pupil, further evaluation is needed. To confirm a suspected Horner's syndrome, the neuro-ophthalmologist employs apraclonidine (alpha-2 agonist) drops in both eyes. A reversal of anisocoria is seen in Horner's syndrome. If the anisocoria is accompanied with ptosis without oculomotor paresis, imaging of the secondary and tertiary pupillary sympathetic pathway is needed. This pathway arises from the lower cervical and upper thoracic (T1-T2) spinal cord, traverses the apex of the lung, ascends along the carotid artery, exiting to become the primary sympathetic pathway that innervates the pupillary dillators.

Oculomotor Pathway Lesions Leading to Strabismus and Eye Movement Abnormalities

A peripheral sixth cranial nerve palsy inhibits lateral eye movements of the ipsilateral eye only. Moving centrally, a lesion to the right paramedian pontine reticular formation (PPRF) and abducens nuclei leads to an inability to make bilateral rightward eye movements past the midline. Lesions to one of the two ascending medial longitudinal fasciculus (MLF) leads to an ipsilateral adduction deficit known as an internuclear ophthalmoplegia (INO). Multiple sclerosis is one of the most frequent causes for an INO in a younger person while blood pressure and vascular disease is the cause in older people. A slightly larger lesion, which encompasses the right PPRF, abducens nuclei, and right MLF, leads to the "one and half" syndrome: ipsilateral gaze palsy ("one") where both eyes cannot look right and ipsilateral INO ("½") where the contralateral left eye can still look left, but left gaze (adduction) by the right eye is defective. A small midline lesion that damages right and left MLFs leads to both a bilateral exotropia (walleye) and bilateral internuclear ophthalmoplegia ("WEBINO"). These lesions lead to slow and often, restricted saccades.

Skew deviation is sometimes seen in *lateral medullary syndrome* (Wallenberg syndrome) which is accompanied by vestibular dysfunction (vertigo, nystagmus, vomiting), ipsilateral ataxia, ipsilateral loss of pain and temperature on the face with ipsilateral Horner's syndrome (miosis, ptosis, anhidrosis), and ipsilateral dysphagia and contralateral deficits to pain and temperature on the body. This constellation of symptoms requires an emergency stroke workup.

Oculomotor Nerve (CN III) Palsies with Pupil and Lid Involvement

Oculomotor nuclei innervate the ipsilateral superior rectus, medial rectus, inferior rectus, and inferior oblique muscles, and the bilateral levator palpebrae muscles. Parasympathetic efferents that control the pupillary sphincter muscle (miosis) and the ciliary muscle (accommodation) also run along the third cranial nerve. Evaluation for a partial third nerve palsy should be considered with new unilateral ptosis, and/or a new deficit in elevation and adduction in one eye. Pupillary involvement may vary from relative sparing (0.5–2 mm involvement, but briskly reactive) to fully involved (a large pupil that is poorly reactive to light and accommodation) in a third nerve palsy. An MRI with MRA and/or CT angiogram is appropriate to evaluate for a possible posterior communicating artery aneurysm. If none is found, a conventional angiogram may then be performed. In an older patient with vascular risk factors such as diabetes, a third nerve palsy without pupillary involvement may indicate a microvascular infarct of the third nerve, which does not require emergent workup. The pupil is spared because the the parasympathetic pathway exists superficially on the oculomotor nerve and is unaffected. Myasthenia gravis, which can present as any oculomotor muscle weakness, often produces ptosis but will not have pupillary involvement. A key feature to remember for ocular myasthenia is that the weakness changes over time (weeks to months), with symptoms often being better in the mornings, and significantly improved after rest such as after a test of sleep for 30 min.

Horizontal Binocular Diplopia

The most common cause for an acute sixth nerve palsy is diabetic microvascular ischemia. The defect typically presents over several hours and can, initially, be mildly uncomfortable or painful. Patients often report noticing diplopia first while driving (distant targets) and with horizontal gaze in one direction. On exam, one eye is incapable of full adduction and shows slow saccades in comparison to the other, fully adducting eye. Ocular misalignment may range from subtle to greater than 30 or more prism diopters. Management includes referral to a neuro-ophthalmologist, ophthalmologist, or orthoptist to place temporary ("press-on") Fresnel prisms on the patient's glasses (see Chap. 39). Temporary prisms need to be updated every 2–4 weeks as symptoms improve and misalignment decreases. Microvascular sixth nerve palsies will improve over weeks-to-months, with most of the improvement occurring within the first and second month. A residual deficit may linger for up to a year. While some patient's deficits may abate completely, others may never fully resolve. Any

Table 37.3 Pseudo-sixth nerve palsies

Thyroid eye disease
Blowout fracture
Spasm of the near reflex (volitional)
Duane's syndrome
Divergence insufficiency
Decompensating phoria
Autoimmune disorders including:
Myasthenia gravis
Miller Fisher variant of Guillain-Barré syndrome

residual uncompensated divergence insufficiency that is stable for 6 months to a year will require permanent prism to be incorporated into the patient's glasses. If double vision does not improve significantly, or worsens over time, other etiologies must be considered and require close follow-up examination (2–4 weeks).

To evaluate for other causes of horizontal binocular diplopia, it is important to examine for papilledema and perform sensory testing for temperature and pain deficits of the trigeminal nerve in the V1 and V2 distribution. Skull base pathology, which may exert traumatic injury on the sixth nerve, can additionally lead to sensory deficits and decreased tearing. Schirmer's testing for asymmetric tearing deficits should therefore also be performed. The differential diagnosis includes infection or tumor infiltration (e.g., Lyme disease, lymphoma), neurosyphilis, solid tumor masses (e.g., meningioma, chordoma, metastases), carcinomatous meningitis, and neurosarcoidosis. Temporal arteritis is a relatively rare cause for cranial nerve palsies but has been reported and must also be ruled out (see Chap. 36), as it is a treatable and potentially fatal condition. Finally, pseudo-sixth nerve palsies must also be considered when evaluating a lateral rectus palsy (see Table 37.3).

New-Onset Vertical Strabismus: Fourth Nerve Palsy vs. Skew Deviation

The crucial determination of a new vertical strabismus is whether or not the hyperdeviated eye is excyclotorted (indicating a fourth neve palsy) or incyclotorted (a pathologic ocular tilt reaction indicating a skew deviation) (see Fig. 40.1). Although an acute vertical diplopia may have several possible causes, as clinicians we initially attempt to differentiate between two very different syndromes: an isolated fourth nerve palsy due to a peripheral lesion (less of an emergency) versus a skew deviation due to a central (more emergency) or vestibular (less emergency) lesion.

Fourth Cranial Nerve Palsy

The fourth cranial nerve exits the midbrain posteriorly, crosses the midline, travels anteriorly, and innervates the superior oblique muscle; having the longest course of any cranial nerve, it is one of the most susceptible to trauma. It may also decompensate later in life or be subject to microvascular ischemia. The Bielschowsky-Parks three-step test is a useful but not highly sensitive (70%), with the first and third steps combined being the most sensitive (84%):

1. Is the hyper deviation in the right eye?
2. Is the diplopia worse on left gaze?
3. Is the diplopia worse on right head tilt?

If the three answers are yes, this is consistent with a right fourth nerve palsy (the pattern is inverted to left-right-left for a left fourth nerve palsy). Additional findings of a right fourth nerve palsy are:

4. Patients will naturally sit with a head tilt leaning away from the side of the fourth nerve palsy.
5. Patients generally have worse symptoms when looking to the lower left.
6. Symptoms are much better when looking to the upper right.
7. There will be a relative excyclotorsion of the right eye.

Fourth nerve palsy patients are referred to a neuro-ophthalmologist, ophthalmologist, or orthoptist for prisms. The expected outcome is that there will be subjective improvement over a period of weeks, with a possible permanent, residual, small strabismus.

With an apparently new-onset fourth nerve palsy, it should be noted that if old photographs show evidence of a pre-existing consistent head tilt, this strongly suggests a long-standing fourth nerve palsy which has decompensated later in life, often in the 4th to 6th decade. Correction for a long-standing fourth nerve palsy is recommended with prism because a consistent head tilt may lead to arthritis of neck vertebrae.

Skew Deviation

A skew deviation is a sometimes acquired, vertical strabismus that invokes a central lesion. It is due to a disruption of the labyrinthine-vestibular pathway of the inner ear to the oculomotor nuclei. This pathway normally keeps vision stable from very quick angular and tilting movements of the head and is known as the vestibular ocular reflex (VOR). The pathway relies on afferents from the semicircular canals for angular, horizontal, and vertical VOR eye movements. In a normal patient, when the head tilts right, both eyes rotate left, while the left eye depresses in the orbit and right eye elevates – keeping both eyes stable to the horizon up to approximately 20° of tilt. Damage to the VOR neural pathway will lead to an imbalance, causing a pathologic ocular tilt reaction. The patient with a skew deviation (e.g., a right hypertropia) will have a compensatory opposite head tilt (left head tilt) as the right eye will be slightly incyclotorted. A simple test to see pathologic incyclotorsion from skew deviation utilizes direct ophthalmoscopy: normally the fovea appears lower than the optic nerve, whereas the fovea appears to be higher than the nerve in an incyclotorted eye.

Other Causes of Diplopia

Monocular Diplopia

Patients may have monocular diplopia in one or both eyes. A pinhole is useful to determine if the abnormality in the affected eye is due to an optical abnormality. Optical light transmission abnormalities include ocular surface abnormalities including dry eye, an abnormal tear film, corneal irregularities (inflammation, edema), recent ocular trauma or surgery, a large astigmatism, keratoconus, lenticonus, displaced lens, or severe cataract. Testing each eye separately with the Amsler grid, the patient is asked about "doubling of the lines, distortions of the grid, or missing areas of the grid." If pinhole does not resolve the diplopia, one must think about a maculopathy caused by retinal abnormalities such as macular degeneration from drusen (calcium deposits), edema or other retinal infiltration, or retinal detachments. Note that *progressive*-type lenses in glasses produce an optical aberration at the transition zone in the lens, which may be interpreted by some patients as double vision. Maculopathies require consultation with an ophthalmologist. In a primary care setting or emergency room, the easiest screen to detect a possible retinal detachment is to look for a pale red reflex when at a distance from the patient with a direct ophthalmoscope. Monocular diplopia is best referred to the ophthalmologist, while binocular diplopia is usually evaluated by a strabismus surgeon or neuro-ophthalmologist.

Anisometropia

Anisometropia is either the presence of myopia in one eye and hyperopia in the other eye with two diopters or greater difference in refractive power or the presence of significantly unequal refractive powers, even without there being a myopic-hyperopic mismatch. Patients may complain of binocular double vision but without any manifest misalignment of the eyes; the diplopia occurs due to the large optical mismatch between the eyes, which causes images of unequal size to be focused on the macula. If the size discrepancy is large enough, the occipital cortex is not able to fuse the discordant images and double vision results, although the eyes are perfectly aligned. Large astigmatisms that are oblique by 90 degrees may also produce a persistent perception of binocular double vision called meridional aniseisokonia.

Thyroid Eye Disease (See Chap. 29)

Thyroid eye disease, or Graves' orbitopathy, involves slowly progressive fibrosis and engorgement of the extraocular muscles over time (typically 12–18 months) due to autoimmune inflammation. It is one of the most common causes of diplopia in adults. The inferior rectus is the most common muscle affected although all the EOMs are susceptible. Grave's thyroiditis may occur at the same time, but does not directly cause ophthalmopathy. Later in the disease, there may be eyelid retraction, lid and periorbital edema, proptosis, and lagophthalmos. Attempts to move a paretic eye through forced ductions may be met with resistance, due to orbital tissue fibrosis. Imaging via CT or MRI will show enlarged EOM bodies with sparing of the tendons. Initial serologic testing includes T3, T4, TSH, anti-TPO antibodies, and Thyroid Stimulating Immunoglobulin (TSI).

Brown's Syndrome

Fibrosis of the sheath of the superior oblique muscle prevents elevation of the eye when adducted (looking nasally), by preventing the oblique tendon from sliding through the pulley-like structure called the trochlea. It may be congenital or acquired through an inflammatory process(trauma, surgery, or infection).

Myasthenia Gravis

Autoimmune antibodies to the neuromuscular junction in myasthenia gravis (MG) can cause weakness of any of the EOMs and lid muscles, potentially mimicking any of the oculomotor disorders. Patients may have a history of fatigue in axial/appendicular muscles, aspiration of liquids, signs of unilateral/bilateral ptosis, and weakness of eye closure. The sleep test (patient closes eyes and naps for >30 min), ice pack test, or edrophonium test are suggestive of MG if symptoms

immediately but temporarily resolve. Initial serum testing includes binding, blocking, and modulating acetylcholine receptor antibodies (50% positive in ocular MG, 87% with generalized MG) and anti-muscle-specific kinase (MuSK). If initially negative, the tests are repeated. Additional tests for serum antibodies associated with MG include anti-low density lipoprotein receptor-related protein 4 (LRP4) and rarely, anti-titin and anti-agrin antibodies. Neuromuscular testing with repetitive stimulation EMG is helpful; however, single fiber testing is more sensitive and specific for ocular myasthenia (performed by neuromuscular diagnostic specialists in neurology). A routine chest CT scan for thymoma is indicated in new cases of MG. The differential diagnosis includes mitochondrial myopathies (e.g., chronic progressive external ophthalmoplegia), congenital cranial dysinnervation disorders (see below), oculopharyngeal dystrophy, and thyroid eye disease.

Divergence Insufficiency Esotropia

Divergence insufficiency describes the inability of the eyes to binocularly fuse targets at distance. It often presents as a slowly developing, comitant, symmetric symptom in all directions of gaze that is not associated with abduction slowing or nystagmus. The mechanism is currently unknown. In its benign form, it is self-limiting, usually causing temporary double vision which can be treated with prism. If papilledema is present, elevated intracranial pressure can affect the abducens nerves, leading to bilateral sixth nerve palsies, which could also prevent normal divergence. The differential diagnosis includes myasthenia gravis, Guillain-Barré syndrome (Miller Fisher variant), and brainstem compression due to an Arnold-Chiari malformation. Orthoptic or 'eye exercises' have limited efficacy and are not recommended for this condition. If the underlying mechanism is non-progressive and benign, prisms applied to corrective lenses is the appropriate treatment.

Convergence Insufficiency

The inability to converge the eyes to a near target is very common in the pediatric population (up to 13% in some studies), which can lead to complaints of eye strain, headache, and avoidance of reading or other near vision activities. In the developing child, the brain may compensate for the inability to converge through visual cortical suppression where visual information from one eye becomes unconsciously ignored, leading to amblyopia and thus should be consulted with a strabismus surgeon (see Chap. 39). Office based convergence exercises ("pencil pushups") have been shown to have some limited but positive efficacy. Patients may have significant strabismus on alternate cover testing but may not report double vision when binocular vision is revealed – leading to variable objective measurements on exam. Convergence insufficiency may also be acquired later in life due to injury of the neural convergence circuitry in the midbrain such as through traumatic brain injury (concussion) or neurodegenerative disease (e.g. Parkinson's Disease or Progressive Supranuclear Palsy).

Sagging Eye Syndrome

Rutar and Demer recently described an acutely presenting defect in orbital connective tissue that connects the superior rectus and lateral rectus muscles in elderly Caucasian populations. This results in a "sagging eye syndrome," which presents as a small diopter, vertical strabismus with divergence insufficiency at distance and excyclotorsion unilaterally or bilaterally. It may develop slowly, over time, or can occur acutely, prompting an acute stroke workup. Saccades are normal as are the movements of the eyes in lateral and downward directions. Diagnosis requires a special sequence orbital MRI with forward fixation for both eyes, which demonstrates the attenuated fascial connection. Treatment for symptomatic sagging eye syndrome is strabismus surgery or prism.

Double Vision in Neurodegenerative Disease

Parkinson's disease and the related progressive supranuclear palsy (PSP) have in common a convergence insufficiency leading to double vision at near targets. PSP patients often present with ocular symptoms first and have an associated reduction in midbrain volume best seen on sagittal MRI; this area houses vertical and vergence oculomotor circuitry, and abnormalities can produce slow vertical saccades and convergence insufficiency. Referral to ophthalmology, neuro-ophthalmology, or an orthoptic specialist for adding prism to reading glasses is helpful to treat the convergence insufficiency.

Congenital Cranial Dysinnervation Disorders (CCDD)

This diverse group of disorders is present at birth. Some are developmental errors in cranial innervation (Duane's syndrome) involving multiple cranial nerves with secondary aberrant innervation. Included in this group are congenital fibrosis of the extraocular muscles (CFEOM), congenital ptosis, Marcus Gunn jaw-winking, Möbius syndrome, crocodile tears, horizontal gaze palsy, and congenital facial palsy.

Ocular Myositis and Mitochondrial Myopathies

Pain on eye movements and diplopia suggest an inflammation of the EOMs, of which there are two major forms: (1) limited oligosymptomatic ocular myositis (LOOM), which may also have conjunctival injection, and (2) severe exophthalmic ocular myositis (SEOM) that may exhibit ptosis, chemosis, and proptosis. Corticosteroids are the mainstay of treatment for both conditions.

Chronic progressive external ophthalmoplegia (CPEO) is the most frequent manifestation of mitochondrial myopathies restricted to the EOMs that presents as a slowly progressive ophthalmoplegia which can occur later in life. Many other mitochondrial myopathies have been identified which have additional symptoms outside of the EOMs and include:

- Kearns-Sayre syndrome (age onset <20, myopathic weakness, heart block, cerebellar ataxia)
- Mitochondrial myopathy and encephalopathy, with lactate acidosis, and stroke-like episodes (MELAS)
- Sensory ataxic neuropathy with dysarthria and ophthalmoparesis (SANDO)
- Myoclonic epilepsy, myopathy with ragged-red fibers (MERRF)
- Mitochondrial neurogastrointestinal encephalopathy (MNGIE)
- Neuropathy, ataxia, retinitis pigmentosa (NARP)
- Progressive external ophthalmoplegia (PEO)

These diseases are maternally inherited, and efforts to treat mitochondrial disease with gene therapy are in active clinical trial development. If other cranial neuropathies are involved (III, IV, and VI) and there is pain on eye movement in all directions, it is possible that the inflammation is not limited to the EOMs but is located in the cavernous sinus, affecting cranial nerves III, IV and VI (e.g., Tolosa-Hunt syndrome).

Relationship of Nystagmus to the Vestibular and Cerebellar Systems

New-onset disequilibrium or dizziness is worrying to both patients and clinicians as patients have difficulty describing their symptoms, which only sometimes match classic textbook case scenarios. Nystagmus is a comorbid sign with many disorders of the oculomotor system. Severe vertigo often caused by a unilateral peripheral vestibular lesion is experienced by the patient as the room "spinning" in one direction. Benign paroxysmal positional vertigo (BPPV) is elicited by certain head movements depending on which semicircular canals contain free-floating canalith crystal (also referred to as an otolith). Symptoms are delayed by seconds and often occur when lying supine and turning to one's side or when the patient returns to an upright position after bending over for an extended period of time (e.g., sitting up after tying one's shoes). The unilateral peripheral vestibular syndrome of Meniere's disease is thought to be caused by viral etiologies, while macrolide antibiotics (erythromycin, gentamycin) may cause permanent unilateral and bilateral vestibular dysfunction.

The patient who complains of general low-grade dizziness at all times, slightly worsened with any head movement, represents a common but often difficult-to-diagnose condition. Such patients may have several syndromes simultaneously, especially those who are older, or have other comorbidities. A careful evaluation by a primary care/internal medicine physician is necessary to evaluate overall health and rule out any systemic problems, such as hyper- or hypotension, anemia, metabolic and nutritional deficiencies are a few possibilities. Patients who complain of disequilibrium may have orthostatic hypotension. Blood pressure dysregulation is associated with a wide number of conditions including dysautonomia, hypothyroidism, Addison's disease, multiple system atrophy, Parkinson's disease, syndrome of inappropriate antidiuretic hormone secretion (SIADH), cerebral salt-wasting syndrome, postural orthostatic tachycardia syndrome (POTS), and autonomic neuropathy (secondary to diabetes or paraneoplastic syndrome). However after a full normal medical workup, persistent disquilibrium may require an evaluation by neurology and/or otolaryngology. Orthostatic hypotension is treated by addressing the underlying medical conditions, medical therapy (e.g., fludrocortisone, midodrine) and compression stockings.

Even though peripheral vestibular pathways feed into midline cerebellar structures, disequilibrium from central cerebellar injury is of a different character than peripheral vestibular damage. Patients describe disequilibrium on active movement, including walking. They may also have discoordination in movement of appendicular and axial structures. Cerebellar tremors are associated with movement and are not manifest at rest. Cerebellar damage classically shows under- and overshooting of targets by limb (finger-nose-finger or finger chase testing on exam) or by eye movements (hypometric or hypermetric saccades). While human cerebellar lesion correlations are documented, the pathophysiologic mechanism is still under investigation.

Suggested Reading

Evaluation and management of diplopia – clinical education focal point excerpt. Am Acad Ophthalmol. https://www.aao.org/focalpointssnippetdetail. aspx?id=8eb21322-ab3c-49f9-a772-b9ba8bd9783f.

Horn AKE, Adamczyk C. Chapter 9 – Reticular formation: eye movements, gaze and blinks. In: The human nervous system, vol. 3. 3rd ed. Amsterdam: Elsevier Academic Press; 2012.

Kattah JC, Talkad AV, Wang DZ, Hsieh YH, Newman-Toker DE. HINTS to diagnose stroke in the acute vestibular syndrome: three-step bedside oculomotor examination more sensitive than early MRI diffusion-weighted imaging. Stroke. 2009;40(11):3504–10.

Kattah JC. Update on HINTS Plus, with discussion of pitfalls and pearls. J Neurol Phys Ther. 2019;43(2):S42–5.

Krauzlis RJ. Chapter 32: Eye movements. In: Fundamental neuroscience. 4th ed. Amsterdam: Elsevier/Academic Press; 2013.

Leigh RJ, Zee DS. The neurology of eye movements, Contemporary neurology series. 5th ed. New York: Oxford University Press; 2015. (HIGHLY RECOMMENDED REFERENCE GUIDE).

Purvin VA, Kawasaki A. Common neuro-ophthalmic pitfalls: case-based teaching. Cambridge: Cambridge University Press; 2009. (HIGHLY RECOMMENDED).

Rutar T, Demer JL. "Heavy Eye" syndrome in the absence of high myopia: a connective tissue degeneration in elderly strabismic patients. J AAPOS. 2009;13(1):36–44.

Schoser BG. Ocular myositis: diagnostic assessment, differential diagnoses, and therapy of a rare muscle disease – five new cases and review. Clin Ophthalmol. 2007;1(1):37–42.

Linus D. Sun

It is estimated that nearly half of the brain's neurons are connected directly to the retina and involved in the processing of vision, attesting to the paramount importance of vision in brain functioning. For more than a century, scientists have investigated the visual system through studies of its complex anatomy, biochemistry, and physiology. Although we are still at the early stages of understanding vision, great progress is being made toward deciphering how the brain interprets shapes, objects, movement, location, and facial recognition.

The optical system of the cornea and lens projects focused images of the external world onto the retina, but experiencing and interpreting conscious, visual phenomena involve structures deep within the brain's cortex and brain stem. Scientists have only begun to decode and build neural network models to simulate and explain how what we experience as vision is processed and interpreted by the brain.

Visual experience begins in the retina. There are approximately 120 million photoreceptors (7 million cones and 110 million rods) in each retina that receive images from the external world. Rod receptors respond to low light; cone receptors are less sensitive to low light but are specialized to distinguish color, which rods are incapable of doing. While peripheral vision is represented in the outer retina, the highest density of photoreceptors, and thus high-resolution vision, is in the center of the macula known as the fovea. Cone receptors are most densely packed in the fovea, where there are few rods, and hence, the central retina is less sensitive to dim light but exquisitely responsive to color discrimination. This anatomic organization has been known by astronomers for many years, using a technique known as "averted vision": stars that are too dim to be detected directly by the fovea may become visible when the observer looks adjacent to the star, placing it on the low-light receptive, black and white (scotopic) portion of the retina, rather than the central, color-specialized fovea (photopic). This phenomenon occurs because of higher rod density in parafoveal areas, which enhances low-light visual acuity.

Highly accurate acuity and color vision is best appreciated in the fovea, where 20/20 or better vision is possible. Foveal color cones are densely packed, approximately 50 per square micrometer, compared to approximately 12 in parafoveal areas. The majority of cone cells respond to red light and a smaller amount to green light; very few actually respond to blue light, which results in vision more heavily weighted toward the yellow-green spectrum. It is this central retinal area that is most sensitive to disruption by calcification (drusen) or fluid collection in macular degeneration.

L. D. Sun, MD, PhD (✉)
Department of Ophthalmology, Edward S. Harkness Eye Institute, Columbia University Vagelos College of Physicians and Surgeons, New York, NY, USA
e-mail: ls2747@cumc.columbia.edu

© Springer Nature Switzerland AG 2019
D. S. Casper, G. A. Cioffi (eds.), *The Columbia Guide to Basic Elements of Eye Care*,
https://doi.org/10.1007/978-3-030-10886-1_38

Vision is enabled by proteins located within photoreceptor cells (rhodopsin, also known as "visual purple," in rods and photopsin in cones), which are activated by light, initiating a biochemical pathway that produces an electrical signal. Rhodopsin and photopsin are part of a group of proteins known as opsins. This group also includes melanopsin, a blue light-sensitive visual pigment that is found in ganglion cells, but not photoreceptor cells, and is involved in pupillary reflex and circadian rhythm activities, rather than conscious visual perception. The photoreceptor cell's electrical signal, through neural transmission, is processed by retinal ganglion cells and inhibitory interneurons. Ultimately, through the retinal ganglion cells this signal is transmitted to the brain for visual perception.

The retina is able to detect and processes light, dark, motion, contrast, and edges. It can sense total light input and adjust its sensitivity to the wide range of light levels we experience. Because the ratio of photoreceptors to ganglion cells is approximately 100:1, a major component of image processing involves compression of signal information as it proceeds toward the inner retina. Color and light are first acquired in the deepest (outer) retinal layer (Fig. 38.1): this information is processed initially via photoreceptors and, subsequently, through a parallel series of interactions between bipolar cells (within the inner nuclear layer), inhibitory amacrine interneurons, and laterally connected inhibitory horizontal cells, which act to suppress surrounding photoreceptors. Final output is through the gan-

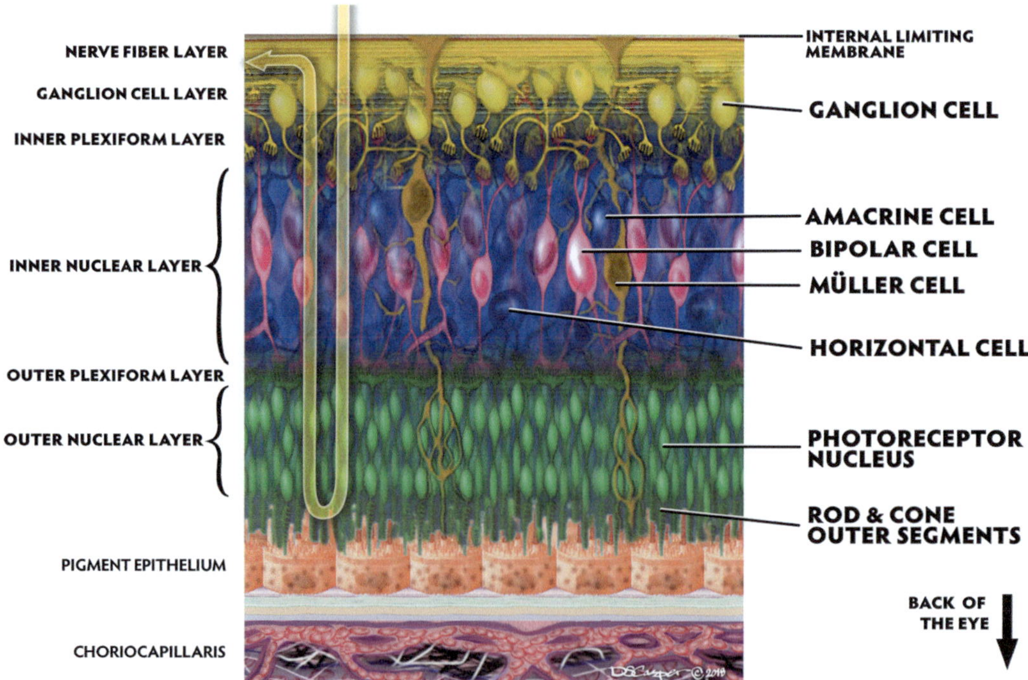

Fig. 38.1 Retinal microanatomy and image processing (long arrow represents the path of information through the retina to the ganglion cell axon). Light enters from the top of the illustration and traverses the transparent retina to reach the posteriorly located rod and cone photoreceptors. There, light is converted to neural signals which are then processed in a chain-like fashion from deep ("outer") retinal structures (bottom) to the superficial ("inner") layers. In the ganglion cell layer, information is organized and output via the nerve fibers, which converge at the optic nerve, which then exits the eye (see Chap. 1). The pigment epithelium layer absorbs excess light which helps to reduce scatter and improve the image, as well as provide nutrients to the photoreceptor cells.

glion cells, whose axons form the retinal nerve fibers that travel radially across the superficial (inner) retinal surface and converge to form the optic nerve, which exits the eye and enters the central nervous system. Through electrophysiological studies, we know that patches of photoreceptors are connected to individual retinal ganglion cells (RGCs) whose activity is referred to as receptive fields. Individual ganglion cells respond to small columns of photoreceptors of the same color, while surrounding photoreceptors inhibit the ganglion cell response. This is known as the "center-surround" receptive field and this type of signal processing is propagated throughout all neurons in the visual system. Thus there is a one-to-one connection between microscopic portions of the retina and individual, visually responsive neurons that exist throughout the brain's visual pathway.

Five classes of retinal ganglion cells have been identified, each of which plays a specific role in visual processing:

- *Midget retinal ganglion cells* comprise 80% of all RGCs and have small receptive fields that are color sensitive, have slower conduction velocities, and project to the *"What" color detail selective layers (or parvocellular pathway)* of the lateral geniculate nucleus (LGN). Some scientists refer to these cells as the P-cell for its connection.
- *Parasol retinal ganglion cells* represent 10% of all RGCs, are connected to more rod and cone cells (thus having larger receptive fields), have faster conduction velocities, and project to the *"Where" motion selective layers (or magnocellular pathway)* of the LGN. They are sometimes referred to as the M-cell for it's connection.
- The *bistratified cell* is intermediate in receptive field size and sensitivities ("on" to blue cone input but "off" to green and red), have large receptive fields, and may be participate in *color vision perception.*
- As mentioned above, a population of *specialized photosensitive ganglion cells* respond to light due to their melanopsin photopigment; they have large receptive fields and are thought to *modu-* *late circadian rhythms* directly via the suprachiasmatic nucleus and control the pupillary light reflex via the Edinger-Westphal nucleus.
- *A specific group of visually sensitive retinal ganglion* cells bypasses the cortical visual processing system. They project directly to the *saccade-driving* superior colliculus in the brain stem and thus subconsciously elicit the fastest reaction time eye movement to a visual stimulus (90–120 ms); if the slower conscious motor-vision network is engaged, the latencies are longer and are typical for human reaction times (170–230 ms).

After exiting the posterior globes and orbits, the optic nerves merge in the optic chiasm, just above the pituitary stalk, and segregate based on vertical hemifields (see Chap. 36). Post-chiasmal optic tracts continue posteriorly to the lateral geniculate bodies of the thalamus, where the majority of the brain's initial visual processing begins (Fig. 38.2).

The lateral geniculate nucleus (LGN) of the thalamus has distinct layers, defined by which eye from which it receives input. Thalamic structures are considered "way stations" for sensory information collected from peripheral organs. There are also extensive connections between the cortex and thalamic nuclei – only about 5% of inputs into the LGN originate in the retina. The remaining 95% are reciprocal connections with the visual cortex, superior colliculus, pretectum, thalamic reticular nuclei, and local LGN interneurons. This suggests that the LGN plays a significant role in visual perceptual processing, which includes stereoscopic vision, vergence to an object of regard, motion, eye positioning, and attention. LGN output travels through the optic radiations in the retrolenticular limb of the internal capsule to what is known as the striate cortex (primary visual cortex, V1). Input arrives in layer 4 of V1, which sends feedforward connections to higher visual areas (V2, V3, V4, V5) in the occipital cortex. Layer 6 in V1 sends its output back to the LGN to complete the feedback circuit. LGN neurons are not "tuned" for detecting edges; the primary visual cortex performs this task.

Each hemi-primary visual cortex receives contralateral visual field input from both eyes (i.e., the right primary visual cortex receives left visual field input from both eyes and vice versa; see Fig. 38.2). Hubel and Wiesel (1960s) received the Nobel Prize in part for their discovery that primary V1 neurons have receptive fields that respond to light edge stimuli oriented at a specific angle. It is highly instructive to witness their original mapping experiments, which are available online (https://youtu.be/KE952yueVLA). Remarkably, millimeter-wide stripes in V1 appear as "columns" in cross-section; these are organized by which eye provides input to those neurons in a particular column (Fig. 38.3). Within a group of several neurons, the orientation preference of adjacent neurons is not random but continuously and topographically organized into a "pinwheel"-like arrangement. While it is thought that early stereopsis is processed in area V2, it is likely that motion, shadow, and vergence cues are combined throughout the brain to produce full stereo vision. This is an area of active investigation in vision neuroscience.

Visual information is first processed in the striate cortex and then streams from V1 to other cortical areas that are concerned with "What" things are and "Where" those things are located

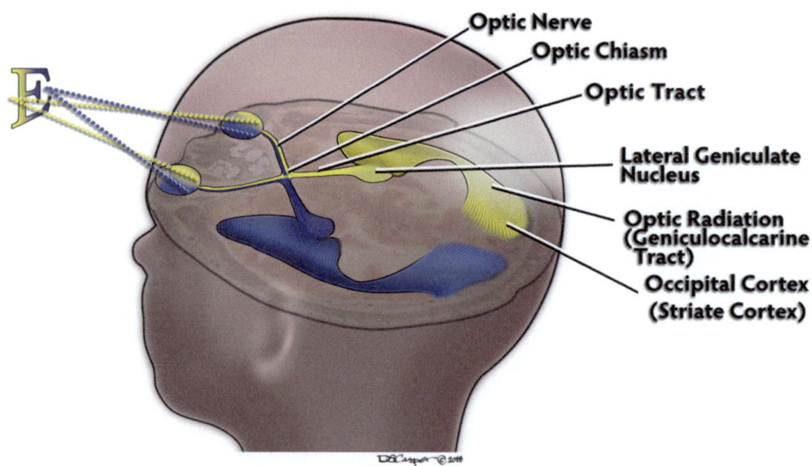

Fig. 38.2 A schematic view of the visual pathway from object to the visual cortex. Image projections are separated along the retinal vertical medians and travel together. Combined nasal and temporal nerve fibers enter the middle cranial fossa as the optic nerves but segregate out into separate temporal and nasal retinal information at the optic chiasm (note that the yellow, left half of the image contributes only to the right visual path intracranially, while the purple, or right side of the image, becomes the left; this is accomplished by temporal fibers remaining on the ipsilateral side, while nasal fibers cross over at the chiasm). Segregated right and left retinal information continues posteriorly in the optic tracts, is further processed in the lateral geniculate nuclei, and then reaches the visual cortex via the optic radiations. Not shown are optic tract fibers which leave the visual pathway prior to the lateral geniculate nuclei and terminate at the Edinger-Westphal nucleus, hypothalamic nuclei, and the superior colliculi to enable pupillary, circadian, and saccadic processing

Fig. 38.3 The complete pattern of ocular dominance columns in the human brain. (**a**) Cytochrome oxidase (CO) activity in layer 4 Cβ montage of the right primary visual cortex after loss of the right eye. The CO pattern in V2 is a montage compiled from three sections passing through layer 4. (**b**) Ocular dominance columns rendered by high-pass Fourier filtering of the image in (**a**). Columns are absent in the blind spot and monocular crescent regions. (From Adams DL, Sincich LC, Horton JC. Complete pattern of ocular dominance columns in human primary visual cortex. J Neurosci. 2007;27(39):10391–403, with permission)

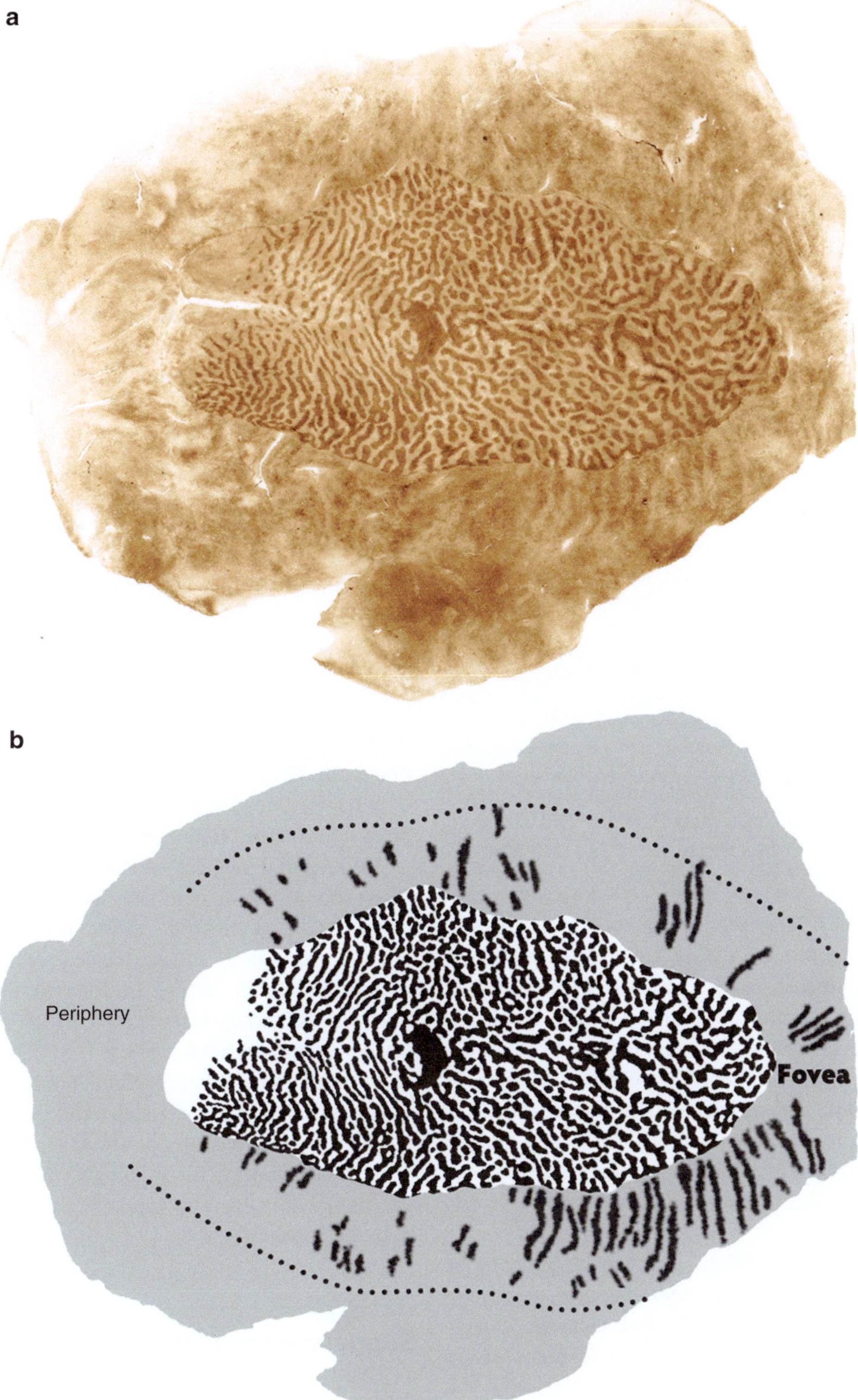

a
b
Periphery
Fovea

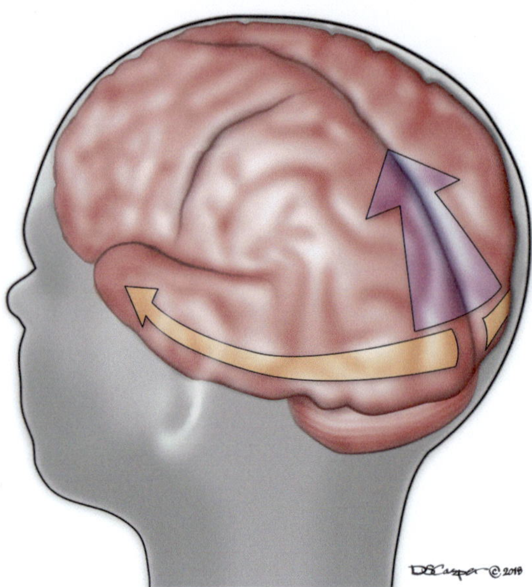

Fig. 38.4 V1 neurons project to two functional pathways: (1) the "What" pathway (horizontal arrow) where slow, color-sensitive parvocellular lateral geniculate nucleus (LGN) neurons project to V1, V2, and V4 and then project ventrally to the inferior temporal cortex; and (2) the "Where" pathway (vertical arrow), where fast magnocellular LGN neurons project to V1, V2, and V3 and then to the medial temporal cortex (MT) for motion processing and to the posterior parietal cortex for attention, localization, and action. (Data from the image found at https://en.wikipedia.org/wiki/Visual_cortex (https://commons.wikimedia.org/wiki/File:Ventral-dorsal_streams.svg) under the GNU Free Documentation License, version 1.2)

(Fig. 38.4). The "Where" pathway runs dorsally, projecting to area V5/MT (medial temporal cortex in humans) and the posterior parietal cortex. This is a specialized pathway where speed and motion in vision are processed. MT lesions (through trauma, neurodegenerative disease, or medication effects) lead to the perception that motion is frozen (akinetopsia) or that objects leave a trail of afterimages (palinopsia). However, these patients maintain the ability to identify objects.

The ventral "What" pathway appears to be involved in conscious identification of objects and features. For example, lesions to areas associated with V4 can cause loss of color vision (cerebral achromatopsia). Associated with V4, and nearby in the inferior temporal cortex, is the fusiform gyrus. Lesions in this area produce an inability to recognize faces, even familiar ones like the patient's parents and siblings (prosopagnosia). In a monkey model, neuroscientists have discovered that facial features are broken down into a series of information nodes that work together as a network to encode memory traces (engrams) of individually recognized faces.

Lesions to the right parietal cortex through large strokes in the middle cerebral artery territory can produce a particularly debilitating condition referred to as the contralateral hemispatial-neglect syndrome. In this condition, patients with a right unilateral parietal cortical defect are "blind" to stimuli in their contralateral left visual field, in either visual or personal sensory space. This can be tested with double simultaneous visual or tactile stimulation of the patient. For example, a patient with a right parietal lesion may forget to put their left arm into a sleeve, or to shave the left side of their face, or, negelct to eat food off the left side of their plate. Navigation and independent living are severely limited in these patients, much more so than in patients with verbal aphasias or hemiparesis. Right sided hemispatial neglect is rare because it is redundantly encoded in the brain bilaterally. While the left side of the world is predominantly encoded in the right hemisphere for most right-handed (left dominant) brains.

Hemispatial neglect (the absence of awareness) should not be confused with hemianopsia. Conscious awareness of vision requires intact visual processing areas located within the temporal-parietal cortex. Lesions to the optic tracts, LGN, and optic radiations, which spare the temporal and parietal cortex (see Chap. 36), result in a hemianopsia. Patients are fully aware of this specific type of visual scotoma, particularly if it is acquired later in life. Over time, however, patients may fill in empty regions by a perceptual illusion that replaces the blind area with the surround.

Suggested Reading

Adams DL, Sincich LC, Horton JC. Complete pattern of ocular dominance columns in human primary visual cortex. J Neurosci. 2007;27(39):10391–403.

Barrett AA. Aristotle and averted vision. R Astron Soc Can J. 1977;71(4):327.

Guillery RW, Sherman SM. Thalamic relay functions and their role in corticocortical communication: generalizations from the visual system. Neuron. 2002;33(2):163–75.

Horton JC, Trobe JD. Akinetopsia from nefazodone toxicity. Am J Ophthalmol. 1999;128(4):530–1.

Hubel DH. Eye, Brain, and Vision (Scientific American Library series : no 22). 1995.

Lal R, Friedlander MJ. Effect of passive eye position changes on retinogeniculate transmission in the cat. J Neurophysiol. 1990;63(3):502–22.

Lindstrom S, Wrobel A. Intracellular recordings from binocularly activated cells in the cat's dorsal lateral geniculate nucleus. Acta Neurobiol Exp (Wars). 1990;50(3):61–70.

McAlonan K, Cavanaugh J, Wurtz RH. Attentional modulation of thalamic reticular neurons. J Neurosci. 2006;26(16):4444–50.

Moeller S, Freiwald WA, Tsao DY. Patches with links: a unified system for processing faces in the macaque temporal lobe. Science. 2008;320(5881):1355–9.

Pelak VS, Hoyt WF. Symptoms of akinetopsia associated with traumatic brain injury and Alzheimer's disease. Neuro-Ophthalmology. 2005;29:137–42.

Poggio GF, Motter BC, Squatrito S, Trotter Y. Responses of neurons in visual cortex (V1 and V2) of the alert macaque to dynamic random-dot stereograms. Vis Res. 1985;25(3):397–406.

Schmid MC, Mrowka SW, Turchi J, Saunders RC, Wilke M, Peters AJ, et al. Blindsight depends on the lateral geniculate nucleus. Nature. 2010;466(7304):373–7.

Part VIII

Pediatrics and Strabismus

Amblyopia

39

Pamela F. Gallin

Amblyopia is a silent disease, the scourge of pediatric ophthalmology, and an end common pathway for many anatomic and strabismic problems. Many do not understand what it is and why it is of paramount importance. Amblyopia is visual deprivation in the brain, specifically the visual cortex (Brodmann Areas 17 and 18). At birth, the visual cortex must learn how to see, as many other cortical areas must learn how to function as well. This learning process requires normal and equal (left vs right) input to the visual cortex via the optic radiations, and any diminution of these signals can produce pathologic abnormalities in the Brodmann Areas that result in diminished visual acuity. This pathology is a structural deficit which, remarkably, can be reversed (usually) until age 7–9. The younger the child is at diagnosis and treatment, the faster and better the visual improvement. When not identified until early elementary school, it takes longer and is more challenging to reverse. Amblyopia is a national health issue and a silent disease, and early identification and immediate and appropriate treatment are critical in arresting this preventable and, if untreated, ultimately irreversible visual deficit.

Amblyopia is defined as a two-Snellen line difference of best corrected acuity from one eye to another. Amblyopia is usually classified as:

1. Amblyopia *ex anopsia* (anterior segment etiology)
2. Congenital (organic; posterior segment etiology)
3. Strabismic amblyopia (ocular misalignment etiology)
4. Anisometropic amblyopia (refractive etiology)

Strabismus and anisometropia (a refractive difference between the eyes of greater than 1.5–2.0 spherical equivalent diopters [in general]) are the most frequent causes of amblyopia, although structural anomalies contribute as well. Photoscreeners are now the standard of care in preverbal children. They are quite accurate and are recommended by the American Academy of Ophthalmology, the American Association of Pediatric Ophthalmology and Adult Strabismus, and the American Academy of Pediatrics. However, photoscreening should be combined with an examination by the pediatrician or healthcare provider in an attempt to find children with strabismus secondary to structural anomalies. An ophthalmologist must perform a full exam, including cycloplegic retinoscopy and indirect ophthalmoscopy. In a nonstrabismic child, it may be quite difficult to diagnose amblyopia. In a preliterate child, amblyopia is often inferred from retinoscopy, fixation preference, and an intraocular examination. Determination of fixation

P. F. Gallin, MD, FACS (✉)
Department of Ophthalmology, Edward S. Harkness
Eye Institute,Columbia University Vagelos College
of Physicians and Surgeons, New York, NY, USA
e-mail: pfg1@cumc.columbia.edu

© Springer Nature Switzerland AG 2019
D. S. Casper, G. A. Cioffi (eds.), *The Columbia Guide to Basic Elements of Eye Care*,
https://doi.org/10.1007/978-3-030-10886-1_39

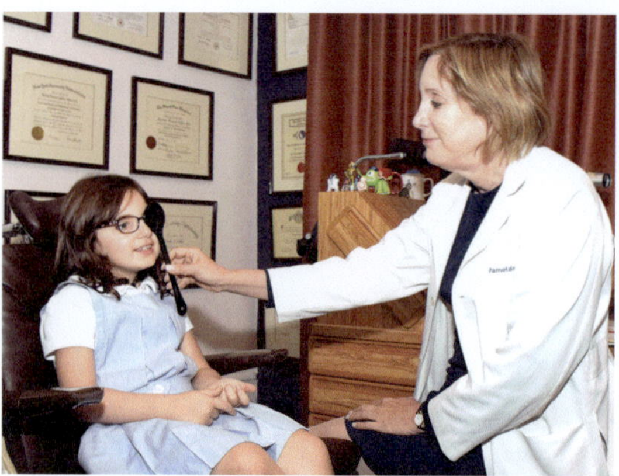

Fig. 39.1 Examination with occlusion of one eye

preference in an infant is exceedingly difficult to assess and requires the skills of an examiner schooled in the assessment of vision in preverbal children. When a child is able to read a Snellen chart of any type (see Fig. 2.1), one can appreciate large or subtle differences of acuity. When acuity differences are minimal, it is important that the second or non-seeing eye be evaluated on more than one occasion to determine that these are accurate data. Often, children are less cooperative when their second eye is tested; conversely, they are sometimes skittish when the first or initial eye is examined (Fig. 39.1). Photoscreeners are an excellent tool for flagging children with potential and existing issues that require further evaluation.

Etiology

The exact etiology of the amblyopia determines the treatment. In the case of structural problems, it is imperative that these anomalies, such as a cataract, be corrected prior to the onset of treatment. In the case of strabismus, it is imperative that the amblyopia be resolved prior to any surgical procedures (with some exceptions). With anisometropia, spectacle correction is necessary to ensure a focused image on the eye that has the greater refractive error. David Hubel and Torsten Wiesel's Nobel Prize-winning work with macaques and kittens showed that amblyopia occurs due to a structural change in the cerebral cortex at a microcellular level. They concluded that during an initial window following birth, normal vision develops in the occipital cortex, in the absence of structural anomalies. If, however, there is asymmetry in the presentation of images to the two eyes, then, on a cellular level, the occipital cortex layers correlating with the less clear eye become severely disorganized. They also showed that if there are cerebral cortical changes due to visual obscuration and the image is subsequently normalized, vision can, in fact, recover to an excellent (but not perfect) level.

There are numerous windows of time in the development of vision. The first window, which determines the onset of vision, is within days and weeks of birth. This is the determining factor in the urgency of congenital cataract extraction. If the visual defect goes unopposed (for any structural, strabismus, or refractive etiologies), poor vision will become entrenched within a few months' time. However, if there is a bilaterally symmetric obstacle, then vision appreciation in cortical cells is "suppressed," and anatomic reorganization begins anew when the obstacle is reversed. The amblyogenic window exists from birth to approximately 7.5–9 years of age. This end point is not exact but is the current, clinically accepted age after which vision improvement can no longer occur.

The basis for amblyopia treatment is to correct existing conditions which have produced the visual inequality (structural, strabismic, or refractive etiologies) and then depress visual input to the preferred eye, thereby forcing the second (i.e., poorly seeing) eye to compensate for this new deficit. If a perfectly focused image on the macula of the poorly seeing eye is present, this method results in cellular reorganization in the occipital cortex and subsequent improvement in vision.

Treatment

Classic (Occlusion)

The classic amblyopia therapy utilizes an occlusive patch of which there are two types readily available in the United States, Elastoplast and Coverlet (Fig. 39.2). The initial treatment regimen is for full-time occlusion. This means that the child wears the occlusive patch on the better eye on a full-time basis, during waking hours, except for 1 h per day. Although a recent paper reported that 2 h per day of occlusion was equivalent to the full-time patching regimen, this author does not subscribe to the results. Furthermore, many parents do less than the reported time of patching.

The child is patched 1 week per year of life. In the event that the child does not return for examination following this interval, then *occlusion amblyopia* may occur. Occlusion amblyopia is an amblyopia that develops in the previously preferred eye due to overpatching the preferred eye; in these cases, the poorly seeing eye becomes the preferred eye, with better acuity than the previous "good" eye. All patients undergoing occlusion therapy must be warned to remove the patch if they miss follow-up visits. Full-time occlusion has numerous difficulties, most significantly the possibility of developing occlusion amblyopia and the requirement for strict cooperation with the prescribed regimen.

One of the many difficulties in patients who occlude full time is that functionally they cannot see in the patched eye, forcing the child to use a relatively non-seeing eye to fulfill daily tasks. This is quite difficult for children and their families, and if the amblyopia is dense, treatment essentially blinds the child. In addition, at times, adhesive from the patch can irritate the skin, requiring either cessation of patching or, at times, medical treatment to excoriated areas.

However, full-time occlusion in almost all amblyopia treatment is the initial treatment of choice. This regimen will yield the largest improvement in acuity in the smallest time interval, due to the fact that the less preferred eye must function on a full-time basis. It is quite extraordinary that the occipital cortex retains plasticity up until the age of at least 7–9 years.

For example, a 6-month-old infant who has a fixation preference (i.e., unequal acuity) due to an esotropia will be patched only 3 days prior to the next visit for fear of rapid development of an occlusion amblyopia in the better eye. Fixation preference in young children is extraordinarily plastic, such that it can change within hours, thus requiring frequent follow-up.

A baby's visual demands are less significant than those of a 5-year-old. Therefore, with the rapid increase in vision and lower visual demands, a baby will become more comfortable with occlusion therapy in a relatively shorter interval than will a school-aged child who is learning to read and is additionally subject to peers' social comments about their appearance with a patch.

With all children, the initial phases of amblyopia treatment are the most difficult. Parents need support and cajoling to understand the effectiveness of this treatment. In the extreme, one can explain that if the treatment is not followed, the child will grow up effectively a one-eyed person, and, in the event of any loss of vision (be it an injury or other pathological process) in the preferred eye, will not be able to function at the

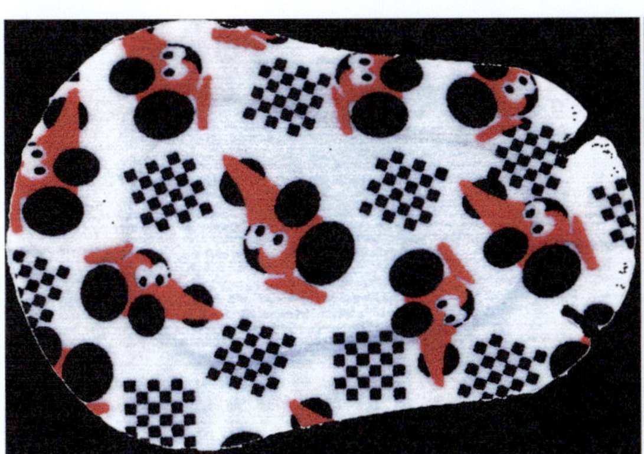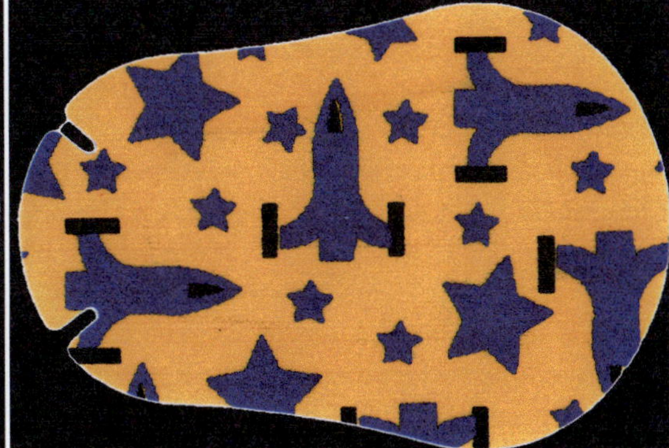

Fig. 39.2 Patches: note – pointy narrow side aligned toward the patient's nose

same level as they would otherwise have, with at least one eye with normal vision.

Often, in the case of anisometropia, children are identified on 4-year-old or kindergarten vision screening examinations. Much to the dismay of their parents, it is determined that the vision in one eye is in the range of 20/80 to 20/100, while the other eye is 20/20. The parents are understandably concerned that this has never been brought to their attention before. These "older" children are difficult to treat and constitute the significant majority of amblyopes detected on incidental eye examinations. It is necessary for them to use a spectacle in the one eye that often has either an oblique astigmatism or significant myopia or hyperopia, relative to the other eye. At times, using such an intermediate-level treatment for one time interval prior to the use of occlusion therapy can facilitate the reversal of amblyopia, thus delaying or eliminating the eventual need for full-time occlusion.

Often, children have difficulty with occlusion therapy because they understandably prefer to use their better-seeing eye. They can be quite vociferous in their protests against occlusion of their better eye. One alternative is to additionally instill 1% atropine drops into the preferred eye, which blurs vision, such that the amblyopic eye becomes the relatively better-seeing eye. In this case, even if the child removes the occluder, they cannot see well due to atropine-induced blur. This can be used to get children to accept their spectacles and a patch in the early, and most difficult phases of treatment, and can be justified in comparison with a simple patching failure.

Some physicians use occlusion therapy on a limited, few-hours-per-day basis as an initial treatment regimen. There is one paper which states that 2 h of patching per day is equal to full time minus 1 h. I find the shorter time to be not equal and also challenging at the beginning of occlusion when it is most challenging for children and their parents. After the vision has begun to "move," then a tapering of occlusion time can be undertaken. There are exceptions as in very young infants, neurologically challenged children, and those with genetic syndromes.

Bangerter Films

An alternative to full-time occlusion therapy (which, as stated previously, is the preferred initial treatment) is Bangerter films, transparent plastic squares introduced by Dr. Alfred Bangerter in 1956 (Fig. 39.3). These semitransparent films are essentially used in anisometropes as they mount directly on a spectacle lens. The Bangerter film functions to switch fixation to the less preferred eye when acuity reaches a specific threshold. As an example, if a patient sees 20/20 in the right eye and 20/60 in the left (amblyopic) eye, a Bangerter film is used on the right spectacle lens to blur acuity to a level two lines worse than the amblyopic eye, in this case, 20/100. For a large target, the child will see with both eyes. For smaller targets they will effectively only see with the left or amblyopic eye.

Bangerter films come in nine densities, which occlude to different levels of image clarity. As therapy results in visual improvement, the film can be weakened such that more light reaches the normal-acuity eye. They are an excellent treatment modality with middle-range amblyopias, and for maintenance until 9 years of age, once excellent acuity has been achieved.

Bangerter films are an excellent adjunct in the treatment of amblyopia. School-aged children often prefer these films as their vision is improv-

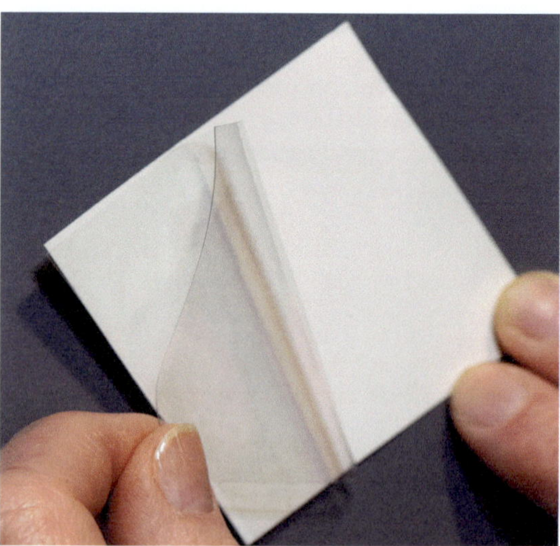

Fig. 39.3 Bangerter film

ing, for a variety of reasons. First, they can see from both eyes for larger targets. Second, it is cosmetically acceptable compared to occlusive patching. School-aged children can be quite brutal when a child wears a patch, and Bangerter films are not cosmetically objectionable. Most children do not notice that their colleague is wearing one. Third, as vision improves, the film can be downwardly titrated. Fourth, when the child has achieved a final vision in the amblyopic eye, a very mild Bangerter film can be used to tip the balance in favor of the preferred eye.

Optical Penalization

Optical penalization is the intentional induction of a pharmacologic or optical blur to the preferred eye.

Pharmacologic

In Europe, a pharmacologic blur through the use of 1% atropine drops in the preferred eye is frequently used. This allows the preferred eye to see clearly only at distance and the amblyopic eye to see at both distance and near. The frequency of visits to the ophthalmologist can be diminished and intervals increased, as the treated eye is much less likely to develop an occlusion amblyopia to the same degree as happens with full-time patching. This can be very useful in preverbal children who are resistant to occlusion therapy. It is an excellent adjunct to spectacles or occlusion therapy.

Optical

Optical penalization was created by Dr. David Guyton to induce an optical blur in the preferred eye, thus switching fixation to the less preferred or second eye. Specifically, using the American Optical Vectographic Stereopsis slide, the cycloplegic refraction is purposely blurred over the preferred eye until fixation is switched to the other eye. This penalization Rx is then prescribed to the patient.

By using penalization spectacles, the patient effectively assigns the amblyopic eye for distance and the preferred eye for near. Again, there is less chance of occlusion amblyopia, and the patient usually tolerates these well. All penalization treatments follow a period of initial occlusion. They are most effective when the acuity is in the 20/80 or better range.

All of these techniques require an understanding of the dynamics of the specific child-parent interaction. Some parents do not want a patch, and other parents resist pharmacologic treatment. It is very important to discuss the need for amblyopia treatment with the parents and have the child begin treatment early on. When the child is older, it is important to provide choices as to which modality the child would prefer, as this often changes over the course of the child's development. Amblyopia treatment must be maintained until the child is approximately 9 years of age and is, of course, exceedingly difficult, as this requires constant treatment. It is an invisible treatment in that there are not any side effects from medication. Furthermore, the treatment needs to be maintained over many years, which is extremely difficult for children. Giving them the option of different treatment modalities at different times frequently makes it more acceptable.

The goal is vision of 20/20 in the amblyopic eye. Even when a child achieves 20/20 acuity, on direct questioning, they may say that it is less preferable to the better eye. This is due to the fact that, on a microcellular basis, cellular reorganization in the occipital cortex is not identical to that of the preferred eye. Stereopsis requires equal vision in each of two eyes and excellent alignment. These criteria need to be met before 2 years of age. Unfortunately, visual challenges are frequently not diagnosed prior to this age.

Patching Failures

Many children are "patching failures." This occurs due to the difficulty of having a child of any age function with a poorly seeing eye, resulting in poor compliance with the planned course of therapy. Many parents find it difficult to institute amblyopia treatment of school-aged children due to their forced reliance on the amblyopic eye, which results in handicapped functioning in school. Furthermore, occlusion therapy often begins at a time when children are just learning to read. Amblyopic children should be given front row seats and be placed in an optimal position (without patch) for any testing, and teachers should be well-informed about the condition and the treatment plan, so that they understand their important role in this process. Their encouragement and participation often helps determine visual outcomes in school-aged children.

There are children who are discovered to have a net refractive difference of more than seven to eight diopters of spherical equivalent between the two eyes. In these children we know that it is quite rare for them, even in an optimal situation, to develop excellent acuity in what is most often a highly myopic eye. An attempt should still be made to improve the acuity of all children, but the specific etiology of the amblyopia directly affects realistic expectations and appropriate counseling of parents.

If, after many months, a child is unresponsive to occlusion therapy and a parent chooses to stop treatment, it is important that a parent and a witness sign the chart, recording that there was a discussion between parent and physician concerning the desired treatment, that the treatment was unable to be complied with, and that the parents fully understand the consequences of treatment cessation.

In the event that an examiner is treating a child for amblyopia and there is no change in the acuity despite the child's compliance with treatment and family cooperation, the examiner should rethink the diagnosis, repeat the exam, and at times consider a neurological evaluation in conjunction with a retinal examination. Visually significant oblique astigmatisms are often difficult to ascertain and are ultimately noted on repeat retinoscopy. Autorefraction can be very helpful in finding small yet significant oblique astigmatisms. An electroretinogram (ERG) and/or visual evoked potential (VEP) in conjunction with other neuroradiologic testing, if deemed appropriate, may identify the presence of subnormal retinal functioning. Any subnormal visual input received by the visual cortex will result in diminished cortical competence, so an aberrant signal due to retinal or retrobulbar dysfunction, even in the face of a corrected refractive error, strabismus, or other anterior amblyogenic pathology, will still produce an amblyopic state not responsive to typical occlusion therapy. Assuming the detected pathology is not amenable to treatment, occlusive therapy would not be indicated.

Conclusion

Amblyopia forms the basis for many pediatric ophthalmic clinical diseases and subsequent visual rehabilitation. However, treatment can be exceedingly daunting. Both parents and children require a great deal of moral support and cajoling. Often, various types of treatment must be substituted to gain the compliance of these children and their families. When properly prescribed and followed, occlusive amblyopic therapy can convert a relatively non-seeing eye into one with remarkably good acuity.

Suggested Reading

Aldestein AM, Scully J. Epidemiological aspects of squint. Br Med J. 1967;3:34–8.

Duke-Elder S. System of ophthalmology. St. Louis: Mosby; 1958.

Gallin P. Amblyopia in pediatric ophthalmology. USA/Germany: Thieme; 2000.

Hubel DH, Wiesel TN. Effects of mononuclear deprivation in kittens. Arch Exp Pharmak. 1964;248:492–7.

Hubel DH, Wiesel TN. The period of susceptibility, the physiological effects of unilateral eye closure in kittens. J Physiol. 1970;206:419–36.

Repka MX, Gallin P, Scholz RT, Guyton DL. Determinants of optical penalization by vectographic fixation reversal. Ophthalmology. 1985;92(11):1584–6.

Wiesel TN, Hubel DH. Single-cell responses in striate cortex kittens deprived of vision in one eye. J Neurophysiol. 1963;26:1003–17.

Strabismus

Steven E. Brooks

Binocular vision gives us the ability to achieve high degrees of depth perception. It improves visual orientation and balance, enhances eye-hand coordination, improves visual acuity, and facilitates normal social interaction. Its relative importance is underscored by the complexity of neural and neuromuscular systems that have developed to control it. Strabismus is the general term used to describe any situation in which the visual axes of the two eyes are not properly aligned. In other words, the eyes are not simultaneously focused on, or directed at, the object being viewed. It is a pathological condition whose severity, implications, and consequences vary greatly.

Because of the broad nature of the definition and situations it encompasses, it is difficult to define overall prevalence or incidence of strabismus in a population. Although many epidemiological studies note a prevalence of 1–4% in the population, this may be an underestimation, since milder or transient forms of strabismus are generally not included and most studies are focused only on prevalence in children. It is critical to recognize, however, that the presence of strabismus can be a sign of potentially serious underlying pathology in the eye, orbit, or brain. In addition, the presence of strabismus may lead to amblyopia and anomalous neural development in the visual cortex of children and produce disabling symptoms in adults. Psychosocial consequences and quality of life issues resulting from strabismus may also be significant.

Classification and Characterization of Strabismus

There are many possible classification schemes for strabismus. At a minimum, it should be described according to several distinct characteristics, including frequency, direction, comitance, time of onset, and whether or not it is primary or secondary. The clinician should be able to detect and describe the misalignment in terms of those characteristics.

Frequency

Strabismus can be manifest constantly, intermittently, or only under conditions in which binocular vision is particularly stressed or disrupted (e.g., by occlusion, systemic illness or stress, or extreme fatigue). Manifest deviations are called tropias, while latent deviations are called phorias. Phorias generally have much less pathological significance than tropias and are much more

S. E. Brooks, MD (✉)
Columbia University Irving Medical Center,
New York, NY, USA

Department of Pediatric Ophthalmology, Jonas
Children's Vision Care, Columbia University Vagelos
College of Physicians and Surgeons, New York-
Presbyterian/Morgan Stanley Children's Hospital,
New York, NY, USA
e-mail: seb2204@cumc.columbia.edu

difficult to detect. By definition, phorias are generally well controlled but can cause symptoms such as eyestrain, blurring, and headache, particularly with fatigue. Strabismus occurring in the context of severely altered mental states (e.g., sleep, general anesthesia, coma) is a normal, usually self-limited occurrence and would not be considered a phoria or intermittent tropia.

Direction

The direction of a deviation can be around any of the three principal axes of eye rotation (horizontal, vertical, and axial) (Fig. 40.1) and is a particularly important feature to document, as it can point to the potential etiology and guide management. The following terms are used to describe the direction of deviation and can be applied in various combinations to describe complex cases. Analogous terms are used for phorias:

- Orthotropia: Normal binocular alignment. No strabismus is present.
- Esotropia: The eyes are overly convergent or crossed.

- Exotropia: The eyes are overly divergent or wall-eyed.
- Hypertropia/hypotropia: One eye is higher than the other. The higher eye is the hypertropic eye, and the lower eye is the hypotropic eye.
- Cyclotropia: One eye is rotated clockwise or counterclockwise relative to the other (Figs. 40.2, 40.3, and 40.4).

The magnitude of a strabismus is often expressed in terms of the angle of misalignment. Instead of degrees of deviation, the more common unit is the prism diopter. One prism diopter is roughly equal to 0.5°; a deviation of 20 prism diopters is equal to about 11°. Cyclotropias, on the other hand, are exclusively expressed in degrees of rotation rather than prism diopters. For the purposes of diagnosing and characterizing strabismus, it is generally not necessary to quantify the deviation, although quantification may be important for monitoring the natural history of a strabismus, surgical or optical management, and response to treatment.

Comitance

A third important element of classification is the manner in which the strabismus varies with gaze position. Deviations that are comitant show little or no alterations with changes in gaze, while incomitant deviations change significantly in the different directions of gaze. For example, if a person has esotropia that increases in magnitude in left gaze, that esotropia would be classified as incomitant. Incomitant deviations more likely suggest pathological processes affecting the orbit, cranial nerves, or central nervous system

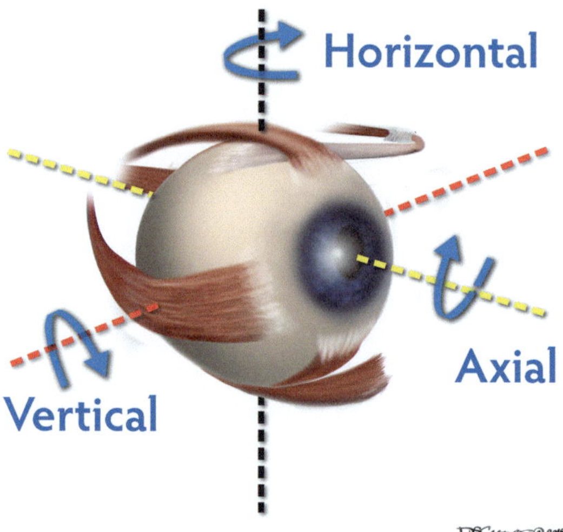

Fig. 40.1 Diagram showing the three principal axes of eye rotation. Rotation about the red axis produces vertical eye movement. Rotation about the black axis produces horizontal eye movement. Rotation about the yellow axis produces incyclo- or excyclotorsional movements. The medial and lateral rectus muscles produce purely horizontal movement of the eye, while the other four muscles produce varying degrees of rotation about all three axes of rotation

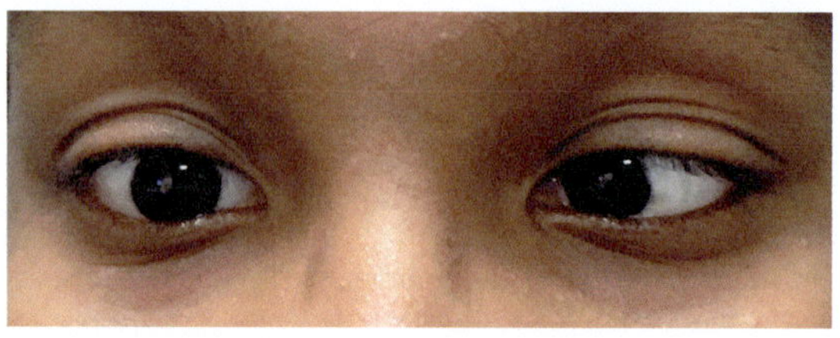

Fig. 40.2 Photograph demonstrating esotropia, or "crossed" eyes

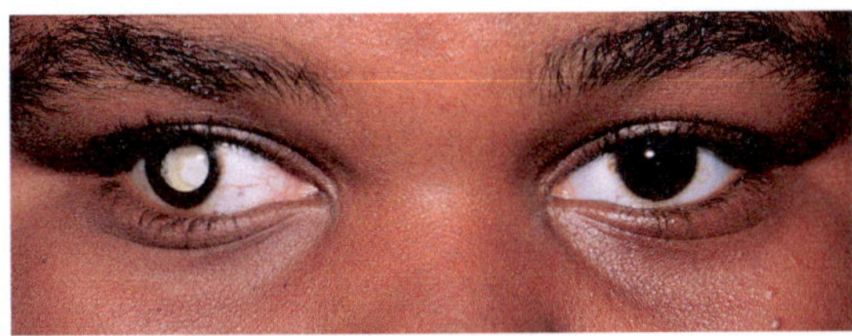

Fig. 40.3 Photograph demonstrating exotropia, associated in this case with leukocoria (a white pupil) in the right eye

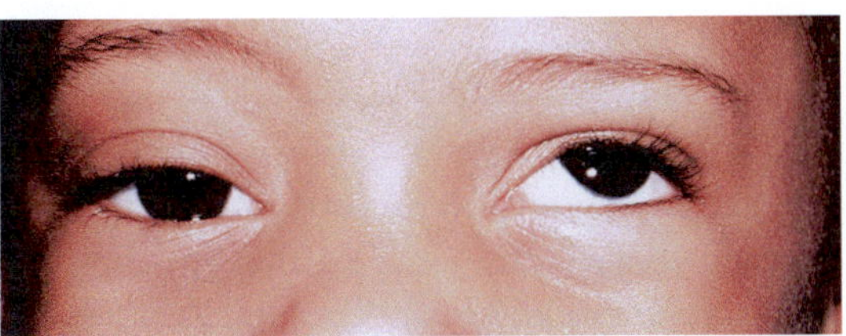

Fig. 40.4 Photograph showing hypertropia of the left eye. Alternatively, if this photograph was taken with the patient attempting to look upward, then the right eye could be considered hypotropic

than do comitant deviations and are therefore of greater concern clinically.

Time of Onset

It is important to discern the time of onset of strabismus. In the most basic terms, strabismus can either be congenital or acquired. Strabismus presenting in the first 4–6 months of life is considered to be congenital or infantile, and these are generally associated with the poorest prognosis for normal binocular vision and demand early intervention to optimize the chances for success. However, congenital strabismus is typically less suggestive of serious underlying disease than is acquired strabismus.

Relationship to Underlying Pathology

Finally, strabismus may be primary or secondary. Primary forms are thought to be due to intrinsic functional defects in the binocular visual system in an otherwise healthy patient. A positive family history is sometimes present, though specific genetic loci have not been identified. Congenital esotropia and intermittent exotropia are two examples of primary strabismus conditions. Secondary forms, on the other hand, are due to specific underlying lesions such as cranial nerve palsy, loss of vision, orbital pathology, or disorders of the neuromuscular junction. Strabismus associated with other underlying pathology is typically incomitant and acquired, although the onset may be quite slow and insidious.

Detection and Diagnosis

Detection and accurate characterization of strabismus are critical to determining appropriate evaluation and treatment (see Chap. 3). The presence of symptoms is particularly helpful in adults, who typically complain of blurry or double vision (diplopia) or cosmetic concerns. In young children, however, symptoms are typically absent, especially if the strabismus has been present for some time. In adults or older children who complain of diplopia, the presence of strabismus may or may not be readily apparent on casual inspection, since the angle may be small or the deviation may be incomitant or intermittent. In such cases, it is useful to confirm that the diplopia is due to strabismus, and not an intrinsic refractive issue in one eye, by noting that it is relieved by occlusion of either eye. Young children with diplopia may not be able to effectively verbalize this symptom, but instead indirectly indicate the symptom's presence by closing or rubbing one eye.

Measurement of visual acuity, an essential part of the physical examination, is not particularly helpful in diagnosing strabismus. It is absolutely critical, however, in evaluating strabismus, because (as will be discussed later) loss of vision in one or both eyes may cause strabismus to develop. In terms of detecting strabismus, tests of binocular visual function are much more informative. There are many specialized tests that may be used, all of which attempt to determine the presence or absence of fusion (the successful synthesis in the brain of the images coming from each eye). Each eye sees the world from a slightly different perspective, due to their separate positions in space. The fusion of these two similar yet slightly disparate images allows the perception of three-dimensionality and depth and also provides a greater amount of visual data, which leads to improved acuity. One of the most commonly used tests to assess binocular vision and fusion is a stereogram. By using glasses or another optical device to provide distinctly separate images to each eye (e.g., using polarized or colored filters), fusion and stereopsis can be measured. Patients with strabismus may have simultaneous perception of the images, but do not perceive any apparent depth or stereopsis. The presence of intact fusion and stereopsis argues strongly against the presence of strabismus.

Perhaps the simplest way to detect strabismus on physical examination is by shining a penlight toward the patient's eyes and noting the position and symmetry of the corneal light reflex in each eye (Hirschberg test). Normally, the light reflexes are well centered on the pupils or symmetrically displaced in the same direction. However, if the corneal light reflex is centered in one eye and significantly displaced in the other eye, then strabismus is likely present. If the light reflex becomes centered in the second eye when that eye is forced to look at the light by covering the other eye, it is even stronger evidence that strabismus is present (cover test). It is important to keep in mind, however, that strabismus may only be present intermittently or in certain gaze positions (see Fig. 3.5).

Assessment of eye movement is a basic component of the physical examination. It is especially important in the presence of strabismus. The observer should attempt to note if either eye is limited in its range of movement (duction testing) and whether or not the eyes move symmetrically into the different positions of gaze (version testing). Abnormalities in ductions or versions produce characteristic patterns of strabismus and may be suggestive of specific underlying lesions (e.g., sixth nerve palsy, orbital floor fracture, or internuclear ophthalmoplegia (often associated with multiple sclerosis in younger patients and stroke in an older population)).

Observation of a patient's head posture can provide important information about the presence and nature of strabismus. Patients with incomitant strabismus may habitually tilt their head or turn their face to one side if it enhances binocular vision. In fact, the presence of a habitual head tilt or face turn in a child should strongly alert the physician to the possibility of strabismus and not be assumed to be musculoskeletal in nature. Furthermore, head posture itself may provide a clue to the underlying problem. For example, patients with unilateral fourth nerve palsy typically tilt their head toward the opposite shoulder, and patients with partial sixth nerve palsy turn their face to the side of the palsy. Interestingly, if a patch is placed over one eye, thereby eliminating any diplopia, the compensatory head tilt will generally improve or resolve, since the purpose of the head posture is to eliminate diplopia. Thus, an abnormal head posture in the setting of strabismus is highly suggestive of binocular vision being intact and is therefore a favorable sign. The absence of a compensatory head posture in the setting of strabismus may indicate unequal vision but is less specific in that regard.

In addition to the history and physical examination, photoscreening devices are available that detect strabismus by using software to analyze symmetry of the corneal light reflexes and characteristics of pupillary red reflexes in digital images. These instruments may be particularly helpful in detecting small angle deviations in children. It is important to keep in mind, whether the angle of deviation is large or small, that the effects on vision are similar. The magnitude of deviation, therefore, is not a particularly good marker of severity in the functional sense (Fig. 40.5).

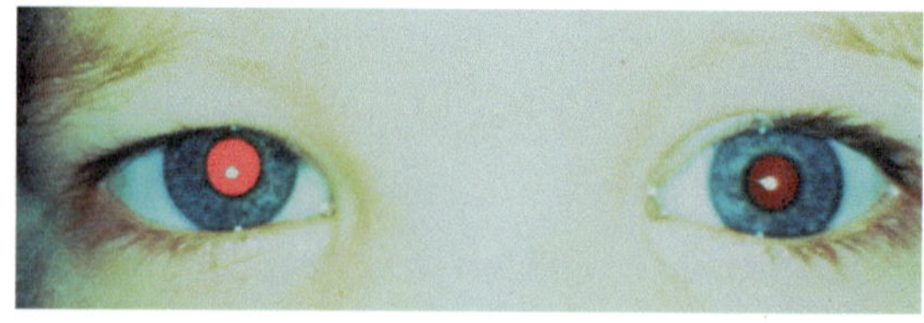

Fig. 40.5 Photo showing an asymmetric red reflex. The dark red reflex on the left is a normal, well-focused red reflex, while the brighter reflex on the right is suggestive of poor fixation on the light. In this case the right eye is slightly hypertropic, as indicated by the corneal light reflex being lower on cornea than on the left eye

Specific Entities and Special Cases of Strabismus

Congenital Esotropia

Eye alignment at birth is often variable but becomes progressively more stable and aligned over the first 4–6 months. For this to occur, sensory and motor pathways must be intact, and neurological development must be normal as well. Impairments in any of these components can prevent or compromise development of normal binocular vision. In addition, for reasons not well understood, some children develop esotropia, or crossed eyes, soon after birth in spite of being otherwise normal. Sometimes there is a positive family history, but often not. The deviation is constant, often quite large, and usually easily detected. It must be differentiated from pseudo-esotropia, caused by the presence of prominent epicanthal skin folds causing the eyes to appear esotropic when in fact they are straight (Fig. 40.6).

Other anomalies of eye movement may be associated with congenital esotropia, including overaction of the inferior oblique muscles (causing vertical deviations in side gaze), latent nystagmus, and dissociated horizontal or vertical deviations. Early intervention is important, and eye muscle surgery in the first year of life is considered to provide the best opportunity for binocular visual development. Even with the best management, however, in these cases, the prognosis for good binocular vision and stereopsis is low.

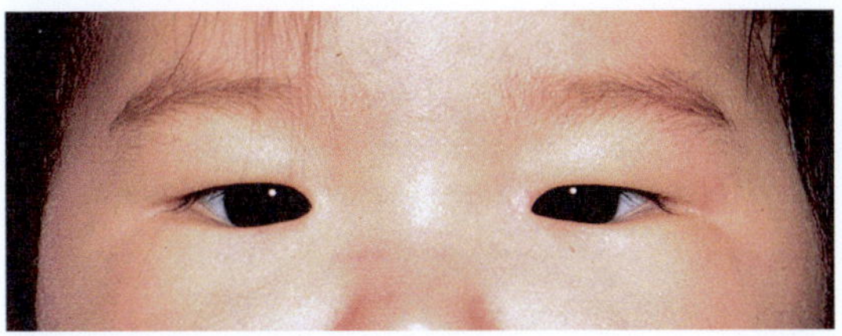

Fig. 40.6 Photograph demonstrating pseudo-esotropia. The presence of prominent epicanthal skin folds obscures the sclera medially, giving the impression that the eyes are crossed. The corneal light reflexes, however, are well centered in each eye, suggesting that the eyes are straight and that esotropia is not actually present

Accommodative Esotropia

Accommodation is voluntary contraction of the ciliary muscle inside the eye to alter the shape of the lens in order to shift focus from distance to near. Accommodation is reflexively linked to pupillary constriction and binocular convergence. Convergence helps to maintain binocular fixation on objects as they get closer. Esotropia can occur, however, if the amount of accommodation required is high, as may be the case, for example, in patients who are highly hyperopic (farsighted) or in patients whose reflex convergence is inherently excessive for any given level of accommodation (e.g., a so-called high accommodative convergence/accommodation ratio). In either case the excess convergence tone may overwhelm fusional control mechanisms and lead to esotropia. This type of strabismus is relatively common, tends to appear in early childhood rather than infancy, and a positive family history is common. Since the problem stems from an optical issue (accommodative effort), the solution is optical. Glasses to correct hyperopia, or bifocals to reduce accommodative demand, generally are very successful. However, because the strabismus tends to be intermittent and most obvious when looking at near objects, there is often a delay in diagnosis, frequently leading to amblyopia that must also be treated.

Sixth Nerve Palsy

The sixth cranial, or abducens nerve, provides motor innervation to the lateral rectus muscle. In doing so it is critically involved in horizontal eye movement and alignment. Damage to the sixth nerve by any mechanism causes lateral rectus weakness on the same side. The palsy may be partial or complete, causing an incomitant esotropia of the affected eye that is worse in gaze toward the affected side and worse at distance than near fixation. Depending on severity, fusion may be possible in gaze toward the opposite side, with a resulting face turn toward the affected side. The simple relationship between the sixth cranial nerve and lateral rectus does not generally allow the specific location of the lesion to be deduced based on the strabismus alone. The differential diagnosis of sixth nerve palsy is quite long, varies with age, and encompasses a wide variety of pathological conditions. It can also occur as a result of raised intracranial pressure, and neurological evaluation, including neuroimaging, is generally indicated (Fig. 40.7).

Fourth Nerve Palsy

The fourth cranial, or trochlear nerve, provides motor innervation to the superior oblique muscle. This muscle is involved primarily in cyclovertical eye movement. Its main actions are to cyclorotate the eye inward (incyclotorsion) and downward, and it also exerts an abducting force, particularly in downgaze (i.e., the normal ocular position for reading). Damage to the nerve causes an incomitant hypertropia of the affected eye, worse with the eye in adduction. The palsy is also associated with excyclotropia and esotropia in downgaze. In unilateral cases, there is often a compensatory head tilt toward the oppo-site side (e.g., a right fourth nerve palsy is associated with a head tilt to the left). A compensatory head tilt is especially common in children with what is assumed to be a congenital form of this problem and can be confused with muscular torticollis.

The congenital form is not typically indicative of serious underlying disease and requires no neurologic investigation. Acquired cases, often bilateral, may occur in the setting of closed head trauma, while unilateral cases are often the result of microvascular injury in diabetes and hypertension. A high index of suspicion should be maintained, and neurologic investigation carried out, in acquired cases and those associated with signs or symptoms suggestive of central nervous system disease (e.g., headache, ataxia, blurred vision, or nystagmus) (Fig. 40.8).

Intermittent Exotropia

This form of strabismus is relatively common but, due to its intermittent nature, may be underdiagnosed. It tends to occur in early-to-

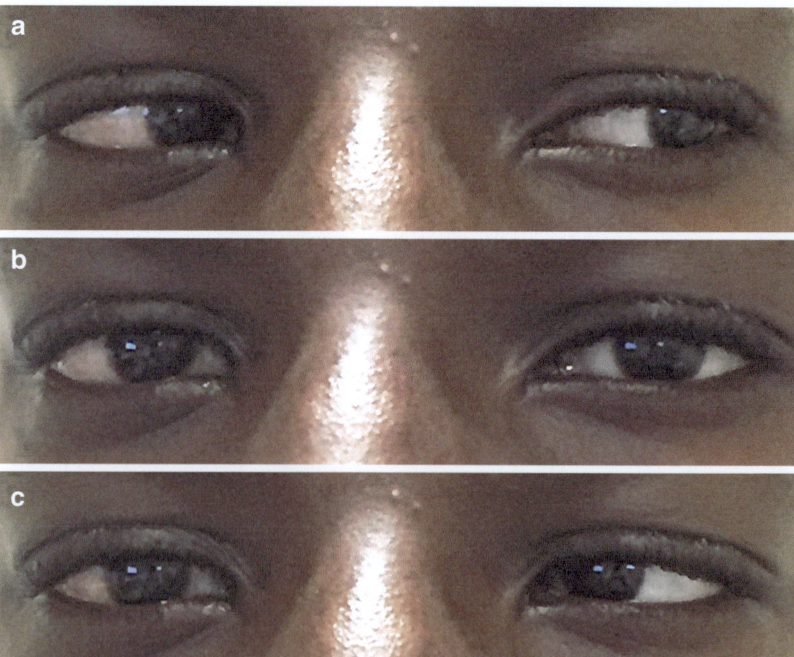

Fig. 40.7 Photographs of a patient with right sixth nerve palsy. (**a**) Shows normal gaze to the left, (**b**) very slight esotropia in primary position, and (**c**) marked esotropia in right gaze due to inability move the right eye laterally. This patient tended to adopt a small face turn to the right, keeping the eyes in a left gaze position, to avoid double vision

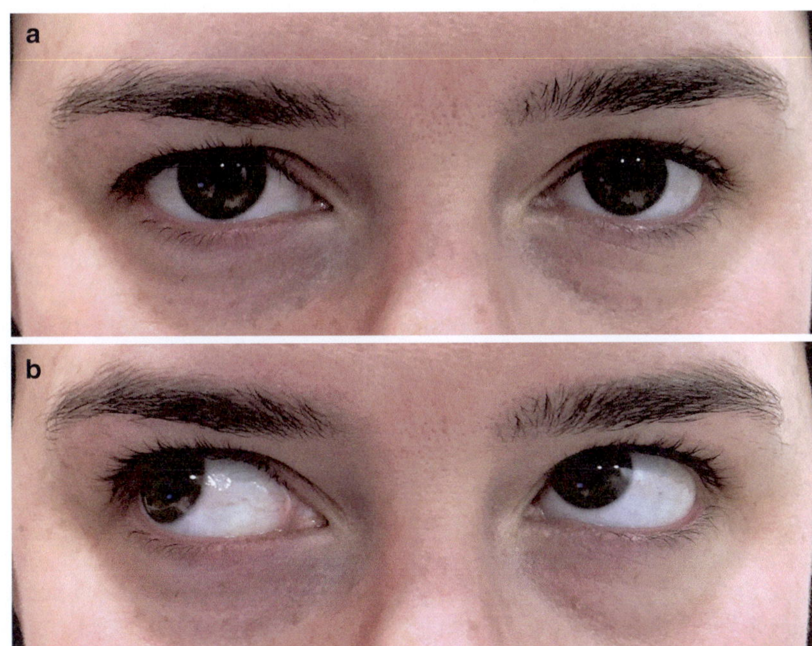

Fig. 40.8 Photos showing a patient with a left superior oblique palsy. (**a**) The eyes appear well aligned in primary gaze. (**b**) A marked left hypertropia is noted in right gaze due to the loss of action of the left superior oblique, a muscle that acts to move the eye in a downward direction, particularly when the eye is in adduction

middle childhood and can vary greatly in magnitude and frequency. A positive family history is not uncommon. It is typically first detected by the parents but often missed by the primary care physician due to its intermittent nature and the tendency for it to be well controlled during times of mental alertness. It tends to be manifest more frequently when patients are tired, sick, or visually inattentive and is generally more prominent with distance fixation. It can be provoked by exposure to bright sunlight and, though not normally symptomatic, frequently causes patients to unconsciously close one eye, perhaps to avoid diplopia. Because it is intermittent and not usually of early onset, this form of strabismus is typically associated with excellent vision and stereopsis and is not usually associated with amblyopia. Treatment includes correction of underlying refractive errors, anti-suppression exercises in some cases, and eye muscle surgery. There is no consensus on the optimal timing of surgical intervention; the decision is based on a number of factors, including evidence of progression, magnitude of the deviation, and age at onset. It is common with intermittent exotropia that surgery may have to be repeated, most often because the exotropia tends to recur.

Thyroid-Related Strabismus

Graves' disease is often associated with significant orbital complications, including enlargement and fibrosis of the extraocular muscles and orbital fat (see also Chap. 29). The inferior rectus is the most commonly involved muscle, followed by the medial rectus. Muscle enlargement with sparing of the tendons is typical and may precede strabismus, which tends to be restrictive in nature. For example, fibrosis and contracture of the inferior rectus muscle causes hypotropia in the affected eye with limited ability to elevate the eye secondary to loss of muscle elasticity. Proptosis is also typically present due to the increase in muscle volume as well as an expansion in the volume of other orbital soft tissues. Diplopia is common, and surgical intervention (e.g., recession of fibrosed muscles) is often required to restore at least a limited range of single binocular vision. Approximately 5% of patients also develop myasthenia gravis (see below), which can also cause strabismus if the extraocular muscles are affected.

Myasthenia Gravis

Myasthenia gravis can affect any of the extraocular muscles. In approximately two-thirds of cases, they are the primary sites of involvement, and occasionally the disease is confined to the ocular muscles. Affected muscles are weakened at the neuromuscular junction by the disruption of normal synaptic transmission mediated by acetylcholine. A hallmark of the strabismus is its variability throughout the day and from examination to examination. It is generally more prominent with fatigue and improves with rest. Ptosis is commonly an associated finding and also may vary during the course of the day and from exam to exam. Patterns of incomitant strabismus that do not fit specific cranial nerve palsies should raise the possibility of myasthenia, regardless of age. A variety of methods, including blood tests and electromyography, are used to diagnose myasthenia. Treatment of the underlying disease is critical. Although not a surgical disease, extraocular muscle surgery may be used to reduce strabismus in late stages if alignment has stabilized and remains unresponsive to medical therapy.

Strabismus Secondary to Sensory Loss

In the setting of severe loss of vision, either unilaterally or bilaterally, strabismus is common. The loss of normal afferent sensory input disrupts vision-dependent binocular control mechanisms, resulting in loss of fusion and destabilization of alignment. It is important to realize that in infants and young children loss of vision in one eye is often neither symptomatic nor apparent. It is critical therefore to rule out visual loss as the cause of strabismus in children until proven otherwise. This requires an examination by a specialist trained to assess vision in young children. It is not sufficient to simply examine the pupils or observe how well a child sees. Coats disease, retinal scars, retinoblastoma, and optic nerve hypoplasia are classic causes of early onset strabismus secondary to low vision. In early childhood, strabismus secondary to sensory loss tends to lead to esotropia, while in older children and adults, it tends to cause exotropia. The reasons for this difference are not clear, and certainly there are exceptions to this general rule. Treatment is aimed primarily at the underlying cause. Though diplopia is rarely present and recovery of single binocular vision is unlikely, surgical intervention is often performed for cosmetic correction. Interestingly, adults with long-standing sensory strabismus who have their sight restored (e.g., following surgery to remove a long-standing dense cataract) are sometimes unable to recover normal binocular vision and, as a result, are bothered by chronic intractable diplopia.

Skew Deviation

Skew deviation is characterized by a vertical deviation stemming from a neurological lesion in the posterior fossa affecting central vestibular otolithic inputs. Small-to-moderate horizontal and cyclotorsional deviations may be present as well, and patients are generally unable to fuse. The skew deviation may alternate, in that the hypertropia will shift depending on which direction the patient is looking. In such cases there is typically a left hypertropia on left gaze and a right hypertropia on right gaze. Pathological head tilts may also be present, given the involvement of the vestibular system, though the tilt does not promote fusion. Because a skew deviation indicates an underlying disruption of central binocular control, neuroimaging is critical, and treatment is aimed at resolving the underlying lesion while symptomatically managing the diplopia.

Management of Strabismus

Optical Techniques

The major goals in the management of strabismus include:

- Elimination of diplopia
- Restoration of single binocular vision
- Treatment of underlying conditions
- Improved cosmetic appearance

Treatment often begins with optical correction of significant refractive errors in order to optimize visual acuity. Full correction of hyperopia is particularly essential in cases of accommodative esotropia and may be combined with a bifocal if the amount of convergence associated with accommodation is abnormally high (e.g., high accommodative convergence/accommodation ratio).

Another important form of optical treatment is the use of prisms in glasses. Prisms redirect images entering the eye to compensate for a deviation and in doing so eliminate diplopia and promote fusion. The best candidates for prism therapy are those with relatively small angle, uniplanar, comitant deviations that do not include significant cyclotropia. Prisms can be incorporated into glasses, though the maximum amount that can reasonably be ground into each lens is limited due to lens edge thickness and development of increasingly troublesome optical aberrations with larger corrections. A second method of using prism is Fresnel (pronounced Frez-nel or Freh-nel) prisms, which are thin membranes that are affixed to the surface of a spectacle lens in the appropriate orientation. They are helpful in a variety of situations, relatively inexpensive, cosmetically acceptable, and easily reoriented or removed and can be used to correct much larger deviations than ground-in prism.

If fusion is not possible, diplopia may still be effectively eliminated. Monocular occlusion, or patching, is perhaps the most common technique. It is generally not employed for that purpose in children, however, as children generally do not experience symptomatic diplopia and may be susceptible to amblyopia caused by occlusion. A major problem with patching, aside from the cosmetic issues it causes, is the loss of peripheral vision. Another method for relieving diplopia that allows the patient to retain most of their peripheral vision involves placement of a semi-translucent filter on one lens of the patient's glasses. This can take the form of a thin plastic membrane that self-adheres to the lens surface (e.g., a Bangerter foil; see Chap. 39), a frosted lens, or even strips of scotch tape. Rather than completely blocking vision as a patch does, incoming light is defocused so that the degraded image is ignored by the brain.

Vision Therapy

The goal of vision therapy is to use optical devices and vision training exercises to establish and strengthen fusional control mechanisms and amplitudes. This form of treatment may be conducted in an office setting or at home and is overseen by an experienced orthoptist or optometrist. It requires that patients be able to first achieve some level of binocular fusion and is therefore most useful in intermittent tropias or symptomatic phorias. Convergence insufficiency exophoria is an example of a condition that is particularly well suited for vision therapy. On the other hand, it is not well suited for sensory deviations, large or incomitant deviations, and deviations secondary to orbital or cranial nerve pathology. Careful co-management between the vision therapist and the ophthalmologist is important.

Surgical Intervention

Extraocular muscle surgery has a prominent role in the management of strabismus, and in some cases, it can eliminate strabismus completely. Procedures used include weakening procedures (e.g., recessions or myotomies), strengthening procedures (e.g., resections, advancements, or plications), or transposition procedures. Surgery may be performed on the muscles of one or both eyes as required by the specific details of the case and is generally titrated according to the pattern and magnitude of the strabismus. In children, surgery is performed under general anesthesia and, in adults, either under general or local anesthesia. Although generally quite safe, the success rate depends on many factors including the complexity of the strabismus, the condition of the muscles and orbital tissues, and the strength of the patient's intrinsic binocular control mechanisms. Prior to surgery it is important to first identify and treat any underlying conditions contributing to the strabismus. In children, treatment of amblyopia generally takes a higher priority than correction of the strabismus, and it is thought that the results of surgery will be improved if amblyopia has been eliminated first. Surgery can be repeated if necessary to achieve the desired outcome. The stability of the result varies on a case-by-case basis but is often quite good (Fig. 40.9).

Botulinum toxin (Botox) has been used with some success to treat strabismus, either as a primary or adjunctive treatment. It works by inducing a temporary paresis of the injected muscle (i.e., by inhibiting acetylcholinergic transmission at the neuromuscular junction) and has been used most effectively in the treatment of eso- or exotropia. The medial rectus is injected to treat esotropia, and the lateral rectus is injected to treat exotropia. A lasting effect on eye alignment once the toxin has worn off is thought to occur due to contracture in the antagonist muscle during the period in which it is essentially unopposed by the pharmacologically weakened muscle. By the same mechanism, Botox can also be used to augment the effect of strabismus surgery; it can be administered to a muscle in the operating room under direct visualization or in cooperative adults under local anesthesia in the office. Although its use in strabismus management is well established, it is not as versatile, nor as widely used as surgery.

Summary and Key Points

Strabismus is a term encompassing a diverse group of pathological conditions in which normal ocular alignment is disrupted. Although it is often a confusing subject for the nonspecialist clinician, it is extremely important because of the potential implications it has for vision and detection of underlying disease. The identification of strabismus should begin with a careful history and examination that includes an assessment of vision, extraocular movements, and ocular alignment. Diplopia, a key symptom in adults, is often absent in children. The presence of a habitual abnormal head posture, such as a head tilt or face turn, is highly suggestive of strabismus, particularly in children. Once detected, the clinician characterizes strabismus in terms of frequency, direction, comitance, time of onset, and whether or not it is primary or secondary. Consultation with an ophthalmologist (pediatric ophthalmologists and neuro-ophthalmologists tend to be most specialized in evaluation and management of strabismus, in children or adults) is warranted in all cases.

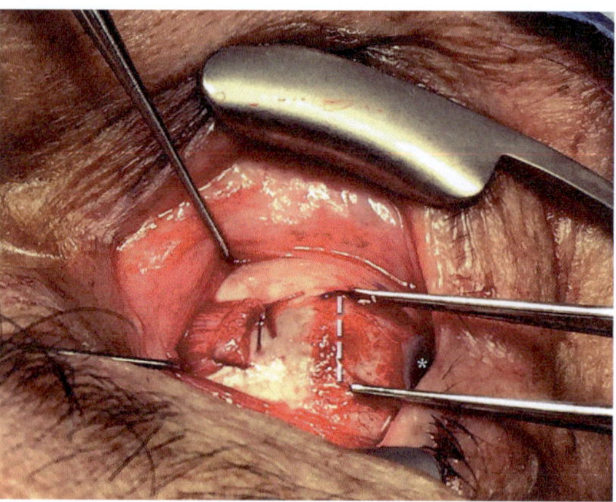

Fig. 40.9 Intraoperative photograph showing a medial rectus muscle that has been recessed (detached from its original insertion which is being grasped at each end by locking forceps) to a more posterior position on the sclera. This procedure is done to reduce esotropia. The asterisk indicates the cornea; the white dashed line is the original insertion point of the medial rectus prior to recession

Suggested Reading

AAO website. https://www.aao.org.

AAPOS website. https://aapos.org.

Chia A, Dirani M, Chan YH, et al. Prevalence of amblyopia and strabismus in young Singaporean Chinese children. Invest Ophthalmol Vis Sci. 2010;51:3411–7.

McKean-Cowdin R, Cotter SA, Tarczy-Hornach K, et al. Prevalence of amblyopia or strabismus in Asian and non-Hispanic white preschool children: multi-ethnic pediatric eye disease study. Ophthalmology. 2013;120:2117–24.

Multi-Ethnic Pediatric Eye Disease Study (MEPEDS) Group. Prevalence of amblyopia and strabismus in African–American and Hispanic children ages 6 to 72 months the multi-ethnic pediatric eye disease study. Ophthalmology. 2008;115:1229–36.

von Noorden GK, Campos EC. Binocular vision and ocular motility. 6th ed. St. Louis: Mosby; 2002. https://www.aao.org/Assets/0c711d7f-503f-4cd9-b4ac-92d6ec31a718/636343503854270000/strabismus-binocular-vision-and-ocular-motility-vnoorden-pdf?inline=1

Intraocular Tumors

41

Brian Marr

Intraocular tumors make up a broad spectrum of malignant and benign lesions that can impact patients' vision and life. It is important to be able to identify these conditions for many of them have systemic implications, whether it be an associated medical condition, syndrome, or malignancy. The eye is composed of many specialized tissues including connective tissue, neural tissue, muscle, and vasculature. The two main intraocular structures are the retina and uvea. The retina is composed of neural, glial, and vascular cells, while the uvea is composed of melanocytes, muscle, connective tissue, and vasculature. Primary intraocular tumors originate from these cell types. Both retina and uvea are highly vascularized tissues and can be affected by systemic diseases. Identification and diagnosis of retinal and uveal conditions are unique in that most of them are identified by direct visualization by a skilled examiner. Presumed diagnoses can be confirmed and documented with the help of highly specialized imaging modalities such as fluorescence angiography, optical coherence tomography (OCT), ultrasonography, and funduscopic photography. Diagnostic biopsies can be done on these tissues; however, the procedure itself may have significant negative visual implications and is used cautiously. More often, biopsies are used for obtaining tissue for genetic testing or when the clinical presentation is atypical. In the last few decades, many advancements have been made in the recognition and treatment of intraocular tumors.

Uveal Tumors

The uvea is divided into three parts: the iris, ciliary body, and choroid. Its function is to provide nutrition and gas exchange to ocular structures and to absorb light. The iris is a specialized part of the uvea designed to restrict and permit light entering the eye. The ciliary body contains epithelial cells that produce aqueous humor and muscles that cause the crystalline lens to change focus during accommodation. The choroid provides blood supply and nourishment to the outer retina and absorbs light.

Iris Tumors

The iris is composed of the iris stroma (the visible anterior portion of the iris), pigment epithelium (the dark pigmented layer behind the stroma), and dilator and sphincter muscles. The iris can develop benign cysts, benign solid lesions, infiltrations, and primary malignant lesions.

B. Marr, MD (✉)
Columbia University Irving Medical Center, New York, NY, USA

Department of Ophthalmology, Edward S. Harkness Eye Institute, Columbia University Vagelos College of Physicians and Surgeons, New York, NY, USA
e-mail: bpm2133@cumc.columbia.edu

© Springer Nature Switzerland AG 2019
D. S. Casper, G. A. Cioffi (eds.), *The Columbia Guide to Basic Elements of Eye Care*,
https://doi.org/10.1007/978-3-030-10886-1_41

Both the iris pigment epithelium and stroma can develop cysts. These benign lesions can be picked up incidentally or become large and symptomatic. The most common is the iris pigment epithelial cyst. These lesions develop from the darker iris pigment epithelium and can be noted on examination as a subtle elevation of the iris or be visible during a dilated examination, simulating an underlying pigmented neoplasm (Fig. 41.1).

Iris Pigment Epithelial Cysts

Iris pigment epithelial cysts can be divided into peripheral, mid-zonal, and marginal. Marginal cysts can be seen at the pupillary rough (the iris – pupil margin). Sometimes called iris flocculi, these lesions can be visible and, rarely, have been associated with aortic dissection. The more common mid-zonal cysts are rarely visualized directly but instead appear as a mass elevating the iris stroma. These lesions should be examined with ultrasound biomicroscopy (UBM) to confirm that they are not solid lesions such as a ciliary body or iris melanoma extending anteriorly (Fig. 41.2). Peripheral iris pigment epithelial cysts can cause angle narrowing in the region of the cyst and also should be confirmed with UBM (see Fig. 20.3).

Iris Stromal Cysts

Iris stromal cysts can be congenital or acquired and are seen directly as translucent cysts with fine vessels within the cyst walls (Fig. 41.3). The acquired lesions are usually after trauma or previous intraocular surgery. Enlarging lesions can abut the corneal endothelium, thereby causing endothelial loss, leading to a local corneal opacity. Occasionally iris stromal cysts can rupture, causing significant anterior chamber inflammation. Symptomatic cysts can be drained, sclerosed using a sclerosing agent, or resected. Asymptomatic lesions are observed.

Iris Nevus

Nevi are elevated collection of melanocytes most commonly seen on the skin but can occur in the

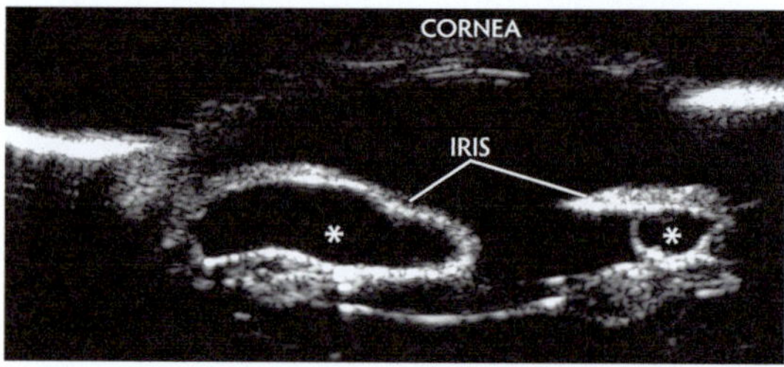

Fig. 41.2 Ultrasonic biomicroscopy (UBM) of an iris pigment epithelial cyst (asterisks) showing a hollow cystic structure underneath the iris

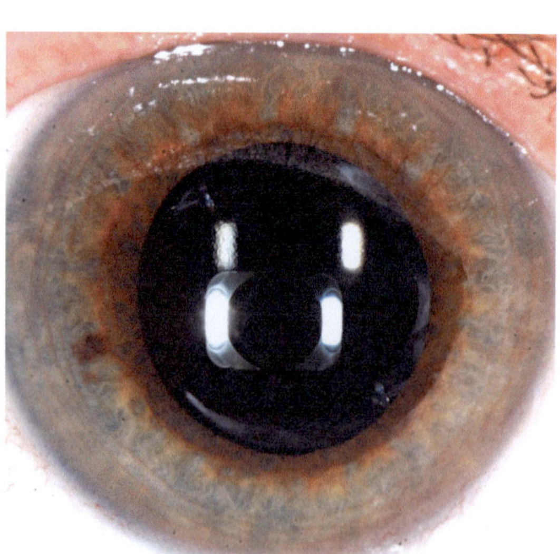

Fig. 41.1 Iris pigment epithelial cyst seen under the iris at 9 o'clock as a brown rounded mass

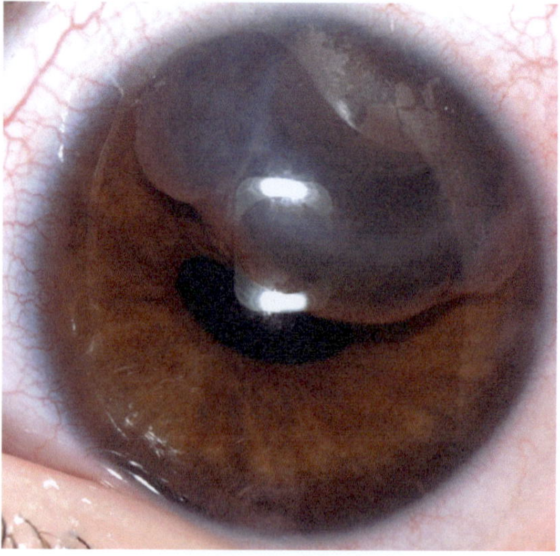

Fig. 41.3 Iris stromal cysts seen from 10:00 to 2:00 distorting the iris and pupil

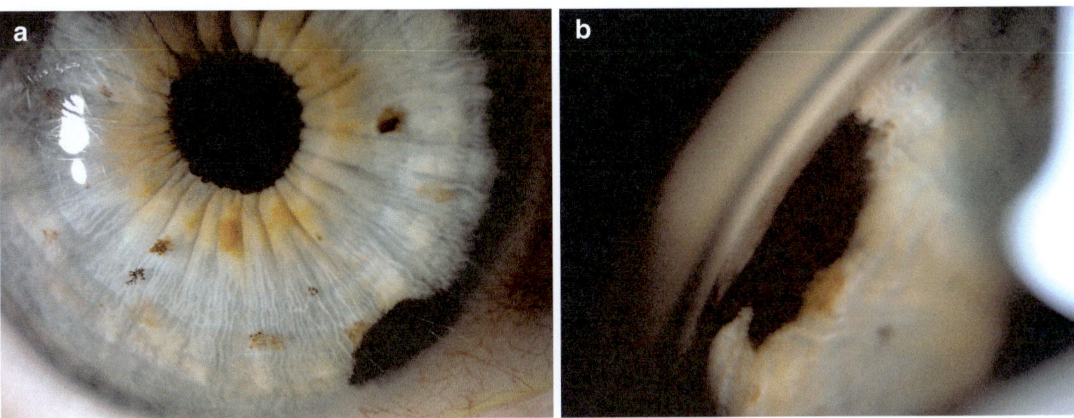

Fig. 41.4 (**a**) Iris nevus seen as a small pigmented elevation on the peripheral iris. (**b**) Gonioscopy of the nevus showing no invasion of the trabecular meshwork or angle seeding

iris, ciliary body, and choroid. Iris nevi appear as stuck-on plaques which can be pigmented or amelanotic and account for 47% of all iris lesions in adults (Fig. 41.4a, b). These lesions should be watched and photographed yearly to monitor for malignant transformation. Risk factors for malignant transformation include young age (less than 40 years old), inferior location, irregular edges, large feeder vessels, diffuse distribution, seeding, and nodular growth.

Lisch Nodules

Lisch nodules are iris lesions that can resemble freckles or nevi but are small and lightly brown-orange-colored, stuck-on nodules that can be seen in patients with neurofibromatosis type I. They can increase in number and size with age, but do not affect vision or the health of the eye. If noted incidentally, patients should be evaluated for neurofibromatosis (Fig. 41.5).

Iris Melanoma

Iris melanoma is rare and accounts for 2% of all uveal melanoma. These lesions can arise from a previous nevus or develop de novo (Fig. 41.6a, b). Characteristics of iris melanoma include large elevated nodular lesions with feeder vessels, iris stromal or angle seeding, or bleeding; melanomas may also present as a diffuse lesion covering the iris and angle, associated with heterochromia and elevated intraocular pressure. Treatment includes radiation with brachytherapy, proton beam ther-

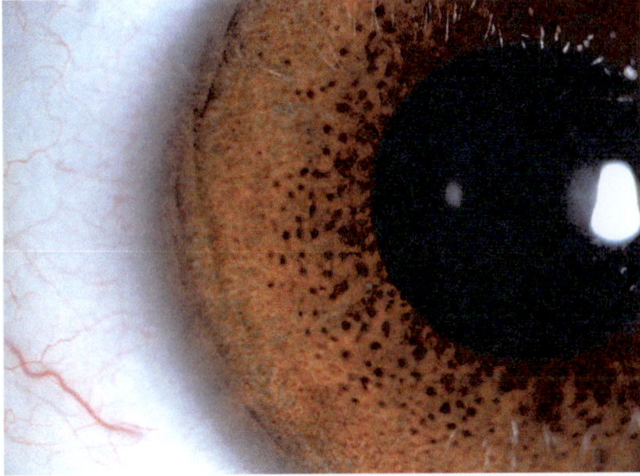

Fig. 41.5 Iris Lisch nodules in an 8-year-old girl. Her parents refused evaluation for neurofibromatosis

apy, tumor resection, or enucleation. The rate of metastatic disease for iris melanoma is 3–11% at 5 years.

Iris Metastases

Metastases to the iris from other systemic cancers are rare and are most commonly seen in patients known to have metastatic breast or lung cancer. They typically appear as white, creamy lesions distorting the normal iris but may present as hyphema or simulate iritis or uveitis with a pseudo-hypopyon (Fig. 41.7). Iris metastases may be observed if the patient is on systemic treatment to assess response. Symptomatic lesions can be treated with external beam radiotherapy or plaque brachytherapy.

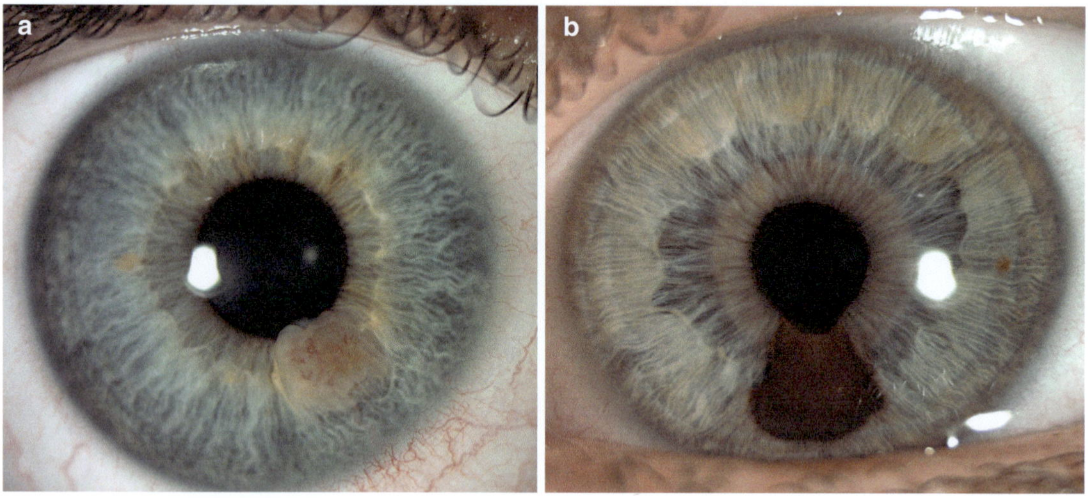

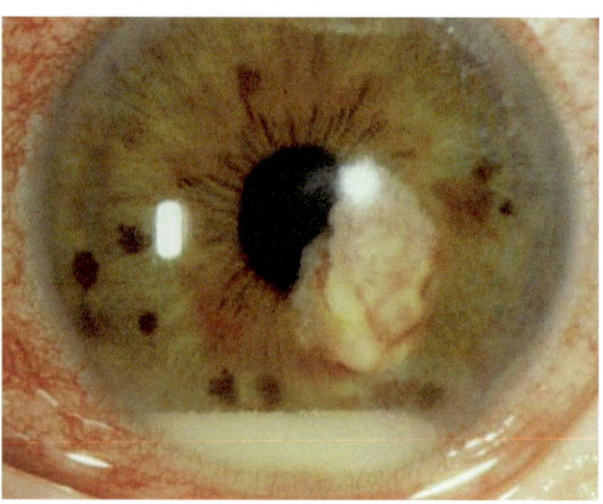

Fig. 41.6 (**a**) Iris melanoma. Note the nodularity and hypervascularity of this amelanotic lesion. (**b**) Melanotic iris melanoma with corectopia and ectropion uvea inferiorly

Fig. 41.7 Iris metastases. Note the white infiltrating lesion at the pupillary margin and pseudo-hypopyon

Ciliary Body, Choroidal, and Pigmented Neoplasms

The choroid is the most posterior portion of the uvea, consisting of pigmented vascular tissue lying between the retina and sclera.

Choroidal Nevi

One of the most common choroidal neoplasms is the choroidal nevus. Choroidal nevi are benign, melanocytic lesions found in up to 6–8% of the US population. They usually appear as an asymptomatic, pigmented, or amelanotic spot in the choroid that may be minimally elevated (Fig. 41.8). Over time, benign choroidal nevi may grow very slowly and can develop overlying drusen, retinal pigment epithelial changes, and, occasionally, choroidal neovascularization. Choroidal nevi have a small risk of transforming into a choroidal melanoma. Clinical features of suspicious lesions include overlying subretinal fluid, orange pigment on the nevus surface, thickness greater than 2 mm, and proximity to the optic nerve (<3 mm). Choroidal nevi are managed by obtaining a baseline photograph of the lesion, with routine follow-up to monitor for changes. Rapid growth of a nevus, in conjunction with the clinical risk factors described, suggests malignant transformation to a choroidal melanoma and requires treatment.

Choroidal Melanoma

Choroidal melanoma is the most common primary intraocular malignancy. It can develop from a nevus or arise de novo. These lesions are identified clinically as elevated pigmented or amelanotic choroidal lesions with overlying subretinal fluid and orange pigment (Fig. 41.9a, b). When evaluated by ultrasound, they have a typical acoustic signature, showing a hypoechoic center and subretinal fluid, and visible intrinsic vascular pulsations may be detected in larger lesions. Fine needle aspiration biopsy can be used when lesions are clinically atypical to confirm the diagnosis, but generally are not required for diagnosis. Biopsies are more widely used for genetic testing and lesion prognostication. The genetics of uveal melanoma are highly conserved compared to its cutaneous counterpart, with only a few common mutations. Early genetic testing has shown that loss of chromosome 3 (monosomy 3) is associated with a higher mortality rate.

Cytogenetics has also detected abnormal copy numbers on chromosomes 3, 6, and 8. Chromosome and mutation status have been shown to correlate to life prognosis; loss of chromosome 3 and inactivating mutations in BAP1, which is located on chromosome 3, are associated with tumors that often metastasize. Other genes involved in uveal melanoma are SF3B1, EIF1AX, GNAQ, and GNA11, which are found to be mutated in intermediate- and low-risk tumors. Despite growing understanding of the genetics of uveal melanoma, metastatic disease still proves difficult to control with current medications and is associated with a high mortality rate. However, globe-sparing treatment of the primary lesion is successful in up to 97% of patients. Treatment for primary uveal melanoma includes plaque brachytherapy, thermal laser, photodynamic therapy, proton beam radiation, and enucleation. Treatment choice is largely determined by lesion size and location.

Melanocytoma

Melanocytoma (magnocellular nevus) is a choroidal nevus variant that typically is found on the optic nerve but can be found in the ciliary body and iris as well. These benign lesions appear as a velvety, blackish elevation. When on the optic nerve, they obscure portions of the nerve head

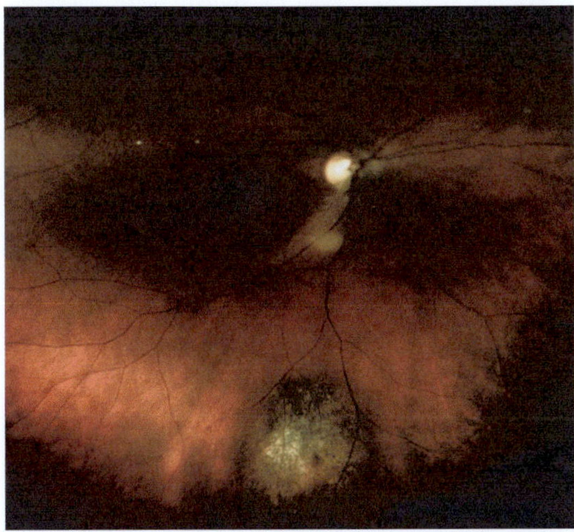

Fig. 41.8 Choroidal nevus. Note the inferior pigmented slightly elevated lesion with overlying drusen

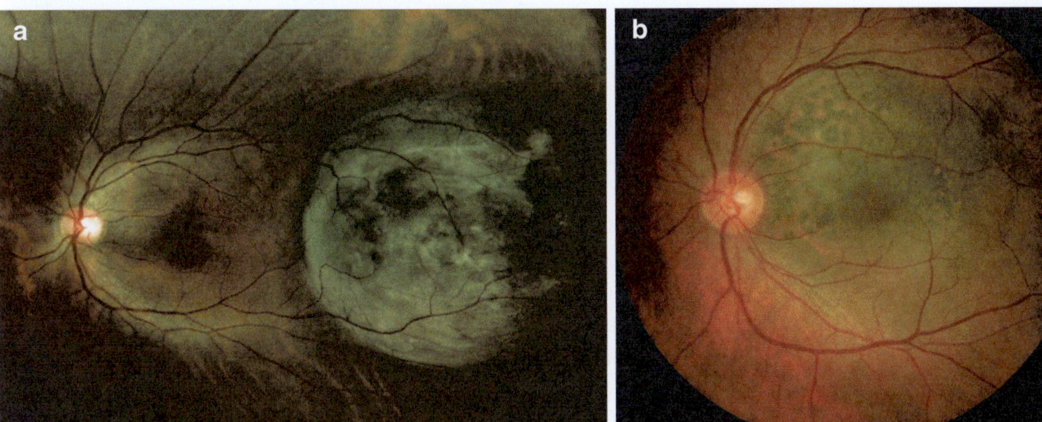

Fig. 41.9 Choroidal melanoma. (**a**) Note the temporally located, elevated melanoma with surrounding subretinal fluid. (**b**) Note the smaller submacular choroidal melanoma with overlying orange pigment

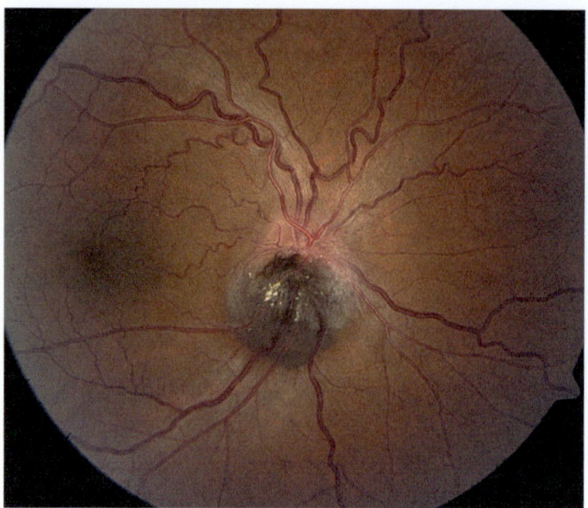

Fig. 41.10 Melanocytoma of the optic nerve

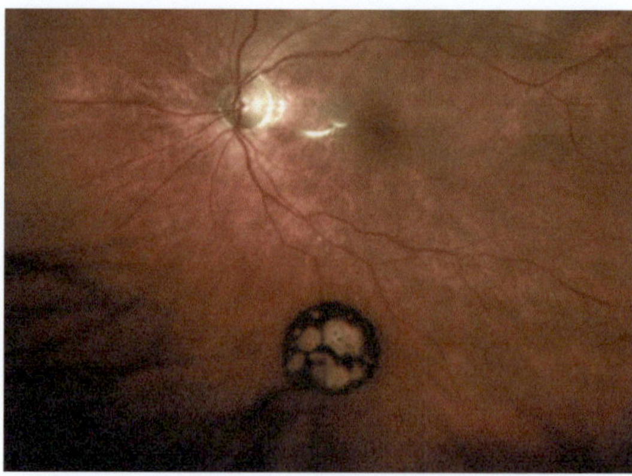

Fig. 41.11 Congenital hypertrophy of the retina pigment epithelium (CHRPE). Note the solitary black flat lesion with a sharp, well-defined margin, surrounded by a pigmented halo and central lacunae

and may have a small choroidal component (Fig. 41.10). It is important to differentiate these lesions from juxtapapillary choroidal melanoma. B-scan ultrasonography is used to confirm that the lesion is isolated to the optic nerve, which is typical for melanocytoma, and that there is no extraocular extension, which would be more typical of melanoma. Melanocytomas are usually stationary lesions with no effect on visual acuity; however, larger optic nerve lesions can produce visual field deficits in up to 25% of patients. Documented growth of these lesions, which is slow, has been seen in 10% of patients and only 1–2% progress to malignancy.

Congenital Hypertrophy of the Retina Pigment Epithelium (CHRPE)

Congenital hypertrophy of the retina pigment epithelium is a benign lesion present at birth and which grows slowly over time. This usually is an incidental finding and produces no symptomatic visual loss, given that they are usually in the periphery. CHRPEs are black, flat lesions with a sharp, well-defined margin surrounded by a pigmented halo. With time, they develop lacunae, which are seen as areas of atrophy within the lesion. There are three general patterns of CHRPE: solitary lesions (Fig. 41.11), multiple lesions (bear tracks), and pisciform lesions.

Familial adenomatous polyposis syndrome has been associated with pisciform lesions. CHRPEs do not progress into malignancy, but rare case reports of adenomas or adenocarcinomas have been reported originating from them (without any documented cases of subsequent metastases), so annual follow-up is recommended.

Adenomas and Adenocarcinomas of the Retinal Pigment Epithelium

Adenomas and adenocarcinomas are rare, pigmented lesions that can be confused with choroidal melanoma. They arise from the retinal pigment epithelium, sometimes in areas of hypertrophy or scarring, and appear as nodular, pigmented lesions with associated retinal feeder vessels and surrounding subretinal fluid and exudate. Symptomatic lesions are treated either with anti-VEGF therapy to reduce fluid and exudate or destructive procedures such as laser, cryotherapy, or plaque brachytherapy.

Combined Hamartoma of the Retina and the Retinal Pigment Epithelium

Combined hamartoma of the retina and the retinal pigment epithelium is a rare, benign posterior pole lesion that is usually first noted in childhood and consists of glial-vascular tissue and sheets of pigment epithelial cells. When found in young children, it usually presents with decreased visual acuity or strabismus. The lesions appear as mossy gray, slightly elevated masses with associated gliosis and traction. Association with neurofibromatosis type II has been documented in a few cases. Combined hamartomas can cause significant vitreoretinal interface disease, and attempts to surgically manage them have limited success. Depending on their location, these lesions can cause slow, progressive decline in visual acuity and are usually managed by supportive care.

Choroidal Metastases

Choroidal metastases are often detected by symptomatic visual loss, usually in patients with a known history of metastatic disease. Occasionally, choroidal metastasis may be the presenting findings of cancer. The most common origins of choroidal metastasis include breast and lung cancer, although other cancers can be found in the choroid as well, to a lesser extent. Clinically, choroidal metastases are creamy, white lesions with ill-defined borders and significant amounts of subretinal fluid. They can appear as solitary or multiple lesions, are usually posterior to the equator of the eye, are located under the retina in the choroid, and demonstrate an irregular surface on OCT. There is a high correlation with central nervous system disease, and CNS imaging should be performed in patients that present with new choroidal metastases. The patient's overall status should be evaluated and staged, and if systemic treatment is administered, lesions can be observed to see if they respond. Otherwise, symptomatic or vision-threatening lesions can be treated with external beam radiation, plaque brachytherapy, or photodynamic therapy.

Medulloepithelioma

Intraocular medulloepithelioma (diktyoma) is a congenital tumor of the nonpigmented ciliary epithelium, usually diagnosed in childhood. Medulloepitheliomas are slow-growing tumors that are detected when they protrude into the visual axis, disrupt the iris, or invade adjacent ocular tissues. They appear as smooth, gray lesions adjacent to the lens, occasionally with an associated lens coloboma. They can be cystic and have an associated fibrovascular membrane. They are classified into nonteratoid and teratoid tumors, with benign and malignant variants. Approximately two thirds of these lesions are, or become, malignant. Extraocular disease has a higher rate of mortality. Malignant lesions usually require enucleation; globe-sparing therapies have been successful in limited cases.

Circumscribed Choroidal Hemangiomas

Circumscribed choroidal hemangiomas are benign vascular tumors that usually occur in the posterior pole. They appear as orange elevations of the choroid and may be difficult to differentiate from surrounding tissue. If located in the macula, they can cause a hyperopic shift, and they can also produce sub- and intraretinal fluid, which can disrupt vision. These lesions can be mistaken for central serous retinopathy or metastatic disease. Asymptomatic lesions are observed. If persistent subretinal fluid disrupts vision, the lesions are best managed with photodynamic therapy or radiation.

Tumors of Retinal and Other Origin

Retinal Hemangioblastoma (Retinal Capillary Hemangioma)

Hemangioblastomas are benign vascular tumors located within the retina and can appear as a solitary lesion (Fig. 41.12). Multiple hemangioblastomas may be associated with Von Hippel-Lindau syndrome (VHL). These lesions are characteristically red or orange masses located within the retina, with associated enlarged feeding and draining vessels. Although smaller lesions can be asymptomatic, larger ones can cause visual loss from leakage of subretinal and intraretinal fluid, associated retinal exudate, and vitreoretinal traction. Symptomatic lesions can be difficult to treat. Destructive procedures such as laser photocoagulation, cryotherapy, and radiation treatment have been used as well as anti-vascular endothelial growth factor (anti-VEGF) medication. Patients with multiple hemangioblastomas should be tested for Von Hippel-Lindau disease with systemic and genetic testing.

Retinal Cavernous Hemangiomas

Retinal cavernous hemangiomas are rare, vascular intraretinal tumors usually located in the posterior pole. They consist of multiple, dilated vascular structures in grape-like clusters (Fig. 41.13). These lesions disrupt vision and, rarely, can bleed and cause vitreous hemorrhage. Retinal cavernous hemangiomas can be associated with cutaneous and central nervous system vascular abnormalities. These have been associated with the KRIT1, CCM1, CCM2, and CCM3 genes and can occur in families. A thorough family history as well as central nervous system imaging should be recommended to patients found to have this benign vascular lesion.

Astrocytic Hamartoma

Astrocytic hamartomas are benign lesions that arise in the retina. They appear as gray-white, elevated, fleshy intraretinal lesions. They may have calcifications within them that are glistening, yellow, blackberry-shaped clusters with very fine intralesional vessels. The normal retinal vasculature can be pulled toward the lesion, appearing as if the lesion has shrunk and pulled vessels closer to it. Local, larger vessels pass through the lesion without feeding it or altering it in any way. Astrocytic hamartomas are usually stationary lesions that do not progress or affect vision adversely. These lesions may be associated with tuberous sclerosis complex, and if found, patients

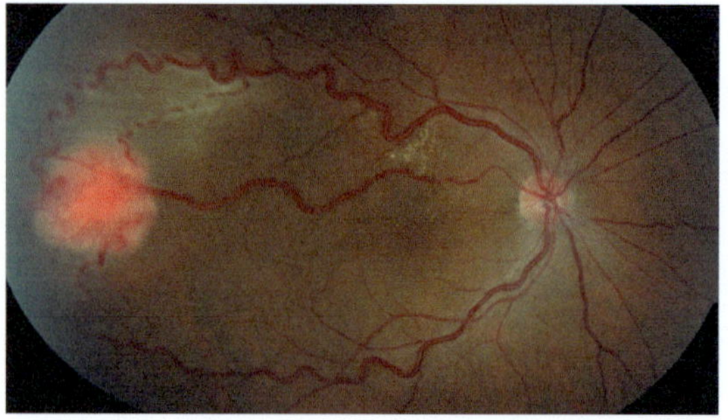

Fig. 41.12 Retinal hemangioblastoma. Note the large feeder and draining vessels with associated subretinal exudate

Fig. 41.13 Cavernous hemangioma. (**a**) Note the dilated, retinal cavernous vascular formations and areas of fibrosis. (**b**) Optical coherence tomography of the cavernous hemangioma demonstrating intraretinal cavernous vascular formations

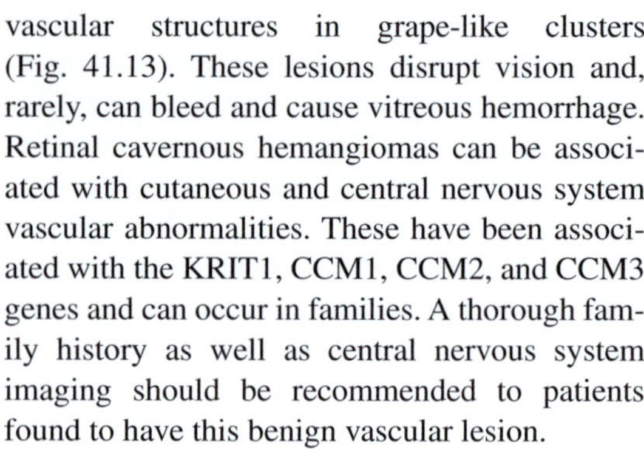

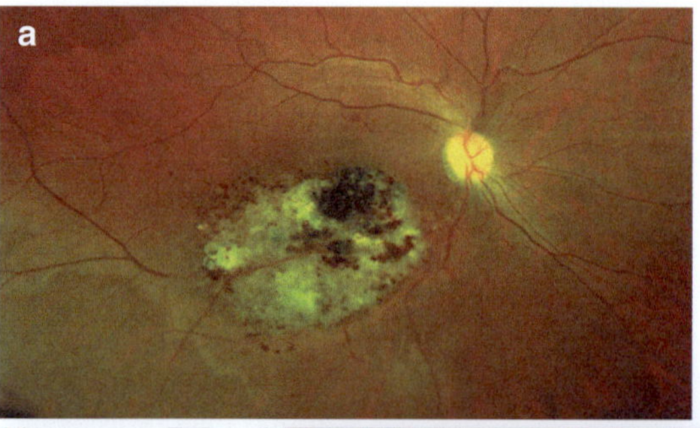

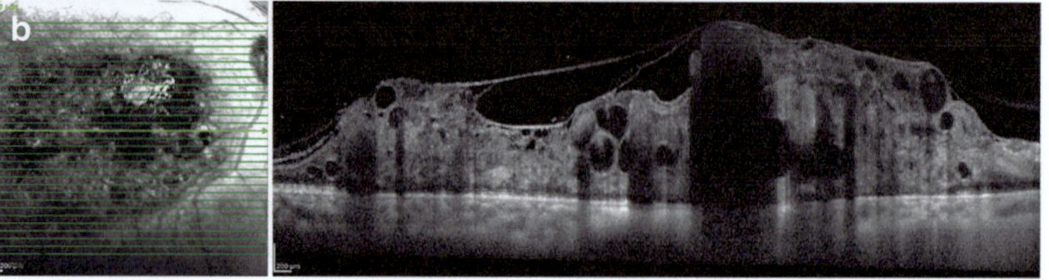

should be questioned and examined for signs of the syndrome.

Intraocular Lymphoma

Intraocular lymphoma can present in two common patterns. The first has been called primary intraocular lymphoma or vitreoretinal lymphoma. This pattern is usually caused by diffuse, large B-cell lymphoma, but there are some exceptions. The vitreous either has floaters or unexplained panuveitis and is commonly misdiagnosed as an inflammatory condition. It can involve the retina, presenting as a whitish glaze to the retina with thickening, or as white, subretinal pigment epithelial infiltrates (Fig. 41.14). This presentation of intraocular diffuse large B-cell lymphoma has a high association with central nervous system disease, and greater than ¾ of patients will have CNS involvement within 3 years. Patients with biopsy-diagnosed vitreoretinal lymphoma should undergo a systemic and CNS evaluation for signs of lymphoma involvement. Patients are treated for symptomatic disease with radiation or intraocular injections of methotrexate and/or rituximab. Ocular control of lymphoma is usually possible, but when the CNS is involved, there is a higher recurrence and mortality rate.

The second pattern of intraocular lymphoma is choroidal involvement, which is usually caused by a low-grade B-cell lymphoma that infiltrates the choroid in a multifocal pattern of yellow choroidal infiltrates. Most patients have minimal visual complaints. This pattern can be mistaken for bird shot chorioretinopathy. Ultrasound findings show a low-reflective choroidal infiltrate and choroidal thickening, occasionally with extraocular extension. The diagnosis is obtained via fine needle aspiration biopsy of the choroid or extraocular disease. The majority of cases are low-grade B-cell marginal zone lymphomas; however, variability in cell type can be seen. Symptomatic cases are treated with external beam radiotherapy.

Retinoblastoma

Retinoblastoma, the most common intraocular tumor of children, is caused by a mutation in chromosome 13 and can occur as a somatic mutation or germline mutation occurring in 1 in 20,000 live births (Fig. 41.15). Approximately 300 cases occur annually in the United States. Somatic retinoblastoma mutations account for unilateral disease and make up two thirds of the cases. Germline retinoblastoma cases are usually associated with bilateral disease and can be transferred genetically to offspring. Patients with germline mutations carry an elevated risk for second cancers (commonly soft-tissue sarcomas) throughout their lifetime. If untreated, retinoblastoma can cause blindness, metastatic disease, and death; early detection and proper treatment have

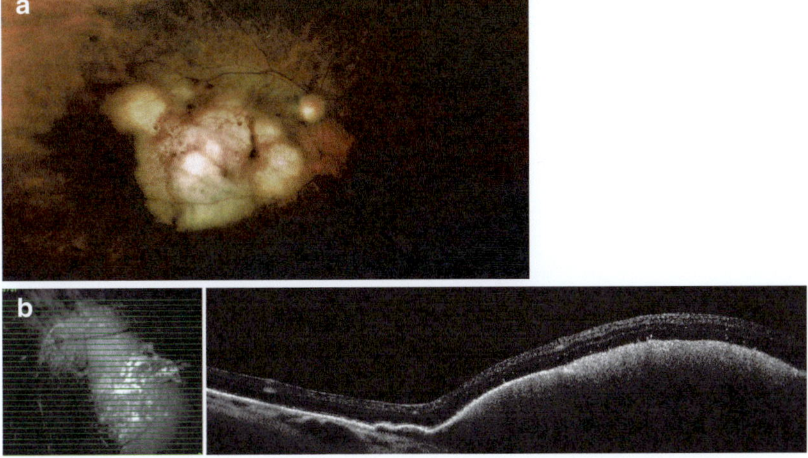

Fig. 41.14 Vitreoretinal lymphoma. (**a**) Note the central, white, subretinal pigment epithelial infiltrate and overlying haze caused by vitreous cells. (**b**) The optical coherence tomography shows infiltrate in the subretinal space

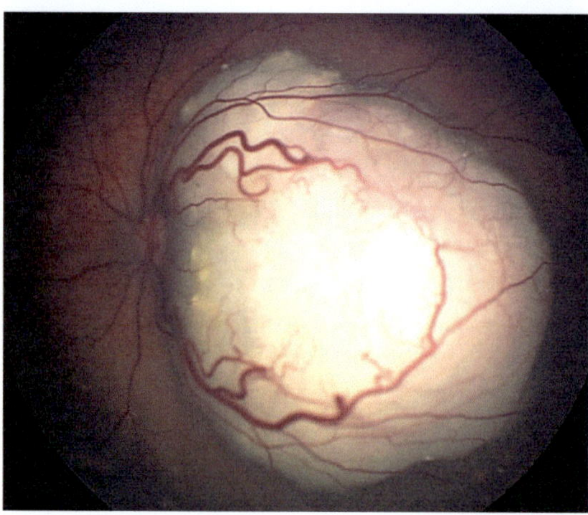

Fig. 41.15 Retinoblastoma. Note the white intraretinal and some retinal lesion with calcification and feeder vessels

prevented death in up to 95% of children in the United States. Retinoblastoma is discussed in more detail in the following chapter (Chap. 42).

Suggested Reading

Augsburger JJ, Schroeder RP, Territo C, Gamel JW, Shields JA. Clinical parameters predictive of enlargement of melanocytic choroidal lesions. Br J Ophthalmol. 1989;73:911–7.

Chan CC, Rubenstein JL, Coupland SE, Davis JL, Harbour JW, Johnston PB, Cassoux N, Touitou V, Smith JR, Batchelor TT, Pulido JS. Primary vitreoretinal lymphoma: a report from an International Primary Central Nervous System Lymphoma Collaborative Group symposium. Oncologist. 2011;16:1589–99.

Dogrusöz M, Jager MJ. Genetic prognostication in uveal melanoma. Acta Ophthalmol. 2017; https://doi.org/10.1111/aos.13580. [Epub ahead of print] Review.

Lois N, Shields CL, Shields JA, Mercado G. Primary cysts of the iris pigment epithelium: clinical features and natural course in 234 patients. Ophthalmology. 1998;105:1879–85.

Saunders T, Margo CE. Intraocular medulloepithelioma. Arch Pathol Lab Med. 2012;136:212–6.

Schachat AP, Shields JA, Fine SL, et al. Combined hamartomas of the retina and retinal pigment epithelium. Ophthalmology. 1984;91:1609–15.

Schefler AC, Kim RS. Recent advancements in the management of retinoblastoma and uveal melanoma. F1000Res. 2018;7. pii: F1000 Faculty Rev-476. https://doi.org/10.12688/f1000research.11941.1. eCollection 2018. Review.

Shields JA. Primary cysts of the iris. Trans Am Ophthalmol Soc. 1981;79:771–809.

Shields JA, Shields CL, Materin MA, Marr BP, Demirci H, Mashayekhi A. Changing concepts in management of circumscribed choroidal hemangioma: the 2003 J. Howard stokes lecture, part 1. Ophthalmic Surg Lasers Imaging. 2004;35:383–94.

Shields JA, Demirci H, Mashayekhi A, Eagle RC, Shields CL. Melanocytoma of the optic disk: a review. Surv Ophthalmol. 2006;51:93–104.

Shields CL, Kancherla S, Patel J, et al. Clinical survey of 3680 iris tumors based on age at presentation. Ophthalmology. 2012;119:407–14.

Shields CL, Kaliki S, Hutchinson A, Nickerson S, Patel J, Kancherla S, Peshtani A, Nakhoda S, Kocher K, Kolbus E, Jacobs E, Garoon R, Walker B, Rogers B, Shields JA. Iris nevus growth into melanoma: analysis of 1611 consecutive eyes: the ABCDEF guide. Ophthalmology. 2013;120:766–72.

Shields JA, Magrath GN, Shields C, Mackool R, Eagle RC Jr, Grossniklaus HE. Dissecting aortic aneurysm 55 years after diagnosis of Iris Flocculi. Ocul Oncol Pathol. 2016;2:222–5.

Sisley K, Curtis D, Rennie IG, Rees RC. Loss of heterozygosity of the thyroid hormone receptor B in posterior uveal melanoma. Melanoma Res. 1993;3:457–61.

Wang W, Chen L. Cavernous hemangioma of the retina: a comprehensive review of the literature (1934–2015). Retina. 2017;37:611–21.

Retinoblastoma

Ariana M. Levin, Jasmine H. Francis, and David H. Abramson

Definition

Retinoblastoma is a rare cancer that develops from cone precursor cells. It is the most common intraocular cancer of children, with about 250–350 new cases per year in the United States. Ninety-five percent of cases occur before age 5 years.

Etiology

Retinoblastoma arises from a loss of function of the RB1 gene (either by loss of heterozygosity or other mechanisms), which is located on the long arm of chromosome 13 (specifically 13q14). Genetic abnormalities range from large deletions to single base changes. The majority of mutations result in premature termination signals. Epigenetic modifications, such as hypermethylation of the RB1 promoter, also occur. Disease development usually requires that both RB1 alleles become inactivated.

Retinoblastoma may originate from a germline alteration, in which case a child has one inactive allele either from a parent or more commonly a de novo mutation, and subsequently develops a mutation in the other allele. A child with non-germline retinoblastoma has developed de novo mutations in both alleles in a cell that will give rise only to retinal cells. Non-germline retinoblastoma tends to present as unilateral disease and later than germline retinoblastoma, as a result of the low statistical probability of developing two de novo mutations in one cell. However, there is some thought that unilateral disease is a form of germline retinoblastoma, but with a low-level mosaicism.

Functioning Rb protein negatively regulates progression through the G1 phase of the cell cycle. RB1 mutations result in aberrant cell division. In addition to its role as a gatekeeper in the cell cycle, Rb protein has also been shown to function in DNA replication, differentiation, and apoptosis.

Screening

Bilateral retinoblastoma and many unilateral cases have germline disease, and therefore screening of relatives is needed – this is true even if genetic testing of a unilateral patient is normal, due to mosaicism. Siblings are clinically screened with a fundus exam by indirect ophthalmoscopy for the first 28 months of life.

Relatives of patients with germline RB1 mutations have an increased risk of secondary cancers in addition to retinoblastoma. For example, in a

A. M. Levin, BS (✉) · J. H. Francis, MD, FACS
D. H. Abramson, MD
Ophthalmic Oncology Service, Department of Surgery, Memorial Sloan Kettering Cancer Center, New York, NY, USA
e-mail: aml2020@med.cornell.edu

© Springer Nature Switzerland AG 2019
D. S. Casper, G. A. Cioffi (eds.), *The Columbia Guide to Basic Elements of Eye Care*,
https://doi.org/10.1007/978-3-030-10886-1_42

rare case of events, the grandmother of a retinoblastoma patient was found to carry an RB mutation subsequent to the diagnosis of her grandchild. Though the grandmother never developed retinoblastoma, her knowledge of her increased risk of secondary cancers enabled her to obtain an early diagnosis and treatment for a sarcoma that she developed at age 59. Screening can also inform parents' considerations of preimplantation genetic diagnosis to avoid the risk of retinoblastoma in future children.

Even though RB1 mutations are identified in >95% of tumors, a small subgroup of tumors that have MYCN amplification (v-myc avian myelocytomatosis viral oncogene neuroblastoma derived homolog, which is responsible for tissue and organ formation during embryogenesis and is involved in cell growth, differentiation, and apoptosis) and no RB1 mutations has been identified in children with unilateral RB diagnosed at an earlier age.

Presentation

Common initial presentations of retinoblastoma are leukocoria (white pupil), strabismus (either exotropia or esotropia), and poor vision. Leukocoria is often noticed by a parent when laying the child down to sleep or as a lack of "red eye" in photographs. The differential diagnosis for leukocoria and strabismus includes congenital cataract, persistent hyperplastic primary vitreous (or persistent fetal vasculature syndrome), retinopathy of prematurity, Coats' disease, toxocariasis, uveitis, and less common conditions. All of these require evaluation and management by an ophthalmologist; thus patients with leukocoria or strabismus should always be referred to an ophthalmologist as soon as possible. Less common presentations of retinoblastoma include heterochromia, painful or red eye, and orbital cellulitis.

A minority of cases arise from a deletion of more than one gene on the long arm of chromosome 13, resulting in 13q deletion syndrome. Children with this aberration may present with developmental delay or dysmorphism before retinoblastoma is detected.

Diagnosis

Diagnosis of retinoblastoma is made based on the child's clinical appearance on a dilated ophthalmoscopic examination. More than half of patients with retinoblastoma are diagnosed due to leukocoria, which is initially noticed by a parent in 80% of cases and by the pediatrician in fewer than 10%. However, the referral lag time for these signs is often weeks.

The diagnosis is supported with imaging. Tumors may be imaged using a wide-angle digital retinal camera to capture images of the retina (Fig. 42.1), B-scan ophthalmic ultrasound (Fig. 42.2) to identify spread of disease into the orbit or optic nerve, and high-frequency ultrasound biomicroscopy (Fig. 42.3) to image the anterior structures of the eye. Optical coherence tomography can also be useful. MRI (Fig. 42.4) is routinely done to confirm the diagnosis, as well as examine the optic nerve, pineal gland, and brain. Fluorescein angiography is rarely used. Biopsy is rarely if ever done because of a concern of spreading tumor outside the eye. CT scanning is avoided in children to minimize exposure to ionizing radiation. In fetuses known to carry RB1 mutations, obstetric ultrasound has rarely detected intraocular tumors.

Staging

The Reese-Ellsworth classification system, developed at Columbia and first reported in 1963, was developed to predict a child's response to lateral

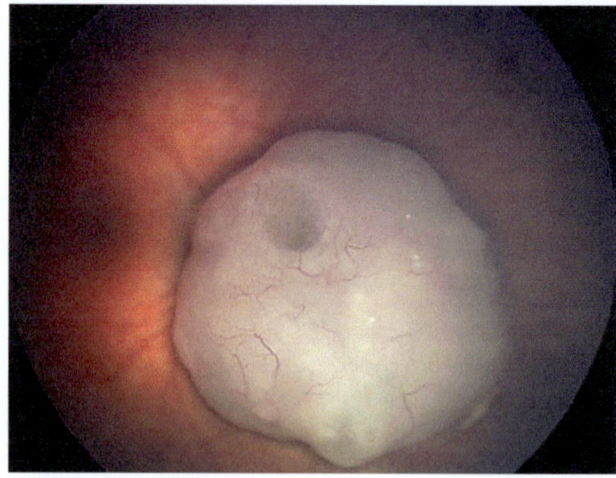

Fig. 42.1 Fundus image of retinoblastoma tumor obscuring the optic nerve

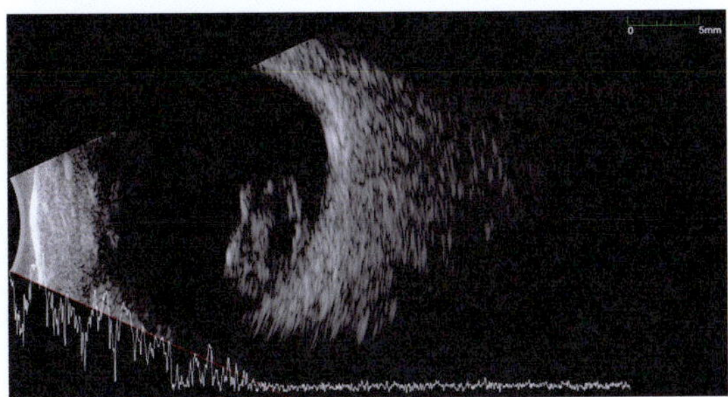

Fig. 42.2 B-scan ophthalmic ultrasound demonstrating echogenic retinoblastoma tumor emanating from the posterior retina

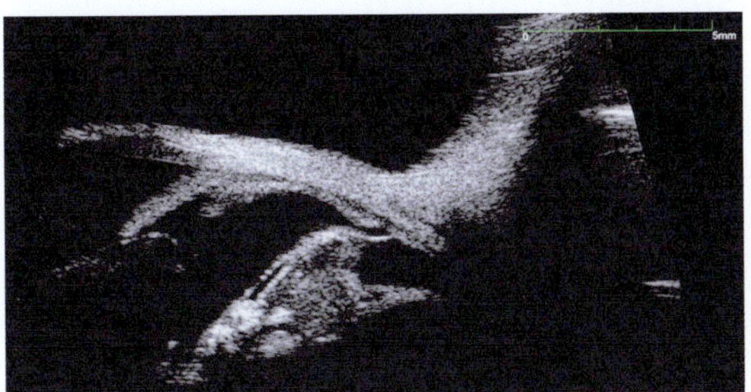

Fig. 42.3 Ultrasonic biomicroscopy demonstrating an anterior retinoblastoma tumor

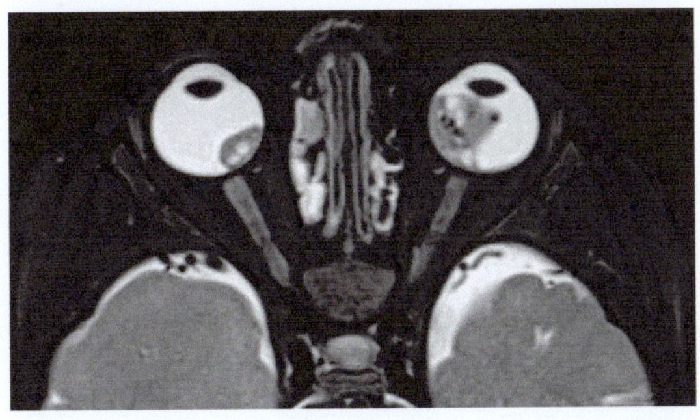

Fig. 42.4 T2-weighted magnetic resonance image demonstrating bilateral intraocular retinoblastoma

photon radiation. However, the use of radiation therapy has since decreased as the use of chemotherapy and conservative treatment has increased. The International Classification for Retinoblastoma predicts responses to systemic chemotherapy, dividing tumors into five groups based on prognostic criteria. Vitreous seeds can be classified based on morphologic characteristics, and this classification has been found to predict response to intravitreal chemotherapy. The TNM staging system is rarely used for retinoblastoma.

Treatment

In the United States, the survival rate of children with retinoblastoma who receive appropriate treatment is greater than 90%. Radiotherapy options include external beam therapy, proton beam therapy, and plaque brachytherapy. The use of external beam therapy has declined due to the associated increased risk of secondary cancers. Plaque brachytherapy may be used to treat small tumors or as an adjuvant therapy.

Surgical removal of the eye (enucleation) is used by some centers for eyes with advanced retinoblastoma or for eyes that failed globe-salvaging treatment. Enucleation involves removal of the entire globe and a portion of the optic nerve, followed by replacement with an orbital implant and prosthesis, both for cosmesis and to promote future normal skull growth and development. A pathologist carefully evaluates the globe for pathological features that may be associated with metastatic disease, including residual tumor cells in the cut end of the optic nerve.

Historically, systemic chemotherapy was used to shrink tumors prior to focal treatments with laser or cryotherapy. As with most systemic chemotherapy treatments, children are carefully monitored for acute and late toxicities, such as pancytopenia and its sequelae, renal dysfunction, secondary malignancies, infertility, and hearing loss. Systemic chemotherapy rarely cures retinoblastoma and relies upon additional focal treatments for efficacy. Due to this and the systemic consequences of cytotoxic drugs, a localized delivery of chemotherapy (such as ophthalmic artery chemosurgery (OAC) and intravitreal chemotherapy) has become first-line treatment in many centers.

Advancements in ophthalmic artery chemosurgery and intravitreal chemotherapy now save eyes that were once destined for enucleation. Ophthalmic artery chemosurgery involves placing a catheter in the femoral artery and guiding this to the ostium of the ophthalmic artery where chemotherapy is delivered. Children less than 3 months of age can receive single-agent chemotherapy to "bridge" them until they are old enough for OAC; children with bilateral disease can be treated with "tandem" therapy, when both eyes sequentially receive chemotherapy during the same treatment session. Intravitreal chemotherapy is administered as an injection directly through the wall of the eye into the vitreous fluid. A number of safety-enhanced techniques are employed, and the risk of extraocular tumor extension is believed to be very small.

Cryotherapy and laser photocoagulation are both focal treatments used to treat small tumors. Typically, more anteriorly located tumors are treated with cryotherapy, while tumors toward the posterior pole are treated with laser. Periocular chemotherapy (injection of chemotherapy agents into the tissues surrounding the eye) was developed to enable local delivery of chemotherapy, but due to its toxicity and relative ineffectiveness compared to other methods, periocular chemotherapy now has limited use.

Secondary Cancers

Patients with germline mutations have an increased risk of developing secondary malignancies, most commonly soft tissue sarcomas and osteosarcomas. Therefore, many patients receive screening for secondary cancers (such as an annual MRI), even after their retinoblastoma is considered cured. The risk of secondary malignancies is higher in patients with recurrent nonsense mutations, compared with low penetrance mutations. Prior treatment with external beam radiotherapy, particularly if administered in the first year of life, further increases the risk of secondary cancers in retinoblastoma patients. Treatment with alkylating agents containing chemotherapy, such as triethylenemelamine, may also increase the risk of subsequent bone tumors and leiomyosarcoma.

Metastasis

In the United States, fewer than 5% of patients develop metastatic retinoblastoma. Metastases are treated with systemic chemotherapy, autologous hematopoietic stem cell rescue, and radiotherapy.

Long-Term Outcomes

Retinoblastoma patients and their families benefit from psychosocial support as they navigate treatment and care of the child. Families may express anxiety about their child's quality of life and schooling; however, they can be reassured that studies have demonstrated that survivors of retinoblastoma can enjoy a quality of life equivalent to their peers'.

Suggested Reading

Abramson DH. Saving life with vision. Annu Rev Med. 2014;65:171–84.

Abramson DH, Frank CM, Susman M, et al. Presenting signs of retinoblastoma. J Pediatr. 1998;132(3 Pt 1): 505–8.

Abramson DH, Shields CL, Munier FL, Chantada GL. Treatment of retinoblastoma in 2015: agreement and disagreement. JAMA Ophthalmol. 2015;133(11): 1341–7.

Balmer A, Munier M. Differential diagnosis of leukocoria and strabismus, first presenting signs of retinoblastoma. Clin Ophthalmol. 2007; Dec;1(4):431–9.

Jenkinson H. Retinoblastoma: diagnosis and management- the UK perspective. Arch Dis Child. 2015;100(11):1070–5.

Lohmann DR, Brandt B, Hopping W, et al. The spectrum of RB1 germ-line mutations in hereditary retinoblastoma. Am J Hum Genet. 1996;58(5):940–9.

Reese AB, Ellsworth RM. The evaluation and current concept of retinoblastoma therapy. Trans Am Acad Ophthalmol Otolaryngol. 1963;67:164–72.

Temming P, Viehmann A, Arendt M, et al. Pediatric second primary malignancies after retinoblastoma treatment. Pediatr Blood Cancer. 2015;62(10): 1799–804.

Weintraub N, Rot I, Shoshani N, et al. Participation in daily activities and quality of life in survivors of retinoblastoma. Pediatr Blood Cancer. 2011;56(4): 590–4.

Wong JR, Morton LM, Tucker MA, et al. Risk of subsequent malignant neoplasms in long-term hereditary retinoblastoma survivors after chemotherapy and radiotherapy. J Clin Oncol. 2014;32(29):3284–90.

Xu XL, Singh HP, Wang L, et al. Rb suppresses human cone-precursor-derived retinoblastoma tumours. Nature. 2014;514(7522):385–8.

Appendices

Appendix 1: A Brief Overview of Present and Future Technologies in Ophthalmic Diagnosis and Treatment

Daniel S. Casper, Lama A. Al-Aswad, Srilaxmi Bearelly, Steven Brooks, Jonathan S. Chang, Royce W. S. Chen, D. Jackson Coleman, Irene Maumenee, Tarun Sharma, Ronald Silverman, Stephen L. Trokel, Stephen P. Walters, and Bryan J. Winn

Introduction

Since the introduction of the direct ophthalmoscope by Hermann von Helmholtz in the mid-nineteenth century, ophthalmology has relied heavily on technological developments for both diagnosis and treatment and has often been at the forefront of medical technological advances. In this appendix, we discuss current uses of imaging in ophthalmology and some of the directions we expect our field to pursue in the future.

Ophthalmic Imaging

Ophthalmic Photography
Until recently, the main advancement in ophthalmic photography was the migration from film to digital image acquisition. High-resolution digital ophthalmic cameras, now universally accepted, spurred the development of extensive advances in camera systems, image storage, and image transmission. Newer digital cameras have also made possible the simple acquisition of external images (Fig. A1.1) as well as fundus images which do not require the use of dilating drops (non-mydriatic cameras). Small, relatively inexpensive non-mydriatic fundus cameras are widely available, and their use is automated enough that medical technicians in non-ophthalmic office settings can quickly learn to obtain excellent fundus images which may then be immediately reviewed and, if necessary, sent electronically to an ophthalmologist for further interpretation.

Recently, widefield image systems have been developed (such as the Optos and Zeiss Clarus)

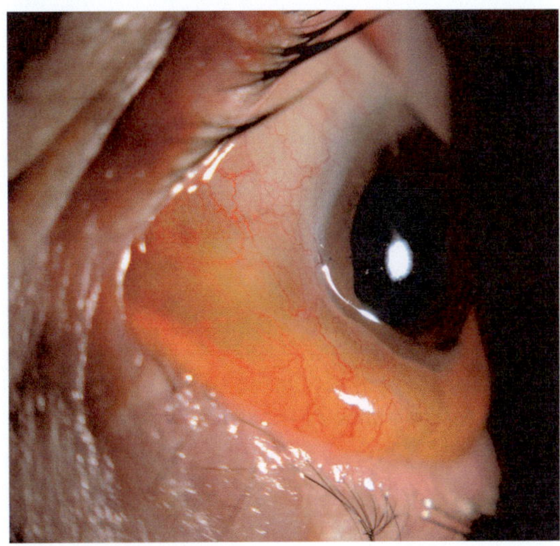

Fig. A1.1 Digital slit lamp photograph showing conjunctival chemosis

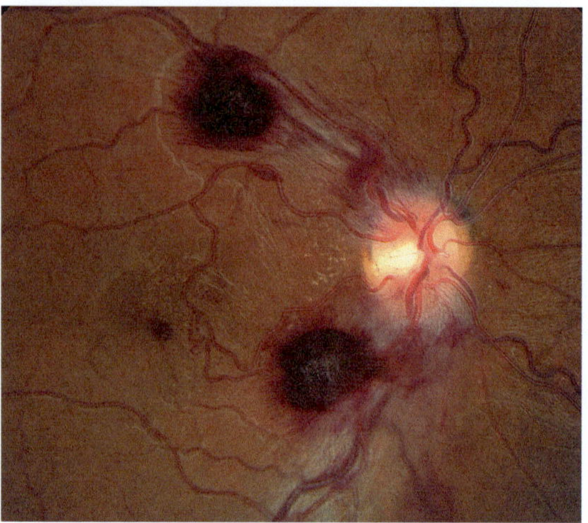

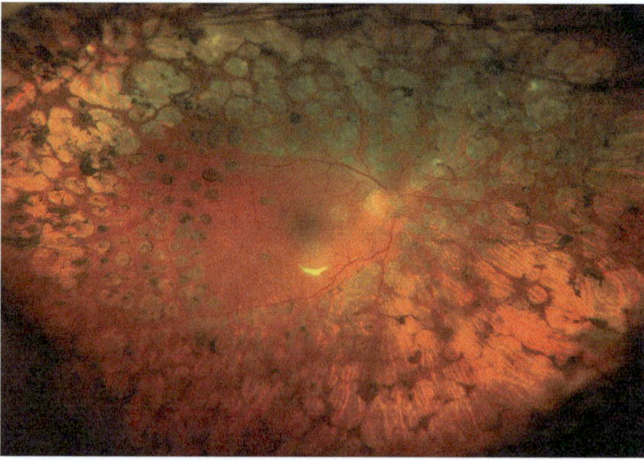

Fig. A1.3 Widefield (Optos) digital fundus image showing peripheral scarring in a diabetic patient after panretinal photocoagulation treatment for proliferative diabetic retinopathy

Fig. A1.2 Digital photograph of the right fundus of a 17-year-old girl with a pilocytic astrocytoma, after multiple resections, VP shunt and Ommaya reservoir placement, and chemotherapy. Her fundus shows mild blurring of the nasal disc margin, with small intraretinal hemorrhages and two oval, slightly elevated subhyaloid hemorrhages believed to be related to underlying thrombocytopenia. Hyaloid membrane reflections are visible, particularly around the upper subhyaloid hemorrhage

which permit acquisition of 200° images, compared to the standard fundus image size of approximately 45° (Figs. A1.2 and A1.3). These images, remarkably, do not require dilation, and widefield angiographic studies, something that was not possible less than a decade ago, have been introduced as well.

Portable, handheld camera systems such as the Volk Pictor and the JedMed Horus can be used to easily view and record the fundus, and interchangeable lenses enable both fundus images and macrophotographs of the external eye. Pictures obtained with these systems can be saved and downloaded for archiving, and some models can record video images, which is useful in documenting optic nerve blood flow, mobile retinal detachments, or other findings.

The introduction of affordable smartphones has resulted in significant advancements in ophthalmic imaging. These ubiquitous cameras simplify and enhance viewing, making them excellent teaching tools, and permit instant storage and image transmission. Smartphone camera technology becomes especially helpful in

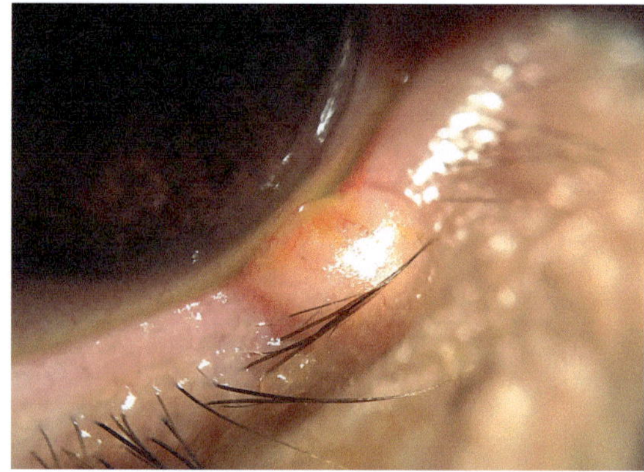

Fig. A1.4 Photograph of lid marginal basal cell carcinoma, taken with smartphone camera and macro adapter clip-on lens

monitoring ocular changes in settings where standard photography would be difficult or impossible, such as remote clinics, in-hospital settings such as critical care units, or other hospital settings where patients cannot be transported to ophthalmic photography suites. Previously, written descriptions and crude sketches were the only means of following such patients; now, easily acquired, accurate photographic images can document pathologies and demonstrate changes over time (Figs. A1.4 and A1.5).

The original smartphone camera systems required handheld lenses (e.g., a 20D or 28D lens typically used for indirect ophthalmoscopy)

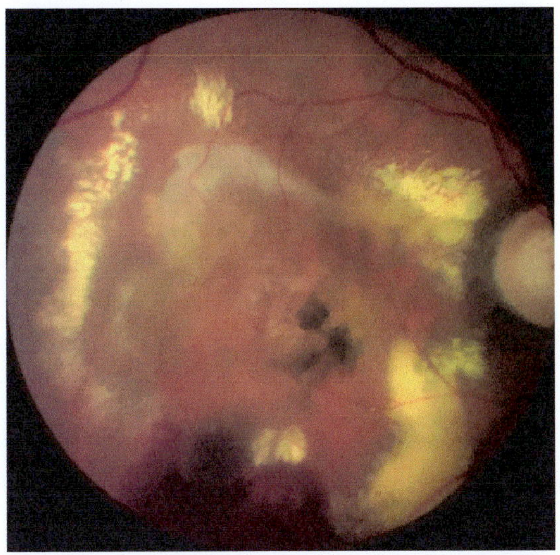

Fig. A1.5 Fundus image taken with the Remidio smartphone camera system, showing polypoidal choroidal vasculopathy, retinal exudates, choroidal neovascular membrane, subretinal hemorrhage, and subretinal fibrosis

to produce a fundus image. Although relatively simple and inexpensive, this approach requires a degree of practice to master proper lens alignment to obtain a clear picture. Newer, more expensive systems have been introduced which adapt smartphones to existing ophthalmoscopes (such as the smartphone adaptor for the Welch Allyn iExaminer PanOptic Ophthalmoscope); others employ dedicated lens systems which attach directly to a smartphone (such as the D-EYE system being developed in Italy; oDocs in New Zealand; the Remidio, developed in India; or the Peek Retina system, developed for Peek Vision, a UK-based charitable foundation) (Fig. A1.5). These systems are currently marketed principally for use with people in remote and rural areas, but it is likely that if successful, they will, even in major urban settings, eventually replace direct ophthalmoscopes as the primary instrument for non-office examination. Many of these systems also take excellent macrophotographs of external lesions; some can be attached directly to slit lamps or to portable units that function as slit lamp substitutes in the field.

Ultrasound (US)

Ultrasound technology utilizes noninvasive, high-frequency sound waves sent by a transducer into body tissues; at tissue interfaces of varying densities, reflecting or "echoing" waves are returned to, and received by, the same transducer. The transducer initially converts electrical waves into sound waves and then, upon receiving reflected echos, converts the sound back into an electrical wave, which is displayed as an image on the screen. As the amount of tissue penetration and image resolution is dependent on transducer frequency, different transducers producing varying ultrasound frequencies are required for different tissues; e.g., ultrasound equipment used for abdominal scanning is not the same as that employed for ocular or orbital scans. The more similar two adjacent tissues are, the less difference there will be in the reflected echo images, and the more different two adjacent tissues are, the greater the contrast in the ultrasound image produced.

US, due to its unique ability to make accurate measurements within the eye even in the presence of opacities such as vitreous or aqueous hemorrhage, has proved valuable in providing high caliber images of the retina, vitreous, uvea, extraocular muscles, and ocular and anterior orbital tumors, among others. It is also better at imaging retro-iridial structures than other optical methods and allows visualization of the irido-corneal angle, as well as intraocular IOL positioning. Newer technologies will enable excellent visualization of vascular flow as well as 3D imaging (see below).

Transducer design is critical in obtaining high-quality ophthalmic ultrasound images. At present, virtually all ophthalmic ultrasound is performed with mechanically scanned single-element probes. This is in contrast to US imaging in other clinical specialties, which almost universally rely on linear array probes. Such linear arrays are composed of numerous (typically >100) transducer elements that can independently transmit US and receive echo data. By precision timing of transmission, a focused beam can be produced and scanned without requiring mechanically moving parts. Linear arrays have been slow to be adapted to eye examination because ophthalmology generally requires higher frequencies than most other clinical specialties, and fabrication becomes more challenging and expensive with increasing frequencies.

Ketterling et al. developed an annular array as an intermediate step between single-element probes and linear arrays, which consists of concentric elements that can receive and send independently. This provides major improvement over conventional fixed-focus US probes by providing an increase in depth of field, although because of the annular arrangement, mechanical scanning is still necessary.

Another new technology is plane-wave imaging. In a recently developed technology called compound coherent plane-wave imaging, all elements fire at once to produce one wave front, and focusing is achieved only on receive. Acoustic intensity is significantly reduced, and there is an increase in image acquisition speed compared to both conventional linear arrays and mechanically scanned probes, making it ideal for imaging transient motions. This technology, plus the recent introduction of linear arrays of 20–30 MHz, enhances the prospect for improved ocular imaging, making it an ideal noninvasive technique to visualize and measure ocular blood flow within individual vessels as small as arterioles as well as tissue capillary beds to investigate tissue perfusion (Fig. A1.6).

Computed Tomography (CT)

The roots of CT technology go back to the introduction of the X-ray by Wilhelm Conrad Roentgen in the late nineteenth century. X-ray imaging of the eye and orbit, primarily structural abnormalities of the skull and orbital bones, was described by Schüller in 1918, followed by Pfeiffer's classic papers on roentgenography of exophthalmos in 1943. Prior to CT, plain X-ray was used extensively for the diagnosis of orbital disease, but CT has almost entirely supplanted plain film studies. Computed tomography, developed by Hounsfield, was first performed on a patient in the early 1970s, and orbital CT was pioneered by Trokel and Hilal in the late 1970s and early 1980s.

CT uses X-ray beams with an array of detectors that surround the body part being scanned. Images are acquired by rapid rotation of the X-ray source around the body. As X-rays pass through tissues, they are partially absorbed, with the degree of absorption depending on tissue density, and, after passing through the patient, are received by detectors. While early CTs received data one slice at a time, imaging speed has increased with the introduction of multislice detector arrays. Unlike X-rays, which have limited capacity to measure subtle variations in density, modern CTs have exquisite capacity to distinguish densities, with a wide dynamic range, enabling representation of soft tissues as well as bone. The grayscale of CT images can be adjusted in post-processing to best show either bone or soft tissues. As with MRI, CT data can be reconstructed to form either 2D or 3D images, with pixel brightness representing X-ray absorption.

CT is now being used in the preoperative planning of complex orbital and facial fractures to create computer-generated, 3D-printed, custom implants, often made of porous polyethylene or polyetheretherketone (PEEK). In addition, CT data can be used to generate real-time image guidance that is helpful for complex cranial, sinus, and orbital surgeries (Fig. A1.7).

CT is advantageous compared to MRI in having higher image acquisition speed. Bone detail on CT imaging is superior to that of MRI, facilitating identification of orbital fractures and surgical planning, although soft tissue image contrast is not quite as good. CT units are more widely available than MRI, and, unlike MRI, CT is suitable where there is a possible presence of a metallic foreign body. Although there are no absolute contraindications, CT does expose the patient to about 100 times as much radiation as a conventional X-ray, and this needs to be taken into account in situations such as examinations in children or those who require repeat or serial evaluations.

Magnetic Resonance Imaging (MRI)

Magnetic resonance imaging was first developed by Damadian and employed on a patient in 1977, and the first imaging of the eye and orbit was performed in the early 1980s. MRI is based

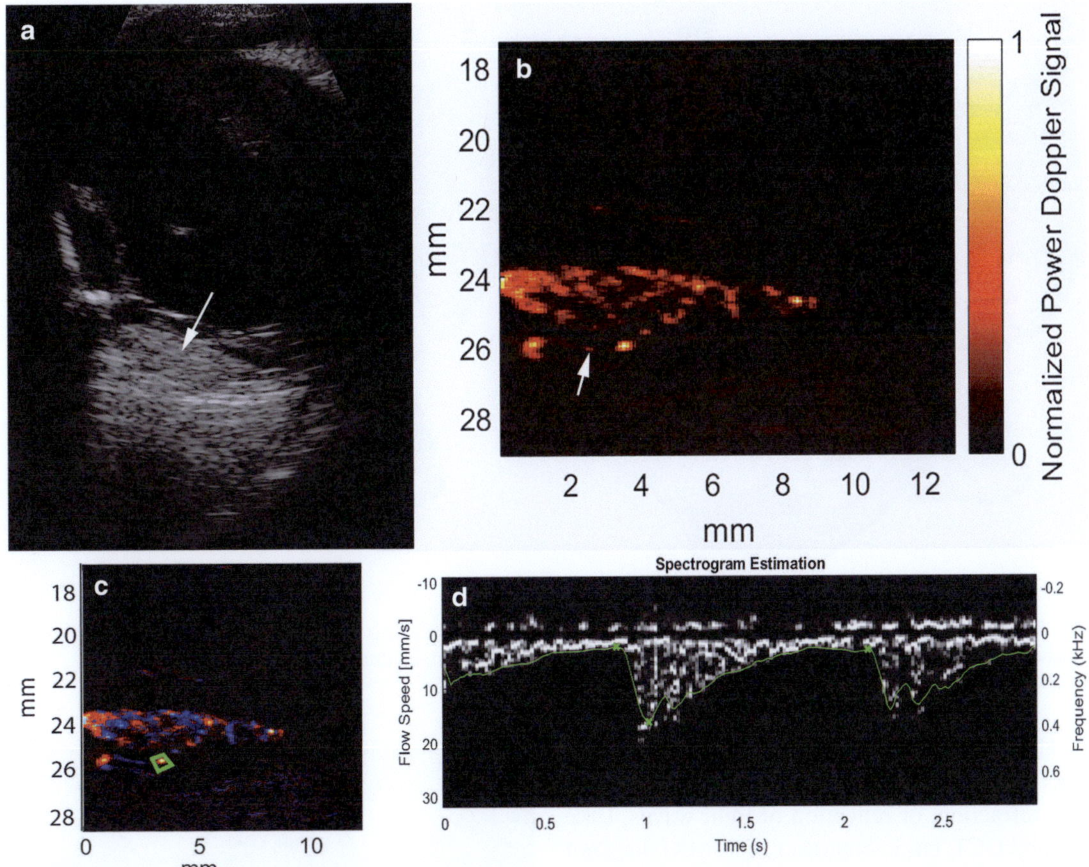

Fig. A1.6 Images of a choroidal melanoma 20 years after treatment by proton beam irradiation demonstrating vascular flow imaging with ultrafast plane-wave ultrasound (US). (a) A conventional 10 MHz B-scan US demonstrated a choroidal mass (arrow). Vitreous debris is present, and the retina is detached, with multiple tractional vitreous membranes that are fixed on kinetic scanning. There are regions of high reflectivity noted at the posterior pole consistent with scarring. (b) An ultrafast plane-wave ultrasound, with data digitally filtered to remove slow-moving and stationary structures and high-resolution blood-flow images. Power Doppler images demonstrated a feeder vessel (arrow) and a vascular network within the tumor. (c) Directionally coded power Doppler, in which reds and blues, respectively, indicate flow toward or away from the ultrasound axis, demonstrates highly variable directionality of flow within the tumor. (d) A spectrogram of the feeder vessel near its point of entry into the tumor (green box in c) shows pulsatile flow. The tumor spectrogram (not shown) showed low velocities and negligible pulsatility

on interaction of hydrogen nuclei (protons) with an externally applied magnetic field that flips the protons (which act like minute magnets) into alignment. After the applied field is terminated, nuclei return to equilibrium, which releases radio frequency energy that induces nuclear magnetic resonance signals in a receiver. These signals are converted into intensity levels, which are displayed as grayscale images.

The images obtained reflect the spatial concentration and relaxation time of specific nuclei. In the case of the eye, there is a wide variation in water content among solid and fluid components and orbital fat, resulting in high contrast in proton density or relaxation-time weighted images.

Indications for MRI include visual loss due to potential presence of an orbital or optic nerve tumor (e.g., meningioma or glioma), vascular orbital lesions such as AV malformations, and inflammatory conditions including optic neuritis, myositis, orbital pseudotumor, and thyroid ophthalmopathy.

a

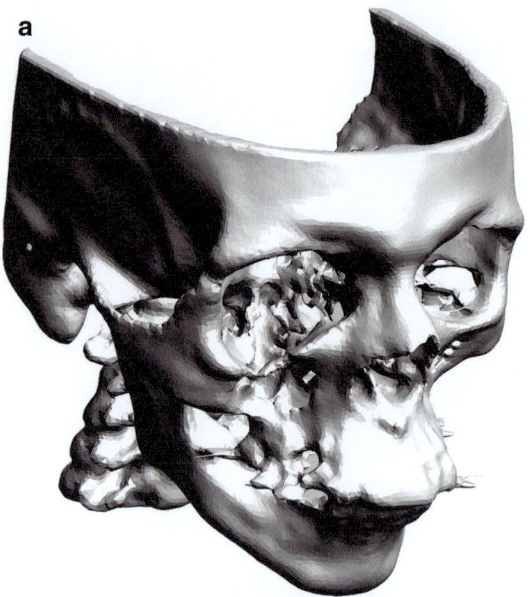

b

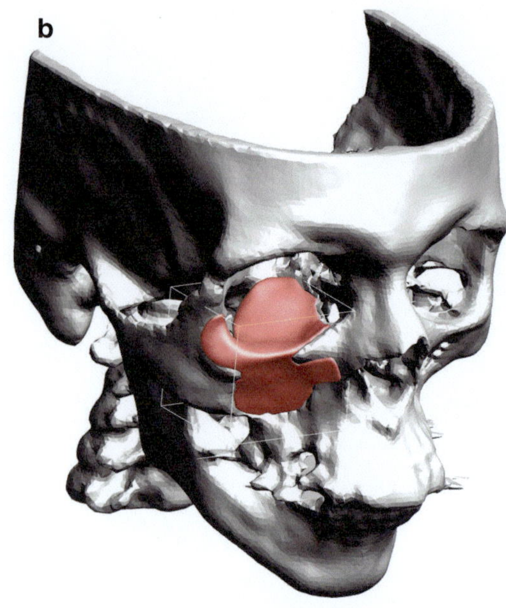

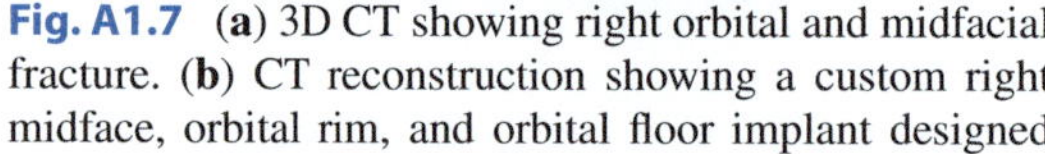

Fig. A1.7 (**a**) 3D CT showing right orbital and midfacial fracture. (**b**) CT reconstruction showing a custom right midface, orbital rim, and orbital floor implant designed using 3D printing based on a subtraction image from the uninvolved, contralateral side

Unlike US and optical coherence tomography (OCT), MRI is unaffected by absorption, scattering, refraction, or reflection of light waves. Like US and OCT, but in contrast to CT, MRI does not involve exposure to ionizing radiation. Although clinical MRI systems have significantly lower resolution and slower acquisition times (several minutes) than US or OCT, high-field systems have recently achieved an impressive resolution of 80 μm (Fig. A1.8). MRI is disadvantageous in terms of portability (it is not portable), accessibility, and expense. Because acquisition time is slow, head and eye motion result in reduced resolution. Cardiac pacemakers and intraocular, intraorbital, or intracranial metallic foreign bodies are absolute contraindications to MRI, as magnetic force can induce uncontrolled, potentially damaging movement of the device or foreign body. Implanted titanium and gold, which are not magnetic, are typically considered safe for MRI.

Traditionally, T1- and T2-weighted imaging sequences have been used clinically for imaging the eye and orbit. Fluid, such as vitreous and CSF, is dark on T1-weighted imaging (T1WI), and these sequences, especially with fat suppression, are very helpful for delineating anatomy.

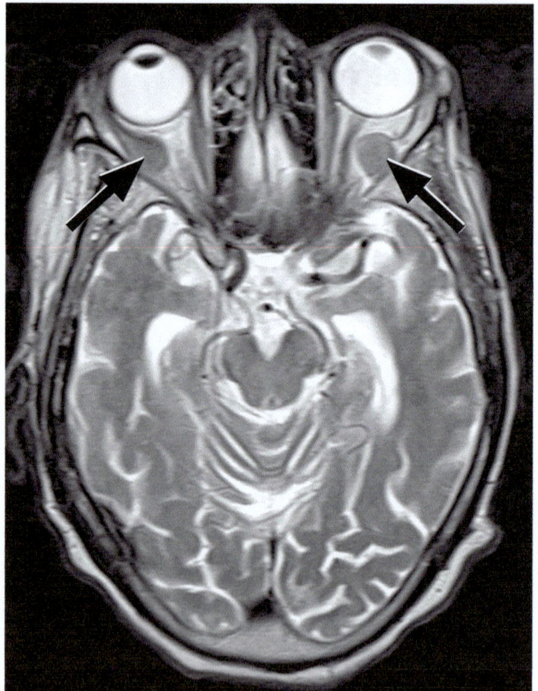

Fig. A1.8 A magnetic resonance image demonstrating bilateral soft tissue masses (arrows) in the lateral recti in a patient with known metastatic neuroendocrine carcinoma. Among other things, the image also clearly shows medial rectus muscles, orbital fat, optic nerves, and the intraocular lenses

Conversely, T2-weighted images (T2WI) highlight tissues with high water content. Most orbital pathological processes are hyperintense on T2WI since these processes (e.g., infection, inflammation, and most tumors) have associated edema. That said, there are certain pathological processes that are hypointense on T2WI due to the lesions containing substances with short T2 relaxation times such as blood clot, fibrosis, melanin, paramagnetic minerals, and amyloid. Some clinical conditions which demonstrate hypointensity on T2WI include melanoma (melanin); retinoblastoma (calcium); invasive fungal disease (manganese, magnesium, calcium, and free radicals); lymphatic malformation and superior ophthalmic vein thrombosis (blood clot); scirrhous metastatic breast cancer, sclerosing orbital inflammation, granulomatosis with polyangiitis, and sarcoidosis (fibrosis); and amyloidosis.

Steady-state free precession (SSFP) imaging is an MRI sequence that uses steady states of magnetizations. Balanced SSFP images such as fast imaging employing steady-state acquisition (FIESTA) utilized by MRI machines (General Electric), TrueFISP (Siemens), and b-FFE (Philips) can be very useful for visualization of the entire pathway of cranial nerves as they provide good contrast between nerves and surrounding cerebrospinal fluid.

Diffusion-weighted imaging (DWI) takes advantage of how water molecules diffuse in tissues. Diffusion restriction occurs in certain pathologic processes such as acute infarction, abscess formation, highly cellular tumors such as lymphomas and high-grade gliomas, as well as toxic, metabolic, and demyelinating conditions, resulting in bright regions on DWI. One special form of DWI is diffusion tensor imaging (DTI) which excels at mapping white matter tracts (such as the visual tract) in the brain.

Improved, high-resolution orbital imaging techniques are being developed. Spatial resolution in the orbit can be greatly improved with the use of surface coil arrays embedded in a facemask worn by patients during the scan. Three-dimensional black-blood MRI is being used experimentally to image the posterior ciliary arteries and may prove beneficial

in the diagnosis of ischemic optic neuropathy related to giant cell arteritis. With this technique, circumferential arterial wall thickening and enhancement of the vessel wall can be imaged, distinguishing arteritic from nonarteritic processes.

Optical Coherence Tomography

Optical coherence tomography is a noninvasive technology, introduced by Fujimoto and his group at MIT and Harvard Medical School in 1991, that enables visualization of microscopic ocular structures in exquisite detail. OCT, originally developed for measurement of eye axial length, is now used extensively in many areas of ophthalmology and has also been adapted for use in other medical areas such as cardiology, oncology, and dermatology. Whereas US employs sound waves to produce images of tissues, OCT uses light waves to produce in vivo optical cross sections and 3D reconstructions of the macula, optic nerve, and anterior segment. Original OCT units utilized a technique known as Time Domain acquisition and could create retinal images with a resolution of 10–15 μ; newer, spectral-domain systems can resolve to 2–3 μ (Fig. A1.9). Conditions such as macular edema and epiretinal membrane, which previously were difficult to diagnose and almost impossible to quantify, as well as subtle changes in optic nerve head anatomy or individual retinal layer thicknesses can now be visualized and measured in high resolution, and this capability has transformed the practice of ophthalmology in the last decade. As an example, fluorescein angiography, an invasive test which used to be the gold standard exam for many retinal conditions, has been almost completely supplanted by OCT.

Optical Coherence Tomography Angiography (OCTA)

OCT angiography (OCTA) is a developing imaging modality that provides information about retinal microvasculature. OCTA visualizes vasculature using motion contrast; unlike traditional fluorescein angiography (FA), no dye injection is required to produce images of the retinal vasculature, which show a high degree of detail, and unlike FA, this noninvasive testing allows

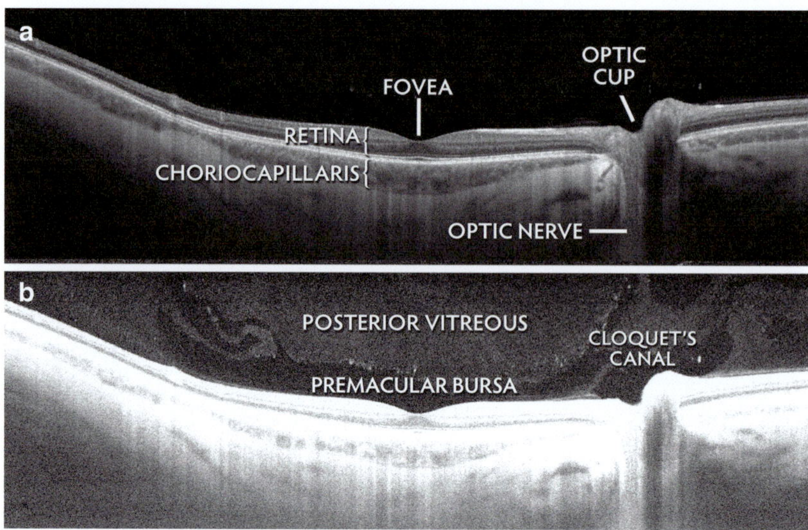

Fig. A1.9 A high-resolution OCT of the retina and optic nerve obtained with the Zeiss Plex ® Elite imaging system utilizing swept-source technology. (**a**) OD posterior pole image showing normal anatomy. (**b**) Brightness and contrast adjustment of image in the same eye allows visualization of posterior vitreous anatomy details which are normally not visible. (Picture courtesy Katherine Broderick)

for three-dimensional imaging of retinal and choroidal vessels. At times, detailed information regarding blood flow can be visualized on OCTA that is not visible on FA. Individual capillary layers can be isolated on an image, which can be helpful for evaluating visual changes and disease progression, particularly in the setting of AMD and diabetic retinopathy (Figs. A1.10 and A1.11).

3D Optical Coherence Tomography

Three-dimensional optical coherence tomography (3DOCT) is a novel application of data generated from spectral-domain and swept-source OCT systems. Because OCT systems are now able to acquire images with high speed, high resolution, and limited motion artifact, high-quality 3D reconstructions can be rendered to evaluate a particular area of interest in the retina. Virtual reality walkthroughs of 3D reconstructions allow for better appreciation of the pathological changes in retinal disease, and serial quantitative analysis of the volumetric data sets may provide more precise measurements of the response to therapeutic agents than conventional OCT images.

Future Directions in Ophthalmic Therapeutics

Glaucoma

Glaucoma and glaucoma treatment can greatly impact a patient's life. Given our aging population, glaucoma prevalence is expected to dramatically increase; therefore, it is of utmost importance that healthcare providers outside of ophthalmology are aware of new developments in glaucoma diagnosis and management. As with other fields, there is constant research and development of novel therapies to help combat this potentially blinding disease.

Eyedrops are a mainstay of treatment and usually the initial therapy for glaucoma patients. Mechanistically, drops lower intraocular pressure by either decreasing aqueous production within the eye or increasing aqueous outflow from the eye. In recent years, prostaglandin analogues have been the predominant first-line therapy, given the low side effect profile, efficacy, and once-daily dosing schedule. Two new FDA-approved medications have recently been developed to treat glaucoma:

Latanoprostene bunod (trade name Vyzulta, Bausch and Lomb) is a prostaglandin analogue, combined with a nitric oxide-donating component. It works by increasing outflow, targeting both uveoscleral and trabecular meshwork outflow pathways. The prostaglandin component increases uveoscleral outflow, as with other prostaglandin eye drops, while the novel nitric oxide component is thought to relax the trabecular meshwork, promoting increased aqueous outflow.

Netarsudil (trade name Rhopressa, Aerie Pharmaceuticals) is one of a completely new class of medications, called Rho kinase inhibitors. It is

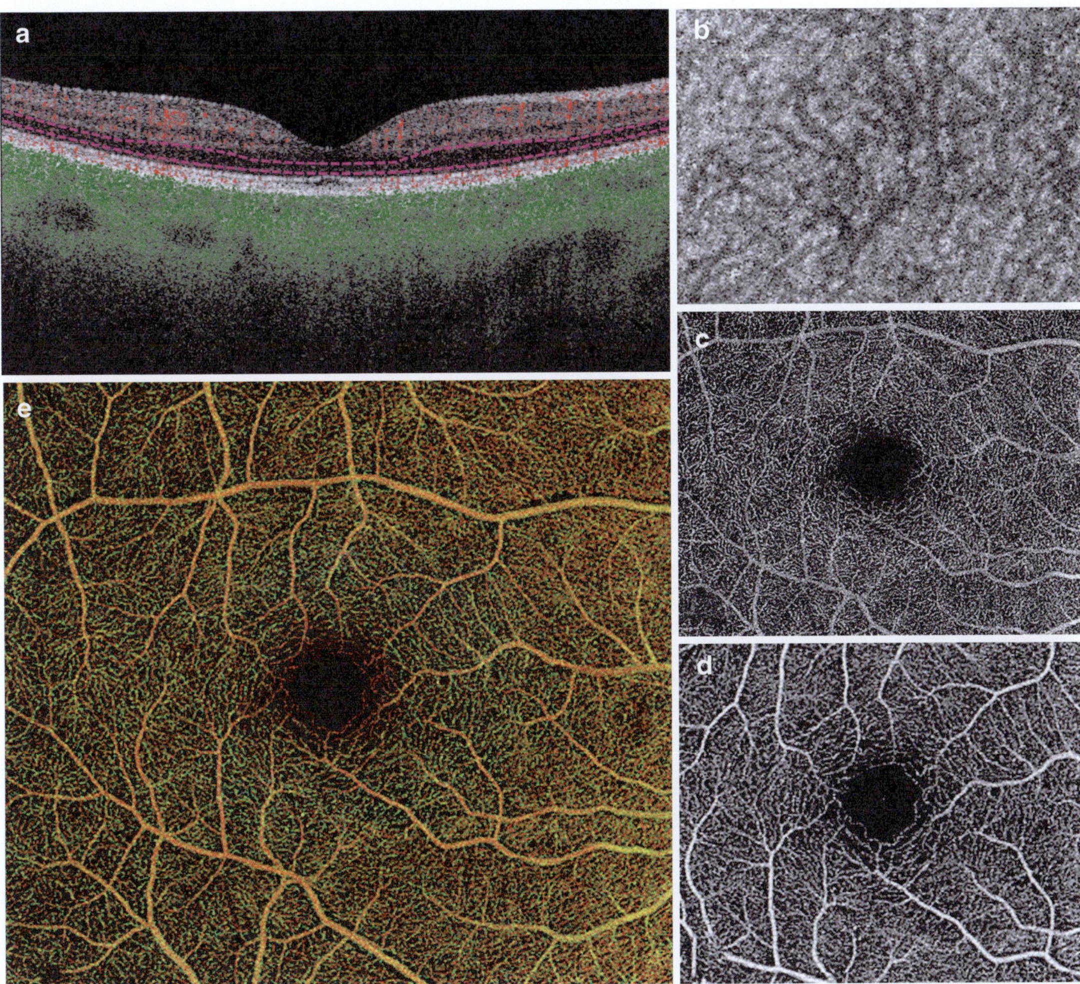

Fig. A1.10 OCT-angiography images of a normal macula. (**a**) Cross section of foveal area images. (**b**) En face image of choroidal layer. (**c**) En face image of deep retinal vascular layer. (**d**) En face image of superficial vascular layer. (**e**) Image of combined vasculature layers visualized in images (**b, c,** and **d**)

also dosed once daily, and is believed to work at the cellular level, increasing trabecular meshwork outflow.

Many patients fail glaucoma medical therapy and will eventually require surgical management. As with other surgical fields, ophthalmology has shifted toward less invasive surgeries, utilizing technologically advanced surgical instrumentation and devices. The development of microsurgical instruments and devices, spearheaded in the area of vitreoretinal surgery, is now expanding into other ophthalmic specialties. Microinvasive or minimally invasive glaucoma surgery (MIGS) has undergone tremendous development and growth in recent years. The goal of newly introduced devices and modified procedures is to achieve clinically significant eye pressure reduction, without the invasiveness and risk of traditional glaucoma surgeries (e.g., trabeculectomy and glaucoma drainage implants). Many new devices have recently been approved, with additional ones pending approval. This includes devices targeting the traditional trabecular meshwork pathway and downstream channels (e.g., the iStent inject by Glaukos and the Hydrus Microstent by Ivantis) and those targeting the suprachoroidal space outflow pathway (including the CyPass Micro-Stent by Alcon, as well as

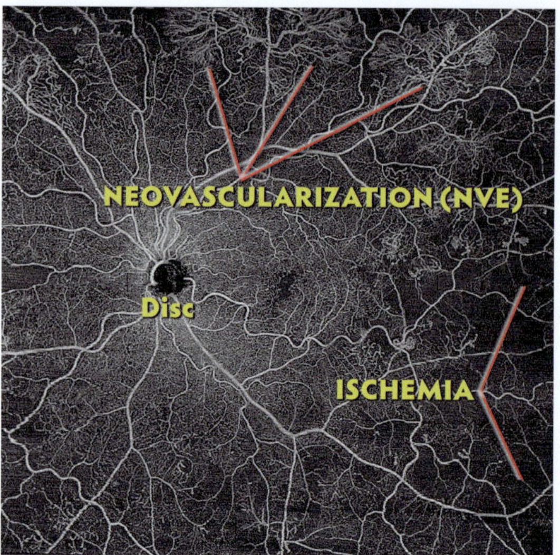

Fig. A1.11 Montage image of high-resolution OCT-angiography images currently being developed (Zeiss Optics, Plex® Elite imaging) showing left eye in patient with proliferative diabetic retinopathy. Areas of both ischemia and peripheral neovascularization are clearly visualized in this new, noninvasive technique

the iStent Supra by Glaukos). Other new MIGS devices drain fluid from the eye to the subconjunctival space, a pressure-lowering mechanism similar to that accomplished by the classic, but more invasive trabeculectomy (e.g., the Xen Gel Stent by Allergan and the InnFocus by Santen Pharmaceutical).

New technology has also focused on clinical monitoring of patients from their homes. Home tonometers to measure intraocular pressure, for example, allow patients to monitor themselves (without the need for anesthetic eyedrops), which can greatly help ophthalmologists manage glaucoma while easing the burden of multiple physician visits. The FDA-approved contact lens called Triggerfish can continuously monitor eye pressure in patients throughout the day, providing meaningful clinical information for glaucoma monitoring and treatment. Many clinicians feel that continuous pressure monitoring, similar to data provided by a cardiac Holter monitor or similar device, provides significantly more useful information than that obtained by single, or even multiple, office-visit pressure readings. This is particularly important in those patients suspected, or known, to have significant diurnal pressure variations, which are most likely missed with routine, in-office glaucoma testing.

Vitreoretinal Diseases

There are many promising future technologies in diagnosis and management in vitreoretinal disease that will change and enhance our ability to treat vision-threatening illness. Optical coherence tomography (OCT) of the macula is a mainstay of current treatment, but images capturing a wider area of the retina are possible in the research setting, and widefield fluorescein angiography is already being employed. The use of real-time OCT during surgical procedures is being investigated. OCT angiography, a noninvasive way of measuring capillary blood flow, is commercially available, and its clinical utility is still being determined (see above). Adaptive optics, an imaging technique that allows actual microscopic images of a patient's individual photoreceptor cells, is available at some institutions in the research setting. These technologies have quickly become the mainstay of diagnostic procedures in retinal disease, allowing for the effects of novel therapeutics to be monitored.

Intravitreal injections of therapeutics are now commonplace in retina clinics, so the future focus has been on more durable treatments requiring fewer injections. Therapeutic alternatives include drug-eluting implants, molecules with a longer intraocular half-life, molecules that target a variety of angiogenic factors, and use of surgically implantable and refillable drug delivery ports. Dry macular degeneration and retinal atrophy are currently untreatable, and there is hope that subretinal stem cell or viral vectors may help regenerate photoreceptors and outer retinal structures. In addition, a number of drug targets within the development pathways of dry age-related macular degeneration are now being investigated in clinical trials. The ARGUS II retinal prosthesis system (produced by Second Sight Medical

Products, Sylmar, CA) currently has a very narrow clinical indication but demonstrates that a functional retinal prosthesis may be possible in the future. Voretigene neparvovec (Luxturna™) is an adenoviral vector-based therapy for the treatment of RPE65-related inherited disease which may pave the way for future gene therapy.

Ophthalmic Gene Therapy

Based on the Human Genome Project data, previously unimagined therapeutic methods have been developed for treatment of genetic diseases. The sequencing results of the human genome have permitted us to decipher gene mutations or variants in an increasing number of genes and their correlated diseases. Pathogenic mechanisms have been analyzed, and identification of abnormal functions of mutated genes has permitted us to derive their normal functions.

Three basic questions have to be answered before applying gene therapy to patients:

1. Which approach can be used to correct the mutated gene?

   Ideally, all causative genes and their mutations have been identified prior to development of treatment for a given disease. Protein actions and interactions have been defined, animal or cell models have been developed, therapeutic approaches have been proposed and tried in cell or animal models prior to clinical trials, and finally, FDA approval for clinical care has been obtained. At present, gene mutations are being identified in isolation, and gene-specific therapies are being developed as mutations are found. However, alternative approaches to therapy may become available as the gene and function complex is more fully understood.

   In order to run a clinical trial, an adequate number of patients need to be identified. Patients with rare diseases ought to be sought worldwide; the patients themselves or their treating physicians should be registered in GPS-based data files so that they can be alerted, when treatment trials are going to be started or when therapy has become approved by the FDA or corresponding organizations in other countries.

   The safety and efficacy of all developed techniques will require continued detailed studies, so that the most specific and long-lasting approach to therapy is available for any of the thousands of human ocular diseases.

2. How do you deliver the therapeutic agent?

   Ideally, therapy would be applied in the least traumatic fashion. Many patients with inherited retinal diseases will develop multiple ophthalmic complications, including keratoconus, posterior subcapsular cataracts, glaucoma, uveitis, or a Coats response. Thus, these are fragile eyes that will need interventions minimalized whenever possible.

3. At what stage of the disease do you undertake treatment?

   Patients should undergo therapy as early as possible, so that as much of a normal retina as possible can be preserved.

Methods of gene transfer include, among others, viral and non-viral gene transfer, RNA interference, oncolytic virotherapy, aptamers, oligonucleotide therapeutics, and targeted genomic interventions. Targeting nucleases to chosen locations in the human genome include meganucleases, zinc-finger proteins, TALENs (transcription activator-like effector nucleases), and clustered regularly interspaced short palindromic repeats (CRISPR) and CRISPR-associated protein 9 (CRISPR/Cas9).

The exciting results of at least temporary and partial, though hopefully permanent, correction of the molecular defect in the dystrophin gene through CRISPRCas9 and other technologies show that the pathway to treatment of localized genetic diseases is open as long as the gene defect is correctly identified. The use of gene transfer methodology has become reality for inherited retinal diseases.

Currently, genetic testing and gene therapy are only recommended for those inherited retinal diseases that are monogenic (i.e., caused by a sin-

Table A1.1 Ongoing gene therapy trials for inherited retinal diseases (Updated, August 2018)

Diseases	Number of patients to be enrolled, trial phase	Interventional drug
Leber congenital amaurosis	12, I/II	Drug: QR-110
	27, I/II	AAV RPE65
	27, I/II	AAV OPTIRPE65
Choroideremia	15, II	AAV2-REP1
	140, III	AAV2-REP1
	30, II	AAV-mediated REP1 gene replacement
Achromatopsia	18, I/II	AAV – CNGB3
	18, I/II	AAV – CNGB3
	24, I/II	AGTC-402
	24, I/II	rAAV2tYF-PR1.7-hCNGB3
X-linked retinoschisis	27, I/II	rAAV2tYF-CB-hRS1
	24, I/II	RS1 AAV vector
Retinitis pigmentosa	12, I/II	AAV2/5-hPDE6B
	24, I/II	AAV-RPGR
	15, I/II	rAAV2tYF-GRK1-RPGR
	36, I/II	AAV-RPGR
Stargardt disease	120, II	Zimura
	46, I/II	SAR422459
	46, I/II	SAR422459
	50, II	ALK-001
Usher syndrome	18, I/II	UshStat

Details of trials are available on the website: *ClinicalTrials.gov*

gle gene), as these defects are most amenable to therapeutic interventions. Routine genetic testing of patients with complex, polygenic disorders like age-related macular degeneration is not warranted. In 2008, Leber congenital amaurosis (LCA) was successfully treated using gene transfer therapy, the first instance of reversal of congenital blindness utilizing a genetic treatment. Other ophthalmic conditions which show promise in gene therapeutics include choroideremia, Usher syndrome, and Stargardt disease (Table A1.1).

Refractive Technologies

The refractive state of the eye is based on the length of the globe, the power of the crystalline lens, and the shape of the cornea. Progress will occur as technology allows control of these structures. The most successful and widely used refractive procedures modify curvature of the cornea. Current technologies require that tissue be removed or material be added to the cornea to change its shape. It is almost certain that technologies that allow the corneal shape to be changed will be developed: Laser-tissue interaction that will allow controlled change of corneal shape without tissue removal or addition of material will likely play a major role in refractive surgery. The current experience with collagen cross-linking has shown that the corneal shape can be influenced by photochemically induced alteration. It will be a small step to create laser-induced cross-linking to allow precise and controlled corneal changes.

In addition, the long sought-after desire to control scleral growth in progressive myopia is now being realized. Compounds have been tested in the laboratory that inhibit sclerocytes and prevent scleral growth. It is only a question of time before this will be tested in a clinical population.

The prevalence of childhood myopia (nearsightedness) has increased dramatically over the past several decades, particularly in developed countries. Because myopia is not only a hindrance to good vision but may also predispose to retinal detachment and glaucoma, it is a significant public health concern. Accordingly, there is considerable interest in developing interventions that can prevent or reduce myopia. Although the underlying pathophysiologic mechanisms are not clear, most cases result from increased axial elongation of the eye. The risk of developing myopia is significantly increased by the presence of myopia in one's parents. A causative role for prolonged amounts of near viewing (e.g., phones, tablets, books) and artificial light are suspected but not well-established. Recent studies, however, have shown the use of topical low-dose atropine 0.01% eyedrops can slow down the progression on myopia in some children, as can the use of specially designed contact lenses that either alter the contour of the cornea at night (e.g., orthokeratology or ortho-k) or provide aspheric optics during the day. The long-term efficacy of these treatments is not yet known. There is ongoing research to better understand the molecular and genetic basis for myopia, as well as the interaction with environmental and behavioral factors.

Artificial Intelligence

Ophthalmology is a visual specialty where disease is often detected and treatments dictated and monitored based on clinical imaging modalities such as photography, optical coherence tomography, ultrasound, and angiography. It is not surprising, then, that the use of artificial intelligence (AI) technology in diagnosis and management of a variety of different eye diseases has become a crucial component in developing diagnostic regimens for such diseases as glaucoma, diabetes, age-related macular degeneration, and retinopathy of prematurity.

Complex AI algorithms have been constructed by a variety of companies, including Google and IBM, utilizing readily available ophthalmic images (such as fundus photographs) to detect ocular diseases. Recently, the Food and Drug Administration (FDA) approved marketing of an AI-based diagnostic system for autonomous detection of diabetic retinopathy (IDx-DR). This promising technology is the first of many new AI modalities which, in coming years, will likely provide valuable data to the practicing ophthalmologist to better diagnose and manage patients.

Telemedicine

Ophthalmology is primarily an outpatient specialty, and, as with similar areas of medicine, is embracing the potential benefits of utilizing telemedicine initiatives to provide enhanced diagnosis and monitoring of a variety of diseases, especially those which are, in their early stages, asymptomatic and treatable. Multiple, well-established tele-ophthalmology screening programs already in use provide ophthalmic diagnostic services to populations which would otherwise have limited access to quality eye care. These programs have aided in the detection and staging of many eye

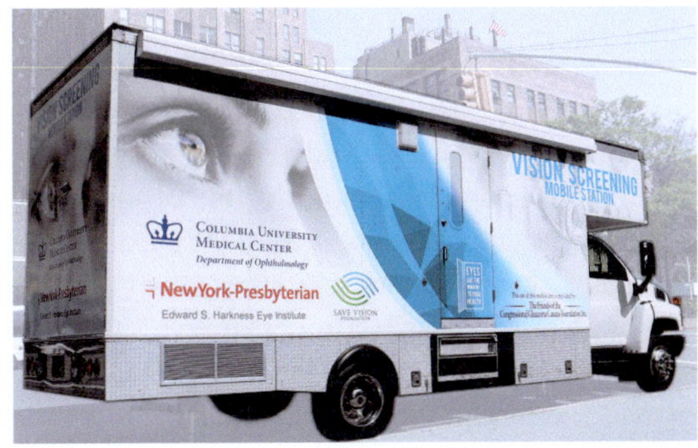

Fig. A1.12 Real-time tele-ophthalmology mobile unit currently employed at the Harkness Eye Institute at Columbia University. The van helps provide free screening for the four leading causes of blindness and their comorbidities in high-risk and low-socioeconomic areas

diseases, including diabetic retinopathy, glaucoma, and retinopathy of prematurity. Fully equipped screening trucks, for example (Fig. A1.12), allow access to care in underserved populations, remotely putting patients in contact with trained ophthalmologists who can screen an array of data which is obtained in the field. Collected data is transmitted to reading sites for analysis, which expedites the detection of disease that may otherwise go undiagnosed and untreated and greatly accelerates the arrangement of appropriate follow-up care.

Appendix 2: Common Ophthalmic Surgeries

Daniel S. Casper and James Auran

Introduction

Although historians have traced the first known cataract treatments to India around 1000 B.C.E., intraocular surgical cataract procedures were not performed until the middle 1700s. The earliest treatments involved variations on a technique known as "couching," whereby a mature, usually opaque lens was, by external means, forcibly relocated to the posterior compartment of the eye, within the vitreous, thus restoring a clear (but poorly focused) visual pathway to the retina. The invasive, surgical procedures first developed in eighteenth-century France were a bold advancement, involving the complete surgical removal of the opaque lens, rather than its repositioning within the eye.

Today, it is remarkable how many different surgical techniques are performed on such a small area of the body and the breadth and depth of the extensive advancements in ophthalmic surgery that have occurred in a relatively short period of time. Two of the most innovative techniques, microsurgery and laser photocoagulation, have only been introduced and refined in the last half century and continually improve at an exceptional rate.

The advancements in ophthalmic surgery that technological developments have enabled cannot be overstated. As an example, laser photocoagulation techniques are currently routinely used in cataract, glaucoma, refractive, vitreoretinal, and oculoplastic procedures, and the same could be said for other surgical innovations as well.

This chapter will present a brief overview of some of the more common ophthalmic procedures which are currently commonly performed.

Anterior Segment

Cataract surgeries account for approximately 3.5–4 million surgeries in the USA per year, and as the population ages, this number is expected to steadily increase. Advancements in cataract surgery have been among the most dramatic in ophthalmology and, in less than 50 years, have advanced from a somewhat crude procedure usually requiring an overnight hospital stay (or longer) and general anesthesia, followed by a 6-week recovery procedure, to a rapid, day surgery that rarely requires more than local anesthesia and usually produces significant visual improvement with hours and full recovery in a week or 2. Although the improvements in surgical technique can be mostly ascribed to advancements in microsurgical instrumentation and binocular intraoperative microscopy, the implementation of artificial intraocular lenses to replace the removed natural lens has completely revolutionized the achievement of excellent postoperative visual acuity.

There are numerous other anterior segment procedures regularly performed. Corneal transplantation (penetrating keratoplasty, or PK), a remarkable operation that replaces an opaque or perforated cornea with a cadaveric donor, usually provides excellent results and does not require lifelong immunosuppression. In spite of this success, newer techniques, which often have better results and a better safety profile, are rapidly replacing the PK in a growing number of cases (see Chap. 15). Surgical removal of conjunctival masses and corneal growths is routinely performed, again with excellent results.

Refractive surgery was popularized by Jose Barraquer in the 1960s and Svyatoslav Fyodorov in the 1970s and utilized different surgical methods to modify the anatomy of the cornea, lens, or sclera, to reduce or eliminate the need for glasses. In the 1980s, Stephen Trokel and Rangaswamy Srinivasan introduced the use of an excimer laser rather than a surgical scalpel to produce a similar effect, in a procedure termed photorefractive keratectomy (PRK), which has spawned a host of similar techniques (LASIK, SMILE, etc.; see Chap. 7) which are used to reduce or eliminate myopia, hyperopia, astigmatism, and presbyopia.

Glaucoma

The classic description of open-angle glaucoma as a disease of high intraocular pressure (IOP) that responds to pressure-lowering therapies has, for the most part, given way to a broader definition of a group of optic neuropathies that frequently, but not always, responds to IOP-lowering measures. As the understanding and definition of glaucoma have evolved, the treatment regimens remain quite similar, with IOP-lowering the mainstay of treatment. Typically, treatment starts with a variety of topical IOP-lowering drops (frequently used in combination) and then, if necessary, the introduction of oral medications (such as acetazolamide) that reduce aqueous fluid formation. When such conservative measures fail, the next step is usually a photodestructive procedure such as trabeculoplasty, designed to improve aqueous outflow through the trabecular meshwork. Should laser trabeculoplasty either fail or lose effectiveness over time, there are a variety of surgical procedures that can be employed to further reduce IOP (see Chap. 19). Usually, these are directed toward enhancing aqueous outflow, such as with trabeculectomy procedures, which establish an enhanced outflow channel, or the use of a variety of implanted valve devices which similarly shunt fluid to the subconjunctival space.

In rare cases, cryotherapy may be employed to intentionally destroy the ciliary body, thus significantly reducing aqueous fluid production; such procedures are usually employed as a last resort, after all other therapeutic measures have failed.

In narrow-angle glaucoma, the mainstay of prophylactic treatment remains the surgical construction of an aqueous fluid bypass channel through the iris. Prior to the introduction of laser treatments, surgical iridectomies were employed, which usually created a sectoral ("keyhole") area of iris tissue removal. With the introduction of laser therapy, small, peripheral iridotomies (see Chap. 10) are utilized to obtain similar results with significantly less morbidity.

Posterior Segment

As microsurgical techniques and binocular visualization have become advanced, posterior ocular surgical procedures have become more common and more complex. Although the previous standard of care for retinal detachment, the buckle procedure (see Chap. 24), continues to be used, newer therapies are being employed as well. Included in this armamentarium are vitrectomy procedures (both in the operating room and in-office), which can remove vitreous gel, fibrous bands, and intraocular hemorrhage, and the use of intraoperative laser to photocoagulate when needed, commonly used with retinal holes, tears, or diabetic detachments. The instruments developed to perform these maneuvers include miniature intraocular fiberoptic "light pipes," micro-cutting and suction instruments, and a variety of microscopic picks and forceps for the excision ("peeling") of intraocular membranes. When the vitreous gel is surgically removed, air, various gases, or perfluorocarbon liquids may be injected into the eye to temporarily replace the gel.

In addition to these commonly performed procedures, a variety of newer techniques have been employed to eradicate intraocular tumors, such as melanoma (see Chap. 33). In the last century, it was not unusual for uveal melanomas to be treated by enucleation (surgical removal of the globe). The options for treatment of intraocular tumors now include the use of surgery, laser destructive procedures, and radiation therapy (both external, which employs highly focused charged-particle or gamma knife treatments, and internal, which utilizes surgically implanted radioactive plaques, either within the eye, adjacent to the tumor, or outside, on the scleral wall opposite the area of pathology).

Periocular/Orbital/Strabismus

Ophthalmic surgical procedures are commonly utilized in the periocular region, for a variety of pathologic processes. Periocular lid tumors (see Chap. 30) are common and frequently require either primary surgical excision or Mohs surgical procedures for their removal. Often, these excisional procedures will result in large areas of tissue removal, sometimes including an entire lid, and extensive local plastic surgical reconstruction is required to assure that the globe has adequate protection, lubrication, and tear drainage and that the surgical result is as cosmetically satisfactory as may be obtained. Old lid scar tissue, particularly if it has caused abnormal lid rotation (either entropion or ectropion; see Chap. 31), will also usually require surgical repair, and in the case of conditions like trichiasis, oculoplastic repair may be sight-saving if performed expeditiously.

Tearing (epiphora) is a common complaint and in some cases is due to blockage of the canalicular drainage system. When outflow obstruction is the cause of chronic epiphora, the treatment is usually surgical, requiring either reconstitution of the normal outflow channels or, if necessary, the construction of a replacement tear outflow pathway (dacryocystorhinostomy).

Lid malpositions are common and may be congenital or acquired. As discussed above, lid malpositions can have significant deleterious effects on corneal protection, lubrication, and epithelial integrity and may present a significant cosmetic issue; the classic example of this is thyroid ophthalmopathy, with proptosis and lid retraction. In severe thyroid eye disease, simple oculoplastic lid repair is insufficient; in such cases, orbital decompression, utilizing fat or bone removal, may be necessary to restore the globe to its proper position and enable adequate lid closure. If the extraocular muscles are asymmetrically affected, which is common, then globe malpositioning results in unacceptable double vision; these patients usually require muscle (strabismus) surgery as well, the same procedures used to properly align the eyes in a child with horizontal or vertical globe misplacement.

Orbital tumors may be benign (e.g., hemangioma), malignant (e.g., adenocystic carcinoma), or benign tumors that behave aggressively and require aggressive actions (optic nerve gliomas, meningiomas). Most such tumors will require direct surgical excision. Occasionally, anterior or middle cranial fossae pathologies will invade the orbit and require a combined neurosurgical-ophthalmologic approach for excision.

Until recently, the rare, centrally mediated condition known as blepharospasm, or, in severe cases, hemifacial spasm, frequently required drastic surgical intervention (usually severing of one or more branches of the seventh (facial) cranial nerve) when more conservative medical therapies offered little, or no, improvement. In these patients, overaction of the periocular muscles results in involuntary, sometimes violent, lid closure, with the inability to reopen voluntarily. In recent years, periocular injection of botulinum toxin (as has also been employed for certain migraine headache patients) may offer dramatic relief of symptoms. Usually, repeated injections are required, as the effects of the botulinum toxin are limited to a few months' time; typically, reinjections are necessary two to four times per year for adequate symptom relief.

Appendix 3: Deciphering the Eye Exam

Daniel S. Casper

After documenting an appropriate medical and ophthalmic history, the ophthalmic exam always requires an assessment of best corrected *visual acuity* (usually indicated on the exam with the letter "V" or "BCVA," and indicating if exam was done with or without correction). Whenever possible, this should be distance vision, although near ("N"), or reading vision, may be included as well. Distance vision is always measured in each eye, individually, and by convention, results are indicated for the right (OD) eye prior to the left (OS). Occasionally, binocular vision (OU) will be indicated as well. If the person already has a spectacle or contact lens correction, this Rx is usually noted (either by "H" for has, or "W" for wearing). If a new Rx is obtained, this is indicated as either a "Manifest" or "Accepts" prescription. 20/20 vision is considered "normal"; 20/40 or better is required for driving vision in NY State; 20/200 or worse is considered legally blind. Complete blindness is referred to as "NLP," for no light perception.

The next part of the examination contains a variable number of tests, dependent on the person's age, history, chief complaint, vision, etc. This almost always includes an assessment of the *pupils* and may also cover an *external exam* (lids, lid position and movement, eye position), extraocular motility, color vision testing, and visual field assessment, either confrontational or formal testing. Frequently, diagrams of lid and/or external eye anatomy are included to document abnormalities.

The *slit lamp examination* provides a magnified, binocular, stereoscopic view of the lids, conjunctiva sclera, cornea, anterior chamber, iris and pupil, and the lens. Specialized accessory lenses may also be used with the slit lamp to provide a view of the anterior chamber angle, where the peripheral cornea and iris meet (gonioscopy), or of the posterior portion of the eye, which is usually performed after the pupillary dilation. *Intraocular pressure (IOP)* is usually measured with an instrument known as a Goldmann tonometer, although there are other instruments which can also assess IOP. Normal IOP is approximately 10–21 mmHg. If necessary, the angle anatomy can be viewed with accessory gonioscopic lenses.

Pupils are dilated for a complete ophthalmic examination, which will render the patient blurry at near and light sensitive for a period of about 5 h. Topical *drops instilled* to obtain dilation typically are tropicamide (an anticholinergic compound related to atropine) and phenylephrine (an α-adrenergic agonist). Cyclopentolate, a stronger anticholinergic, is usually used in children. Stronger medications (such as atropine) are used in rare occasions.

Ophthalmoscopy, or the dilated examination, usually includes an assessment of lens clarity, the vitreous, retinal arterioles and venules, optic nerve, and retina. This is accomplished with a binocular indirect ophthalmoscope and usually with the slit lamp and accessory lenses. Frequently, the ratio of the optic nerve central cup to the outer nerve profile (cup-to-disc or C/D ratio) is indicated, with the normal usually being about 0.3 or less. An enlarged C/D ratio is suggestive of optic nerve damage, often indicative of open angle glaucoma.

Appendix 4: Standard Topical Eyedrop Bottle Cap Colors

Daniel S. Casper

The American Academy of Ophthalmology and the FDA have formulated a uniform set of eyedrop bottle cap and label colors based on drug mechanism, to aid in both patient compliance and in identification of medications. First developed in 1983, the system is regularly updated as new ophthalmic drug categories (e.g., prostaglandin inhibitors) are introduced.

It has been argued that this system has some severe limitations, particularly for patients who are vision impaired or have cognitive deficits. In addition, the system presupposes that the appropriate cap is placed on the matching bottle; as caps may be interchangeable, this is not always the case. It has been suggested that an enhancement of this system, with different shape caps, and unique, standardized threading systems for each category, would likely reduce many of the current problems.

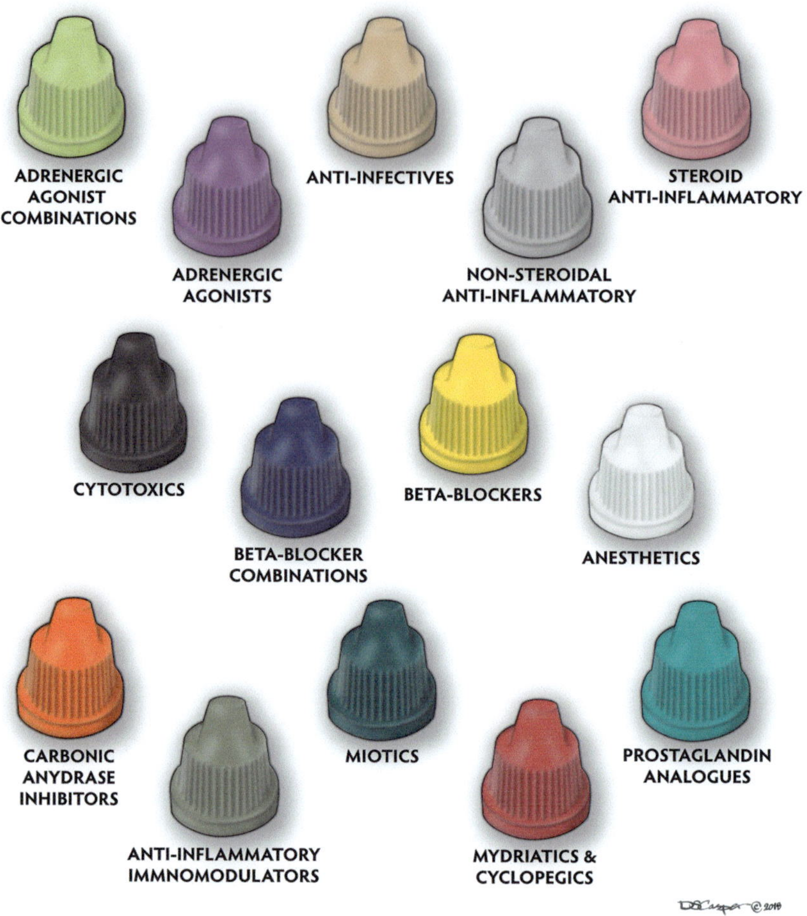

References

1. https://www.aao.org/about/policies/color-codes-topical-ocular-medications
2. https://www.aao.org/editors-choice/color-communication-confounds
3. Brandt, JD. Human factors and ophthalmic drug packaging: time for a global standard. J Ophthalmol 2015;08, 035. https://doi.org/10.1016/j.ophtha.2015.08.035

Appendix 5: Terminology

Daniel S. Casper

AC IOL	Anterior chamber intraocular lens
Accommodation	A three-part reflex related to visualization of near objects, involving the in-turning (convergence) of both eyes, ciliary muscle contraction producing a change in the crystalline lens convexity, and pupillary miosis
ACG	Angle closure glaucoma
AF	Autofluorescence
AION	Anterior ischemic optic neuropathy
ALT	Argon laser trabeculoplasty
Amblyopia	A partial or complete loss of vision in one or both eyes, secondary to abnormal development in the visual cortical area; the ocular anatomy is normal, and the lesion is a neurologic one. Also referred to as "lazy eye"
Amsler grid	A simple diagnostic test employing a grid of horizontal and vertical lines which is used to test and monitor the central visual field for distortions (metamorphopsias) or blind spots (scotomas)
Aniridia	Absence of the iris; congenital or acquired
Aniseikonia	A significant difference in the perception of image size between the two eyes, usually due to a large difference in refractive errors/corrections
Anisocoria	Unequal pupil size
Anisometropia	Unequal refractive powers of the two eyes
Anophthalmos	Absence of eye; congenital or acquired
AO/HRR	American Optical/Hardy-Rand-Rittler color plates
APD, RAPD	Afferent pupillary defect, or reverse afferent pupillary defect (also referred to as a "Marcus Gunn pupil")
Aphakia	Absence of the normal intraocular crystalline lens
ARMD; AMD	Age-related macular degeneration
Astigmatism	A refractive error producing distorted images focused on the macula due to either a non-spherical corneal curvature or irregularity in the structure of the crystalline lens
Band keratopathy	A central corneal degeneration with deposition of calcium, which may be idiopathic or associated with a variety of systemic (e.g., hypercalcemia) or local conditions
Blepharitis	A common, noncontagious inflammation of the eyelids, usually involving the lid margins. It is frequently chronic in nature but may present acutely as well. It may be associated with dermatologic conditions such as rosacea or seborrhea or may be a local reaction to bacterial infection, Meibomian gland dysfunction, or other causes.
Blepharospasm	Involuntary eyelid twitching or closure, a form of dystonia, which may be an isolated condition or associated with hemifacial spasm. When severe, it may result in functional blindness of the affected eye.
Capsule opacification	Post-cataract surgery opacification of the posterior capsule ("PCO," a common postoperative condition which results in decreased acuity and is usually remedied with the use of a YAG laser treatment). Previously referred to as a "second" or "secondary" cataract

Cataract	Any opacity of the natural crystalline lens. Depending on location, size, and density, there may be anywhere from minimal to severe vision impairment. Although most cataracts are a normal, age-related phenomenon, cataracts may be caused by trauma, inflammation, medication, or systemic disease.
C/D ratio	Cup-to-disc ratio
Chemosis	Edema of the conjunctiva, leading to a swollen and gelatinous appearance which, in severe cases, may interfere with lid closure
Choroiditis	A type of uveitis (i.e., inflammation of the uveal tract) involving the posterior portion of the uvea, the choroid
Chorioretinitis	Inflammation of both the uveal choroid and the neural retina, a type of uveitis. It is most commonly associated with systemic infections such as toxoplasmosis, syphilis, sarcoidosis, tuberculosis, or other conditions.
Cogan lid twitch	Brief overshoot of the upper lid upon return to primary gaze after a period of downgaze. It is often, but not solely, seen in myasthenia gravis.
Comitant	Ocular deviation in which the misalignment is consistent in all fields of gaze
Conjugate	Yoked eye movements that maintain binocular fixation
Corectopia	Eccentric placement of the pupil away from the central iris
Crystalline lens	The natural lens in the eye
CSME; CME	Clinically significant macular edema
Cyclitis	A type of uveitis (i.e., inflammation of the uveal tract) which involves the middle uveal portion, the ciliary body
Cyclotorsion	Rotation (clockwise or counterclockwise) of the eye around the anteroposterior visual axis
Dacryoadenitis	Inflammation and enlargement of the lacrimal glands, which may be of infectious or inflammatory origin. It may present acutely or be a chronic condition. When chronic, it is often associated with systemic conditions (e.g., sarcoidosis or idiopathic orbital inflammation {pseudotumor}).
Dacryocystitis	Infection of the lacrimal sac, located at the medial canthus, usually due to obstruction of the nasolacrimal drainage system. Dacryocystitis may be acute or chronic and, if severe and untreated, may result in orbital cellulitis.
DES	Dry eye syndrome
Diopter	Unit used to measure lens or prism power
Diplopia	Double vision; seeing the same image of regard at two different positions at the same time
Drusen	(1) Various types of lipid material which collect beneath the retinal pigment epithelium and may be associated with age-related macular degeneration; (2) mucoprotein and mucopolysaccharide accumulations in the optic nerve head (the disc) that may simulate disc edema
Duane syndrome	A congenital strabismus involving limitation of horizontal eye movements, usually also associated with globe retraction, lid fissure narrowing, and limitation of convergence (there are various variations of Duane syndrome)
Ductions	Range eye movements or each eye (including adduction, abduction, elevation, and depression). "Forced duction testing" refers to an examiner forcibly moving an anesthetized eye to determine if any restrictive component of motion limitation is present.
Ectropion	An outward turning of the eyelid(s), usually the lower lid, which may be secondary to normal aging changes, cicatricial lesions, or paralytic processes. If the lower punctum is everted, chronic tearing may occur; if the underlying eye is exposed, dryness may be the main complaint.

Endophthalmitis	Intraocular inflammation or infection, most commonly occurring after intraocular surgery or trauma, although it may be seen with systemic infection via hematogenous spread (e.g., fungal infections) as well. Severe visual impairment, or even loss of the eye, may occur.
Enophthalmos	A posterior displacement (sinking) of the eye into the orbit, the opposite of exophthalmos, seen after bony orbital fracture, globe phthisis, orbital fat atrophy, and other causes
Entropion	An inward turning of the lid(s), which usually results in corneal irritation or abrasion from the misdirected lashes (trichiasis). Entropion is most frequently caused by scarring or orbicularis muscle spasm. If severe enough, it can be vision threatening (e.g., trachoma).
Enucleation	Removal of the entire globe, but preservation of surrounding adnexal tissues
Epiphora	Excessive tearing, overflowing the lower lids. It is caused by either excess lacrimation or nasolacrimal blockage which produces insufficient tear drainage.
Epiretinal membrane (macular pucker, cellophane maculopathy)	A proliferation of fibrocellular tissue on the internal retinal surface at the vitreoretinal interface, usually as an idiopathic finding in older patients, in association with some diseases such as diabetes, or after posterior intraocular surgeries or trauma
Episcleritis	Inflammation of the external layer of the eye which is located between the outermost conjunctiva and the inner sclera. It is a common, benign condition that typically has no known etiology but may be associated with systemic conditions, usually inflammatory. It can easily be misdiagnosed as infectious conjunctivitis.
ERM	Epiretinal membrane
Esotropia	A type of strabismus where one or both eyes turn inward
ET	Esotropia
Evisceration	Removal of all intraocular contents, but preservation of the outer ocular layer (the sclera) and attached extraocular muscles, as well as adjacent orbital tissues
Excyclotorsion	An outward rotational movement of the globe (from the observer's point of view, clockwise rotation for the left eye, counterclockwise rotation for the right eye); the inferior oblique muscle is primarily responsible for excyclotorsion.
Exenteration	Surgical removal of the eye and all adjacent tissues (usually including lids, orbital fat, extraocular muscles, nerves, blood vessels)
Exophthalmos	Protrusion of one or both eyes anteriorly from the orbit (also referred to as proptosis), usually due to increased orbital volume from tumor, lymphoid infiltration, hemorrhage, edema, abscess, or other causes (some clinicians reserve exophthalmos for endocrine-related bulging only and employ the term proptosis when caused by other conditions)
Exposure keratopathy	Damage to the outer layers of the cornea from chronic exposure, which may be caused by cicatricial, neurologic, or orbital causes of defective lid closure
Eyelid lag	Delayed downward movement of the eyelid in downgaze; often, but not always, associated with thyroid eye disease
FA	Fluorescein angiogram
Fixation	Direction of the eyes on an object of regard

Flashes   Brief bursts of light seen in one eye which appear as spots, jagged lines, arcs, or lightning bolts and are usually due to vitreous traction, a small area of vitreous adherence to the retinal surface that results in tugging on the retinal surface with the resultant production of these visual phenomena also known as phosphenes or photopsias

Floaters   Minute opacities in the vitreous body, usually due to normal age-related changes in the vitreous composition (known as syneresis) which move with eye movements and cast shadows on the retina, seen as mobile spots, linear strands, blotches, webs, etc. Floaters may also be a sign of retinal tears or holes or blood or inflammatory cells in the vitreous.

GCA   Giant cell arteritis (temporal arteritis)

Glaucoma   A family of diseases which exhibit damage to the optic nerve (optic neuropathy), often, but not always, associated with increased intraocular pressure

GPC   Giant papillary conjunctivitis

GVF   Goldmann visual field

Hemianopsia (or hemianopia)   Vision deficit in one half of the visual field in one or both eyes. It may be congruous (the bilateral defects are identical) or incongruous (the deficits in the two eyes differ). Also, it may be homonymous (a nasal deficit in one eye and a temporal in the other) or heteronymous (deficits in either both nasal fields {binasal deficit} or in both temporal fields {bitemporal}).

Heterochromia   Different color irises, or significant color variation in a single iris

Horner's syndrome   A unilateral disruption in the sympathetic pathway from the superior cervical ganglion to the orbit, causing ptosis, miosis, and decreased sweating on the ipsilateral side. Although often benign, a new Horner's syndrome may indicate serious pathology in the neck or chest, which must be investigated.

HVF   Humphrey visual field (automated perimetry test)

Hyperopia   Farsighted

Hyperopic shift   A change in the eye's refractive error toward hyperopia (or reduced myopia) due typically to crystalline lens changes, macular elevation (edema), or a mass behind the eye, pushing anteriorly against the posterior sclera

Hyphema   Blood in the anterior chamber. It may be layered out inferiorly in the space between the iris and the corneal endothelium, diffusely spread through the entire chamber, or a dense clot which fills the entire chamber (an "eight-ball hyphema"). Hyphema is common after trauma or surgery, although it may occur spontaneously with a variety of systemic (e.g., hematologic abnormalities or with anticoagulation therapy) or ocular (e.g., iris melanoma or rubeosis iridis) conditions.

Hypopyon   A collection of white blood cells in the anterior chamber, often layered out inferiorly, usually accompanying iritis or more severe forms of uveitis. It may be seen with severe ocular infections (e.g., keratitis or endophthalmitis) or in association with systemic diseases such as Behçet's syndrome.

Hypotony   Eye with abnormally low intraocular pressure

ICG   Indocyanine green angiogram

Incomitant   Ocular misalignment which varies depending on the direction of gaze

Incyclotorsion   An inward rotational movement of the globe (from the observer's point of view, counterclockwise rotation for the left eye, clockwise rotation for the right eye); the superior oblique muscle is responsible for incyclotorsion.

Injection	Dilated vessels, usually referring to conjunctival, episcleral, or scleral vessels
INO	Internuclear ophthalmoplegia, a disorder of horizontal conjugate gaze, caused by a lesion in the medial longitudinal fasciculus (MLF), often associated with multiple sclerosis or brainstem infarction
IOL	Intraocular lens implant
IOP	Intraocular pressure
Iris bombe	A buildup of aqueous fluid in the posterior chamber secondary to posterior synechiae, which prevents normal fluid egress through the pupil and results in a forward displacement of the iris, which can lead to or worsen a narrow-angle glaucoma attack
Iritis	Inflammation of the iris. It may be idiopathic, caused by trauma (including, commonly, eye surgery), infections, or in association with systemic autoimmune conditions.
J	Jaeger near vision reading scale
Keratitis	Inflammation of the cornea. It may be caused by infection, trauma (including chemical injury or contact lens overwear), exposure, and dryness, or in association with systemic diseases, particularly autoimmune.
Keratoconus	A corneal disease manifested by progressive thinning and resultant distortion, leading to a bulging misshaping of the cornea, resulting in blurred vision. Severe cases have classically been treated by corneal transplantation, but newer medical techniques which employ cross-linking of collagen fibers can retard or stop progression.
Lagophthalmos	Incomplete eyelid closure, resulting in ocular exposure in the interpalpebral fissure. Often a result of seventh cranial nerve palsy
LASIK	Laser in situ keratomileusis (refractive surgical procedure)
Lattice degeneration	A common thinning of the peripheral retina. Lattice itself does not normally require any treatment, but complications (such as retinal breaks or tears, which can lead to retinal detachment) may need intervention.
Lazy eye	Another term for amblyopia, often mistakenly used to refer to ocular misalignment (strabismus)
Leukocoria	A white-appearing pupil (usually due to some opacity behind the iris), potentially an indication of a severe intraocular condition such as retinoblastoma, retinal detachment, or retinopathy of prematurity, among others
LP Vision	Light perception visual acuity
Marcus Gunn jaw winking (trigemino-oculomotor synkinesis)	An upward jerking of the superior eyelid seen in infants, associated with chewing movements of the jaw, due to an aberrant connection between trigeminal motor fibers and the oculomotor nerve branches to the levator muscle. Marcus Gunn jaw winking may be congenital or acquired.
Marcus Gunn pupil	(See APD, RAPD)
Metamorphopsia	A disturbance of visual acuity, usually caused by macular distortion or disease, and tested for with an Amsler Grid. Images may appear twisted, wavy, absent, or improperly sized (micropsia or macropsia)
MGD	Meibomian gland disease
Monovision	The technique of using one eye for focusing at distance and the other at near, among the presbyopic-aged population. Usually accomplished with either a single contact lens on one eye or purposely mismatched bilateral contact lenses

Myopia	Nearsighted
Myopic shift	A change in the refractive power of the eye toward myopia (or reduced hyperopia) typically due to certain types of cataracts or diabetes-induced changes in lens shape
NAION	Nonarteritic ischemic optic neuropathy
Narrow angle	An abnormal anatomic configuration where the iris is bowed forward toward the posterior surface of the cornea, which may result in decreased aqueous fluid outflow with increased intraocular pressure and an acute narrow-angle glaucoma attack
NLP vision	No light perception visual acuity (i.e., complete blindness)
NPDR	Nonproliferative diabetic retinopathy (formerly called "background retinopathy")
NVG	Neovascular glaucoma
NVI	Neovascularization of the iris; rubeosis
Nyctalopia	Night blindness
Nystagmus	Usually involuntary repetitive ocular movements in horizontal, vertical, or rotatory fashion. It is usually binocular, may be fast or slow, and may be congenital or acquired. It is frequently associated with decreased visual acuity. It may be idiopathic, related to medications or substance abuse, or associated with intracranial pathologies.
OCT	Optical coherence tomography
Ocular hypertension	Intraocular pressure greater than 21 mmHg, without evidence of glaucoma (such as an abnormal optic nerve or visual field defects) or other ocular diseases which could result in increased pressure. A thicker than normal cornea will also usually indicate an artifactually elevated intraocular pressure.
Ocularist	A practitioner specialized in the creation of ocular prostheses for cosmesis in patients who have unilateral or bilateral anophthalmos
OD	Right eye (oculus dexter)
Orthoptist	Practitioner specialized in evaluation and treatment of eye movement and binocular vision disorders
OS	Left eye (oculus sinister)
OU	Both eyes (oculus uterque)
Pannus	Pathologic conjunctival blood vessel encroachment across the limbus onto the normally avascular cornea
PC IOL	Posterior chamber intraocular lens
PCO	Posterior capsular opacification (previously inaccurately referred to as a "second cataract")
PDR	Proliferative diabetic retinopathy
Phoria	A latent ocular deviation that is seen only when one eye is covered and binocular fusion is broken
Phosphenes	Brief bursts of light seen in one eye which appear as spots, jagged lines, arcs, or lightning bolts and are usually due to vitreous traction, a small area of vitreous adherence to the retinal surface that results in tugging on the retinal surface with the resultant production of these visual phenomena, also known as flashes or photopsias
Photopsia	The impression of brief bursts of light, usually due to areas of vitreous adherence to the retinal surface, retinal detachment, or non-ocular causes such as migraine auras or other intracranial pathologies

Phthisis, or Phthisis bulbi An end-stage, blind, atrophic eye which generally has no visual potential

PK Penetrating keratoplasty (corneal transplant)

POAG or COAG Progressive (or chronic) open-angle glaucoma

Posterior pole The posterior portion of the inside of the eye, including the optic nerve head (the disc) and the adjacent macula and temporal arcades. This roughly correlates to the typical view of the inside of the eye seen with an indirect ophthalmoscope if the patient is looking at the examiner.

PRK Photorefractive keratectomy (refractive surgical procedure)

Proptosis Protrusion of one or both eyes anteriorly from the orbit (also referred to as exophthalmos; some clinicians reserve the term proptosis for non-endocrine-related globe protrusion and exophthalmos for endocrine-related bulging only)

PRP Pan-retinal photocoagulation (laser treatment utilized for neovascularization).

Pseudotumor Pseudotumor *cerebri* (more recently termed idiopathic intracranial hypertension) is a condition of unknown etiology in which the intracranial pressure is elevated, which may cause a variety of symptoms, most commonly headache and visual loss related to optic nerve compression. *Orbital* pseudotumor is an unrelated condition involving inflammation of one or more orbital compartments (e.g., extraocular muscles, lacrimal gland, orbital fat), typically caused by infection or autoimmune disease. The term "pseudotumor" reflects the historical diagnosis of tumor, prior to current imaging techniques, when the diagnosis was based on tumorlike findings; the absence of tumor was then discovered upon surgical exploration.

Ptosis Drooping lid(s) or globe

PVD Posterior vitreous detachment (or separation). A normal process, usually occurring after age 65, whereby the posterior vitreous surface (the hyaloid) pulls away from the inner retinal surface, due to natural age-related shrinkage of the vitreous body. Flashes of light, and the appearance of "floaters" is common after PVD, but rarely there may be an associated tear of the retina, which may cause a retinal detachment or tear of a blood vessel, which would result in intraocular hemorrhage.

Recurrent erosion An apparent idiopathic corneal abrasion that may result after previous corneal trauma or may occur in certain individuals without any prior history of damage to the cornea. In the first case, it is believed that the epithelial healing process is, for unclear reasons, abnormal, leading to spontaneous "re-abrasion." In the latter, it is usually found that there is an underlying corneal dystrophy that predisposes to erosions (e.g., anterior basement membrane dystrophy).

RD Retinal detachment

RGP lenses Rigid gas permeable contact lenses

RRD Rhegmatogenous retinal detachment (i.e., detachment due to a tear or hole in the retina)

Rubeosis (rubeosis iridis) Neovascularization of the iris surface. It is usually associated with ischemic conditions of the retina, such as diabetes.

Saccade Simultaneous rapid eye movements in the same direction which quickly change fixation

Schisis	Splitting of the retinal neurosensory layers. Depending on the location of the splitting, schisis may be asymptomatic or associated with visual loss.
SCL lenses	Soft contact lenses
Scotoma	A blind spot in the visual field
Skew deviation	An unusual acquired torsional and vertical strabismus due to poorly understood pathology related to vestibular abnormalities, and with various clinical presentations. It can mimic fourth cranial nerve palsy.
Snellen letters	Visual acuity-testing letters ("optotypes") designed to project an image of a certain size on the retina at a certain distance, thus standardizing acuity testing. Other acuity charts, such as the LogMAR, Tumbling E, Landolt C, and ETDRS charts, are also used.
Steroid responder	The abnormal response noted in approximately one-third of the population, where steroid medications cause an elevation of intraocular pressure. This may represent a transient increase in pressure (ocular hypertension) or may lead to development of glaucoma.
Strabismus	Misalignment of the eyes, which frequently will produce double vision
Symblepharon	An adhesion of the eyelid portion of the conjunctiva (palpebral) to the conjunctiva lining the globe (bulbar). This typically occurs after trauma or in association with certain diseases (e.g., pemphigoid, trachoma, Stevens-Johnson syndrome).
Synechiae, anterior	Adhesion(s) of the anterior surface of the iris to the posterior, endothelial surface of the cornea. Typically seen after trauma (including ocular surgery) or ocular inflammation such as iritis. May be associated with a secondary angle-closure glaucoma
Synechiae, posterior	Adhesion(s) of the posterior surface of the iris to the anterior lens surface, typically occurring secondary to intraocular inflammation such as iritis or iridocyclitis. May be associated with a secondary angle-closure glaucoma
Syneresis	A natural degeneration of the gelatinous vitreous body, resulting in liquification of portions of the gel, with the development of vitreous "floaters" and subsequent shrinkage
TED	Thyroid eye disease
Trichiasis	A pathologic in-turning of the lashes toward the eye, usually resulting in irritation to the cornea's surface, which may result in eventual abrasion and chronic infection (e.g., in trachoma). Trichiasis may be congenital or acquired (usually from lid trauma, infection, or autoimmune conditions). When sever, corrective surgery is usually necessary.
TRD	Tractional retinal detachment (i.e., detachment due to fibrotic contraction, rather than the presence of a retinal hole or tear)
Tropia	A manifest ocular misalignment when the person is viewing an object with both eyes uncovered
Uveitis	An inflammation of the eye, affecting the uvea, the vascular, middle tunic of the globe. It may be anterior (iritis), middle (cyclitis), or posterior (choroiditis) or affect the entire uvea (panuveitis). Uveitis occurs after trauma and in association with many autoimmune systemic diseases. When severe, it can lead to blindness, particularly if left untreated.
VA	Visual acuity (usually refers to distance acuity)
VEGF	Vascular endothelial growth factor (an angiogenesis promoter)
Vergence	Opposite binocular eye movements to maintain binocular vision, e.g., convergence at near or divergence at distance

Vitreoretinal traction   An area of abnormal adhesion between the vitreous and the underlying retina which may cause distortion of the retina with secondary visual changes such as blurring or light flashes; in severe cases, may cause the retina to develop a tear (vitreomacular traction, or VMT, is a subset that is confined to the macula)

VF   Visual field

Xanthelasma   A benign, plaque-like deposition of lipid material in the superficial eyelid tissues, producing a yellowish discoloration

XT   Exotropia

YAG (laser)   Ytterbium argon green laser treatment, usually to perform peripheral iridotomy

Index

© Springer Nature Switzerland AG 2019
D. S. Casper, G. A. Cioffi (eds.), *The Columbia Guide to Basic Elements of Eye Care*,
https://doi.org/10.1007/978-3-030-10886-1

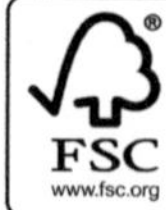